ESSENTIALS OF ENVIRONMENTAL HEALTH MANAGEMENT

ESSENTIALS OF ENVIRONMENTAL HEALTH MANAGEMENT

JANVIER GASANA

Aglob Publishing

Hallandale Beach, Florida

Aglob Publishing
P.O. Box 4036,
Hallandale Beach, Fl. 33008

E-Mail: info@aglobpublishing.com

www.aglobpublishing.com

```
              Library of Congress Cataloging-in-Publication Data

 Gasana, Janvier.
    Essentials of environmental health management / Janvier Gasana.
        p. ; cm.
 Includes bibliographical references.
    ISBN 0-9708560-4-0
   1.  Environmental health.
    [DNLM: 1.  Environmental Health. 2.  Environmental Exposure. 3.
 Environmental Pollution. 4.  Occupational Health.  WA 30 G246e 2003]
 I.
 Title.

    RA565.G37 2003
    616.9'8--dc21

                                                    2003004619
```

Printed in the United States of America

10 9 8 7 6 5 4 3 2 1

FORWARD

The environment has always been of great concern to mankind, whether it was the natural environment, from which human beings derived virtually all needs, or the environmental habitats man created for shelter or for work. As permanent settlements developed and populations increased, maintaining a constant food supply, water supply, adequate shelter, and basic sanitation become more problematic. Where environmental conditions changed (i.e. rainfall) or were not controlled, starvation, disease, and a lowering in the quality of life occurred. Throughout history, numerous examples exist of civilizations, which declined due to environmental factors. The fall of the Roman Empire, in part, has been attributed to the use of lead canisters to store wine. The Black Plague was due to poor sanitation practices in Europe and led to the demise of one-third Europe's population.

As civilization moved into the 19th and 20th centuries, many technological advancements caused increased agricultural and industrial productivity. In the late 1800's the basis of disease transmission became understood, as did the means to control transmission by water treatment and waste disposal practices. At the turn of the century many U.S. states had active public health programs. With the advent of modern medicine and antibiotics, infant and adult mortality were greatly reduced in the first half of the 20th century, particularly in the developing nations. As a result, the population of developing nations and that of the world exploded.

Only within the past three or four decades has significant attention been devoted to correcting environmental problems in nature and within the workplace. By the 1960's many natural ecosystems had been threatened or destroyed by industrialization, pollution, population expansion and agricultural practices. In North America, The Great Lakes ecosystem and its fisheries were greatly damaged by chemical pollution. Urban centers such as Los Angeles, New York, and Chicago had all developed serious air pollution conditions unsafe for human health, largely due to the automobile. Chemical exposures and safety practices in industrial environments were also having human health impacts. Society was awakened to the reality that our environmental quality rather than improving, appeared to be declining. In response, a number of laws were enacted in the 1970s to protect the environment and improve working conditions.

The environmental and occupational health sciences, which encompass the traditional sciences such as chemistry, physics, biology and medicine, were also created and shaped in recent decades to solve environmental and workplace problems. A multidisciplinary approach, using several sciences, was required. The wide-ranged nature and complexity of the problems was often beyond the scope of a single scientific discipline.

The combination of legislation and a broad based citizen concern led to great improvements in environmental quality by the late 1970s in many industrialized, developed nations, such as the United States. However, it was also discovered that the tremendous demand placed upon non-renewable (energy and mineral) resources and renewable resources (water, land, air, biota) by a few industrialized nations representing a small fraction of the world's population could cause major environmental, economic and political problems in the decades ahead. As a result some, but limited, conservation measures were implemented.

Today such environmental concerns remain, from overpopulation to nuclear war, from hazardous wastes to radon in homes, from acid rain to destruction of the ozone layer, from the loss of the world's tropical forests to the loss of wildlife, from the toxic effects of chemicals to providing a safe working environment. Many of the problems we now face have become increasingly complex and interrelated. For example, the growing of food grains in the United States, which are exported to feed millions of people in third world nations rely, in part, on groundwater which is diminishing in the central and western United States. The fertilizer and pesticides we use to produce higher crop yields consume non-renewable energy are polluting high quality groundwater used also for drinking water, and may affect the ozone layer of the planet which protects life on earth from harmful ultraviolet radiation. Our agricultural practices themselves may eventually lead to the loss of topsoil and productivity, cause greater crop vulnerability to insects, and wide-scale ecosystem damage. A combination of drought and improper agricultural methods led to the desertification of large areas in Central Africa, the end result being the starvation of hundreds of thousands of Africans including Ethiopians. For something as simple as growing food, it has been difficult to predict all the possible impacts. It has been even more difficult, where problems have been identified and solutions known, such as those with agriculture, to implement environmentally sound approaches in a timely fashion.

Environmental health concerns continue to be central to the modern practice of public health. Workplace and ambient exposures in air, water, and soil continue to meld, and individuals, communities, and even the world now claim the attention of the environmental health professionals. This book attempts to provide the reader with an overview as well as the fundamentals of the environmental and occupational health sciences. Current and future problems will be identified as will the mathematical and public health basics needed to understand and solve such problems.

This book is organized into four main sections, which are the following:

1. The basic principles.
2. The exposure pathways.
3. The environmental and occupational settings.
4. The assessment and monitoring methodologies.

The basic principles cover the introduction, toxicology including environmental calculations, epidemiology, disease, and law.

The exposure pathways explore the impact of air quality, water quality, solid and hazardous waste, the control of rodents, insects and pests, food quality, energy including radiation and noise.

The environmental and occupational settings examine the role of the world population with regard to community level exposures, urbanization and health, deforestation and desertification, ozone depletion and chlorofluorocarbons, global warming, climate change, greenhouse effect, acid rain, biodiversity and environmental justice. The section also covers the problems at the community level including natural disasters, the impact of injury and violence on the health of the public and the problems encountered in the work place.

The assessment and monitoring methodologies describe the techniques used for assessing the risks resulting from the exposure of the population to these hazards and monitoring the environmental /occupational hazards in order to protect the health of the public and the environment.

Environmental/ occupational hazards and methods for their control are presented with particular emphasis on public health efforts. Upon completion of the book the reader will hopefully have a better understanding of the environmental and occupational sciences and their direct connection to public health and environmental quality. More importantly, the author hopes the reader will see the world somewhat differently and apply what she / he has learned in order to help preserve and enhance our world for the generations to come.

ACKNOWLEDGMENTS

To my grandmother, Asterie, a traditional healer, who taught me the art of caring for my fellow humans and who at 100 years of age, although blind, still sees more than I do.

I am grateful to many of my fellow medical, public health and environmental health professionals for sharing their talents and expertise with me.

I owe a deep debt of gratitude to one of my graduate assistants, Luisa Fernanda Santos, MD for her outstanding editorial work that made this textbook a reality. The sleepless nights and frustrations that go with editing a book did not stop her from bringing it to fruition. She deserves more than mere thanks.

I extend sincere thanks to my other graduate assistants, Christine Daley, for her excellent preparation of almost half of the chapters of this book and Diana Goldbort for editing most of the chapters.

I also want to express my appreciation to Janisse Rosario, MPH; Pie Kamoso, MD, MPH; and Debra Miller, MPH for preparing a good number of the chapters of this book.

Special thanks are due my colleagues in the Department of Public Health for their unconditional support and belief in me from the time they met me, especially Dr. Virginia H. McCoy and my very good friend Dr. William Keppler.

The book brings together the experience of more than 15 years of teaching the course entitled "Principles of Environmental and Occupational Health Sciences" all the way from Africa (at the Rwandan Medical School), to Chicago (at the University of Illinois), and to North Miami (at Florida International University). It is the result of working with the many students who took that course that I could compile a text that emphasizes the public health aspect of environmental and occupational health sciences. I feel that I learned more from them than they did from me. I wish to thank every single one of these graduate students and / or graduate assistants for providing me with the opportunity to write this book.

I also wish to thank my lovely wife Bella and my children Adelard, Adelin, Eusebio, and Parfait for their never ending encouragement, love, and support throughout this challenging period of my scholarly development. They put up with an absentee husband and father and waited with patience to see this work realized.

CONTENTS

SECTION I. BASIC PRINCIPLES

CHAPTER 1. INTRODUCTION

CHAPTER 2. TOXICOLOGY

CHAPTER 3. EPIDEMIOLOGY

CHAPTER 4. DISEASE

CHAPTER 5. LAW

Section II. Exposure Pathways

Chapter 6. Air Quality

Chapter 7. Water Quality

CHAPTER 8. SOLID / HAZARDOUS WASTE AND RODENTS, INSECTS, AND PESTS

Chapter 9. Food Quality

Chapter 10. Energy, Radiation, And Noise

Section III. Environmental And Occupational Settings

Chapter 11. Global Issues

CHAPTER 12. LOCAL ISSUES

Chapter 13. Injury

CHAPTER 14. THE WORKPLACE

SECTION IV. ASSESSMENT AND MONITORING METHODOLOGIES

CHAPTER 15. RISK ASSESSMENT

CHAPTER 16. MONITORING

Contents

SECTION

I

BASIC PRINCIPLES

CHAPTER

1

INTRODUCTION

I.   BIOGEOCHEMICAL CYCLES

II. DEFINITION OF HEALTH AND THE ENVIRONMENT

III. LINK BETWEEN ENVIRONMENT AND HEALTH

IV. LINKS BETWEEN ENVIRONMENTAL AND OCCUPATIONAL HEALTH

V.   HISTORY OF ENVIRONMENTAL HEALTH

VI. ENVIRONMENTAL HEALTH ADMINISTRATION

I. BIOGEOCHEMICAL CYCLES

A. INTRODUCTION

The study of environmental health is concerned primarily with the effects of the environment on human health. But, there is no easy way to really comprehend and appreciate these effects until one has also examined the effects of human activities on the environment. In order to do this, one needs some understanding of the nature of the environment and how it functions when the human population is considered as simply another species of animal, accepting and working with the natural systems and laws.

All living organisms need essentially the same things for survival; whether we call these things life support systems or simply food and shelter, we really mean the basic elements needed to sustain life and growth. Although the mechanisms of growth and maintenance of any organism are extremely complex, the major constituents of the materials needed for these processes are actually limited in number, namely, carbon (**C**), oxygen (**O**), hydrogen (**H**), nitrogen (**N**), sulfur (**S**), and phosphorus (**P**). There are, of course, many other chemicals needed as well but in comparatively small or even trace amounts. These six elements, alone and in combination, comprise nearly all of what is necessary for our life support, whether it be the air we breathe, the food and water we consume, or the materials we use to protect us from physical stresses.

Nature has devised very specific means of regulating these elements by what are called the **biogeochemical cycles**. It is the recycling of nutrients from inorganic to organic and back again in a living system. The basic cycle is shown in Figure 1.1.

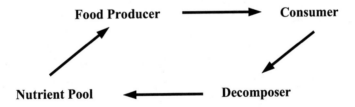

Figure 1.1. Components of a Basic Biogeochemical Cycle.

The energy-containing mass of the producers, called **autotrophs**, is consumed by the **heterotrophs**, who themselves may be consumed by **higher-level heterotrophs**. All of what is commonly called the waste products of this constant process of growth and consumption, as well as the mass of material remaining when the organism dies, is broken down. Some of the material is returned to the environment in a form usable once again by the producer, but some also is lost for periods of minutes to millenia due to various chemical processes and environmental conditions. The decomposers (bacteria, fungi, and various higher level organisms) are thus crucial to this system.

Two issues, which are integral to this basic cycle, will be addressed in subsequent chapters. The first is the basic necessity missing from Figure 1.1, **energy**, and the second, related to the first, is the **loss of efficiency** (or **energy**) at each level of the cycle. The component understood to be present in the basic cycle (and in each of the cycles to be discussed in detail) is the **sun**. Energy from the sun does not recycle but is always going in one direction, from a state of maximum, usable energy to a state in which the energy is dissipated as what is considered waste heat. Each level of producers and consumers in the basic cycle is a less efficient user of energy than the one below. The principal reason for this is that beyond the producer level, organisms cannot use the energy of the sun directly, but must obtain their energy through metabolizing and releasing the chemical energy present in the material of the producers. With each increase in level of complexity and size of the organisms, more energy is used to obtain and metabolize the food needed for maintenance, growth, and reproduction and more waste heat is generated.

Many of what we refer to as "pollutants," "stressors," or perhaps just "irritants" in this book can be seen to actually be an integral part of one of the biogeochemical cycles and a necessary source of nutrition and/or energy to some level of organism. Although imbalances and thus accumulation of pollutants may occur naturally as a result of catastrophic events, what we consider pollution is most often caused by human interference with and/or ignorance of nature's system of checks and balances.

In general, the cycles are divided by where the largest usable reservoir of the element is found. The **carbon** and **nitrogen** cycles are thus considered **gaseous cycles** in which the atmosphere constitutes a major reservoir. The **phosphorus** and **sulfur** cycles are **sedimentary cycles** in which major portions of the element may be found in the lithosphere (the solid part or crust of the earth) and so lost to the cycle. The third major type of cycle is that of the compound **water** and involves all three divisions of the ecosphere: the **hydrosphere**, **lithosphere**, and **atmosphere**.

B. GASEOUS CYCLES

Carbon Cycle. The carbon cycle (Figure 1.2.) is considered cycle in that C is returned to the environment about as fast as it removed. The basic movement is that of carbon dioxide (CO_2) from atmosphere to producers. The carbon-containing compounds produced consumed by those unable to use CO_2 directly and CO_2 is returned to atmosphere via respiration. CO_2 is also returned via the action of decomposers by combustion of carbon-containing materials: wood, peat and oil, and weathering of carbonate-containing rocks.

The geological component of the carbon cycle contains more than 99% of the total carbon on the earth. The extensive and ecologically excessive combustion of these fossil fuels constitutes an interference in the carbon cycle that is perhaps irrevocable. Although it would appear that the atmosphere would be poisoned by the quantity of CO_2 and carbon monoxide (CO) that are being produced due to combustion, this is not the case. It is believed that the ocean serves as a reservoir for most of the CO_2 produced in excess of that needed for photosynthesis without noticeable effect as of yet. Also, the increase in the amount of area of the world now under cultivation has of course increased the demand for CO_2. The amount of CO_2 in the atmosphere has increased since the Industrial Revolution however, and is projected to continue to increase unless changes are made in both the forms and consumption of energy. The largest known projected effect of this increase is an increase in the average world temperature.

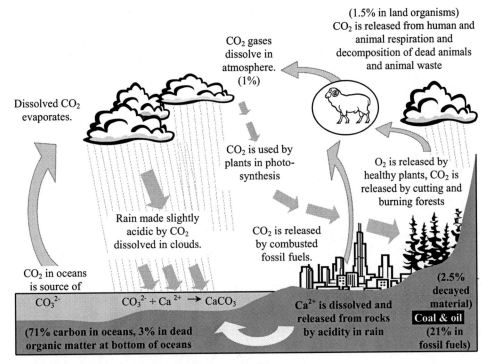

Figure 1.2. Carbon Cycle. (Source: Moore, 1999).

Nitrogen Cycle. The nitrogen cycle is depicted in Figure 1.3. It is also an essentially perfect cycle in that use from and return to the environment is essentially equal. Unlike CO_2, the gaseous form of nitrogen, N_2, cannot be used directly by most producers but must be "fixed" or converted to usable forms. The principal forms of usable nitrogen are nitrate (NO_3) and ammonia (NH_3). Although these can be produced by natural physico-chemical processes (e.g., lightning, volcanic activity) the greatest amount of naturally occurring fixation is accomplished by the biological processes of the symbiotic and free-living nitrogen fixers. Principal among these are the species of the root-nodule bacteria Rhizobium present in the leguminous plants. Certain other bacteria, fungi, and algae are also nitrogen fixers. The inorganic NO_3 is incorporated into organic forms (urea, protein, and nucleic acids) and is returned as waste products or dead organisms. This material is utilized by a variety of decomposers who produce NH_3 as a byproduct of their metabolism. Although there are some organisms that can use NH_3 directly, the majority requires that it be converted to NO_3. This process is called nitrification and again is specific to certain groups of bacteria. In the nitrification process, NH_3 or ammonium salts (NH_4^+) are converted to nitrite (NO_2) and the NO_2 is oxidized further to NO_3. This process obviously requires oxygen and as such is termed aerobic. If a source of oxygen is not present, the reverse (anaerobic) reaction, or denitrification may occur, even to the point of production of gaseous N_2. Again, specific bacteria and fungi accomplish these processes, as a means of satisfying their own energy needs. The process of nitrification is obviously crucial to the survival of all organisms dependent on plant life for food. The industrial fixation of N_2 to fertilizer is actually approaching the quantities fixed biologically. Tremendous quantities of energy (fossil fuel) are used in this process. If NO_3 is not quickly assimilated by plants, it may percolate through the soil to ground water or enter surface waters via runoff.

This fertilization of other systems than those intended by the farmer has resulted in serious water pollution problems. As of yet, nature has not compensated for this increase in "artificial" nitrification by increased or different pathways of denitrification. Another possible effect of over-fertilization is the denitrification of NO_3 to gaseous nitrous oxide (N_2O), as an intermediate step in the production of N_2. This reaction has serious implications in that N_2O plays a part in the destruction of the stratospheric ozone layer. This layer is needed to protect the earth from the ultraviolet rays of the sun, exposure to which has been found to cause skin cancer.

A second interference in the nitrogen cycle is that of combustion of fossil fuels in the presence of air, for example, in automobiles. This combustion yields NO_2, a health hazard in itself and also an important precursor in the formation of O_3 at ground level.

All terrestrial ecosystems continuously lose some nitrogen when nitrates and organic matter are washed, or, **leached**, out of the soil into groundwater and streams. In most cases, the nutrients are then eventually carried into the oceans. In a few places on Earth, leached nutrients have collected in natural geological deposits. Streams flowing out of the Andes Mountains in Chile travel across one of the driest deserts in the world, leaving behind deposits of nitrate through evaporation.

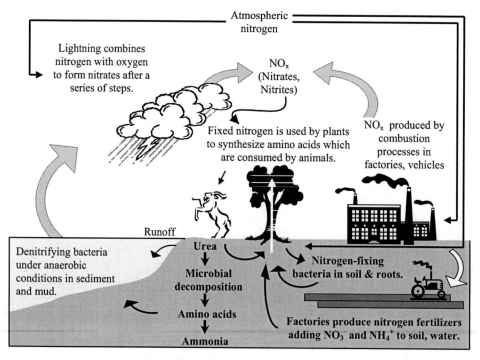

Figure 1.3. Nitrogen Cycle. (Source: Moore, 1999).

C. SEDIMENTARY CYCLES

The sedimentary cycles are characterized by fewer self-correcting mechanisms than are the gaseous cycles and so stagnation can occur, primarily in sedimentation in the oceans and deep fresh water lakes. Although sulfur has a gaseous phase, for example, sulfur dioxide (SO_2), and the carbonaceous deposits are considered the largest accumulation of carbon, the delineation of the cycles is by the largest, usable reservoir.

Sulfur Cycle. The sulfur cycle (Figure 1.4) is similar to that of nitrogen in that the inorganic, oxygenated form of sulfur, sulfate (SO_4^{-2}) is that used by the producers. The biological or organic form of sulfur is primarily the sulfhydrol group (-SH) present in protein. This organic matter is mineralized to the inorganic SO_4^{-2} by bacteria and fungi via aerobic decomposition. Under anaerobic conditions, elemental sulfur or sulfides such as hydrogen sulfide (H_2S) may be produced. The sulfur within the organic matter may also be "lost" by the formation of fossil fuel deposits.

Combustion of fossil fuels may thus return sulfur to the atmosphere as SO_2, a health hazard. Atmospheric H_2S and SO_2 may be oxidized to sulfur trioxide (SO_3), which combines with H_2O to form sulfuric acid (H_2SO_4) by which it returns to the producers via "acid rain." Although acid rain has become a pollution problem, this soluble form of sulfur is important to many ecosystems.

Sulfur is precipitated and lost in the sediments due to the presence of iron and calcium in fresh, and salt water. Ferrous sulfide (FeS), and ferric sulfide (Fe_2S_3) and calcium sulfate ($CaSO_4$) are either highly or relatively insoluble depending on pH, and thus sulfur and other nutrients needed for the formation of these substances may be trapped for various periods of time.

Phosphorus Cycle (Figure 1.5). Phosphorus is also needed by the producers in its oxygenated inorganic form, phosphate (PO_4^{-3}). This form is highly soluble and is taken up by plants in its dissolved state. The organic phosphorus plays a significant role in growth and metabolism (e.g., phosphate energy transfer compounds, nucleic acids, phospholipids). The difference between this cycle and the others discussed above is that organisms at higher levels than the bacteria and fungi return the phosphorus tied up in organic compounds to the inorganic state.

Phosphorus is lost to the cycle in a manner similar to sulfur in that it is easily precipitated out with cations of aluminum, calcium, iron, and magnesium. However, the physiological role of phosphorus also contributes to this loss. Phosphorus is bound up in bones and teeth, both of which are highly resistant to decomposition. These bound forms of phosphorus may become deposited in deep sediments, eventually forming phosphate containing rock. The return of this phosphorus to the natural cycle is dependent upon geological upheavals and/or erosion upon which the rock is exposed to weathering and leaching.

A far greater source of return of phosphorus at present, however, is via mining of phosphate bearing rock and "guano" deposits resulting from phosphorus excretion by marine birds. Phosphorus is an essential element for plant growth and is often the "limiting factor" upon which successful production of crops depends.

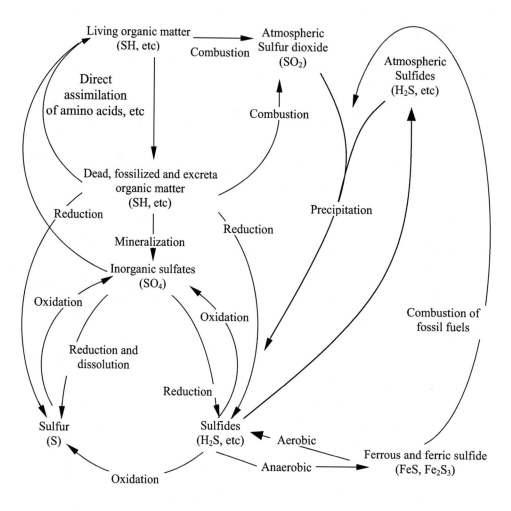

Figure 1.4. Sulfur Cycle. (Source: Kormondy, 1976).

The depletion of phosphate rock for fertilizer production more quickly than it can be deposited could lead to a worldwide of political situations similar to those caused by the growing awareness of those countries possessing the greatest fossil fuel deposits as phosphorus becomes an increasingly scarce, but vital 'resource'. In addition, increasing phosphorus-containing runoff from fertilization can lead to water pollution.

D. WATER CYCLE

The water cycle is shown in Figure 1.6. Besides being the major constituent of all organisms and the medium for biological activity, it is a significant instrument of nutrient distribution and plays a major role in the cycles discussed below. Water also plays an important role in energy transfer and distribution.

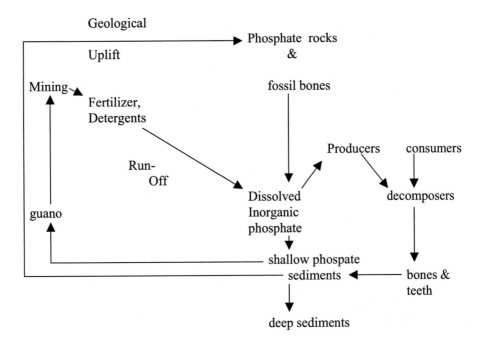

Figure 1.5. Phosphorus Cycle. (Source: Kormondy, 1976).

Figure 1.6. shows the general pattern of the hydrologic cycle in 10^{17} kgm and the distribution of water in 10^{17} kgm; amounts in parentheses are annual rates. The ecological cycle involves uptake by photosynthesis and imbibition and loss by respiration and transpiration. The primary movement of water is to and from the earth's surface and the atmosphere via precipitation and evaporation. An imbalance exists in that greater precipitation than evaporation occurs over the land and greater evaporation than precipitation occurs over the ocean, resulting in run-off from the land.

Although animal respiration and plant transpiration are crucial to our survival, they actually do not have a significant effect on this overall movement of water. The fact that only 5% of the earth's water is actually free, indicates how carefully we should be using this resource. The cycling process is capable of "cleaning" the water as it travels from surface waters, through the atmosphere, and through living organisms and/or geological strata. At the moment, however, we are straining this natural system of purification and distribution perhaps beyond recovery.

Although it is difficult for us to relate many of the interferences with these cycles to direct human health effects, many of the diseases which are now the principal causes of death can be traced back to such manmade imbalances. In short, there are five basic "laws" of ecology, which might prove helpful to the reader in trying to relate the tremendous amount of varied material in the area of environmental and occupational health sciences.

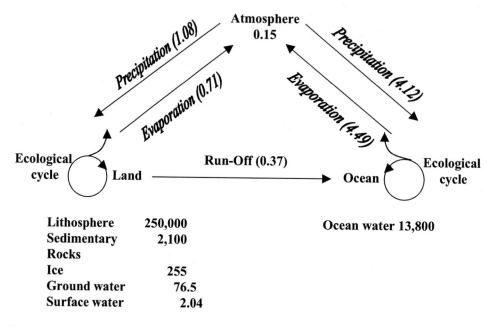

Figure 1.6. Water Cycle (Source: Kormondy, 1976).

These five basic "laws" of ecology are the following:

1. Everything is connected to everything else, either through positive or negative feedback mechanism.
2. There is no such place as "away".
3. We never get something for nothing.
4. Construction happens slowly, destruction happens quickly.
5. Nature knows best!

II. DEFINITION OF HEALTH AND THE ENVIRONMENT

A. DEFINITION OF HEALTH

In the Constitution of the World Health Organization, health is defined as "a state of complete physical, mental and social well-being and not merely the absence of disease or infirmity". This is the most commonly quoted modern definition of health. The concepts of disease, disability, and death tend to be much easier for health professionals to address than this idealistic concept of health. As a result, health sciences have largely been disease sciences since they focus on treating illness or injury rather than enhancing health.

B. DEFINITION OF ENVIRONMENT

Similarly inclusive definitions of environment in the context of health have been proposed. Environment is defined as "[All] that which is external to the individual human host. [It] can be divided into physical, biological, social, cultural, any or all of which can influence health status in populations." This definition is based on the notion that a person's health is basically determined by genetics and the environment. From the parents of an individual come genetic factors (genes), consisting of the DNA in each body cell. The genes exist when the embryo is first formed and do not generally change during the course of one's life. If a gene does change (as in the case of a mutation), it may lead to loss of function, cell death, and occasionally to cancer, as a result of very specific mutations.

C. SUSCEPTIBILITY TO ENVIRONMENTAL EXPOSURE

Some studies have suggested that genes provide a built-in "clock of self-destruction," as the body can only function properly for a limited time. The limit for most individuals is within the range of 70 to 100 years. An individual's genetic material is one of the major factors that determine how he or she is affected by environmental exposure. While everybody will have problems if subjected to high enough exposures to an environmental hazard, some people are affected at lower exposures because they have preexisting or concomitant risk factors or conditions, and some people are affected at quite low exposures because of an inherited susceptibility.

D. OTHER IMPEDIMENTS TO HEALTH

Poverty, poor living and working conditions, and lack of education have been repeatedly identified as major impediments to health. Over the years it has become clear that substantial improvements in health cannot be achieved without improvements in social and economic conditions. Providing relevant health services in the context of these conditions is addressed in the Health for All policy of the World Health Organization (WHO), established at a conference in Alma Ata in 1978. The final declaration stated that a goal of governments, international organizations, and the world community should be "the attainment by all people of the world by the year 2000 of a level of health that will permit them to lead a socially and economically productive life." It was explicitly noted that this could be attained only through a fuller and better use of the world's resources: "Health is only possible where resources are available to meet human needs and where the living and working environment is protected from life-threatening and health-threatening pollutants, pathogens and physical hazards".

Environmental pollution and degradation have a huge impact on people's lives. Every year hundreds of millions of people suffer from respiratory and other diseases associated with indoor and outdoor air pollution. Hundreds of millions of people are exposed to unnecessary physical and chemical hazards in the workplace and living environment. Half a million die as a result of road accidents. Four million infants and children die every year from diarrheal diseases, largely as a result of contaminated food or water. Hundreds of millions of people suffer from debilitating intestinal parasites. Two million people die from malaria every year while 267 million are ill with it at any given time. Three million people die each year from tuberculosis and 20 million are actively ill with it. Hundreds of millions suffer from poor nutrition. Almost all of these health problems could be prevented.

E. PERSONAL VERSUS AMBIENT ENVIRONMENT

In another definition, people's "personal" environment, the one over which they have control, is contrasted with the working or ambient environment, over which they may have essentially no control. Although people commonly think of the working or ambient environment as posing the greater threat, environmental health experts estimate that the personal environment, influenced by hygiene, diet, sexual practices, exercise, use of tobacco, drugs, and alcohol, and frequency of medical checkups, often has much more influence on well being.

F. GASEOUS, LIQUID, AND SOLID ENVIRONMENTS

The environment can also be considered as existing in one of three forms-gaseous, liquid, or solid. Each of these is subject to pollution, and people interact with all of them (Figure 1.7). Particulates and gases are released into the atmosphere, sewage and liquid wastes are discharged into water, and solid wastes, particularly plastics and toxic chemicals, are disposed of on land.

G. CHEMICAL, BIOLOGICAL, PHYSICAL, AND SOCIOECONOMIC ENVIRONMENTS

Another perspective suggested by Moeller (1997) considers the environment in terms of the four avenues or mechanisms by which various factors affect people's health.

1. **Chemical** constituents and contaminants include toxic wastes and pesticides in the general environment, chemicals used in the home and in industrial operations, and preservatives used in foods.

2. **Biological** contaminants include various disease organisms that may be present in food and water, those that can be transmitted by insects and animals, and those that can be transmitted by person-to-person contact.

3. **Physical** factors that influence health and well-being range from injuries and deaths occurring as a result of accidents, to excessive noise, heat, and cold, to the harmful effects of ionizing and nonionizing radiation.

4. **Socioeconomic** factors, though perhaps more difficult to measure and evaluate, significantly affect people's lives and health. Statistics demonstrate compelling relationships between morbidity and mortality and socioeconomic status. People who live in economically depressed neighborhoods are less healthy than those who live in more affluent areas.

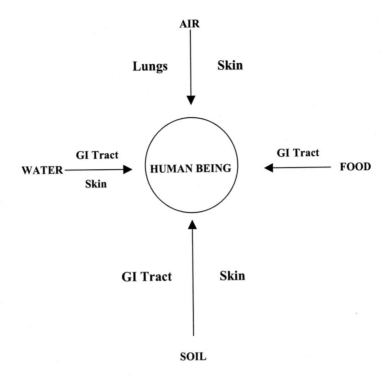

<u>Figure 1.7.</u> Routes of Human Exposure through the Gaseous, Liquid, and Solid Environments. (Source: Moeller, 1997).

Clearly, illness and well being are the products of community as well as of chemical, biological, and physical forces. Factors contributing to the differences range from the unavailability of jobs, inadequate nutrition, and lack of medical care to stressful social conditions, such as substandard housing and high crime rates.

The contributing factors, however, extend far beyond socioeconomics. Studies have shown that those without political power, especially disadvantaged groups who live in lower-income neighborhoods, often bear a disproportionate share of the risks of environmental pollution. One common example is increased air and water pollution due to nearby industrial and toxic waste facilities. In many cases it appears that personnel in various governmental agencies, including those at the federal level, have intentionally selected lower-income communities as sites for the most hazardous types of industrial operations, including waste disposal facilities and waste incinerators. Disadvantaged groups also suffer more frequent exposure to lead paint in their homes and to pesticides and industrial chemicals in their work.

Recognizing these and related problems, the President on February 11, 1994, signed an Executive Order on environmental justice, with the goal of ending this form of environmental inequity and discrimination. Included among the objectives was a reaffirmation that all communities and individuals, regardless of economic status or racial makeup, are entitled to a safe and healthful environment and that, in the future, the risks associated with hazardous industrial facilities will be distributed equitably across population groups. As part of the siting of any potentially hazardous operation, regulators will be required to identify and critically examine all potentially adverse impacts on the health and environment of minority and low-income populations. The Order also required that disadvantaged populations have an opportunity to participate fully in decisions that affect their health and environment.

None of the above definitions of the environment is without its deficiencies. Classification in terms of inner and outer environments, or in terms of gaseous, liquid, and solid environments, for example, fails to take into account the significant socioeconomic factors cited above, or physical factors such as noise and ionizing and non-ionizing radiation. Consideration of the full range of existing environments is essential to understanding the complexities involved and to controlling the associated problems.

III. LINK BETWEEN ENVIRONMENT AND HEALTH

A. INTRODUCTION

The environment, which sustains human life, is also a profound source of ill health for many of the world's people. In the least developed countries, one in five children do not live to see their fifth birthday - mostly because of avoidable environmental threats to health. That translates into roughly 11 million avoidable childhood deaths each year. Hundreds of millions of others, both children and adults, suffer ill health and disability that undermine their quality of life and hopes for the future. These environmental health threats - arguably the most serious environmental health threats facing the world's population today - stem mostly from traditional problems long since solved in the wealthier countries, such as a lack of clean water, sanitation, adequate housing, and protection from mosquitoes and other insect and animal disease vectors.

Contaminated water -contaminated by feces, not chemicals- remains one of the biggest killers worldwide. Lack of adequate water, sanitation, and hygiene is responsible for an estimated 7 percent of all deaths and disease globally, according to one recent estimate. Diarrhea alone claims the lives of some 2.5 million children a year.

Overcrowding and smoky indoor air - from burning biomass fuels for cooking or heating - contribute to acute respiratory infections that kill 4 million people a year, again, mostly children younger than age 5. The World Bank estimates that between 400 million and 700 million women and children are exposed to severe air pollution, in most instances, from cooking fires.

Malaria kills 1 million to 3 million people a year, approximately 80 percent of them children. Other mosquito-borne diseases, such as dengue and yellow fever, affect millions more each year and are on the rise, prompting the World Health Organization to declare the mosquito "Public Enemy Number One".

In the world's wealthiest regions, such as Europe, North America, and Japan, although environmental risks overall tend to be lower, they have by no means disappeared.

Asthma is rising dramatically throughout the developed countries, and environmental factors appear to be at least partly to blame.

Millions of people in Europe and North America are still exposed to unsafe air, and some air pollutants are proving more recalcitrant to control than many expected.

Meanwhile, biological contamination is by no means a thing of the past, as shown by the 1993 outbreak of **Cryptosporidium** in the United States.

The extension of travel and trade is providing new opportunities for the spread or re-emergence of infectious diseases. In the past two decades, some 30 "new" infectious diseases have emerged.

In all regions of the world, populations face the threat of climate change and other global environmental problems, such as stratospheric ozone depletion. Worldwide, fossil fuel emissions continue to rise, bringing with them the risk of climate change and both immediate and long-term health effects. However, it is important to note that although the activities that are driving these changes, such as intense fossil fuel consumption, have largely been concentrated among the wealthiest nations, the impacts are likely to be greatest in the poorest regions that do not have the resources to adapt to them. Similarly, in the wealthiest countries, disadvantaged populations often endure the highest exposures and have the fewest resources to deal with them.

B. TYPES OF ENVIRONMENTAL HEALTH HAZARDS

Environmental health hazards arise from both natural and anthropogenic (man made) sources. These include **biological hazards** (e.g., bacteria, viruses, parasites, and other pathogenic organisms), **chemical hazards** (such as toxic metals, air pollutants, solvents, and pesticides), and **physical hazards** (e.g., radiation, temperature, and noise). Health can also be profoundly affected by **mechanical hazards** (e.g., motor vehicle, sports, home, agriculture, and workplace injury hazards) and **psychosocial hazards** (e.g., stress, lifestyle disruption, workplace discrimination, effects of social change, marginalization, and unemployment).

On a global scale, environmental factors including overcrowding, migration, poor sanitation, and the broad use of pesticides intimately involved in the transmission of infectious agents have had a profound effect on the occurrence of disease. When infectious diseases are reduced, other environmental factors causing human diseases (e.g., chemicals, ionizing radiation, ultraviolet light) become increasingly important as determinants of ill health.

Some traditional hazards, which are still predominant in less developed countries and rural areas, and modern hazards, are becoming more important with increasing urbanization and industrialization. This is the case of traditional hazards such as the agents of reemerging infectious diseases and modern hazards such as outdoor air pollution from industry and automobiles.

1. Biological Hazards

Biological hazards include all of the forms of life (as well as the nonliving products they produce) that can cause adverse health effects. These hazards are plants, insects, rodents, and other animals, fungi, bacteria, viruses, and a wide variety of toxins and allergens. A recently discovered type of biological hazard has been called **prion** (disease-producing protein particle), which has been related to a number of diseases including Creutzfeldt-Jacob ("**mad cow**") disease.

Environmental health is largely determined by the health effects of exposure to microorganisms and parasites, whose occurrence and spreading depend on environmental factors.

Microorganisms of concern in environmental health include **bacteria**, **viruses**, and **protozoa**, such as amoebas. Most microorganisms and parasites that cause human illness need to grow inside the human body to cause it harm. Bacteria and protozoa may live and multiply outside other living cells and they can survive and multiply for long periods in food items or water, as long as there are enough nutrients for them and the pH and temperature are within viability limits. Viruses, however, cannot multiply outside of other living cells, although some can survive for long periods and remain infective. To sustain their life cycle, viruses need to enter either human cells or the cells of an animal, insect, or plant.

Many diseases caused by microorganisms are spread directly from one person to another. These diseases, considered person-to-person environmental health hazards, include tuberculosis (which is greatly increased by poor housing and crowded conditions) and many infectious childhood diseases. The five major infectious killers in the world are acute respiratory infections, diarrhea, tuberculosis, malaria, and measles.

When a disease can spread from one person to another it is called an infectious or communicable disease. The spread can be direct, by contact between two persons, as happens with sexually transmitted diseases, or it can be transmitted by air, as with the common cold or tuberculosis. One infected person exhales the microorganism that causes the disease and another person inhales the contaminated air. The spread can also take place through vehicles other than air, in materials that have been contaminated by an infected person, e.g., food contaminated with worms (helminths) from another person. Finally, vectors (animals or insects that carry the microorganism or parasite and infect a person via a bite, e.g., malaria via mosquitoes) can spread disease as well.

Certain bacteria and parasites produce toxins that can cause disease through the poisonous action of the toxin, rather than an infection. Much food poisoning is this type of bacteria-produced toxic reaction. The difference between infection and a toxic reaction is important.

Diseases that are caused by the toxins that bacteria produce are not contagious. That is, they do not spread from person to person, but are limited to the people who consume the contaminated food. Thus there is no subsequent risk to other people when the toxin causes the disease. Nonetheless, the precautionary measures taken to prevent both bacterial infection and bacterial toxins are similar (clean food preparation and adequate cooking).

2. Chemical Hazards

Approximately 10 million chemical compounds have been synthesized in laboratories since the beginning of the 20th century. About 1% of these chemicals are produced commercially and used directly (e.g., as pesticides and fertilizers); most chemicals are intermediates in the manufacture of end products for human use. There is virtually no sector of human activity that does not use chemical products, and these products have indeed created many benefits for society, such as the treatment of disease with pharmaceutical products and the use of fertilizers to increase food production.

All chemicals are toxic to some degree, with health risk being primarily a function of the severity of the toxicity and the extent of exposure. However, most chemicals have not been adequately tested to determine their toxicity.

3. Physical Hazards

Physical hazards are forms of potentially harmful energy in the environment that can result in either immediate or gradually acquired damage when transferred in sufficient quantities to exposed individuals. Physical hazards may arise from forms of energy that occur naturally or are man-made. A variety of different energy types can pose physical hazards, for example, sound waves, radiation, light energy, thermal energy, and electrical energy. The release of physical energy may be sudden and uncontrolled, as in an explosive loud noise, or sustained and more or less under control, as in working conditions with long-term exposure to lower levels of constant noise.

Noise, radiation (including light), and **temperature** factors are the most common examples of physical hazards. They can cause health effects in natural exposure situations, such as when ultraviolet (UV) radiation from the sun causes eye cataracts or when heat waves kill the frail, the young, and the elderly. For environmental health management, human-made exposure situations are of the greatest importance, such as the loud noise that millions of people are exposed to in their workplaces. Other examples include the ionizing radiation isotopes spread from the accident at the Chernobyl nuclear power plant, which exposed 5 million people to excessive doses and made large land areas uninhabitable for many years.

4. Mechanical Hazards

Mechanical hazards are those posed by the transfer of mechanical or kinetic energy (the energy of motion). The transfer of mechanical energy can result in immediate or gradually acquired injury in exposed individuals. The terms injury and trauma are often used interchangeably to refer to the harm that may result from mechanical hazards. The events and circumstances that result in injury have commonly been referred to as **accidents**. Those working in injury control no longer use this term. It implies that injuries are random, unpredictable, chance types of events. Environmental health specialists believe that most injuries are predictable and preventable, and can be studied using epidemiological methods, just like any illness or health effect.

Culture's attitudes toward injury are important. Where injury deaths are culturally viewed as determined by fate, there will not be a receptive response to an injury control initiative.

Socioeconomic factors are also important to consider when addressing the problem of mechanical hazards. Injury rates are linked with poverty within both developed and developing nations. Much of the world's population lacks the resources to provide optimal safety in their immediate environment. The necessity of obtaining food for the family by riding a broken-down bicycle through crowded, poorly maintained streets without a helmet is an example of this. Governments and industry are tempted to compromise safety for economic reasons, leading to tragedies such as the collapse of a public building. Many transportation accidents involving trains, ferries, and buses are the result of inadequate resources provided for the safe upkeep and regulation of roads, rails, and vehicles.

5. Psychosocial Hazards

Uncertainty, anxiety, and a lack of a feeling of control over one's own life situation or environment lead to what is popularly called stress. The word stress is sometimes used to describe a stimulus: a specific event or situation that causes a mental or physiological reaction. Stress can thus be defined as a human response to stressors. This definition of stress indicates the state of pressure that a person experiences. Another definition emphasizes the fact that stress is a process, resulting from the interaction between humans and the environment. The stress process consists of two stages: the first involves deciding whether an event (stressor) indeed poses a hazard; the second involves appraising the possibilities of dealing with the situation. As long as an individual can cope with the stressors, there is no problem. However, when coping strategies are no longer adequate, adverse stress reactions will occur.

For many people in both developed and developing countries, stress is a part of daily life, and it may lead to a variety of serious health effects, including depression, suicide, substance abuse, violence against others, psychosomatic diseases, and general malaise. Psychosocial hazards are those that create a social environment of uncertainty, anxiety, and lack of control. This may include the anxiety about mere survival from violence, as in the case of war-torn countries, or the uncertainty about future health effects of radiation exposure, for example, after the Chernobyl accident.

The modern perception of stress is that it is a negative or adverse reaction. The evolutionary perspective is different in that stress is considered to be an important mechanism to prepare the human organism for urgent action, both physically and mentally. The physiological characteristics of the stress reaction include increases in heart rate, blood pressure, respiration, and blood transport to skeletal muscles and a simultaneous decrease in digestive activity. Increased production of stress hormones, such as epinephrine and cortical, also play an important role in this reaction. All of these reactions prepare the individual for defensive actions-attack or flight. They thus improve the individual's chance of survival and can influence the success of a given species. However, if an individual is continuously exposed to environmental stressors and has no adequate coping strategies, adverse health effects are a likely outcome. Cardiovascular diseases such as arterial hypertension and ischemic heart disease may be associated with stress. Other medical conditions such as peptic ulcer disease, bronchial asthma, and rheumatoid arthritis are influenced by psychological factors, although the prevalence of these diseases is less that of cardiovascular diseases.

C. INTERACTION BETWEEN PEOPLE AND ENVIRONMENT

Human health depends on a society's capacity to manage the interaction between human activities and the physical, chemical, and biological environments (Figure 1.8.).

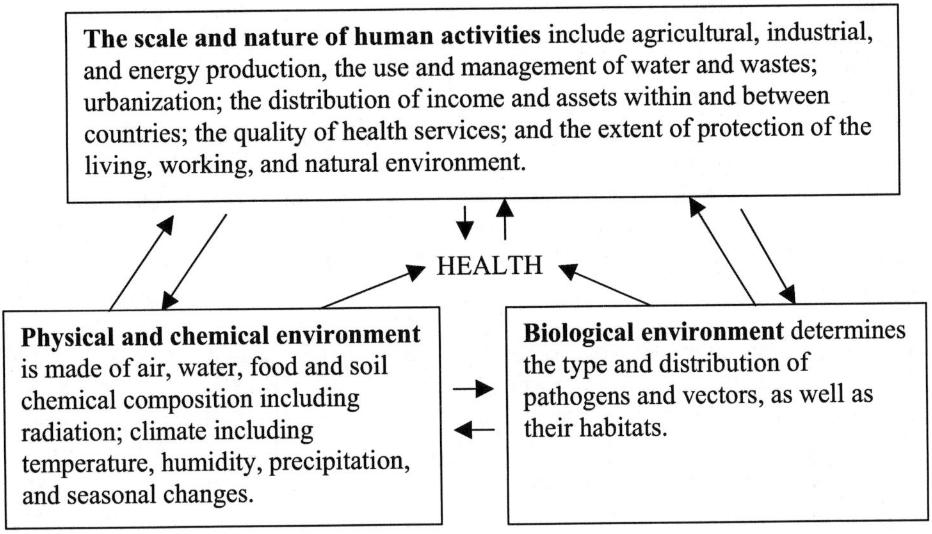

The scale and nature of human activities include agricultural, industrial, and energy production, the use and management of water and wastes; urbanization; the distribution of income and assets within and between countries; the quality of health services; and the extent of protection of the living, working, and natural environment.

HEALTH

Physical and chemical environment is made of air, water, food and soil chemical composition including radiation; climate including temperature, humidity, precipitation, and seasonal changes.

Biological environment determines the type and distribution of pathogens and vectors, as well as their habitats.

Figure 1.8. Interaction between Human Activities and the Physical, Chemical, and Biological Environments. (Source: Yassi, 2001).

The society must do this in ways that safeguard and promote human health, while at the same time protecting the integrity of the natural systems on which a healthy environment depends. The physical and biological environments include everything from the immediate home and work environments to regional, national, and global environments. This includes maintaining a stable climate and continued availability of safe environmental resources (soil, fresh water, clean air). It also includes continued functioning of the natural systems that receive the waste produced by human societies without exposing people to pathogens and toxic substances and without compromising the well being of future generations.

The idea of an inextricable link between human health and the environment has long been recognized. Over 100 years ago, Chief Seattle, an indigenous leader in Washington Territory during the western expansion of the United States, spoke movingly of our relationship to earth in a much-quoted speech: "We are a pan of the web of life and whatever we do to the web we do to ourselves." Thus, when we think of health as a state of complete physical, mental, and social well being, we must recognize that this also implies a context of ecological well being.

Socioeconomic factors control how resources are used. Whether a person is hungry, adequately fed, or overfed, depends not only on the state of his or her natural resources but also on the socioeconomic factors that influence such things as how agricultural practices result in use or misuse of those resources and whether safe, nutritious, and affordable food is available. Health also depends on how people feel about their society- including how much trust and social cohesion exists in their community. The following definition of environmental health is thus applicable: "Environmental health comprises those aspects of human health, including quality of life, that are determined by physical, biological, social, and psychosocial factors in the environment. It also refers to the theory and practice of assessing, correcting, controlling, and preventing those factors in the environment that can potentially affect adversely the health of present and future generations".

One extreme position of the ethical dilemma between promoting human health and protecting the environment is that any control limiting the exploitation of resources may inhibit an individual's or a community's attempts to enhance their standard of living, therefore infringing on their rights and freedoms as well as decreasing their ability to maintain health. At the other extreme is the position that any action to protect the environment and maintain the integrity of the ecosystem is justified regardless of the impact on human activity and health. The United Nations has stated that ensuring human survival should be taken as a first-order principle, one that takes precedence over all others. The first order assigned to meeting human survival is consistent with the United Nations Universal Declaration of Human Rights, which states that "all people have the right to a standard of living adequate for the health and well-being of themselves and their family, including food, clothing, housing, health care, and the necessary social services." Respect for nature and control of environmental degradation is a "second-order" principle, which should guide all human activities, except when these activities conflict with the first principle. In reality, most such conflicts are more apparent than real and arise from a faulty understanding of the human-environment interaction, or a dysfunctional social and economic system.

D. DRIVERS OF CHANGE

Environmental change and its attendant health impacts are driven by many factors, including economic growth, population growth and movements, urbanization, transportation, and war, to name just a few. There are three broad trends - the intensification of agriculture, industrialization, and rising energy use - stand out in terms of their profound impacts on the physical environment and their enormous potential for influencing human health. Given current development patterns, all are essential for economic development and improved welfare. Yet, all lead to pressures on the environment, such as pollutant emissions and resource depletion, which in turn can increase human exposure to threats in the environment.

Intensification of agriculture is essential for producing more food but, when not well managed, creates substantial risks, such as exposing workers and communities to toxic pesticides, contaminating groundwater supplies, and creating pesticide-resistant pests. Land clearing, irrigation, and dams can bring increases in vector-borne diseases such as malaria and schistosomiasis, both of which exact a huge toll in rural areas of the developing world.

Industrialization is the linchpin of economic growth and, like urbanization to which it is closely related, is associated with major gains in health. Yet, along with rising standards of living - at least for a majority of the population - industrialization often means increased exposure to heavy metals, persistent chemicals such as polychlorinated biphenyls (PCBs), and other toxic chemicals. This is especially true for workers and the poor who often live close to factories. Such exposures are likely to be increasingly pronounced in the developing world, where the most rapid industrialization is occurring.

Rising energy use is needed to fuel industrial growth but brings many attendant problems. Local air pollution from industrial and vehicle emissions has proved difficult to manage even in developed economies. Fossil fuel use also has the potential to alter the Earth's climate, with a predicted range of health impacts from severe storms, to drought, to flooding, to an increase in insect-borne diseases such as malaria. Energy demand, which is already huge in the developed countries, is rising fastest in the developing world.

E. POVERTY, HEALTH, AND THE ENVIRONMENT

What accounts for the strikingly different health profiles in various regions of the world? Access to adequate health care, for both prevention and treatment, is vital. Individual behavior and lifestyle choices also matter; they go far in explaining the rising incidence of chronic diseases and injuries. Sedentary lifestyles, high-fat diets, and consumption of alcohol and tobacco - and particularly these factors in combination - all contribute substantially to the increasing incidence of cancer, heart disease, and stroke.

In addition, individual susceptibility determines how one reacts to various health threats. Genetics, for instance, renders some people more susceptible to the effects of certain cancer-causing agents than others. Beyond an individual's particular characteristics or behaviors, one's age also affects health. Both the very young and the very old tend to be more vulnerable to a host of diseases - getting sick more often and dying more often when they are sick.

Disease and death are thus abetted by many factors. Yet of all factors that combine to degrade health, poverty stands out for its overwhelming role. Indeed, WHO has called poverty the world's biggest killer. Statistically, poverty affects health in its own right: just being poor increases one's risk of ill health. Poverty also contributes to disease and death through its second-order effects; poor people, for instance, are more likely to live in an unhealthy environment.

The interactions of disease agents, individual susceptibility, behavior (which often reflects education), and local environmental condition all bear heavily on health outcomes.

Efforts to reduce extreme poverty and increase disposable income levels around the world continue. But this objective will not be achieved quickly or easily. In the interim, understanding how poverty affects both the environment and health can enable policymakers to identify new strategies for action.

IV. LINKS BETWEEN ENVIRONMENTAL AND OCCUPATIONAL HEALTH

A. IMPORTANCE OF THE WORKFORCE

The workforce of a country is the backbone of its development. A healthy, well-trained, and motivated workforce increases productivity and generates wealth that is necessary for the good health of the community at large. Injured and sick workers, quite apart from being a major source of morbidity to themselves and their families, affect the economy as a whole, as do lost workdays due to illness and injury. The environment in the workplace generally involves levels of higher human exposure to environmental hazards and more injuries than in the residential environment. Every year approximately 100 million work injuries and 200,000 occupational deaths are reported in addition to the millions of cases of illnesses due to chronic exposure to noise, infectious agents, biomechanical hazards, and toxic chemicals. The workforce therefore requires particular health protection to maintain productivity, social equity, and personal security.

B. ENVIRONMENTAL AND OCCUPATIONAL HEALTH HAZARDS

The main reason for linking the occupational and general environments when addressing health concerns is that the source of the hazard is often the same. A common approach may work effectively in varied settings, particularly when it comes to the choice of chemical technologies for production. One example is the use of water-based paints instead of paints containing potentially toxic organic solvents. Another example is choosing nonchemical over chemical pest control methods.

Substituting one substance for another that is less acutely toxic may make good occupational health sense. However, if the new substance is not biodegradable or if it damages the stratospheric ozone layer, it is not an appropriate exposure control solution; it only moves the problem elsewhere. Chlorofluorocarbons (CFCs), widely used as refrigerant instead of the more acutely dangerous substance, ammonia, is the classic example of what is now known to have been an environmentally inappropriate substitution, for CFCs are the main cause of damage to the stratospheric ozone layer.

C. COMMON APPROACHES AND HUMAN RESOURCES

The scientific knowledge and training required to assess and control environmental health hazards are generally the same skills and knowledge required to address health hazards within the workplace.

Toxicology, epidemiology, occupational hygiene, ergonomics, and safety engineering are basic sciences that underlie assessment in these two fields. It thus may make good sense for the same professions to monitor both areas, especially in countries with scarce resources.

D. THE WORKPLACE AS A SENTINEL FOR ENVIRONMENTAL HAZARDS

Environmental health hazards have often been first identified from observations of adverse health effects in workers. The workplace is where the impact of industrial exposures is best understood. To conduct an epidemiological study it is necessary to define the exposed population, the nature and level of the exposure, and the specific health effect. It is generally easier to define the members of a workforce than it is to determine the membership of a community, particularly in a community that is transient. As well, the outcome of high levels of exposure typical of the workforce is almost always easier to delineate than more subtle changes attributable to low-level exposure.

Information on occupational health effects of many toxic exposures (including metals such as lead, mercury, arsenic, and nickel, as well as known carcinogens such as asbestos) has been used to calculate the health risk to the wider community. For example, as early as 1942, reports began to appear of cases of osteomalacia with multiple fractures among workers exposed to cadmium in a French factory producing alkaline batteries. During the 1950s and 1960s, cadmium intoxication was considered to be strictly an occupational disease. However, from the knowledge gained about the workplace came the recognition that the osteomalacia and kidney disease that was occurring in Japan at this time, "Itai itai" disease, was due to cadmium contamination of rice from irrigation water containing cadmium from a mine and metal refinery. Research in occupational epidemiology made a substantive contribution to the understanding and recognition of the environmental health effects.

E. THE CONCEPT OF TOTAL EXPOSURE

It is not enough to assess the exposure to a hazard from just one source. The sum of all exposures needs to be measured to assess health impacts and establish dose - response relationships.

Pesticide exposure is a classic example where occupational exposure may be supplemented by substantive environmental exposure. This may come through food and water source contamination and through non-occupational airborne exposure.

In Central America, for example, some cotton growers using pesticides not only have little access to protective clothing but also live very close to the cotton fields; many live in temporary housing with no walls for protection from aerial pesticide spraying. Workers also wash in irrigation channels containing pesticide residues, resulting in increased exposure. Thus to understand the relationship between their pesticide exposure and the health effects that may be reported, all sources of exposure to pesticide should be taken into consideration.

Other examples of exposure that may occur at the workplace as well as in the ambient environment are exposure to particulate matter from engine emissions (from industrial machines or traffic), benzene (as a solvent or from cigarette smoke), and polycyclic aromatic hydrocarbons (from products containing tar or from diet).

F. ASSESSMENT OF THE PROBLEM

A large share of the social, economic, and environmental decline in many parts of the world today results from increased production of materials and wastes, greater consumption of resources as a result of the expanding expectations of a growing population, and the use of ever more sophisticated technologies to satisfy continually increasing demands for goods and services. Many of these practices have global ecological effects, and the combination of local and global effects will inevitably affect human health.

One of the primary goals of environmental health professionals is to understand the various ways in which humans interact with their environment. A primary step is to study the process or operation that leads to the generation of an environmental problem and to determine how best to achieve control. Components of such an analysis include: 1. determining the source and nature of each environmental contaminant or stress, 2.

assessing how and in what form that contaminant comes into contact with people, 3. measuring the resulting effects, and 4. applying controls when and where appropriate.

Instead of focusing on air pollution or water pollution facility by facility environmental health professionals should gather data on all the discharges from a given facility all the sources of a given pollutant, and all the pollutants being deposited in a region regardless of their nature, origin, or pathway.

Even though tracing the source and path of a contaminant is important, an essential part of the process is to determine the effects on human health. Working with an interdisciplinary team, environmental health professionals must establish quantitative relationships between the exposure, the resulting dose, and its effects. On the basis of such data standards can be recommended for acceptable limits of exposure to the contaminant or stress.

To assess the effects of exposures correctly, environmental health workers must take into account not only the fact that exposures can derive from multiple sources and enter the body by several routes, but also that elements in the environment are constantly interacting. In the course of transport or degradation, agents that were not originally toxic to people may become so, and vice versa. If the concentration of a contaminant in the ambient (outdoor) environment (for example, a substance in the air) is relatively uniform, local or regional sampling may yield data adequate to estimate human exposure. If concentrations vary considerably over space and time (as is true of certain indoor pollutants) and the people being exposed move about extensively, it may be necessary to measure exposure of individual workers or members of the public by providing them with small, lightweight, battery-operated portable monitoring units. Development of such monitors and the specifications for their use requires the expertise of air pollution engineers, industrial hygienists, chemists and chemical engineers, electronics experts, and quality control personnel. Once the levels of exposure are known, they can be compared to existing standards, and controls can be applied when and where warranted.

At the same time, environmental health professionals must recognize that advances in technology have produced highly sophisticated and sensitive analytical instruments that can measure many environmental contaminants at concentrations below those that have been demonstrated to cause harm to health or the environment. For example, techniques capable of measuring contaminants in parts per billion are common. The mere act of measuring and reporting the presence of certain contaminants in the environment often leads to concern on the part of the public, even though the reported levels may be well within the acceptable range. The accompanying fears, justified or not, can lead to expenditures on the control of environmental contaminants instead of on other, more urgent problems. Those responsible for protecting people's health must be wary of demands for "zero", pollution: it is neither realistic nor achievable as a goal in today's world. Rather, given the host of factors that are an integral part of our daily lives, the goal should be an optimal level of human and environmental well-being.

G. SYSTEMS APPROACH

Attempts to control pollution in one segment of the environment can often result in the transfer to or creation of a different form of pollution. Such interactions can be immediate or they can take place over time; they can occur in the same general locality or at some distance.

The incineration of solid wastes can cause atmospheric pollution; the application of scrubbers and other types of air-cleaning systems to airborne effluents can produce large amounts of solid wastes; and the chemical treatment of liquid wastes can produce large quantities of sludge.

The discharge of sulfur and nitrogen oxides into the atmosphere can result in acidic deposition at some distance from the point of release; the discharge of chlorofluorocarbons can lead to the destruction of ozone layer in the upper atmosphere; and the discharge of carbon dioxide can lead to the global warming.

At the same time, it must be recognized that many uses of chemicals have brought major benefits to humankind. The chlorination of drinking water, for example, has led to significant reduction in the rates of many infectious diseases. In a similar manner, the use of chlorofluorocarbons has led to low-cost refrigeration and longer-term storage and transportation of milk and food, as well as of vaccines and antibodies. In other cases, however, widespread and indiscriminant uses of chemicals, most notably as insecticides and pesticides and in various types of industrial operations, have led to a global legacy of enormous chemical contamination. Unless environmental health professionals recognize the severity and widespread nature of these problems, attempts to deal with them will be inadequate, piecemeal, and destined to fail.

Clearly, what is done to the environment in one place will almost certainly affect it elsewhere. A systems approach ensures that each problem is examined not in isolation, but in terms of how it interacts with and affects other segments of the environment and our daily lives.

H. CONSISTENCY IN SETTING STANDARDS

Environmental health standards are usually much stricter than occupational health standards. The rationale for the difference is that the community includes many subgroups that are relatively sensitive, including the very old, the ill, young children, and pregnant women, whereas the workforce is at least healthy enough to work. Also, it is often argued that risk is more "acceptable" to a work force, as these people are benefiting by having a job and are therefore more willing to accept the risk. Many ethical and scientific debates rage around the question of standards and their degree of protection and for whom. Linking occupational and environmental health can be a positive contribution to sorting out these controversies. In this regard, tightening the connection between occupational and environmental health may facilitate greater consistency in setting standards.

I. INCENTIVES FOR PREVENTION

Although the workplace is usually the site of more intense exposures, the impact of these hazards on the general public has often been a major force in stimulating cleanup efforts, both inside the workplace and in the surrounding community. For example, the discovery of high levels of lead in workers' blood by an industrial hygienist in a lead foundry in

Bahia, Brazil led to investigations of lead in the blood of children in nearby residential areas.

The finding that the children had high lead levels was a major impetus in the company to take action to reduce occupational exposures as well as lead emissions from the factory, although workers in the foundry are still exposed to substantially higher exposures than would be tolerated by the general community.

J. INTERVENTION AND CONTROL

Because the complexity of the problems in environmental health requires multidisciplinary approaches to their evaluation and control, the techniques for addressing environmental problems often differ from those applied in medical practice.

There are various models for improving the state of human health and the environment. These are: 1. the clinical intervention model, 2. the public health intervention model, and 3. the environmental stewardship model.

In the clinical intervention model, the goal of the physician is to prevent a specific disease from leading to death. The public health intervention model, in contrast calls for preventing the development of disease. Far superior to either is the environmental stewardship model, where the goal is to protect humans by preventing environmental degradation and its resulting impacts on health.

Even after a problem is understood, environmental health personnel need strong support from other groups if their goals are to be achieved. A prime necessity is the assurance of legislators that the requisite laws and regulations, as well as financial resources, are available.

Public health educators need to ensure that the public participates in development of the programs, and that the associated regulations and requirements are fully understood by the industrial organizations and other groups who are expected to comply. Also needed is the input of program planners and economists to assure that available funds, invariably limited in quantity, are spent in the most effective manner.

V. HISTORY OF ENVIRONMENTAL HEALTH

A. EXPOSURE TO NATURAL AND MAN-MADE TOXINS THROUGHOUT HISTORY

Humanity has experienced many mass exposures to natural and anthropogenic toxins throughout history. A few important human exposures have been primarily environmental. Many more have been occupational or industrial in origin, which have subsequently resulted in environmental contamination. They have resulted in illness and death for a great many people. The frequency of these exposures has been increasing with the industrialization of the world. Many disasters involving hazardous substances are never recorded, especially in less developed countries. The public has become more aware of the environment and its pollutants since the publication of the book "**Silent Spring**" by Carson (1962). Table 1.1 shows a list of well-known environmental and industrial episodes.

Table 1.1. List of Known Environmental and Industrial Episodes. (Source: Greenberg, 1997).

Year	Place	Details of Environmental and Industrial Episode
79 AD	Pompeii	Volcanic gas (Mt.Vesuvius) heat, particulates, gases (Nox and sulfur); many deaths.
994 AD	Aquitania, France	Ergot alkaloids are thought to be responsible for the deaths of 40,000 people.
1692	Salem, MA	Ergot alkaloids are thought to be the cause of bizarre behavior.
1700	Italy	Cotton dust [Outbreak of respiratory complaints (byssinosis)]
1767	Devonshire,UK	Lead-contaminated cider caused colic; later, gout was associated with this same episode.
1700s	England	PAHs caused excess scrotal cancer in men who were exposed to chimney sweeps.
1800s	New Jersey	Mercurous nitrate used in the felting process of the hatting industry lead to mercurialism.
1800s	Europe	Yellow phosphorous used in the manufacture of matches led to "phossy jaw"
1838	France	Bread and wine with arsenious acid caused an estimated 40,000 cases of polyneuropathy
1846	Canada	Lead from soldered cans contaminated foodstuffs in Franklin expedition
1900s	Stafforshire, UK	Arsenic-contaminated sugar was used in beer manufacturing
1900s	US and India	B-Naphthylamine use in dye industry resulted in an increase of bladder cancers
1910	Manchester,UK	PAHs; Scrotal cancer in cotton textile factory, and chimney sweeper/paraffin workers.
1915-18	Ypres, Belgium	Chloride, phosphorous, and mustard gases; 10,000 deaths. (1.2 M deaths in WW I).
1920-90s	Worldwide	Asbestos exposure resulted in a market increase in asbestos-related disease and cancer
1928	Cleveland, Ohio	Deaths by nitrocellulose-containing x-ray film burned. Cyanide, NO_2, CO in pyrolysis.
1930	US, Europe, and S. Africa	Triorthocresylphosphate (TOCP) resulted in ginger jake paralysis, a neurotoxic disease affecting many people.
1930	Meuse Valley, Belgium	Smog from a thermal inversion resulted in illness and death for many from photochemical smog.
1937	US	Diethylene glycol used in elixir of sulfanilamide resulted in renal failure
1939-54	Japan	Cadmiun-contaminated water contributed to Itai-Itai disease.
1939-45	Europe, WW II	Cyanide and CO exposure occurred; > 1 M died from Zyklon B (HCN) gas exposure.
1952	Boston, MA	CO and cyanide from a fire at the Coconut Grove nightclub caused 498 deaths.
1944	Salerno, Italy	Carbon monoxide from a stalled train resulted in more than 500 deaths
1948	Donora, PA	Smog from thermal inversion of photochemical air pollution; 20 died and 1000s were ill
1950s	Minimata Bay, Japan	Organic mercury poisoning resulted from the consumption of fish that had eaten plankton that had organified inorganic mercury.
1950-80s	Rocky Flats, Colorado	Beryllium disease detected in +200 workers in ceramics plant that supported the nuclear weapons trigger plant.
1951	Atlanta, GA	Methanol-contaminated whiskey in "moonshine" with ocular toxicity and acidosis.
1952	London, UK	Photochemical smog epidemic caused the deaths of 4000, with countless others ill.
1953	New York City	Smog from photochemical air pollution resulted in an excess of 200 deaths
1954	Marshall Islands	Ionizing radiation from fallout with nuclear testing program developed thyroid cancer
1956	Turkey	Hexachlorobenzene; 3000 cases of porphyria cutanea tarda; "perma yara or pink sore".
1959	Meknes, Morocco	Cooking oils was contaminated with turbojet lubricant containing Triorthocresylphosphate
1960	UK / Germany	Thalidomide as an antiemetic in pregnancy resulted in 5000 cases of phocomelia
1960-70	Louisville, KY	Vinyl chloride use in PVC polymerization workers resulted in hepatic angiosarcomas
1962	London, UK	Smog from photochemical air pollution, >700 deaths, > 3000 fewer than 1952 episode
1962	Osaka, Japan	Smog from photochemical air pollution resulted in an estimated 60 excess deaths

Year	Place	Details of Environmental and Industrial Episode
1968	Japan	Rice cooking oil contaminated with polychlorinated biphenols caused sensory neuropathy
1969	France	Copper sulfate neutralized with hydrated lime (Bordeaux mixture) caused granulomatous disease among sprayers of mixture.
1971	Iraq	Grain with meHg; hospitalization 6530 persons / 59 deaths; grain with a red dye
1973	Michigan	PBBs instead of magnesium oxide mistakenly sent as livestock feed additive; +25000 cattle, pigs, chicken killed to prevent exposure.
1973-75	James River, Virginia	Chlordecone insecticide allegedly caused an increase in neurologic abnormalities among 148 workers.
1970s	California	1, 2 dibromo-3-chloropropane DBCP in soil as a nematocide; increased infertility, azospermia / oligosperma.
1975	El Paso, Texas	Children living within a 6.6 km radius of a smelter had levels of at least 60ug/dl
1975	Kellogg, Idaho	Lead levels in children who lived near a smelter were greater than 40ug/dl in 98% of 1 to 9 years old
1975	Jamaica	Parathion-contaminated flour caused death to 17 and illness in 62 others
1975	Ann Arbor, MI	Pancuronium administration resulted in an epidemic of respiratory and cardiac arrests
1976	Seveso, Italy	Dioxin released after explosion in chemical manufacturing plant, with increased incidence of chloracne in those in zone
1978	Jonestown, Guyana	Cyanide-laced beverage resulted in 911 deaths in a mass suicide-execution
1978	Youngstown, Florida	Chlorine leaked from a punctured tank car carrying 90 liquid tons. This resulted in 8 deaths with 130 total exposures
1978	Love Canal, New York	Toxic wastes placed in trenches resulted in increased public concern for practical or discernible health effects
1978	Bennington, Vermont	Campylobacter jejuni in the community water supply affected more than 3000 people with a typhoidlike illness
1979	Jackson, MI	Methanol-contaminated moonshine was found in a prison
1979	Taiwan	Polychlorinated biphenyl-contaminated rice cooking oil resulted in sensory neuropathy.
1981	US	Benzyl alcohol caused a gasping syndrome in children
1981	Spain	Contaminated rapeseed oil caused an outbreak of pneumonitis in 19,828 cases, 59% hospitalized, 16% whom died.
1982	San Jose, CA	MPTP, a meperidine analog, injected intravenously resulted in acute parkinsonism
1982	US	Cyanide-contaminated acetaminophen tampering incident resulted in 7 deaths
1982	Iraq and Iran	Mustard gas used in the Iraq-Iran war caused hundreds of casualties
1983	Times Beach, Missouri	Hazardous waste contamination after application of roadways resulted in public concern and no health consequences.
1984	Pakistan	Sugar contaminated with endrin, chlorinated hydrocarbon pesticide, caused seizures in 192 people - 10%case-fatality rate.
1984	Bhopal, India	Methyl isocyanate released from the Union Carbide plant resulted in 2000 deaths and 200,000 injuries.
1985	California and Oregon	Aldicarb found in watermelons resulted in cholinergic symptoms, more than 1000 cases reported to state health departments.
1986	Lake Nyos, Cameroon	Carbon dioxide release from the lake caused more than 1700 deaths
1986	Chernobyl, Soviet Union	Ionizing radiation with fire in nuclear power; 32 deaths; radioactive cloud over more than 10,000 square miles; 5 M people affected.
1987	Prince Edw. Island, Canada	Domoic acid and excitatory amino acid; 107 patients with GI symptoms, headache, and memory loss; four deaths with neuronal loss
1988	Pittsburgh, PA	3-Methylfentanyl (China White) epidemic in intravenous drug abusers
1989	US	L-tryptophan associated with eosinophilia-myalgia syndrome
1990	Texas	Hydrofluoric acid leak from a petrol plant

Table 1.1. Continued.

B. CONTROL OF ENVIRONMENTAL QUALITY THROUGHOUT HISTORY

The role of environmental quality as an important determinant of public health has been recognized for many centuries. Archaeologic evidence dating as far back as 4,000 years has revealed drainage systems, bathrooms, and water delivery systems at the ancient Indian sites of Mohenjo-Daro in the Indus Valley and Harappa in the Punjab. Later, Hippocrates noted the necessity of the balance between man and his environment in his book **Airs, Waters and Places.** In the book, Hippocrates first expressed the causal relationships between environmental factors and disease, and listed the factors that contribute to endemic disease in a population: climate, soil, water, mode of life, and nutrition.

In the United States, early public health efforts were developed largely to address serious environmental health issues such as contaminated milk and drinking water, disease vectors, sanitation, and an unsafe food supply. The 1850 **Report of the Sanitary Commission of Massachusetts** recognized the importance of environmental health and protection with the recommendation that "in laying out new towns and villages, and in extending those already laid out, ample provision be made for a supply, in purity and abundance, of light, air, and water; for drainage and sewerage, for paving, and for cleanliness."

Public health experts in Massachusetts also recommended regular surveys of health conditions and discussed the need for environmental sanitation, the regulation of food and drugs, and control of communicable disease. The report thus characterized the focus of the first boards of health that were developed in major cities to concentrate on environmental sanitation.

In the 1850s in London, John Snow conducted his classic study of a cholera outbreak in which he studied the spatial pattern of disease in the population. He traced the risk to the drinking water source, and stemmed the outbreak by removing the handle of the infamous Broad Street pump. This study, along with the discovery of microorganisms in the late nineteenth century, steered environmental health into microbiology and the control of infectious disease to combat epidemics of scarlet fever, diphtheria, typhoid fever, and tuberculosis.

Through the early twentieth century, the sanitary movement was largely driven by the public health community, which played a central role in the provision of sanitary water supplies, sewage disposal, and the establishment of food purity and safety programs. By the 1940s and 1950s, concerns over the effects of chemicals in the food supply led to the development of standards for pesticides and pesticide residues in the Federal Food, Drug and Cosmetics Act.

Similarly, water pollution control efforts resulted in the passage of the Federal Water Pollution Control Act in 1948. At the same time, incidents such as the emergency smog event in Donora, Pennsylvania in 1948 and the London Fog of 1952 galvanized public support for legislation addressing air quality and the control of industrial emissions, resulting in the passage of the Clean Air Act in 1955.

The early 1970s in the United States brought not only the first Earth Day and the creation of the Environmental Protection Agency (EPA), but also a fundamental change in the administration and implementation of environmental health and protection services.

The legislative flurry that followed the EPA's creation resulted in the formation of many state-level environmental protection agencies that took primary responsibility for environmental regulatory programs. No longer were state health departments the lead agency for the programs of clean air, drinking water, sanitation, food safety, and solid waste programs. The transition from a health-based approach for environmental health and protection programs to a regulatory approach has seen vast improvements in the quality of the environment; however, it has also contributed to the erosion of an essential public health infrastructure for environmental health. The shift of responsibilities has resulted in a detachment of public health organizations from many aspects of environmental regulation and decision making.

VI. ENVIRONMENTAL HEALTH ADMINISTRATION

A. INTRODUCTION

Public and scientific concern regarding quality of the environment and related public health and ecological considerations continue to be intense. This poses a challenge to administer environmental health and protection services that balance public demands with sound, science-based principles.

Environmental health and protection services are integral components of the continuum of health services, essential to the efficacy of the other components of the health services continuum (Table 1.2). Other health services include personal public health services (population-based disease prevention and health promotion) and health care (diagnosis, treatment, and rehabilitation of patients under care on a one-on-one basis). Table 1.2 lists the major components of the health services continuum and gives examples of issues related to each.

Administration of modern environmental health and protection programs is as complex as the nature and causes of the problems, and involves both the public and private sectors.

Program administration impacts public health, environmental quality, and the economy. Program administration requires properly qualified personnel, an informed and supportive citizenry, environmental health and protection leadership, a sound scientific basis, the data necessary to measure and understand problems and trends, a number of vital support services, rational public and private sector policies and workable legislation, and budgets prioritized to deal with the more significant problems as determined by sound epidemiology, toxicology, risk assessment, and public health assessment, as well as public demands and expectations.

The emergence of the federal Environmental Protection Agency and many state environmental agencies during the 1970s changed the structure and function of many environmental health programs in the United States. State health agencies were no longer the sole governmental entities that addressed public health issues involving air quality, drinking water, food safety, and solid waste management. Recently, significant policy shifts are contributing to a reemergence of public health organizations as leaders on important environmental health issues.

Table 1.2. Major Components in Health Services Continuum. (Source: Morgan, 1997).

Component	Examples of Issues	Component	Examples of Issues
Environmental Health and Protection	Clean air Clean water Toxic chemicals Safe food Radiation Solid wastes Occupational health Hazardous wastes Risk assessment Risk communication Risk management Global degradation Land use Noise Disease vectors Housing Ecological dysfunction Unintentional injuries Access	**Disease Prevention**	Infectious diseases Clinical prevention PKU screening Glaucoma Diabetes Osteoporosis Cancer Suicides Oral health Heart disease and stroke Maternal and child health Access
Health Promotion	Substance abuse Family planning Nutrition Health education Violence Obesity Tobacco Mental health Physical activity and fitness Access	**Health Care**	Diagnosis Primary response Case management Outpatient services Clinics Treatment Surgery Long-term care Acute care Rehabilitation Cost containment Health insurance Mental health and treatment Developmental disabilities Alcohol and drug treatments Managed care Access Environmental health

Recognition of the critical role of the environment in human development, health, and disease has long been fundamental to the development of prevention strategies. There is the traditional epidemiologic triad, depicting the interaction of **host** factors, **environment**, and **disease** agents in the causation of human disease. The triad illustrates the critical importance of a healthy environment in preventing disease, and has provided a time-tested model for public health practice. The epidemiologic triad was developed during a period when infectious diseases were the primary concern in environmental health. Although the control of infectious waterborne and food borne outbreaks remains an essential component of environmental health, prevention efforts have shifted toward the identification and control of adverse health effects from toxic pollutants in the environment.

B. ORGANIZATION OF ENVIRONMENTAL HEALTH SERVICES

1. National Level

The decline of the role of the public health organization and the rise of the EPA as the primary regulator of the environment began with the first Earth Day in 1970. At this time, programs that had traditionally been the purview of governmental public health agencies were reorganized into environmental regulatory agencies at both state and national levels. The U.S. Public Health Service, which was previously responsible for many environmental programs, witnessed a diminishing authority and a steady decline in resources for environmental health programs. The diminishing role of public health was highlighted in the 1988 Institute of Medicine (IOM) report, **The Future of Public Health**, which concluded that "the removal of environmental health authority from public health agencies has led to fragmented responsibility, lack of coordination, and inadequate attention to the health dimensions of environmental problems".

2. State Level

Because most of the actual implementation of environmental services occurs on the state level, the major federal environmental laws have provided the states with a blueprint for their organization. "Mini-EPAs" have become the dominant model for state-level environmental protection agencies.

3. Local Level

Local environmental health and protection services are administered by an even greater diversity of agencies than the federal and state programs. At the local level, governmental health departments and other agencies vary considerably and may represent a town, city, county, or district - virtually any administrative unit smaller than a state. At the local level, the goals of environmental health and protection agencies are varied and are specific to the local jurisdiction. These goals may include pollution prevention, zoning and planning, economic development, and public health. Many programs are administered with the guidance of local statutory mandates that address not only the media-specific concerns of air, water, and waste, but also noise and nuisance concerns, as well as land use and redevelopment.

C. ENVIRONMENTAL HEALTH COMPETENCIES

The environmental health specialist of today and the future must be a highly skilled, well-educated and trained generalist possessing a multitude of competencies as an effective member of the public health team. A sample of these competencies is presented in 13 specific areas as follows: administrative and supervisory skills, environmental chemical agents, environmental biological agents, environmental physical agents, air, water and liquid wastes, food, solid wastes, hazardous waste, population and space utilization, indoor environment, environmental injuries, and occupational health.

1. Administrative and Supervisory Skills

a. Knowledge and comprehension of environmental and public health laws, regulations, ordinances, codes, and their application.
b. Knowledge and comprehension of administrative techniques used in the management of environmental health programs.
c. Knowledge and comprehension of the systems approach to the analysis of environmental health problems.

2. Environmental Chemical Agents

a. Knowledge and comprehension of potential chemical contaminants of food.
b. Knowledge and comprehension of potential chemical contaminants of potable water supplies.
c. Knowledge and comprehension of transport requirements for hazardous chemicals.
d. Knowledge and comprehension of the techniques and procedures for identifying environmental chemicals.
e. Knowledge and comprehension of the means of disposal for environmental chemicals.
f. Understanding of decontamination of objects or substances that have been contaminated with environmental chemicals.
g. Knowledge and comprehension of field tests used to determine the presence and concentration of environmental chemicals.
h. Knowledge and comprehension of detergent and disinfectant chemistry.
i. Ability to evaluate detergents in an "in-use" situation.
j. Knowledge and comprehension of economic poisons and how they affect the human ecology of the region.
k. Knowledge and comprehension of principles and practices in the formulation application of economic poisons.
l. Knowledge and comprehension of bait formulations used in pest control.
m. Knowledge and comprehension of the safety features needed to prevent accidents with environmental chemicals.
n. Knowledge and comprehension of disinfectant detergents and their use

3. Environmental Biological Agents

a. Knowledge and comprehension of the epidemiology of vector-borne diseases.
b. Knowledge and comprehension of the natural habitat and control of common microorganisms and insects of public health and economic significance.
c. Knowledge and comprehension of basic life cycles of microorganisms, insects, rodents of public health significance.
d. Ability to identify a variety of microorganisms and insects of public health or economic significance in the field.
e. Knowledge and comprehension of environmental factors related to vector control.
f. Ability to identify scope of field problems and to determine control activities required.

g. Knowledge and comprehension of advantages and limitations of microbicides insecticides and their effect on the ecology of the region.
h. Knowledge and comprehension of the operation of sprayers and other pest control Equipment.
i. Knowledge and comprehension of the epidemiology of microbial, insect, and rodent-borne diseases.
j. Knowledge and comprehension of environmental procedures used in microbial, insect, and rodent control.
k. Knowledge and comprehension of biological control of microbes, insects, and rodents.

4. Environmental Physical Agents

a. Knowledge and comprehension of public health and ecological effects of noise the individual and community.
b. Knowledge and comprehension of instrumentation and procedures involved in noise measurements.
c. Knowledge and comprehension of existing laws pertaining to nuisances and noise abatement.
d. Knowledge and comprehension of practical applications of control measures.
e. Ability to implement surveys designed to define the extent of noise problem.
f. Ability to evaluate results of surveys and to establish long-range and short-range goals for control.
g. Knowledge and comprehension of work-related noise stress.
h. Knowledge and comprehension of radiation theory and principles.
i. Knowledge and comprehension of dangers of radiation.
j. Knowledge and comprehension of use of radiation and radioisotopes.
k. Knowledge and comprehension of effects of radiation.
l. Knowledge and comprehension of safety precautions.
m. Knowledge and comprehension of monitoring techniques and instrumentation in radiation detection.
n. Knowledge and comprehension of techniques of storage and disposal of radioactive materials.
o. Knowledge and comprehension of techniques of transportation of radioactive materials.
p. Knowledge and comprehension of techniques of decontamination.
q. Knowledge and comprehension of legal requirements of transportation, use and disposal of radioactive materials.

5. Air

a. Knowledge and comprehension of the different air pollutants and their sources.
b. Knowledge and comprehension of the relationship of weather conditions to air pollution.
c. Knowledge and comprehension of effects of air pollutants on the biosphere.
d. Understanding of the relationship of air pollution to topography.

e. Knowledge and comprehension of microflow of air.
f. Knowledge and comprehension of functional operation of air pollution control devices.
g. Knowledge and comprehension of preventive measures in air pollution control.
h. Knowledge and comprehension of corrective measures in air pollution control.
i. Knowledge and comprehension of the practical applications of air pollution control procedures and techniques.
j. Knowledge and comprehension of the principles of combustion engineering.
k. Knowledge and comprehension of air, air sampling techniques, and the ability to conduct air sampling.
l. Ability to implement surveys to clarify and identify the extent of problems.
m. Ability to evaluate results of surveys in light of long-range and short-range programs within the community.
n. Ability to design and implement cost-benefit analysis of control programs.
o. Knowledge and comprehension of air toxics.

6. Water and Liquid wastes

a. Knowledge and comprehension of water sources.
b. Knowledge and comprehension of potable water quality and standards (physical, chemical, biological, and radiological).
c. Knowledge and comprehension of water-borne diseases and how they are transmitted.
d. Knowledge and comprehension of sampling and testing of potable water.
e. Interpretation of laboratory analysis of water samples.
f. Knowledge and comprehension of legal aspects of water quality control.
g. Knowledge and comprehension of different types of water usage.
h. Understanding of the protection and selection of individual water supplies.
i. Understanding principles of water treatment.
j. Knowledge and comprehension of physical and biological composition of sewage including common and exotic industrial wastes.
k. Knowledge and comprehension of types of industrial wastes and their significance.
l. Knowledge and comprehension of the effects of sewage discharge on water quality.
m. Understanding of the epidemiology of sewage-associated diseases.
n. Knowledge and comprehension of the technology and basic engineering principles related to water flow.
o. Understanding the principles of individual sewage disposal.
p. Knowledge and comprehension of principles of municipal sewage treatment.
q. Knowledge and comprehension of small sewage treatment units.
r. Knowledge and comprehension of the measurement of absorptive quality of soils.
s. Knowledge and comprehension of the principles of nonwater sewage disposal.
t. Knowledge and comprehension of the techniques used in problems of emergency situations related to water and sewage.
u. Knowledge and comprehension of the techniques and potential hazards of sludge disposal.

7. Food

a. Knowledge and comprehension of food technology and its relationship to health.
b. Knowledge and comprehension of principles of food manufacturing, processing, and preservation.
c. Knowledge and comprehension of food-borne diseases and their control
d. Knowledge and comprehension of epidemiological techniques and procedures.
e. Knowledge and comprehension of design, location, and construction of food establishments and their equipments.
f. Knowledge and comprehension of principles of food establishment operations, housekeeping, and maintenance.
g. Knowledge and comprehension of equipment design, operation, maintenance, and cleaning techniques.
h. Knowledge and comprehension of methods of motivating industrial management to understand, accept, and carry out its responsibilities in the food environment, personnel training, and personal supervision.
i. Knowledge and comprehension of legal requirements of food technology.
j. Knowledge and comprehension of inspection, survey techniques, and significance data.
k. Knowledge and comprehension of the examination and licensure of food establishment managers.
l. Knowledge and comprehension of techniques used by different cultural and ethnic groups in food growing and preparation.
m. Knowledge and comprehension of institutional food-handling practices.
n. Ability to obtain public support for food programs.
o. Knowledge and comprehension of characteristic and properties of milk.
p. Knowledge and comprehension of dairy bacteriology.
q. Knowledge and comprehension of milk production and processing.
r. Knowledge and comprehension of legal standards of food and milk composition.
s. Knowledge and comprehension of techniques used to investigate dairy farms.
t. Knowledge and comprehension of milk processing operations and control.
u. Ability to inspect pasteurization plants.

8. Solid Wastes

a. Knowledge and comprehension of the types of solid waste generated in the community.
b. Knowledge and comprehension of the types of waste generated by common industrial processes.
c. Knowledge and comprehension of various methods of storage, collection, disposal of solid waste.
d. Knowledge and comprehension of public health and ecological aspects wastes.
e. Knowledge and comprehension of the use of systems analysis in waste management.
f. Knowledge and comprehension of economics of solid-waste disposal.
g. Ability to evaluate [tie results of solid-waste surveys and to establish long-range and short-range goals.

h. Ability to implement surveys to determine the extent of the solid waste problem.
i. Ability to design, implement, and evaluate programs related to waste disposal vs. public health problems.

9. Hazardous Waste

a. Knowledge and comprehension of the health and safety concerns related to hazardous waste sites.
b. Knowledge and comprehension of the effects of exposure to toxic chemical in hazardous waste site.
c. Knowledge and comprehension of the route of entry to the body of hazardous chemicals, including inhalation, skin absorption, ingestion, and puncture wounds (injection).
d. Understanding of the potential health effects due to acute and chronic exposure to various chemicals at the hazardous waste site.
e. Knowledge and comprehension of the symptoms of exposure to hazardous chemicals such as burning, coughing, nausea, tearing eyes, rashes, unconsciousness, and death.
f. Knowledge and comprehension of the potential chemical reactions that may produce explosion, fire, or heat.
g. Understanding of the psychological effects of oxygen deficiency in humans related to an increase in specific chemicals in the immediate environment.
h. Understanding of the health effects of ionizing radiation related to alpha radiation, beta radiation, gamma radiation, and X-rays.
i. Knowledge and comprehension of techniques used to dispose of radioactive material.
j. Understanding of the potential types of hospital and research facility waste that may cause biological hazards for the individual and may be spread through the environment.
k. Knowledge and comprehension of the various safety hazards that may be found at hazardous waste sites.
l. Knowledge and comprehension of the potential electrical hazard that may occur from overhead power lines, downed electrical wires, and buried cables that have been subjected to potential damage from hazardous waste situations.

10. Population and Space Utilization

a. Knowledge and comprehension of the population explosion and its effect on the present and future needs of our society.
b. Knowledge and comprehension of the health hazards related to congestion.
c. Knowledge and comprehension of individual space needs.
d. Knowledge and comprehension of the effects of different cultures on population control.
e. Knowledge and comprehension of the use of community planning and zoning on space utilization.
f. Knowledge and comprehension of establishment of priorities for the proper use of existing space.

11. **Indoor Environment**

a. Knowledge and comprehension of cultural, economic, and sociological aspects of individuals and multiple dwelling units.
b. Knowledge and comprehension of housing conditions needed for health, comfort, and well-being.
c. Knowledge and comprehension of impact of transportation on housing.
d. Knowledge and comprehension of real estate laws and prevailing practices.
e. Knowledge and comprehension of the various agencies involved in supervision and licensing of community shelters.
f. Knowledge and comprehension of techniques used to evaluate individual and multiple dwelling units.
g. Knowledge and comprehension of local, state, and federal housing program.
h. Knowledge and comprehension of zoning laws and their effect on the use individual and multiple dwelling units.
i. Knowledge and comprehension of the relationship of minority groups and poverty to housing use.
j. Knowledge and comprehension of indoor air pollution problems.

12. **Environmental Injuries**

a. Knowledge and comprehension of public health and ecological aspects of environmental injuries problems.
b. Knowledge and comprehension of the instrumentation, material, and procedures involved in determining the causes of accidents.
c. Knowledge and comprehension of epidemiological techniques used for studying accident problems.
d. Ability to motivate voluntary corrective action on the part of the public.
e. Ability to evaluate accidents and their causes.

13. **Occupational Health and Safety**

a. Knowledge and comprehension of the general principles of worker exposure.
b. Knowledge and comprehension of the legal aspects of the occupational environment.

D. EXAMINATION CONTENT AREAS FOR THE REGISTERED ENVIRONMENTAL HEALTH SPECIALIST (REHS)/REGISTERED SANITARIAN (RS)

The REHS/RS exam is based on the following content areas. Next to each subject heading is the approximate percentage of questions in that content area on the exam.

1. **General Environmental Health   12%**

Knowledge of health inspection procedures, disease-causing agents, epidemiology, sampling techniques, field tests and methodology, land use planning, construction plans, permit/license process, and public education.

2. Statutes and Regulations   5%

Knowledge of legal authority, law concerning inspections, agency administrative actions (embargo, seizure, nuisance abatement, etc.), federal environmental health acts, laws, agencies, and regulations.

3. Food Protection   13%

a. Knowledge of inspection/investigation procedures of food establishments.
b. Knowledge of food safety principles, protection, quality, and storage.
c. Knowledge of temporary food service events.
d. Knowledge of proper food transport.

4. Potable Water   8%

a. Knowledge of sanitary survey principles regarding potential or existing water systems and watersheds.
b. Understand testing/sampling methods, water supply systems, water treatment processes, and diseases associated with contaminated water.

5. Wastewater   9%

a. Knowledge of inspection/investigation procedures of wastewater systems.
b. Knowledge of soil characteristics and analysis methods, land use issues, wastewater treatment systems and processes, and disease-causing organisms associated with wastewater.

6. Solid and Hazardous Waste   9%

Knowledge of waste management systems, waste classifications, landfill methods, hazardous waste disposal methods, and health risks associated with poor waste management.

7. Hazardous Materials   4%

Knowledge of inspections/investigations of hazardous materials, self-protection procedures, and types of hazardous materials.

8. Vectors, Pests, and Weeds   7%

Knowledge of control methods for vectors, pests, and weeds; life cycle; different types of vectors, pests, and weeds; diseases and organisms associated with vectors, pests, and weeds; and public education methods.

9. Radiation Protection   3%

Knowledge of inspections/investigations of radiation hazards, types of radiation, common sources of exposure, protection methods, health risks of radiation exposure, and testing equipment/sampling methods used to detect radiation.

10. Occupational Safety and Health   3%

Knowledge of inspection/investigation procedures of occupational settings, common health and safety hazards at worksites, and general OSHA principles.

11. Air Quality and Noise   4%

Knowledge of inspection/investigation procedures to assess ambient air quality and environmental noise, air pollution sources, air/noise sampling methods and equipment, air/noise pollution control equipment and techniques, and health risks associated with poor air quality and excessive noise.

12. Housing   5%

Knowledge of inspection/investigation procedures of public/private housing and mobile home/recreational vehicle parks, health/safety risks of substandard housing, housing codes, heating, ventilation, and cooling systems, child safety hazards such as lead, and utility connections.

13. Institutions and Licensed Establishments   9%

Knowledge of the health hazards and sanitation problems commonly associated with correctional facilities, medical facilities, licensed establishments (tanning salons, massage clinics, tattoo parlors, and cosmetology salons) child-care facilities and schools, common disease-causing organisms and transmission modes, epidemiology, heating, ventilation, and cooling systems.

14. Swimming Pools and Recreational Facilities   6%

a. Knowledge of inspection/investigation procedures for swimming pools/spas, recreational areas/facilities, amusement parks, temporary mass gatherings (concerts, county fairs, etc.).
b. Knowledge of common organisms and resultant diseases associated with swimming pools/spas, water treatment systems, water chemistry, safety issues, and sampling/test methods.

15. Disaster Sanitation   3%

a. Knowledge of disaster preparation, site management of disaster situations, and post disaster management.

b. Knowledge of emergency response procedures, chain of command, supply needs, temporary shelter/facilities and services, and remediation methods.

VII. BIBLIOGRAPHY

Bruce, J.P., Lee, H.S., & Hates, E.F. (Eds.) (1995). Climate Change: Economic and Social Dimensions of climate Change (pp. 97-99). Cambridge University Press, Cambridge, U.K.

Burke, T.A. (1996). Back to the Future: Rediscovering the Role of Public Health in Environmental Decision-Making. In Cothern, R. (Ed.), Handbook for Environmental Risk Decision Making (pp. 93—l0l). Boca Raton, FL: CRC Press—Lewis Publishers.

Burke, T.A., et al. (1995). Strengthening the Role of Public Health in Environmental Policy, Policy Studies Journal 23, no. 1: 76—84.

Burke, T.A., et al. (1997). The Environmental Web: A National Profile of the State Infrastructure for Environmental Health and Protection. Journal of Public Health Management and Practice 3, No.2: 1—12.

Canadian Public Health Association. (1992). Human and Ecosystem Health – Canadian Perspectives, Canadian Action. Ottawa, Ontario, Canada.

Carson, R. (1962). Silent Spring. Cambridge, MA: Riverside Press.

Clinton, W.J. (1994). Executive Order 12898, 11 February. Federal Actions to Address Environmental Justice in Minority Populations and Low-Income Populations. The White House, Washington, D.C.

Committee on the Future of Environmental Health, National Environmental Health Association. (1993). The Future of Environmental Health, Part One. Journal of Environmental Health 55 (4): 28-32.

Easterling, J., Bennett. (1994, May 22-26). Environmental Justice: Implications for Sitting of Federal Radioactive Waste Management Facilities. Paper presented at the International High-Level Radioactive Waste Management Conference, Las Vegas.

Federal Food, Drug and Cosmetics Act. (1999, September). 21 U.S.C. 301, Chapter 9, subchapter IV, section 3431. http:// www4.law.cornell.eduluscodell/eh9,html. Accessed 15.

Gordis, I.L. (1996). Epidemiology. Philadelphia: W.B. Saunders Co.

Gordon, L. (1990, August). Who Will Manage the Environment?. American Journal of Public Health, 80: 904-905.

Gordon, L. (1997). Environmental Health and Protection. In Southfield & Keck, C.W. (Eds). Principles of Public Health Practice (pp. 300 – 317). Albany, NY: Denham Publishers, Inc.

Gordon, L. (1997). Principles of Environmental Health Administration. In Morgan, M.T. (Ed), Environmental Health 2nd Edition. (pp. 273-288). Englewood, CO: Morton Publishing Company.

Graham, J.D., Chang, B.H., & Evans, J.S. (1992). Poorer is Riskier. Risk Analysis 12, (pp. 333-337).

Greenberg, M.I., Phillips, S.D. (1997). A Brief History of Occupational, Industrial, and Environmental Toxicology. In Greenberg, M.I. (Ed). Occupational, Industrial and Environmental Toxicology (pp. 1-5). St. Louis, MO: Mosby.

Health Resources and Services Administration, Public Health Service, U.S. Department of Health and Human Services. (1991). Educating the Environmental Health Science and Protection Work Force: Problems, Challenges, and Recommendations. Bureau of Health Professions, Rockville, MD.

Institute of Medicine. (1988).The Future of Public Health (Washington, DC: National Academy Ness).

Koren, H., Bisesi, M. (1995). Handbook of Environmental Health and Safety: Principles and Practices. 3rd Edition. Vol. I (pp. 1-106). Boca Raton, FL: Lewis Publishers.

Kormondy, E.J. (1976). Concepts of Ecology. 2nd Edition. Prentice—Hall, Inc., Englewood Cliffs, N. J.

McMichael, A., Kjellstrom, T. and Smith, K. (2001). Environmental Health. In Merson, M., Blake, R., and Mills, A. (Eds). International Public Health (pp.379-437). Gaithersburg, MD: Aspen Publishers.

Moeller, D.W. (1997). Environmental Health. (pp.1-13). Cambridge, MA: Harvard University Press.

Moore, G. S. (1999). Living with the Earth Concepts in Environmental Health Science. (pp. 1-31). Boca Raton, FL.: Lewis Publishers.

Morgan, M. T. (1997). Environmental Health. Englewood, CO: Morton Publishing Company.

Murray, C. L., & Lopez, A. D. (1996). The Global Burden of disease: Volume I World Health Organization, Harvard School of Public Health, and The World Bank, Geneva, P. 311.

National Association of County and City Health Officials. (1988, September). Preliminary Results from the 1997 Profile of U.S. Local Health Departments. Research Brief Series I.

Pee, E. (1997). History and Development of Public Health. In Scutchfield & C.W. Keck C.W. (Eds.), Principles of Public Health Practice (pp.10—26). Albany, NY: Delmar Publishers, Inc.

Penman, H. L. (1970, September). The Water Cycle. Scientific American 223(3): 98—108.

Platt, A.E. (1996). Infecting Ourselves: How Environmental and Social Disruptions Trigger Disease. World watch Paper 129 (World watch Institute, Washington, D.C., P. 6.

Robe. (1990). Environmental Health Policy. In Pickett, O., & Hanlon, J. J. (Eds.), Public Health Administration and Practice (pp. 317-330). St. Louis, MO: Times Mirror Mosby College Printing.

Rosen, O. (1993). A History of Public Health. Baltimore: Johns Hopkins University Press.

Russell, E. (1990, Summer). Environmental Concerns for the Year 2000. The Bridge 20, No. 2, (pp. 3-10).

Ruttenber, A.J. & Kimbrough, R.D. (1995). The Pathophysiology of Environmental Diseases. In Blumenthal, D.S. & Ruttenber, J. (Eds). Introduction to Environmental Health, Revised 2nd Edition (pp. 35-69). New York, NY: Springer Publishing Company.

Schecter, A.J. (1998). Environmental Health. In Wallace, R.B. (Ed). Maxcy-Rosenau-Last Public Health & Preventive Medicine (pp. 411-792). Stamford, CT: Appleton & Lange.

Scientific American. (1970, September). Entire issue.

Shattuck, I.L., et al. (1850). Report of the Sanitary Commission of Massachusetts Boston: Harvard University Press.

Williams, L.K. & Langley, R.L. A Short History of Environmental Health. In Williams, L.K. & Langley, R.L. (Eds). Environmental Health Secrets. (pp. 1-4). Philadelphia, PA. Hanley & Belfus.

World Bank Washington, D.C. (1992). World Development Report. Development and the Environment P. 53.

World Health Organization. (1995). The World Health Report: Bridging the Gaps. WHO, Geneva, P.1.

World Health Organization. (1996). The World Health Report: Fighting Disease, Fostering Development. WHO, Geneva, P. 48.

World Health Organization. (1997). Health & Environment in Sustainable Development.. Five Years After the Earth Summit. WHO, Geneva, P. 1.

World Health Organization. (1997). The World Health Report: Conquering Suffering, Enriching Humanity. WHO, Geneva, P. 15.

WRI, UNEP, UNDP, & WB. (1998). 1988-1999 World Resources A Guide to the Global Environment. Environmental Change and Human Health. (pp. 1-35).

Yassi, A., Kjellstrom, T., Kok, T., Guidotti, T. L. (2001). Basic Environmental Health. (pp. 1-103). New York, N.Y: Oxford University press.

CHAPTER

2

TOXICOLOGY

I. BASIC ENVIRONMENTAL CALCULATIONS

A. PHYSICAL CONCEPTS AND MEASUREMENTS

The International System of Units (SI) defines various units of measurement as well as prefixes for multiplying or dividing the units by decimal factors (Tables 2.1 and 2.2).

The SI rules specify that its symbols are not followed by periods, nor are they changed in the plural. Thus, it is correct to write, "The tree is 10 m high," not "10 m. high" or "10 ms high."

1. Time

The SI unit is the **second,** s or sec, which used to be based on the rotation of the Earth but is now related to the vibration of atoms of cesium-133. SI prefixes are used for fractions of a second (such as milliseconds or microseconds), but the common words **minutes, hours,** and **days** are still used to express multiples of seconds.

2. Length

The SI unit is the **meter,** m, which used to be based on a standard platinum bar but is now defined in terms of wavelengths of light. The closest English equivalent is the **yard** (0.914 m). A **mile** is 1.61 kilometers (km). An inch is exactly 2.54 centimeters (cm). A **nautical mile** is 1.15 miles, or 1.85 km. A **knot** is the speed of a nautical mile per hour, or 1.15 miles per hour.

3. Area

Area is length squared, as in **square meter, square foot**, and so on. The SI unit of area is the **are**, a, which is 100 square m. More commonly used is the **hectare**, ha, which is 100 acres, or a square that is 100 m on each side. (The length of a U.S. football field plus one end zone is just about 100 m.). A hectare is 2.47 acres. An **acre** is 43,560 square feet, which is a plot of, say, 220 ft by 198 ft.

4. Volume

Volume is length cubed, as in **cubic centimeter**, cm^3, **cubic foot**, ft^3, and so on. The SI unit is the **liter**, L, which is 1000 cm^3. A **quart** is 0.946 L; a U.S. liquid **gallon** (gal) is 3.785 L. A **barrel** of petroleum (U.S.) is 42 gal, or 159 L. A **drum** (not a standard unit of volume) of the type generally used by the chemical industry and often found in chemical waste dumps is 55 gal, or 208 L.

5. Mass

Mass is the amount of matter in an object. **Weight** is the force of gravity on an object. To illustrate the difference, an astronaut in space has no weight but still has mass. On Earth, the two terms are directly proportional and often used interchangeably.

Table 2.1. The Metric System. (Source: Marieb, 2001).

Measurement	Unit and abbreviation	Metric equivalent	Metric to English conversion factor	English to metric conversion factor
Length	1 kilometer (km)	1000 (10^3) meters	1 km = 0.62 mile	1 mile = 1.61 km
	1 meter (m)	= 100 (10^2) centimeters = 1000 millimeters	1 m = 1.09 yards 1 m = 3.28 feet 1 m = 39.37 inches	1 yard = 0.914 m 1 foot = 0.305 m
	1 centimeter (cm)	0.01 (10^{-2}) meter	1 cm = 0.394 inch	1 foot = 30.5 cm 1 inch = 2.54 cm
	1 millimeter (mm)	0.001 (10^{-3}) meter	1 mm = 0.039 inch	
	1 micrometer (um)	0.000001 (10^{-6}) meter		
	1 nanometer (nm)	0.000000001 (10^{-9}) meter		
	1 angstrom (A)	0.0000000001 (10^{-10}) meter		
Area	1 square meter (m^2)	10,000 square centimeters	1 m^2 = 1.1960 square yards 1 m^2 = 10.764 square feet	1 square yard = 0.8361 m^2 1 square foot = 0.0929 m^2
	1 square centimeter (cm^2)	100 square millimeters	1 cm^2 = 0.155 square inch	1 square inch = 6.4516cm^2
Mass	1 metric ton (t)	1000 kilograms	1 t = 1.103 ton	1 ton = 0.907 t
	1 kilogram (kg)	1000 grams	1 kg = 2.205 pounds	1 pound = 0.4536 kg
	1 gram (g)	1000 milligrams	1 g = 0.0353 ounce 1 g = 15.432 grains	1 ounce = 28.35 g
	1 milligram (mg)	0.001 gram	1 mg = approx. 0.015 grain	
	1 microgram (ug)	0.000001 gram		
Volume (Solids)	1 cubic meter (m^3)	1,000,000 cubic centimeters	1 m^3 = 1.3080 cubic yards 1 m^3 = 35.315 cubic feet	1 cubic yard = 0.7646 m^3 1 cubic foot = 0.0283 m^3
	1 cubic centimeter (cm^3 orcc)	0.000001 cubic meter		
	1 cubic millimeter (mm^3)	0.000000001 cubic meter	1 cm^3 = 0.0610 cubic inch	1 cubic inch = 16.387 cm^3
Volumes (Liquids / gases)	1 kiloliter (kl or kL)	1000 liters	1 kL = 264.17 gallons	1 gallon = 3.785 L
	1 liter (l or L)	1000 milliliters	1 L = 0.264 gallons	1 quart = 0.946 L
	1 milliliter (ml or mL)	= 0.001 liter = 1 cubic centimeter	1 ml = 0.034 fluid ounce 1 ml = approx. ¼ teaspoon 1 ml = approx. 15-16 drops (gtt.)	1 quart = 946 ml 1 pint = 473 ml 1 fluid ounce = 29.57 ml 1 teaspoon = approx. 5 ml
	1 microliter (ul or uL)	0.000001 liter		
Time	1 second (s)	1/60 minute		
	1 millisecond (ms)	0.001 second		
Temperature	Degrees Celsius (°C)		°F = 9/5 °C + 32	°C = 5/9 (°F – 32)

Table 2.2. Additional Derived Units of the SI System. (Source: CGPM, 1975).

Quantity	Definition	Unit	Symbol	Formula
Force	(mass X acceleration)	Newton	N	$kg\ m/s^2$
Pressure	force per area	Pascal	Pa	N/m^2
Energy	(force X distance)	Joule	J	Nm
Density	mass per volume	kilogram per cubic meter	P	m/V
Area	(length X length)	square meter	m^2	m^2
Volume	(length X length X length)	Cubic meter	m^3	m^3
Velocity	distance per time	Meter per second	v	m/s
Concentration	quantity per volume	mole per cubic meter	mol/m^3	$mol*/m^3$

* The symbol **mol** is used for kilogram mole; **mole** is used for gram mole.

The SI unit of mass is the **kilogram**, kg, which is based on a standard platinum mass. A **pound** (avdp), lb, is a unit of weight. On the surface of the Earth, 1 lb is equal to 0.454 kg. A **metric ton**, also written as **tonne**, is 1000 kg, or about 2205 lb. In the English system, a **short ton** is 2000 lb and a **long ton** is 2240 lb. A tonne is therefore between the two English tons but closer to the long ton. Here we are using the term "tonne" because it is the metric unit.

6. Temperature

The SI unit is the **kelvin** (K). In measuring differences in temperature, such as the rise in temperature from the melting point of ice to the boiling point of water, one kelvin is the same as 1 degree Celsius (°C). However, Celsius temperature (not temperature difference) is related to kelvin temperature as follows:

Celsius temperature (°C) = kelvin temperature (K) - 273 K

Freezing point of water	Boiling point of water
0°C or 273 K	100°C or 373 K
Difference =	100°C or 100 K

In describing very high temperatures, such as the millions of degrees in stars or nuclear reactions, the 273-degree difference between the two scales is too small to matter, so either the kelvin or the Celsius scale can be used. Fahrenheit temperature (°F) is not used in scientific writing, although it is still popular in English-speaking countries.

7. Concentration

Concentration is the quantity of a substance in a given volume of space or in a given quantity of some other substance. "Quantity" can be expressed in units of mass or volume, or even in molecules.

percent	=	parts per 100 parts
ppm	=	parts per million parts
ppb	=	parts per billion parts

Concentration is therefore always a ratio:

$$\frac{\text{quantity of substance X,}}{\text{volume of space}} \quad \text{or} \quad \frac{\text{quantity of substance X}}{\text{quantity of substance in which X is dispersed}}$$

For example, 1 kg of ocean water contains about 65 mg of the element bromine. The concentration of bromine in the ocean is therefore:

$$\frac{65 \text{ mg bromine}}{1 \text{ kg of ocean water}}$$

But a kilogram is million milligrams, so we can write:

$$\text{concentration} = \frac{65 \text{ mg bromine}}{1 \text{ million mg ocean water}}$$

When both quantities are expressed in the same units, the units can be dropped (they cancel out), and we can say simply that the concentration of bromine is 65 parts per million (ppm) by weight (or mass).

Quantities of gases are usually expressed in units of volume. For example, the concentration of carbon dioxide, CO_2, in air is 350 ppm by volume. Because the volume of a gas is proportional to the number of molecules it contains, the concentration of a gas "by volume" really means "by number of molecules." Thus, there are 350 molecules of CO_2 per million molecules of air. The concentration of dusts in air cannot be expressed in volume units, however, because dusts are not gases. The concentration of particulate matter in air is expressed in mass per unit volume. For example, the maximum exposure to the pesticide 2,4 -D allowed by OSHA for an 8-hour work shift is 10 mg per cubic meter (10 mg/m^3) of air.

Concentrations expressed in parts per million or per billion by volume or mass seem quite small. In terms of molecules, however, such concentrations are very large. For example, if there is 10 ppb by weight of the pesticide DDD in water, each gram of water contains 20×10^{12}, or 20 trillion molecules of DDD. That concentration is high enough to kill some species of trout.

8. Energy

Energy is a measure of work or heat, which were once thought to be different quantities. Hence, two different sets of units were adopted and still persist, although we now know that work and heat are both forms of energy.

The SI unit of energy is the **joule**, J, the work required to exert a force of one newton through a distance of 1 m. In turn, a newton is the force that gives a mass of 1 kg an acceleration of $1 m/sec^2$. In human terms, a joule is not much - it is about the amount of work required to lift a 100-g weight to a height of 1 m. Therefore, joule units are too small for discussions of machines, power plants, or energy policy.

Larger units are:

megajoule, MJ = 10^6 J (a day's work by one person),
gigajoule, GJ   = 10^9 J (energy in half a tank of gasoline).

Another unit of energy, used for electrical work, is the **watt hour**, Wh, which is 3600 J. A **kilowatt hour**, kWh, is 3.6 MJ.

The energy unit used for heat is the **calorie**, cal, which is exactly 4.184 J. One calorie is just enough energy to warm 1 g of water 1°C. The more common unit used in measuring food energy is the **kilocalorie**, kcal, which is 1000 cal. When **Calorie** is spelled with a capital C, it means kcal. If a cookbook says that a jelly doughnut has 185 calories, that is an error - it should say 185 Calories (capital C), or 185 kcal. A value of 185 calories (small c) would be the energy in about one quarter of a thin slice of cucumber.

The unit of energy in the British system is the **British thermal unit**, Btu, which is the energy needed to warm 1 lb of water 1°F.

1 Btu = 1054 J = 1.054 kJ= 252 cal.

The unit often referred to in discussions of national energy policies is the **quad**, which is a quadrillion Btu, or 10^{15} Btu.
Some approximate energy values are:

1 barrel (42 gal) of petroleum = 5900 MJ,
1 tonne of coal = 29,000 MJ,
1 quad = 170 million barrels of oil, or 34 million tonnes of coal.

9. Efficiency of energy use

Imagine that you want to heat 1 kg of water from, say, 10°C to 90°C by using the heat from a fuel such as gasoline. The heat that must be absorbed by the water to reach the required temperature is 80 kcal, but let us say that you actually have to use 100 kcal to do the job. Since energy cannot be destroyed, where did the other 20 kcal go? Not into the water, obviously. The pot that contained the water absorbed some heat and so did the air in the room. The efficiency of your operation, therefore, was:

Efficiency = $\dfrac{\text{energy absorbed by the desired process}}{\text{total energy actually supplied}}$ x 100% = $\dfrac{80 \text{ kcal}}{100 \text{ kcal}}$ x 100% = 80%
(1st law)

The assumption that the energy not absorbed by the water was merely wasted, but not destroyed, is really a statement of the first law of thermodynamics. This is the reason why the efficiency described by the above equation is called the **first law efficiency**.

Now imagine that you take the same amount of energy (100 kcal) and use it to run a heat engine, such as a gasoline engine, to make the engine work. The engine extracts the heat from the fuel and converts it to work. But heat can be extracted from a body only by flowing from a higher temperature to a lower temperature. (That is a statement of the second law of thermodynamics). If the engine ran in an environment in which the outside temperature was absolute zero (zero kelvin, or - 273°C), the engine theoretically could convert all the heat into work. But suppose, to pick convenient numbers, that the engine operated at 1000 K and the outside temperature was 500 K. The outside temperature would then be only halfway down from the operating temperature (1000 K) to absolute zero, and the engine could convert only half of its heat to work, yielding only 50 kcal of work. Anything better than that would be impossible; anything less would be inefficient. Therefore, the measure of efficiency is:

Efficiency = $\dfrac{\text{the minimum amount of useful energy (work) needed at a given temperature to do a desired task}}{\text{the amount of useful energy or work actually supplied}}$ x 100%
(2nd law)

The efficiency calculated in this way is called the **second law efficiency**.

10. Power

Power is a measure of energy per unit time. The SI unit is the **watt**, W, which is a joule per second. Other common units are the **kilowatt**, kW, which is 1000 watts, and the **megawatt**, MW, which is 1 million watts. The older English unit is the **horsepower**, which is about three quarters of a kilowatt. The watt rating of a light bulb is its power rating. A 100-watt bulb generates 100 watts of power when it is lit. Your electric bill is a charge for energy, not power - you pay for the wattage multiplied by the time. If the bulb is lit for a day, you pay for 100 watts x 24 hours, which is 2400 watt hours or 2.4 kilowatt hours. A factory that generates electricity is called a power plant, not an energy plant, because it is rated according to the power it can produce (usually expressed in megawatts).

B. BASIC DIMENSIONS / UNITS AND CONVERSIONS

1. Symbol

A **symbol** is a specific designation, such as a letter of abbreviation, chosen to represent a certain item. For example, the letter **d** may be chosen to designate **diameter**, **A** to denote **area**, and **V** to indicate **volume**.

2. Dimension

Dimension is a term given to the three basic units, mass [M] length [L], and time [t] in which all physical units may be expressed. In some cases, temperature [T] and amount of substance [mol] are also included as basic dimensions. For example, the dimensions of the items mentioned above are: d (diameter) = [L], A (area) = $[L^2]$ and V (volume) = $[L^3]$. The symbol = [   ] means "has dimensions of." No matter which system of units is used - the SI, the American engineering system, the British system, or the metric system - the dimensions on each side of a complete equation must be the same. It is therefore very useful to indicate the dimensions of each term in engineering problems to ensure that each item has the correct dimensions. The conversions of weights and measures including length, area, volume, velocity, time, weight, discharge, pressure, power, work, energy, heat and temperature are presented in Table 2.3.

3. Units

Units are specific standards of measurements within a given system, such as the *Système International D' Unités (SI)* or the *American Engineering System (AES)*. For example, the aforementioned items could have the following units:

Item	SI units	AES units
Diameter, d	Meter (m)	Feet (ft)
Area, A	Square meter (m^2)	Square feet (ft^2)
Volume, V	Cubic meter (m^3)	Cubic feet (ft^3)

It is very important to be consistent in the use of symbols and units. Even within a discipline, great inconsistencies may occur, causing unnecessary misunderstandings and confusion. In an applied field such as environmental engineering, which draws on several scientific and engineering disciplines, the problem is compounded. In this book, the symbols used consistently are those common in the environmental health field.

4. International System Of Units (SI)

The Système International D'Unités (SI) was established by the General Conference of Weights and Measures in 1960. It is popularly known as the metric system, although certain modifications of the metric system were made for the SI system. The metric system has been used for a long time in Europe and many parts of the world. The British system of measurement has been used in Britain and its former colonies throughout the world, including North America. In the United States, a variation of the British system referred to as the American Engineering System (AES) has been adopted. An example of a unit in the AES is the U.S. gallon, which is smaller than the Imperial gallon of the British system. The governments of many nations which have not used the metric system in the past have decided to switch to the SI system, because of the advantages of using a unified system in international trade and commerce. In many countries, this changeover is now occurring and causing considerable, but surmountable difficulties.

Table 2.3. Weights and Measures.

Length

Miles	Yards	Feet	Inches	Centimeters
1	1760	5280	...	...
...	1	3	36	91.44
...	...	1	3	30.48
...	...	...	1	2.54

1m=100cm=3.281ft=39.37in

Area

Square Miles	Acres	Square Feet	Square Inches	Square Centimeters
1	640	...	...	...
...	1	43560	...	...
...	...	1	144	929.0
...	...	...	1	6.452

1sqm=10.76sqft

Volume

Cubic Feet	Imperial gallon	U.S. Gallons	Cubic Inches	Liters
1	6.23	7.481	1728	28.32
...	1	1.2	277.4	4.536
...	...	1	231	3.785
...	...	...	57.75	0.946
...	...	...	61.02	1

1 Imperial (UK) gal weighs 10 lbs.; 1 U.S. gallon weighs 8.34 lbs.
1 cu ft of water weighs 62.43 lb.; 1 cu m weighs 2283 lb.
1 cu m=10^3l and weighs 1000 kg

Velocity

Miles per Hour	Feet per Second	Inches per Minutes	Centimeters Per Second	Kilometer Per Hour
1	1.467	1056	...	1.609
...	1	720	30.48	...
...	...	1	0.423	...

Time

Days	Hours	Minutes	Seconds
1	24	1440	86,400
...	1	60	3,600
...	...	1	60

Weight

Tons	Pounds	Grams	Grains	Metric Tons
1	2000	...	...	0.9078
...	1	454	7000	...
...	...	1	15.43	...

1 long ton = 2240 lb   1ppm= 1mg/l= 8.34 lb. per mg

Discharge

Cubic Feet per Second	Million Gallons Daily	Gallons per Minute
1	0.6463	448.8
1.547	1	694.4

1 in. per hour per acre = 1.008 cfs   1 cu m/sec = 22.83 mgd = 35.32 cfs

Pressure

Pounds per Square Inch	Feet of Water	Inches of Mercury
1	2.307	2.036
0.4335	1	0.8825
0.4912	1.133	1

1 atm = 14.70 psia = 29.92 in Hg = 33.93 ft water = 76.0 cm Hg

Power

	Horsepower	Foot-Pound per Second	Kilogram-Meters Per Second
Kilowatts	1.341	737.6	102.0
Horsepower	1	550	76.04

Work, Energy, and Heat

Kilowatt-Hours	Horsepower-Hours	British Thermal Units	Calories
1	1.341	3412	8.6×10^3
0.7457	1	2544	6.4×10^3

Temperature

$C = 5/9\,(F-32)$ $F = 9/5\,C+32$

C	0	5	10	15	20	25	30	35	40	45	50	55	60
F	32	41	50	59	68	77	86	95	104	113	122	131	140

II. GENERAL PRINCIPLES OF TOXICOLOGY

A. INTRODUCTION

The mere administration of a compound either for therapeutic purposes or accidentally initiate the field of toxicology. Even if there are no evident toxicological manifestations based on gross observation, yet the study of any abnormal physiological functions of the body either on organ, cellular, or subcellular levels will indicate such toxic effect.

All chemicals are toxic to some degree, with health risk being primarily a function of the severity of the toxicity and the extent of the exposure. However, most chemicals have not been adequately tested to determine their toxicity. Toxicity of a substance is defined as its inherent capacity to cause injury to a living organism.

In 1976 the United Nations Environment Program (UNEP) established the International Registry of Potentially Toxic Chemicals (IRPTC), which has a computerized central data file containing data profiles for hundreds of chemicals.

In 1980, the WHO, UNEP, and International Labor Organization (ILO) set up the International Program on Chemical Safety (IPCS) to assess the risks that specific chemicals pose to human health and the environment.

Hence, the field of toxicology is very wide and is involved in multidisciplinary areas. To clarify this angle, an entomologist, would like to learn about toxic effects of compounds on insects, an agricultural scientist like to study the toxic effects of compounds on plants and their effects on the yield of crops. Likewise, a veterinian would like to know the toxic effects of compounds on large and small animals and of little importance how much of such compounds will be present in the consumable meat. The health scientist will like to know of compounds in consumable food, meat, vegetables and water.

The physician has more wide varieties of concern in learning toxicology, if she is an in-plant doctor, the toxic substances used in such industry will be her main concern plus any synergistic effect on other drugs used in therapy of such workers. The physician who practices in health community should be aware of environmental toxicants which might interact and affect his therapy to wide variety of patients. The physician in plant operations for drug companies is more concerned about Phase II and Phase III clinical trials of safety of new drugs and compounds and any synergism from food contaminants or environmental pollutants. On the other hand, the physician concerned with approval of labeling of compounds wish to be able to gather as much information on compounds of food additives which definitely will contribute to toxic manifestations in the consumer.

B. TYPES OF TOXICOLOGY

There are, of course, different kinds of toxicologists. Some toxicologists are actively looking for new or better poisons to be used as insecticides, fungicides, rodenticides or herbicides. Specific and selective agents are being sought that will kill undesirable species without harming the beneficial organisms. This group is often called **Economic Toxicologists.** Some toxicologists are seeking better analytical methods to detect poisons in the body that might have been the cause of death. This group consists mainly of chemists who have become **Forensic Toxicologists.** The **Environmental Toxicologist** looks for causal relationships between exposure to chemicals in the environment and the effects on quality of life with emphasis on long-term low-level exposures to chemicals intentionally placed in the environment as well as the acute and chronic problems of chemicals which inadvertently, or through human negligence, are imposed on the population at large. **Clinical Toxicologists** deal with the diagnosis and cure of those individuals who have been poisoned, but also study the toxic side effects of drugs. **Veterinary Toxicologists** work with special problems of toxicity in animals with emphasis on pets and food-producing animals.

However, all of the toxicologists share one particular responsibility, the prediction of the potential toxicity of a new drug or chemical before it is initially administered to humans. A more awesome responsibility is the prediction of the dose that will be safely tolerated and the estimation of the margin between this dose and that necessary to produce the desired beneficial effect. In the absence of this margin of safety, benefit-risk ratios must be weighed.

C. CHEMICAL CLASSIFICATION

There are two major classes:

1. Inorganic chemicals

Inorganic chemicals (containing none or very few carbon atoms). Inorganic substances are halogens, corrosive materials (ammonia, calcium oxide) and metals (cadmium, copper, lead, manganese, mercury).

2. Organic chemicals

Organic chemicals (having a structure based on carbon atoms). Organic compounds are hydrocarbons (methane, propane), halogenated hydrocarbons (fluorine, chlorine, bromine), alcohols (methanol, ethanol), glycols and derivatives [ethylene glycol (anti-freezing agent)] and organic solvents (benzene)

D. ROUTES OF EXPOSURE

Chemicals can be released into the environment in many ways:

1. Natural geological processes (volcanoes),
2. Mining and dredging, and
3. Wastes from industrial, agricultural, commercial, domestic, manufacturing sources.

E. TYPES OF TOXICITY

Toxicity is any harmful effect of a chemical or a drug on a target organ. There are two types of toxicity:

1. Systemic toxicity – an effect on the body system after a chemical has been absorbed and spread by the blood throughout the body.
2. Local reaction – which affects only the organ where the chemical first made contact with the body.

F. Reproductive and Developmental Toxicity

There are also other effects such as genotoxicity and carcinogenicity caused by Chemicals. Chemical, physical, and biological agents can interact with DNA, resulting in structural and/or functional changes that might lead to the alteration of genetic codes and information.

Information on toxicity can be obtained from different sources. Product identity is crucial in hazard identification. The Chemical Abstracts Service (CAS), a section of the American Chemical Society, assigns a CAS registry number to every chemical. The Registry of Toxic Effects of Chemical Substances (RTEC) number is also important, as it is linked to a list of scientific articles on the health effects of chemicals. It is operated by NIOSH (National Institute for Occupational Safety and Health).

G. General Approach To Toxicology

Initial toxicological investigations must of course be performed in laboratory animals and the findings extrapolated to humans, an extrapolation which is often based only upon the accumulated experience of empirical observation rather than a knowledge of specific mechanisms. This approach has been largely successful, but must not be the basis for an undue degree of complacency. Errors in this field lead to misjudgments that can result in human tragedy, and complete reliance upon a previously successful empiricism is exceedingly dangerous. Both development of more sensitive and specific indicators of toxic effects as well as achievement of a better understanding of the fundamental mechanisms underlying toxic effects will allow for the early warning signs of toxicity to be identified.

H. Historical Background

Among the principles that guide the work of toxicologists, two need to be mentioned. The first was elucidated by Paracelsus who taught that all things are potential poisons and that their toxicity is governed by the amount administered. Toxicologists are strong advocates of the importance of dose-response relationships. In this regard the immune system has dealt with some dirty tricks and hard lessons, for it is only through an understanding of immune mechanisms that many "hypersensitivities' have become recognized as special cases of complex dose-response relationships.

A second principle is that there are underlying biological similarities among living organisms that allow us to extrapolate findings from one system to another. While this provides a major opportunity in the practice of toxicology, there are many potential pitfalls related to specific differences in species, strains, or sexes; differences often linked to genetic variance, and at times related to specific qualitative and quantitative variances between immune systems.

I. SPECIFIC PROBLEM AREAS

The concept to be proposed is that no chemical agent is entirely safe, and likewise no chemical agent should be considered as being entirely harmful.

The words safe and hazardous are always misleading. In order to define either, one has to ask the question: Safe to Whom?, or Hazardous to Whom? No substance is a poison as such, yet practically any substance can act as a poison. Several factors determine whether a substance will exhibit a toxic action. These factors can be divided into three major categories with several minor classes involved.

1. Factors Associated with the Exposure Phase

When a biological object is exposed to a substance, a biological or toxicological effect can occur only after absorption of the substance, with the exception of radioactive compounds, and direct contact effects. Figure 2.1 outlines the various phases for a compound action. Referring to the factors associated with the exposure phase, the following classes need to be identified:

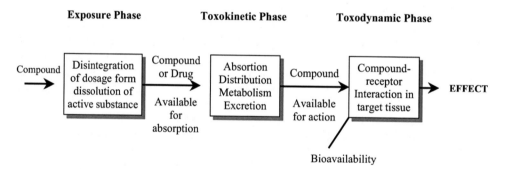

Figure 2.1. Diagram Representing the Three Phases of a Compound Action on Biological System.

a. The Nature of the Substance

Lipophilic substance (substances soluble in fat) can be readily absorbed through the skin; while hydrophilic substances (water soluble) are poorly absorbed through the skin. Greasy or sticky substances adhere to the skin and fine dust adheres to it. Water-soluble substances can be removed simply by washing, while solids and greasy substances are often difficult to remove. With inhalation, the physical properties, especially the degree of dispersion is important as well as the size of the particle. Aerosols with particles larger than 10 µm precipitate in the upper respiratory tract, while particles between 1-10 µm penetrate deep to the lower bronchiolar tree and even the alveoli.

Certain solvents in which the compound may be dissolved can be the cause of toxic effects, as in the case of vinyl chloride (used in the past as an aerosol), or the fluorocarbons (used in most of pressurized atomizers). Detergents used in dissolving the compound can readily spread over the surfaces and can help in determining the effectiveness of exposure. The degree of fineness of mists is another factor in determining risks in exposure to pesticides.

b. The Reaction of the Compound with the Surrounding Environment

The parent compound per se may be of no health or hazardous effects, however, when it reacts with the immediate environment such as water vapor in the air or oxygen, may be transferred to a more hazardous new compound. Sulfur trioxide, on contact with water vapor will react forming sulfuric acid which has more severe corrosive and harmful effects. Reaction of oxygen with nacent oxygen, produced by photochemicals and ultraviolet light will produce ozone, a highly irritant and harmful compound. Silicone tetrachloride, a substance used in plastic production, is liquid under pressure, when released in the air, will react with the water vapor, producing hydrochloric acid, and silicone dioxide, both of which are highly toxic to biological organisms.

c. The Dose of the Compound

The dose is determined by the concentration (how much of the compound), to which a biological system is exposed, and by the duration of exposure. Factors such as ventilation, functioning ventilators, and the effectiveness of occlusion of dust—producing machines all play a role in determining the dose. The number of working hours, including overtime, and the time of the day can affect the dose. The concentration of pollutants in the environment is often higher at the end of the day than in the morning when the work commences. To limit exposure, work breaks should be spent away from the contamination. Under certain conditions, the exposure period may be shortened by job alteration.

d. General Occupational Hygiene

Working clothes may become contaminated during the job. These clothes should be removed, and not taken home. Dangerous substances at the workplace, should be secured to prevent systemic toxicity. Household chemicals such as detergents, solvents, cosmetics and medicines should be secured to prevent accessibility to children and others who may accidentally consume it. Small children always have a tendency to put anything they can lay their hands on, in their mouth, and this is often the cause of poisoning in small children.

e. Individual Occupational Hygiene

Clear instructions to the workers should be given, to limit dust formation and the degree of contact between the pollutant and the skin. Correct use of tools, dust masks, vapor masks, gloves and other protective procedures should be given, to the individual worker, not only by verbal instructions, but also by particular practical sessions. Placing persons on dangerous jobs, with less knowledge would be a lack of social feeling or intelligence on the part of those in charge.

f. Execution of Controls

Levels of pollutants should be monitored regularly, and the concentrations of different compounds used should be determined. In some instances continuous monitoring is required. Threshold Limit Values (TLVs) should be mentioned. These TLVs differ from one country to the other, but in the future it is hoped that an international agreement will be placed for these TLVs values. In dealing with radioactive materials, the worker should be wearing radioactive-sensitive badges or devices.

g. Official Regulations

By implementing suitable policies, the authorities can promote a change from dangerous to less dangerous procedures. Sometimes, it is possible to avoid the use of dangerous substances completely, e.g. the replacement of elemental yellow phosphorous with phophorous sulfide ($P_4 S_3$) in the heads of friction matches: the replacement of tetraethyl lead, as antiknocking agent in motor fuel with the less toxic tetramethyl lead; limiting the use of DDT, etc.

h. The Functional Condition of the Contact Organs

The effectiveness of absorption, is greatly dependent on the condition of the contact organ or system. For example, the amount of compounds absorbed by the respiratory system, not only depends on the concentration of the compound in the air, but also on the amount of the substance retained in the lungs. Even, the amount of retained compound, is not an adequate measure of the amount of the substance absorbed. Retention of a substance in the lungs is the product of the respiratory volume per minute and the difference in concentration of the inhaled and exhaled air. This indicates, that the amount of retained compound is dependent on the frequency of respiration, on the work load, age of the employee, and on the humidity and temperature of the environment.

Moistness of the skin caused by perspiration, intensity of blood supply, and the status of the barrier layers of the skin, affect the amount of the compound uptake by the skin. If the sebaceous layer in the skin is affected, lipophylic and hydrophilic substances could be absorbed through the skin.

The pH of the contents of the gastrointestinal tract is a determining factor in the amount of absorbed materials through this route. This factor also affects the method of treatment, e.g. the use of neutralizing antiacids decreases the absorption of weak acids, but increases the absorption of weak organic substances such as organic amines. The use of absorbents such as activated charcoal, or precipitating agents, such as milk, may decrease absorption. In those cases where bioactivation, or bioinactivation of a poisonous compound takes place in the liver, the route of entry of compound plays an important role in the toxic end manifestations and severity of such compound. As an example, substances that are rapidly inactivated in the liver, are more toxic when they are absorbed after inhalation or through the skin than if they are ingested orally. On the other hand, those that are activated in the liver are more toxic after oral ingestion than after other routes of administration. An example of this latter case is the parathion, an organophosphate insecticide, it is not very toxic as such, however, it is changed to paraoxon, a very potent irreversible inhibitor of acetylcholinesterase.

2. Factors Associated with the Toxokinetic Phase

This phase includes: **Absorption, Distribution, Metabolism** and **Excretion**.

a. Absorption: Influence of Route of Administration on Toxicity

Chemicals can be introduced into the complex biological organism by a variety of routes. The nature of the chemical and the physical properties of each compound largely determine the route by which intentional or accidental exposure occurs. The physicochemical nature of a substance determines the rate of biological inactivation, rate of excretion or accumulation and sequestration in the biological system. It definitely affects the half-life and the time that a compound will reside in the body. Highly lipophylic compounds, e.g. DDT, perthane, and methoxychlor, tend to accumulate in the body, hard detergents are not inactivated while soft detergents undergo biodegradation in the biological processes. In the human, the most common routes of exposure could occur through the skin; inhalation or ophthalmic. However, oral ingestion of substances can occur, due to contaminated hands, or accidentally. The most common routes of testing compounds in laboratory animals, is by injection, parenteral routes, or by adding it to the food or drinking water (oral route). The route used for the administration of a compound can modify the toxicity of the agent.

(1) Percutaneous Route

The simplest and most common exposure of man or animals to foreign chemicals is by exposure through accidental or intentional contact of the chemical with the skin. The chemical must traverse the epidermal cells, or enter through the follicles to cross the skin, and get accessibility to the body. The pathway through the epidermal cells is probably the main avenue because this tissue constitutes the majority of the surface area. The transfollicular pathway provides access to the deeper layers of the skin via relatively permeable cells of sebaceous glands and the follicular wall.

For many years, it was thought that the outer layers of the skin form a barrier to transfer of chemicals. This is no longer an acceptable concept. Percutaneous absorption is defined as the transfer of a chemical from the outer surface of the skin, through the horny layer, the epidermis, the corneum and into the systemic circulation. The isolated epidermis of the rat skin has been found to be a poor barrier to transfer of water. In man and animals the deeper layer of skin (Stratum Corneum) possesses barrier properties to water, which equal that of whole skin.

The barrier properties of the whole skin vary with the site of application and the properties of the chemical applied, both in the same species and different species. As an example, pig skin appears to have a higher diffusion rate for water than that of rat or guinea pig. Two organophosphate insecticides were tested for their relative toxicities by percutaneous route (Table 2.4). The toxicities are expressed as lethal dose 50 (LD_{50}).

Table 2.4. Relative Percutaneous Toxicities of Two Organophosphate Compounds Tested In Eight Animal Species. (Source: McCreesh, 1965).

Species	Compound A*	Compound B*	B/A
Rabbit	1.0	5.0	5.0
Pig	10.0	80.0	8.0
Dog	1.9	10.8	5.7
Monkey	4.4	13.0	3.0
Goat	3.3	4.0	1.3
Cat	0.9	2.4	2.7
Mouse	6.0	9.2	1.5
Rat	17.0	20.0	1.2

* All values expressed as ratio of the LD_{50} of that compound to the rabbit LD_{50} of Compound A.

Also, the integrity of the skin can be altered by application of chemicals, which produce a breakdown in the surface layer, e.g. formic acid. Methyl and ethyl alcohol, hexane, and acetone when applied to the skin, and washed off may be used as solvents for the normal lipids in the skin resulting in a moderate change in permeability. Simple organic amines, such as propyl, butyl and pentyl penetrate rat skin at a rate that linearly increases with concentration.

The physicochemical properties of the compound are a principal factor in percutaneous absorption. In general, gases penetrate quite freely through the epidermal tissues, liquids less freely, and solids which are insoluble in lipids or water are probably incapable of penetrating the skin. Penetration of materials through the skin is time-dependent. The more contact of the compound is with the skin, more percutaneous absorption occurs, even if such compound is in the solid state and is possible to dissolve in the skin secretions (sweat and sebum). Some lipid compounds which can be absorbed through the skin, are phenol, phenolic derivatives, hormones such as estrogens, progesterones, testosterone, and desoxycorticosterone, vitamins D and K and organic bases such as strychnine and nicotine. Salts of some alkaloids may pass freely through the skin.

The presence of a vehicle may act as a carrier for percutaneous absorption or sometimes may inhibit the process. For example, d-tubocurarine passes through the skin of mouse tail in presence of special vehicles such as acetone or dimethyl sulfoxide (DMSO). Such parameters as pH, extent of ionization, molecular size, water and liquid solubility are all involved in the transfer of compounds through the skin.

Biological factors such as local temperature, blood flow, dryness of skin, or excessive perspiration, will affect the toxicity of potent chemicals by the percutaneous route. There are two basic methods in measuring the percutaneous absorption of a compound:

(a) Measure the accumulation of the chemical in the experimental animal, by analytic methods (e.g. blood levels of the compound by chemical analysis or isotope tracing techniques) or measurements of a pharmacological effect (such as anesthesia, vasodilatation, or convulsions in case of strychnine).

(b) Measure the rate of disappearance of the compound from the site of application with precautions taken to prevent evaporation or mechanical loss (e.g. isolated skin, or perfused skin).

(2) Inhalation Route

Exposure to chemicals in the atmosphere will reach the host through the respiratory system, unless a device is used to filter the contaminated air of such before being inhaled. For a particular compound to reach the alveoli of the lungs, it must exist in a gas or sufficiently small particle size that is not removed by the airway passages in the respiratory tract. This route is important in industrial and environmental exposure to contaminants.

In industrial working environments, the atmosphere in which people work, is more or less contaminated with a wide variety of chemicals due to their use in such industries. Therefore, it was necessary to establish some standards regarding the limits of contamination of the atmosphere which would be considered safe. The data necessary to establish a maximum safe concentration of a chemical in the atmosphere for humans who are exposed over an eight-hour working day are only rarely obtainable. Those values that are available for specific chemicals represent estimations based on information obtained by experience in industry and by experiments on humans and animals.

The American Conference of Governmental Industrial Hygienists has compiled a list of the Threshold Limit Values (TLVs) consisting of approximately 400 compounds based on the best available current data on hazards of these compounds. These values are periodically revised as new information becomes available. TLVs refer to airborne concentrations of substances and represents conditions under which it is believed that nearly all workers (healthy adults) may be repeatedly exposed in the working environment day after day without adverse effects. They are guides, and are not intended to assure that there will not be an occasional hypersensitive individual who will respond negatively to the recommended TLV of any agent. The criteria for establishment of a TLV are protection against impairment of health, reasonable freedom from primary irritation, pharmacologic effect, or nuisance-induced stress. TLVs for contaminants in the air that exist as gases or fumes are expressed as ppm (parts per million parts of air by volume at 25°C and 760 mm Hg pressure) or as mg of particle matter per cubic meter of air. TLVs for respirable dusts, such as talc, cement or asbestos, which are suspended in the air, are in terms of m.p.p.c.f. (millions of particles per cubic feet of air). Compounds that are suspected of having a carcinogenic action in man, such as benzidine, B-naphthylamine or B-propriolactone have no TLV value, and exposure or contact of humans at any concentration by any route should be avoided.

Threshold limit values represent values obtained as time-weighted averages, meaning that the concentration of the atmospheric pollutant may vary above and below the listed value during an eight-hour exposure so that the TLV represents the average concentration over the period of time of measurement. A maximal value (or ceiling value C) is also provided that should not be exceeded. TLVs serve a useful purpose in that they represent a gross classification of the relative harmfulness or safeness between a large variety of compounds that become atmospheric pollutants in industry. Their use for any other purpose is grossly erroneous, if one accepts that all harmful effects of chemicals are graded responses that are dose-dependent and that there is no exact concentration of a chemical above which that chemical is harmful or below which it is safe. The only way by which any value can be established which would represent a safe value for human exposure is through sufficiently extensive experience and then such a value would not represent a "limit' but would only represent an estimated safe level for exposure. TLVs are not intended for use in evaluation of community air pollution. There is evidence that air pollution in communities increase morbidity rates of cardiac and pulmonary diseases, as well as other systemic diseases. The EPA has set what is known as Primary Ambient Air Standards to protect the public health, as well as Secondary Ambient Air Quality Standards to protect the welfare of the public (such as agriculture, clothing, housing, etc.). Other factors determining the risk in inhalation route includes functional and reserved functional capacity of lungs, clearance rates, previous state of the alveoli, and air passages, habits such as smoking, concurrent heart disease, genetic deficiencies such as α_1-antitrypsin deficiency, and others.

Despite the vast array of materials producing lung disease, the responses of the lung to toxic agents may be divided into the following general categories:

(a) Irritation of the air passages, resulting in constriction of the airways. Edema often occurs and secondary infection frequently compounds the damage.
(b) Damage to the cells lining the airways, which results in necrosis, increased permeability and edema. The edema is intraluminal instead of interstitial.
(c) Production of fibrosis, which could be massive and cause obliteration of the respiratory capacity of the lung. Local fibrosis of the pleura can occur restricting the movement of the lung and producing pain through irritation of the pleural surfaces.
(d) Constriction of the airways through allergic responses resulting in extrinsic allergic alveoli is or through antigen-antibody responses.
(e) Oncogenic or carcinogenesis causing tumors in the lungs.

(3) Oral Route

The oral route is probably the third most common means by which a compound enters the body. The gastrointestinal tract in the animal may be viewed as a tube going from the mouth and ending at the anus. Although it is in the body, its contents are exterior to the body fluids. Chemicals in the gastrointestinal tract could produce an effect only on the surface of the mucosal cells that line the tract unless absorption occurs, hence the effects are observed on other systems. Caustic or primary irritant agents, such as sodium hydroxide, strong acids or phenols in adequate concentrations will cause necrotizing effects leading to scarring and obstruction.

Factors involved in gastrointestinal absorption include:

(a) **Gastric emptying time and contents of the stomach**. The chemical in the stomach, comes in contact with pre-existing stomach contents (such as food particles and gastric mucin) and secretions (such as pepsin, renin, and gastric lipase) in addition to hydrochloric acid. If the compound reacts with any of these gastric contents, the amount of free chemical would be altered thereby leading to an altered absorption rate of the agent. Products of the reaction may be more or less translocated, or more or less toxic than the parent compound. Ingested compounds will be transferred from the stomach to the intestine, where there is change in the pH and the chemical is mixed further with additional agents, such as food residues, bile, and additional enzymes in the pancreatic juices. The toxicity of the compound is affected by the frequency it is taken and stomach contents. A compound may be more toxic if taken on an empty stomach, than after a meal with full contents diluting its concentration.

(b) **Active transport** indicates that there are specific mechanisms involved for passage of contents even against a concentration gradient. This mechanism only applies to foods and food products.

(c) **Passive diffusion**, implies that the compound will move from the highest concentration gradient to the lower gradient, depending on pH and pK_a, which is the dissociation gradient into ionized and non-ionized portion is equal at such pH value.

(d) **Chemistry of the compound**, such as solubility in water, molecular size, oil/water coefficient ($Kp= C_{oil} / C_{water}$), and ionization coefficient (pK_a).

(4) Ophthalmic Route

It defines the passage of compounds through the eye. Besides direct necrotic effects on the conjunctiva, some compounds could be absorbed through the conjunctival sac and may cause systemic toxicity. This route contributes a small part in toxicology and is mainly used to test topical toxicity of compounds. Again absorption through the membranes depend on the pH and pK_a of the compound as well as its solubility.

(5) Parenteral Routes

Introduction of chemicals into the organism by means of injection from a syringe through a hollow needle to specific sites. In animal testing, it is the most common procedure used in administration of compounds. By this means, the natural body orifices are bypassed and specific amounts or doses of chemicals may be introduced. Such routes consists of: **intradermal**, through the skin; **subcutaneous**, beneath the skin; **intramuscular**, in the muscle; **intravenous**, into the blood of the veins; or **intrathecal**, into the spinal fluids. Specific agents may on frequent occasions be administered into the blood in the arteries (intra-arterial), into tumors, or into chest fluid (intrapleural). In laboratory animals, the injection of chemicals into the abdominal fluid (intraperitoneal) is a very common procedure. In the laboratory it is even possible to inject into single cells (intracellular) by use of micropippette. Intrathecal administration of compounds bypass the blood - brain barrier. Intraperitoneal injection of chemicals represent a selective site of administration in which an absorbable chemical which will first be translocated to the liver via the portal circulation. Therefore, compounds will be subjected to special metabolic transformations existing in the liver as well as the possibility of excretion of the compound in the bile before it gains access to remainder of the animal.

Exposure to chemical hazards may occur via **placental transfer** from a pregnant woman to the fetus, **inoculation** and **direct penetration** to target organs, and from mother to child through **breastfeeding.**

b. Distribution of Compounds

After passage of the compound from whatever route, the real distribution of the compound depends on its circulation to the tissues by the blood. In the plasma there are proteins (mainly albumin) which bind part of the compound (**Bound Portion**) and this part will not be available to tissues, and a free portion (**Unbound Portion**) which can enter the tissues.

c. Metabolism

Some of the compound undergoes changes by enzymes of the body mainly in the liver microsomal system in the form of oxidation, reduction, conjugation...etc. Sometimes the metabolite (end product) may be more toxic than the parent compound, but in most cases the reverse occurs. Example of the first type is the change of parathion (organophosphate insecticide) - of low toxicity per se - to paraoxion (a highly toxic metabolite) and ethyl alcohol (toxic compound) to CO_2 and water (non - toxic metabolite).

d. Elimination (Excretion)

Most compounds disappear from plasma at a rate that is proportional to the amount of compound present. The rate is expressed in terms of a rate constant K.

Half - life $(T\ 1/2) = \dfrac{0.693}{K}$ = time required to reduce the compound content of the body to half its initial value.

e.g. if K= 0.10 day $^{-1}$, 10% of the remaining compound is eliminated per day, therefore

$T\ 1/2 = \dfrac{0.693}{0.1} = 6.9$ days

For 90% elimination the formula is 2.3/K and that for 10% elimination it is 0.105/K.

e. Cumulation

When a compound enters repeatedly into the body until the fraction lost per interval of time is equal to the amount entering in the same time interval, one says that there is accumulation of the compound.

e.g.   If K= 0.1 days $^{-1}$, 50% of the steady state (Figure 2.2) level is reached in 6.9 days and 90% in 23 days.

The use of compound concentration in blood and urine can help determine the kinetics in a one compartment open model.

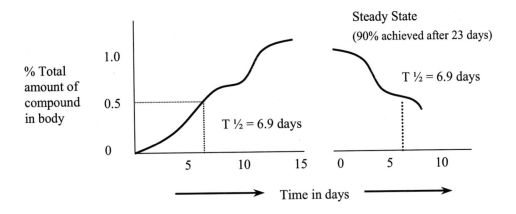

Figure 2.2. Cumulative and Steady States.

3. Factors Associated with the Toxodynamic Phase

This phase, as explained previously, includes the effect of the compound on the target organs. It depends on several factors:

a. The Nature of the Substance

This determines the concentration of the compound at the target tissues and hence the nature and degree of effects. Not only the parent compound is concerned, but also the metabolite.

b. Differences in Individual Sensitivity

Age, sex, pregnancy, nutritional state, and general state of health are all factors that may play a role in this phase. High-risk populations such as people with allergy, respiratory diseases, heart diseases, or children and pregnant women, may show more toxic effects to compounds at concentrations, which do not affect normal healthy individuals. Differences in genetics, e.g. deficiency in glucose-6-phosphate dehydrogenase will cause the red blood cells (erythrocytes) to be more susceptible to effects of trace metals such as lead. Deficiency in α_1-antitrypsin may cause the lungs to be more susceptible to fibrogenic effects of dusts such as asbestos and talcum.

c. Combination of Substances

At the target tissues, effect of two compounds may cause increased response by simple addition (**Additive Effect**) or more than additive effect (**Potentiating Effect**). Some compounds may interfere with the metabolism and excretion of other compounds adding more toxic effects.

d. Previous Exposures

At the target tissues, effect of compounds may last for years, and new compounds could affect the end result of apparent toxicity. As an example, carcinogens and mutagens cause damage to chromosomes and alter genetic properties. Initiators or promoters have been identified in carcinogenesis. Allergic hypersensitivity originating from previous exposure could add to new effects of present compounds.

e. Regular Medical Examination

The regular medical examination is necessary for workers regularly exposed to toxic substances.

f. General Epidemiological Investigation

As an example, Itai Itai disease, occured in Japan, was shown to be caused by high concentrations of cadmium in rivers near a zinc mine. Food materials such as rice and drinking water in that region contained up to 1 ppm cadmium and about 2 mg cadmium was ingested daily per person. Another example is the Minimata disease in Japan due to high concentrations of mercury compounds (50-80 mg/Kg) in fish. The toxodynamic effect caused by compounds could be studied and a cause-effect relationship established, such is needed for preventive measures. To summarize the previous discussion, the following basic information is presented (Figure 2.3):

The conceptual model:

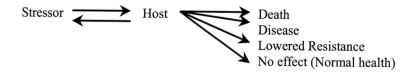

Figure 2.3. Interaction between Host and Environment.

g. Dose-Response Relationship

The characteristics of exposure and the spectrum of effects come together in a correlative relationship referred to as dose-response. This is represented in Figure 2.4. One of the responses used in acute toxicity studies the lethal effects or mortality. One of the parameters used is the LD_{50} or the lethal dose which kills 50% of the experimental population within 24 hours. This can be presented diagrammatically as in Figure 2.5.

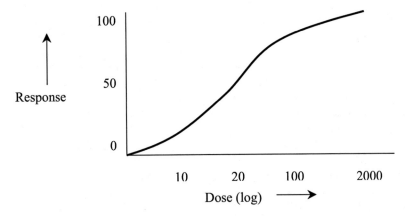

Figure 2.4. Dose-Response Relationship.

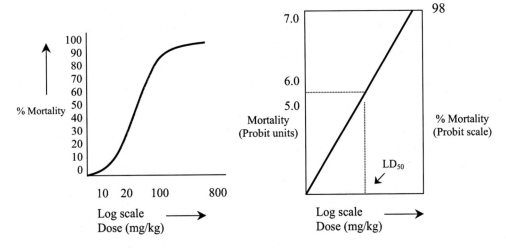

Figure 2.5. Lethal Dose$_{50}$ (LD $_{50}$).

A general accepted classification of compounds with regard to their toxic potency is presented in Table (2.5).

Table 2.5. General Classification of Toxic Compounds Potency and Toxicity.

Definition	Dose
Extremely toxic	1 mg/kg or less
Highly toxic	1-50 mg/kg
Moderately toxic	50-500 mg/kg
Slightly toxic	0.5-5 gm/kg
Practically non-toxic	5-15 gm/kg
Relatively harmless	> 15 gm/kg

With regard to the toxic effects at the target organs, some useful definitions and examples are presented below:

1. **Target Organ** is the tissue or tissues or areas where major effects (e.g. vinyl chloride and the liver) are manifested.
2. **One-Stressor-Multiple Targets:** e.g. lead and its effects on blood, kidney, liver, brain, peripheral nerves.
3. **Multiple-Stressors-One Target Organ:** e.g. asbestos, coal dust, bacteria, and fungi acting together on the lungs.
4. **Body Burden** is defined as the total amount of a compound in the body. It is defined as the total amount of compound in a specific (most affected) target organ.
5. **Sequestration** is the deposition of a compound for prolonged periods of time in specific tissues e.g. lead in bone, chlorinated hydrocarbons in fat.

h. Toxicity Testing

In general, data accumulated from animal studies on a specific compound is part of the toxicity testing. In pharmaceutical industries this is required by the FDA as pre-clinical studies done before any clinical studies.

The latter includes 4 clinical phases: I-IV. There is no regulation of such testing in industry. Therefore, there is a big gap to collect data regarding a specific compound for industrial or household use.

Today we have a considerable amount of chemicals in use but only information (quite limited) on only few of them. The new regulation (**Toxic Substance Control Act**) insists on having toxicity studies data on compounds formulated since 1979, however, there are no requirements for old substances. Even if an old substance is modified, it does not fall under the new regulation.

Data are now being collected by NIOSH (National Institute for Occupational Safety and Health) regarding several compounds. These data include animal studies, epidemiological reports, or reports on any catastrophy or accidents with such compounds.

Correlation between animal toxicity and human toxicities have several limitations. These are the following:

1. Species-species differences.
2. Differences among members of the same species.
3. No species even subhuman primates is exactly like the human in its response to all chemicals.
4. Immunological mechanisms which occur in man (sensitization) may not be shown in animals.
5. Carcinogenicity, if it occurs in laboratory animals, is assumed to be transposable to humans. However, several compounds are found to cause cancer in humans without being able to cause cancer in any animal species, e.g. arsenic.

The effects of toxic chemicals on animals may range from rapid death to sublethal effects to situations in which there are apparently no effects at all. Often the first step in the prediction of effects is to conduct a series of laboratory studies involving a single chemical and a single animal species.

Generally, the animals are exposed to a range of doses and/or concentrations and over different periods of time. Because of legal and ethical limitations, most such studies are conducted using rats or mice rather than humans.

To examine the effects associated with exposure over various time periods, toxicological studies have generally been divided into three categories (Table 2.6):

Acute toxicity studies - either a single administration of the chemical being tested or several administrations within a 24-hour period.

Short-term (also known as **subacute** and **subchronic**) **toxicity studies** - repeated administrations, usually on a daily basis, over a period of about 10 percent of the life span of the animal being tested (for example, about three months in rats and one to two years in dogs); however, shorter durations such as 14-day and 28-day treatments have also been used by some investigators.

Long-term toxicity studies - repeated administrations over the entire life span of the test animals (or at least a major fraction thereof). For mice, the time period would be about 18 months; for rats, 24 months; for dogs and monkeys, 7 to 10 years.

(1) Acute Toxicity Studies

Analyses of the data derived from acute toxicity studies generally begin with the plotting of a curve that shows the relationship between the dose or concentration of a toxic chemical and the number or percentage of test animals that demonstrate an effect. Such curves often exhibit the distribution of sensitivities shown in Figure 2.6. This type of curve is representative of that observed for a large number of variables, including death, change in body weight or size of the animals at a given age, where death is used as an endpoint, such tests fall into the category of acute toxicity studies. The peak of the curve indicates the dose that produces effects in 50 percent of the animals. Either an increase or a decrease in dose will result in proportionately fewer animals responding. This is another way of saying that some animals will exhibit the response at a lower dose, whereas for other animals higher doses are required to demonstrate the same effect. The portion of the curve between "minimum" and point B represents the response of the most susceptible animals; the portion between B and "maximum" represents the response of the most resistant animals. The midpoint (peak) of the curve (denoted on the graph as x) indicates the dose that produces effects in the largest percentage of the animals. Since the curve follows a normal or Gaussian distribution, statistical procedures can be used to evaluate the resulting data.

Although the Gaussian distribution is interesting, data resulting from toxicological studies are generally plotted in the form of a curve relating the dose or concentration to the **cumulative** percentage of animals exhibiting the given response. The curves in Figure 2.7 show this type of plot for two different chemicals, A and B. The curve to the left represents the more toxic of the two compounds, since the dose (or concentration) required to produce death in 50 percent of the exposed population is lower. The LD_{50} designates the dose that is lethal to 50 percent of the exposed animals; the curve to the left represents the more toxic of the two chemicals.

Table 2.6. Toxicity Testing.

Type	Duration of Testing	Administration	LD$_{50}$ Determinations	Evaluation of State of Health
Acute	24 hrs to 1 week	Involves one administration of the compound.	*Needs two species, one rodent and one non-rodent; *Needs two routes of administration, one route similar to method intended to be used later in practical life.	Topical effects usually use rabbit skin (in-vivo)
Prolonged	up to 3 months	*Involves daily doses. *Needs 3 dose levels *Route of administration according to intended route of use.	Need two species, usually rats and dogs	*Blood chemistry, urine analysis, hematology, function tests, performed on all animals *All animals weighed weekly *All animals (alive or dead) are subjected to complete autopsy, including histology of all organ systems.
Chronic	1—2 years	Daily doses	*Species-- 2 species, one non—rodent may use humans for a single dose trial studies *2 dose levels *Route of administration according to intended route of use	*Animals weighed weekly *Complete physical examination weekly *Blood chemistry, hematological tests on all animals at 6- month intervals, and on all ill or abnormal animals more frequent *End of period, autopsy including histological examination of all organ systems.

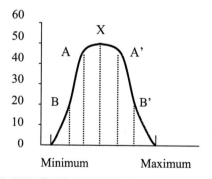

Figure 2.6. Distribution of Animal Responses to a Toxic Chemical as a Function of Dose (Source: Moeller, 1997).

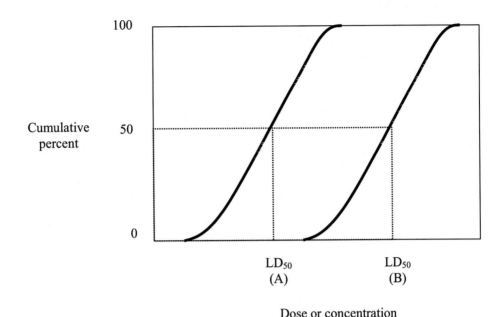

Figure 2.7. Cumulative Percentages of Animals Showing Responses to Toxic Chemicals (Source: Moeller, 1997).

Such graphs are commonly referred to as **dose-response** curves and are plotted using an arithmetic scale on the vertical axis and a logarithmic scale on the horizontal axis. One advantage of this format is that a major portion of the curve is linear, for this portion the response (in this case, death) is directly related to the dose or concentration of the chemical agent. Figure 2.7 also illustrates the approach for determining the lethal dose for half (the so-called LD_{50}) of the exposed animal population within a certain period of time. This endpoint is easily measurable; it either occurs or it does not.

In previous years, determination of the LD_{50} was one of the primary goals of many acute toxicity studies. This is far less true today, particularly in light of the diminished need for this type of information for the regulation of toxic chemicals.

Another contributing factor is the increased interest in both cancerous and non-cancerous diseases, as well as possible behavioral effects, that may be caused by chemical exposures. Other benefits of acute toxicity studies are that they can provide information on the probable target organs for the chemical and its specific toxic effect as well as guidance on the doses to be used in the more prolonged (long-term) studies.

Acute toxicity studies can also provide information on the synergistic and antagonistic effects of certain combinations of chemicals. Such information is very important in the evaluation of environmental exposures, which typically include simultaneous exposures to more than one chemical.

(2) Short-Term And Long-Term Tests

Under normal circumstances, the animals selected are the rat and the dog because of their appropriate size, ready availability, and the preponderance of toxicologic information on their reactions to a wide range of chemicals. Differences in response by gender require that equal numbers of male and female animals be used, and that a control group be maintained for comparison purposes. In addition, the chemical should be administered by the same route of exposure that is anticipated for humans.

To assure that the studies encompass the full range of anticipated outcomes, most investigators select three dose ranges - one sufficiently high to elicit definite signs of toxicity but not high enough to kill many of the animals; one sufficiently low that it is not expected to induce any toxic effects; and an intermediate dose. One of the outcomes of such studies is guidance on the "acceptable intake" of a chemical.

Under normal circumstances, the animals selected are the rat and the dog because of their appropriate size, ready availability, and the preponderance of toxicologic information on their reactions to a wide range of chemicals.

Another piece of information that is needed, however, is an indication of the "no-effect level, (NOEL)" or the "no observed adverse effect level, (NOAEL)."

For this purpose long-term studies are generally employed. As with short-term studies, generally one or more species of animals are used, with the rat being preferred. The routes of administration are similar to those in short-term studies.

The information collected includes body weight, body size, and food consumption, supplemented by general observations, laboratory tests, and postmortem examinations.

General observations include appearance, behavior, and any abnormalities; laboratory tests generally include hematologic examinations, supplemented by analyses of blood and urine; postmortems include gross pathological examinations, including histologic examinations, supplemented by determination of the weights of individual organs such as the liver, kidneys, heart, brain, and thyroid.

(3) Outcomes

Studies of these types provide data on toxicity with respect to the target organs, the effects on these organs, and the associated dose-effect and dose-response relationships.

One determination that is often made on the basis of **acute toxicity studies** of suspected carcinogens is the maximum tolerated dose (MTD), the highest dose just below the level at which toxic effects other than cancer can occur.

The basic reason for using the MTD as an endpoint is to estimate the carcinogenic potential of a chemical in the shortest possible time using the fewest exposed animals. Again, acceptable levels of intake for humans would be extrapolated from the MTD, taking into account appropriate safety factors. The concept of the MTD has been criticized by some toxicologists who believe that the high doses introduce artifacts that exaggerate carcinogenicity in humans. Because of the controversy, scientists do not currently agree on the usefulness and applicability of this test. A variety of complicating factors make it unlikely that the establishment of an acceptable level or intake of a chemical for humans will provide adequate guidance in setting a corresponding limit for the environment. Exposed population groups may include some members who are unusually susceptible. In addition, detrimental effects may have occurred but not been observed. These include changes in reproduction, increased susceptibility to disease, and decreased longevity. Furthermore, there is no justifiable reason to assume a constant relationship, for different chemicals or different species, between the dose required to kill and that needed to impair an organism.

J. HEALTH ENDPOINTS

While acute and short-term tests were a mainstay during earlier toxicological studies, with only death or tissue damage as recognized endpoints, today the evaluation of human exposures tends to be directed at studies encompassing a full range of effects, including those on behavior and other noncancer endpoints. According to the National Research Council, the more prominent endpoints include the following:

1. Carcinogenesis

Chemical carcinogenesis is recognized today as a multi-stage process, involving at least three steps: **initiation**, **promotion**, and **progression**. Although formerly it appeared that various chemical compounds and physical agents were either purely initiators or purely promoters, more recent interpretations suggest that some chemicals and agents are both initiators and promoters.

Current theory posits that the development of cancer involves the activation or mutation of oncogenes, or the inactivation of suppressor genes, and that this causes a normal cell to develop into a cancerous cell.

Because of the expense and time required for related tests using animals, toxicologists have for years experimented with the development of short-term, in vitro tests (experiments conducted outside the body) as an alternative.

One of the most widely applied is the Ames test. This test for mutagenicity in bacteria is based on evidence that deoxyribonucleic acid (DNA) is the critical target for most carcinogens, and on the observation that mutagenic chemicals are often also carcinogenic.

2. Reproductive Toxicity

Toxic effects on reproduction may occur anywhere within a continuum of events ranging from germ cell formation and sexual functioning in the parents through sexual maturation in the offspring. The relationship between exposure and reproductive dysfunction is highly complex because exposure of the mother, father, or both may influence reproductive outcome. In addition, critical exposures may include maternal exposures long before or immediately prior to conception as well as exposure of the mother and fetus during gestation.

3. Developmental Toxicity (Teratogenesis)

The type of illness involving the formation of congenital defects has been known for decades and is an important cause of morbidity and mortality among newborns.

Developmental effects encompass embryo and fetal death, growth retardation, and malformations, all of which can be highly sensitive to chemical exposures.

For some years no connection was suspected between such effects and chemicals; toxicologists had a tendency to assume that the natural protective mechanisms of the body, such as detoxification, elimination, and the placental barrier, were sufficient to shield the embryo from maternal exposure to harmful chemicals. These concepts changed dramatically after the clinical use of **thalidomide**, a sedative first employed in Germany in the late 1950s to relieve morning sickness in pregnant women.

4. Neurotoxicity

Although fewer than 10 percent of the approximately 70,000 chemicals in use have been tested, almost 1,000 have been identified as known neurotoxicants in humans and other animals. The multitude of impacts on humans range from cognitive, sensory, and motor impairments to immune system deficits.

For this reason classification of chemical neurotoxic action is constantly evolving, and the application of data from studies in animals to estimation of the risks of neurologic disease in humans is very complicated. Often there are major differences between the degree of neurotoxic response observed in animals and that found in humans.

5. Immunotoxicity

Various toxic substances are known to suppress the immune function, leading to reduced host resistance to bacterial and viral infections, and to parasitic infestation, as well as to reduced control of neoplasms.

The importance of these effects is well illustrated by the concern about AIDS, in which the infected person often dies owing to inability to resist an organism that would not be a problem in a healthy individual.

Certain toxic agents can also provoke exaggerated immune reactions leading to local or systemic reactions. In recent years some scientists have postulated that certain people have "multiple chemical sensitivity" which can lead to a type of "chemical AIDS."

Animal studies have indicated an immunosuppressive action of dioxins and the dioxin like PCBs, and some human studies have reported increased rates of infection in exposed subjects.

6. Endocrine Toxicity

In people with relatively high exposure to dioxin like compounds (but lower than occupationally exposed people), evidence indicates altered levels of circulating thyroid hormones and decreases in circulating testosterone levels. Animal studies also show that organochlorine exposure is associated with decreased androgen concentrations and feminization of male offspring as well as decreased levels of the thyroid hormones, triiodothyronine and thyroxine.

III. PRINCIPLES OF ENVIRONMENTAL TOXICOLOGY

A. CONCEPTS

The major toxicologic doctrine is that the dose makes the poison. The total body burden in mg/kg of a particular chemical or its toxic metabolic byproducts is often given as a measure of the dose of a chemical or toxic agent. Often the amount of a chemical present in a sensitive or target organ system determines its damaging effect.

The body's ability to metabolize, degrade, and ultimately excrete a toxic chemical is also critical to understanding toxicity. Some chemicals may become activated and hence more toxic in the course of being "detoxified." Such reactions usually take place in the liver, where enzymes such as the monooxygenases of the P_{450} microsomal system attack putatively toxic molecules.

The body normally makes toxic molecules water-soluble or binds them to a conjugate such as glutathione to assist in detoxification. Some hormone-mimicking chemicals, such as dioxin, have toxic effects at very low doses, whereas others, such as cadmium, may have paradoxical-appearing effects. Such effects may result when a toxic chemical present in low concentrations induces its own detoxifying enzymes so that a very low dose may appear beneficial rather than toxic. Beneficial effects at ultra-low doses of toxic substances are known as "**hormesis**", a concept gaining increasing acceptance among toxicologists.

B. THE ENVIRONMENTAL SETTING

The ultimate toxicity of a substance can be attributed to its concentration in susceptible living organisms in the environment. However, the effective toxicity of a chemical, such as oil residues or a toxic metal, is greatly affected by its availability.

For instance, polychlorinated biphenyls (**PCBs**) in the sediments of the Great Lakes may be present in high concentration, but because of sequestration and slow bacterial degradation they do not pose as much of an immediate problem as do some waterborne chemicals, such as the gasoline additive methyl tert-butyl ester (**MTBE**), which can pose problems to water quality at low (ppb) concentrations.

Similarly, chemicals such as **trichloroethylene**, which adsorb to soil particles, may have less effective toxicity than others that are unbound or otherwise free to migrate and concentrate in a fluid medium. In such instances, the bioavailability of a specific chemical in the environment, its persistence, and the existence of particularly vulnerable populations (elderly, young, or immuno-compromised people) determine its penultimate toxicity.

C. TROPHIC LEVELS AND TOXICITY OF A CHEMICAL

Chemicals entering an ecosystem typically are first assimilated and wholly or partially metabolized by organisms at the lowest trophic levels and then passed up the food chain.

Food chains may be simple or complex, depending on the number and linkages among members. Typically, the seven trophic levels begin with **primary producers**, traverse through **primary to quaternary consumers**, and end with **saprophytes** and **decomposers**. Thus, the mercury salts that entered Minamata Bay in Japan from a chemical processing plant were first methylated by anaerobic bacteria (producers) in the bay silt layer. The methyl mercury-contaminated bacteria were then assimilated by plankton and higher organisms in the next trophic level (primary consumers), until they in turn were ingested by shellfish and fin fish (secondary and tertiary consumers, respectively).

When consumed by humans (quaternary consumers), the shellfish and fish, now contaminated with highly magnified concentrations of bioavailable organic mercury, exerted a profound neurotoxic effect, exceeding that predicted by the seawater levels of elemental mercury alone.

Typically, toxic molecules are bioconcentrated by approximately one order of magnitude (i.e., 10-fold) with each trophic level traversed. At the highest trophic levels, notably carnivores such as polar bears and eagles, the final concentration or fat-soluble chemicals may be magnified by a million or more times above ambient environmental levels.

In the instance of dichlorodiphenyltrichloroethane (DDT), water concentrations in eastern U.S. estuaries in the 1960s were typically in the range of less than 0.05 parts per billion (50 parts per trillion). In cormorants or mergansers, birds that feed on surface fish, tissue levels reached 20-25 parts per million.

In the 1960s and 1970s, bald eagle populations were adversely affected through the bioaccumulation of dioxins, dibenzofurans, biphenyls, and organochlorine pesticides such as DDT and its breakdown product, DDE. Although these contaminants have been successfully reduced in some areas of the world, notably in the northwestern United States and Canada, significant levels remain elsewhere (Maine and the Great Lakes).

Reproductive success of eagles has been proportionately improved in areas where organochlorine contaminants have been reduced, whereas elsewhere, such as lakes in Florida contaminated by estrogen-mimicking pesticides, reproductive damage continues.

D. POLLUTANTS AND ECOSYSTEMS

The traditional notion of pollution focuses on point-source origins of contamination. Point sources may be smoke stacks, outlet pipes, or sewage lines. The great preponderance of ecologically significant pollution, however, is not of point-source origin.

General sources of pollution from the aggregate impact of human activities, be they cars, combustion engines generally, or wood product and agricultural burning, contribute significantly more than point sources. The present spate of carbon dioxide represents an extreme example of a relatively nontoxic gas that contributes significantly to environmental degradation.

More classic sources of pollution, such as the excessive combustion of fossil fuels, remain a serious locus of contamination. For instance, in 1991 during the Gulf War, the burning of oil fields increased fourfold the mutagenic particulates in the air over Riyadh, Saudi Arabia.

E. DAMAGES BY POLLUTANTS

To exposed human populations mutagens pose risks of cancer and potential reproductive damage. In general pollutants can damage ecosystems at any of several levels. Human activities as a whole, such as clear-cutting, can destabilize ecosystems, whereas toxic contaminants, such as those contributed by oil spills, tend to poison organisms at specific trophic levels.

At the lowest trophic levels of primary producers, chemicals that are toxic to the metabolic machinery of bacteria and other protists or to the chlorophyll synthetic apparatus of single-cell plants, such as algae, can disrupt the energy balance of the ecosystem as a whole.

Excessive copper ions in water, for instance, can be toxic to green and blue-green algae. Specific herbicides intended to poison the photosynthetic apparatus also may be toxic to single-cell organisms. Chemicals such as glyphosate or bromoxynil also have photosynthetic toxicity, but the persistence of such herbicides in the environment is fortunately short.

At slightly higher trophic levels, chemicals that impair flagellar motility or prevent the efficient incorporation of silica or calcium into dinoflagellate skeletons, including many heavy metals, are of concern. The damage produced by excessive metal ions often is manifest at low trophic levels and leads to disturbances in the available food base for higher organisms. Low-level contamination with neurotoxic chemicals, such as triclopyr, the active ingredient in Garlon herbicide, can impair swimming ability in andromadous fish such as salmon or steelbead trout at levels as low as 50 parts per billion in water.

The presence of excessive nitrogen and phosphorous may lead to overproduction of single-cell organisms, resulting in **eutrophication** of a marine or fresh-water ecosystem. In such circumstances, the biologic oxygen demand soars and the available oxygen is depleted, causing die-offs and further decay and oxygen depletion.

At the highest trophic levels, chemical contaminants that bio-accumulate, often because of their fat solubility, can impair reproduction (e.g.. PCBs, DDT) or immunologic function (e.g., dioxins, PCBs, and certain organophosphate pesticides).

F. MAJOR FACTORS LIMITING ENVIRONMENTAL TOXICITY

Chemical or metallic xenobiotics are toxicologically limited by their persistence, accumulation, migration, and stability. The factors that determine persistence may include sunlight (photo-degradation), bacterial degradation (soil microorganisms), and the presence of an ongoing source of contamination. The likelihood of bioaccumulation of any given xenobiotic is increased by its fat solubility and the number of trophic levels that it will traverse before encountering the penultimate consumer.

Factors that affect the movement of a specific chemical include proclivity to bind strongly to soil particles (e.g., trichloroethylene), atomic weight (in the case of heavy metals), and molecular size. In general, the smaller the molecule, the faster its diffusion through any constant medium (Fick's law). Unstable compounds, such as organophosphate pesticides, tend to hydrolyze and degrade relatively rapidly compared to more stable compounds such as PCBs or DDT.

G. TOXICITY AT ULTRA-LOW DOSES

Among the chemicals of greatest environmental concern, 2,3,7,8-tetrachlorodibenzodioxin stands out because of its ability to cause reproductive harm, immunologic damage, and possibly cancer at ultra-low doses (measured in picograms per liter). This ability is linked to dioxin's ultra-tight binding to microsomal enzymes and its concentration in the thymus and other glands of central importance for immune function.

H. HEAVY METALS IN THE ENVIRONMENT

Heavy metals such as lead (Pb) and cadmium (Cd) tend to accumulate in the subsoils, where they are dispersed after airborne emission or mine tailings (Pb) or sewage sludge deposition (Cd). Soil contamination from inadvertent addition of soil amendments containing such heavy metals can ruin farmland by contaminating the soil to the point that vegetables cannot be grown without toxic accumulations.

When present in soils, they may become a major source of human contamination, either through leaching into drinking water and through pica activities in which significant amounts of lead are ingested by children in contaminated materials.

The resulting body burdens of Pb and Cd have their major affects on porphyrin synthesis (lead-induced porphyria), aplastic anemia (bone marrow toxicity), and neurologic functions (lowered IQ and attention deficits).

I. MAJOR FATES AND IMPACTS OF RADIOISOTOPES

Radioisotopes, whether indigenous or byproducts of commercial or military activities, may pose substantial threats to human health. The two most common examples are radon gas and tritium. Radon is produced as one of the "radon daughters" in the decay pattern of radionucleotides in the radium group. Radon daughters are typically alpha particle emitters. When dispersed in the lungs, alpha particles can cause direct cell damage and DNA mutations that may lead to lung cancer. Radioactive iodine (I^{131}) is a major cause of thyroid cancer, notably in victims of the Chernobyl reactor accident.

J. DURATION OF TOXICITY OF ENVIRONMENTAL CONTAMINANTS

Many pesticides and other biologic control agents are intentionally constructed to have long half-lives in the environment. Such persistence is a logical quality when the objective is to obtain long-lived protection against reinfestation. For this reason, chlordane, which has a half-life in soil of over 20 years, was an "ideal" termite control agent. But a persistent agent is an ecologic hazard when it bioaccumulates or otherwise enhances toxicity overtime. Among such pesticides are dieldrin and DDT, which have protracted half-lives of 10-15 years under some environmental conditions.

Their byproducts, notably DDE in the case of DDT, have even longer persistence. Some recent research suggests that the effective toxicity of such chemicals in soils diminishes overtime even though their soil concentrations remain constant. A likely explanation for this paradoxic finding is that with time some xenobiotics bind tightly to soil particles and thereby become less bioavailable.

K. Occupational Contaminants and Environmental Problems

Occupational contaminants become environmental problems through escape to the surrounding environment and, secondarily, through direct transport by workers to their homes. In the first instance, chemicals such as toluene diisocyanate can contaminate neighborhoods when emissions are inadequately controlled at factories.

Similarly, dioxins escaping from pulp mills are often a major source of dioxin contamination in surrounding waterways. The EPA maintains a web site [epa.gov.] with more specific information about specific toxic sites.

IV. PRINCIPLES OF OCCUPATIONAL TOXICOLOGY

A. The Occupational Setting

The occupational setting is a unique environment. Unlike environmental exposures, the worker is typically exposed for 8 hours/day, 5 days/week. Contract or construction workers are a notable exception because exposures of 10-12 hours/day, 7 days/week, may be sustained for short periods. Dermal and inhalation exposures predominate, and the conditions of work often intensify exposure by increasing respiration rate, providing repetitive exposures, and permitting the build-up of dosages received over the work week.

Several conditions unique to occupational settings provide unusual dosage situations: dermal or pulmonary exposures that sensitize workers may permit very low doses to have adverse effects by generating hypersensitivity.

A classic example is toluene diisocyanate, which can sensitize via inhalation at the part-per-billion range. Additional factors that provide exceptions or modifications of the general rule of dose-dependent toxicity include concomitant exposures that synergize toxicity, metabolic activators of the P450 enzymes in the liver that convert nontoxic chemicals to toxic intermediates, and non-workplace exposures to alcohol or cigarette smoke that exacerbate workplace toxins such as ketones or asbestos, respectively.

B. Exposure Conditions of Particular Concern

Classic instances of unanticipated, high-risk exposure settings include operations in confined spaces. For instance, workers who scrubbed out the interior of vinyl chloride reaction chambers were among the first to show evidence of liver angiosarcomas or brain astrocytomas.

Work environments without adequate ventilation provide another setting in which exposures can be high. For example, a few, highly exposed Turkish shoemakers who worked with solvents containing high concentrations of benzene developed acute myelocytic leukemia.

Other workplace settings in which high concentrations of solvent vapors, gases, or other chemicals can build up include trenching operations, tile-setting, hazardous waste clean-up, and storage tank cleaning.

C. REGULATORY PRINCIPLES

Historically, permissible workplace exposures to individual chemicals were set first by industry through the Association of Governmental Industrial Hygienists (ACGIH) and later by the Occupational Safety and Health Administration (OSHA). Permissible exposure limits (PELs) were adopted. Both entities ostensibly specify air concentrations that a worker can breathe for an 8-hour shift without "material impairment" of health or physiologic functioning. TLVs are constantly reevaluated as new data become available, but PEL values used by government agencies to establish legally enforced limits often are incorporated only after protracted review and delay.

General conditions of employment are based on legislation and regulations, including those of the Department of Transportation, Environmental Protection Agency (EPA), OSHA, and state agencies. Enabling statutes and regulations establish the general proposition that workplaces should be free of potentially hazardous exposures to toxic substances; that the conditions of work should not impair health; and that any potential exposure to a reproductive or carcinogenic agent should be minimized or avoided altogether. Terms used to describe the health-based limits on toxic exposure in the workplace usually refer to exposure limits established by governmental bodies that designate safe workplace conditions.

One limitation of this approach is the general lack of consideration of interactive effects. For regulatory purposes, exposures are averaged on an additive basis; the partial fraction of a TLV for chemical A may be added to the TLV for chemical B and so on, as long as the total TLV fractions do not exceed unity. For example, if the TLV for A is 200 ppm and the average exposure is 100, the fractional TLV is 100/200 or1/2; if the remaining exposures add up to TLV fractions of less than 1/2, the total workplace exposure is considered within permissible limits. The weakness of this approach becomes evident when it is recognized that some chemicals exacerbate the adverse effects of others, even at concentrations below the TLV (e.g.. nontoxic levels of isopropanol potentiate the liver toxicity of carbon tetrachloride).

Technical Terms Used in Occupational Health for Acceptable Exposure Levels are the following:

1. National Institute of Occupational Safety and Health (**NIOSH**)-OSHA-recommended levels: advisory time-weighted averages (**TWAs**), usually based on an average of exposures over 1 or 8 hours.

2. OSHA permissible exposure limit (**PEL**): highest permitted level in an 8-hr workday.

3. NIOSH threshold limit value (**TLV**): maximal average encountered value during an 8-hr workday that can be safely experienced: usually the same or lower than OSHA PEL.

4. OSHA short-term exposure limit (**STEL**): maximal short-term concentration permitted, as reflected by a 15-minute sampling measurement; maximal permissible exposure over a 15-minute period.

5. No observable effect level (**NOEL**): the exposure level in humans, usually extrapolated with a safety factor of 10 from animal data, that is not expected to produce a detectable adverse effect; of no observable adverse effect level (**NOAEL**).

6. Lowest observable effect level (**LOEL**): the lowest level of exposure capable of producing a detectable effect.

7. Health-based exposure level (**HBEL**): an exposure level pegged to conditions necessary to ensure the maintenance of well being.

D. ILLNESSES EXPERIENCED IN THE OCCUPATIONAL SETTING

Many respiratory diseases, such as chronic obstructive pulmonary disease (COPD) and asthma, can be induced or exacerbated by airborne toxins in the workplace.

Other target organs that are commonly affected include the liver (chemical hepatitis), kidney, urogenital tract, and brain or central nervous system (CNS).

Reproductive toxicity is a recently recognized addition to the traditional list of occupational diseases and illnesses. Unique workplace-related injuries or illnesses include angiosarcoma of the liver, a rare tumor experienced by vinyl chloride workers; hemorrhagic cystitis (evidenced by bloody urine) experienced by chlorinated amine workers; abnormal secondary sexual characteristics (e.g., breast enlargement) experienced by male handlers of diethylstilbestrol (DES); and azoospermia experienced by workers heavily exposed to the soil sterilizant, dibromochloropropane (DBCP).

E. MONITORING OR SURVEILLANCE PROCEDURES

Effective monitoring requires a suitable test or detection system for an incipient disease process. So-called "**sentinel**" diseases were used in the recent past (e.g., testicular cancer as an indicator of workplace carcinogens), but most current surveillance systems rely on biomarkers. Monitoring for early signs of disease by using the most sensitive validated test available or measuring specific exposure markers for agents or metabolites, where appropriate, is also desirable. More refined monitoring, such as looking for serologic signs of illness or genetic damage, is also possible.

Monitoring should be distinguished from screening. The target of screening is usually a specific disease entity for which there is an efficacious intervention, such as screening for early signs of liver disease in solvent workers. Monitoring implies a regular, timely testing system that examines a general population for signs and symptoms of varied diseases or disorders linked to workplace exposure.

F. KEY TOXIC EXPOSURES

Among the most important toxicologic factors influencing workplace illness are reactive chemicals, metals, nonbiogenic fibers and dusts, organophosphate pesticides, special pharmaceuticals, and radioactive chemicals (isotopes) and nuclides.

The first category includes monomers used in the plastics industry, such as vinyl chloride. Metals of concern include lead (Pb), mercury (Hg), beryllium (Be), arsenic

(As), cadmium (Cd), and to a lesser extent, zinc (Zn). Fibers capable of producing lung fibrosis and/or malignancy include fiberglass and the various forms of asbestos. Dusts include free crystalline silica. Organophosphate pesticides of particular concern include methyl parathion; organochlorines include chlordecone (Kepone), lindane, DDT, polychlorinated dibenzofurans (PCDFs), chlordane, and heptachlor.

Radioactive isotopes used in medical imaging or therapy, such as technetium or iodine-131 pose potential hazards to technicians and medical personnel. Pharmaceuticals used in chemotherapy or immune suppression are of particular concern because of their mutagenicity, carcinogenicity, or bone marrow toxicity.

G. SPECIAL CASES OF WORKERS

By virtue of preexisting disease or illness, genetic susceptibility, age, or reproductive status many workers are at special risk from occupational toxic substances. Although it is desirable to protect all workers (both male and female) of reproductive age from exposure to any reproductive toxin, such protection may be especially necessary for women in the early stages of pregnancy (first trimester).

Genetically susceptible workers, such as those with α_l-antitrypsin deficiency superoxide dismutase variants, xeroderma pigmentosum haplotypes, and other genetic conditions that reduce the ability to repair or defend against toxic effects of highly reactive chemicals, need to be identified and afforded appropriate protections in hazardous environments in such a way that they are not subject to employment or social discrimination or stigmatization.

H. CHRONIC OR PERSISTENT TOXICOLOGIC EFFECTS

Toxic insults that produce lasting and irremediable harm are of greatest concern to the occupational health provider. Among the most serious irreversible effects, there are the following :

1. Asbestosis and Mesothelioma;
2. Emphysema (induced by smoke or particulates);
3. Permanent Sensitization States (e.g., those induced by toluene diisocyanate); and
4. Permanent neurologic or neuropsychologic disability (e.g., organic solvent-or lead-induced encephalopathy).

V. BIBLIOGRAPHY

Ariens, E.J., Simmonis, A.M., & Offermeir (1976). Introduction to General Toxicology. New York, N:Y: Academic Press.

Baucom, C.D. (2001). Mathematical Formulas for Environmental Engineering Calculations. In L. Williams, & R. Langley (Eds.), Environmental Health Secrets (pp. 230-237). Philadelphia, PA: Hanley & Belfus, Inc.

Cassarrett, & Doull. (1996). Toxicology: The Basic Science of Poisons, 5th Edition. New York, NY: Macmillan Publishing, Co. Inc.

Douiso, J.T. (1982). Pharmacokinetics Workshop. Austin, TX: Anderson Reports.

Gochfeld, M. (1998). Toxicology. In R. Wallace (Ed.), Public Health and Preventive Medicine (pp. 415-427). Stamford, CT: Appleton & Lange.

Greenberg, M.I., & Phillips, S.D. (1997). A Brief History of Occupational, Industrial, and Environmental Toxicology. In M. Greenberg, R. Hamilton, and S. Phillips (Eds.), Occupational, Industrial, and Environmental Toxicology (pp. 1-5). St. Louis, MO: Mosby-Year Book, Inc.

Henry, J.G. & Heinke, G.W. (1989). Environmental Science and Engineering. Appendix A (pp. 673-678). Englewood Cliffs, N.J.: Prentice Hall.

Hughes, W. (1996). Introduction to Environmental Toxicology. In W. Hughes (Ed.), Essentials of Environmental Toxicology: The Effects of Environmental Hazardous Substances on Human Health (pp. 3-7). Levittown, PA: Taylor & Francis.

Hughes, W. (1996). Introduction to Environmental Toxicology. In W. Hughes (Ed.), Essentials of Environmental Toxicology: The Effects of Environmental Hazardous Substances on Human Health (pp. 12-16). Levittown, PA: Taylor & Francis.

Hughes, W. (1996). Toxicological Concepts. In W. Hughes (Ed.), Essentials of Environmental Toxicology: The Effects of Environmental Hazardous Substances on Human Health (pp. 19-23). Levittown, PA: Taylor & Francis.

Lappé, M.A. (1999). Principles of Environmental Toxicology. In R. Bowler, & J. Cone. (Eds.), Occupational Medicine Secrets (pp. 7-13). Philadelphia, PA: Hanley & Belfus, Inc.

Lappé, M.A. (1999). Principles of Occupational Toxicology. In R. Bowler, & J. Cone. (Eds.), Occupational Medicine Secrets (pp. 15-20). Philadelphia, PA: Hanley & Belfus, Inc.

Logan, D.C. (1994). Toxicology. In R. McCunney (Ed.), A practical Approach to Occupational and Environmental Medicine, 2nd Edition (pp. 333-345). Boston, MA: Little, Brown and Company.

Loomis, T.A. (1976). Essentials of Toxicology, Philadelphia, PA: Lea and Febiger.

Lu, F.C. (1996). Biotransformation of Toxicants. In F. Lu (Ed.), Basic Toxicology: Fundamentals, target Organs, and Risk Assessment, 3rd Edition (pp. 27-39). Bristol, PA: Taylor & Francis.

Marieb, E.N. (2001). Human Anatomy and Physiology 5th Edition. San Francisco, CA: Addison Wesley Longman, INC.

McCreesh, A.H. (1965). Percutaneous Toxicity. Tox. Appl. Pharmacol.7:20—26.

Moeller, D.W. (1997). Toxicology. Environmental Health (pp.14-32). Cambridge, MA, and London, UK: Harvard University Press.

Nadakavukaren, A. (2000). Toxic Substances. Our Global Environment: A Health Perspective, 5th Edition (pp.225-268). Prospective Heights, IL: Waveland Press, Inc.

Patty, F.A. (1978). Industrial Hygiene and Toxicology. New York, NY: Interscience.

Stine, K.E., & Brown, T.M. (1996). Measuring Toxicity and Assessing Risk. In K. Stine, & T. Brown (Eds.), Principles of Toxicology (pp. 1-5). Boca Raton, FL: CRC Press, Inc. Lewis Publishers.

Stine, K.E., & Brown, T.M. (1996). Toxicokinetics. In K. Stine, & T. Brown (Eds.), Principles of Toxicology (pp. 11-15). Boca Raton, FL: CRC Press, Inc. Lewis Publishers.

Turk, J & Turk, A. (1988). Environmental Science. 4th Edition. Appendix A (pp. 673-677). Philadelphia, PA: Saunders College Publishing

Yassi, A., Kjellström, T., de Kok, T., & Guidotti, T. L. (2001). Nature of Environmental Health Hazards. In A. Yassi, [et al](Eds.), Basic Environmental Health (pp. 61-79). New York, NY: Oxford University Press, Inc.

CHAPTER

3

EPIDEMIOLOGY

I. <u>BACKGROUND</u>

A. <u>INTRODUCTION</u>

An important use for epidemiology is surveillance of persons exposed to known or suspected toxic substances, both within and outside the workplace. Epidemiologic methods can clarify cause - effect relationships as a prelude to preventive programs and can be used to evaluate control measures.

The ambient levels and body burdens of many toxic substances can be measured only with difficulty and often at great expense. At times, a substance itself is not toxic, but its metabolic breakdown products are. Measurements rarely begin at the time of first exposure to a presumed toxic substance. The dose-response relationships may be uncertain, variable, and poorly understood. Sometimes, although there may be intuitive grounds for believing that long-term low-level exposure is hazardous, it is impossible to demonstrate clinical, physiologic, or pharmacologic effects. There may be a long incubation time between first exposure and the onset of clinically apparent effects. For example, the latency period for both tobacco-related and asbestos-related lung cancer is 20 to 30 years. There may be a low incidence of adverse effects among those exposed, perhaps one in a thousand or even less. If only small numbers are exposed, it may be many years before the health hazard is even suspected, let alone identified. Sometimes people are exposed to multiple environmental toxins, making it difficult to incriminate a particular agent. A case of lung cancer may be due to workplace exposure or to smoking. The gastrointestinal or hepatotoxic effects of a pesticide may be aggravated by alcohol consumption or by exposure to volatile solvents used in a basement home-hobby workshop. Meticulously detailed histories of all exposures, whether work-related or not, are needed to identify such confounding effects, and even then it may not be possible to state with confidence that a condition is due to a particular exposure.

The affected populations may be transient workers. Many people work for a time in an industry with certain exposures, then move to another with different risks. Migratory agricultural workers exposed to a multiplicity of pesticides are very difficult to study for this reason. High dropout rates from some industries and from cohort or follow-up studies undermine the stability of numerators and raise questions about which number to use for the denominator. Some of these difficulties are overcome if there is a large population available for study, and if a record linkage system and a mortality database such as the National Death Index can be used.

A challenging problem is that the population being studied may be members of a labor union, but the necessary information about exposures can come only from management, which might resist disclosure in order to protect trade secrets. Mutual suspicions between these traditional adversaries, especially if complicated by intervention of the media or government regulatory agencies, can introduce political and emotional issues that add further to the difficulty of objective epidemiologic study.

In addition, there is the possibility that the power of suggestion is the cause of at least some symptoms and signs. "Behavioral epidemics" are well documented: They can include obvious physical signs like skin rashes, as well as headaches, nausea, and similar symptoms that are often labeled "emotional" in origin. There have been several epidemics of vague symptoms among office workers in modern sealed buildings, in which air is recirculated through the heating and cooling system to conserve energy. It can be difficult to determine whether these epidemics are behavioral or environmental in origin.

Because of all these difficulties, analysis of mortality data by occupational categories has often been relied on for surveillance, but this is a blunt instrument: occupational details on death certificates are scanty and do not provide any information about exposures, which have to be inferred. Death may not occur until many years and several occupational changes after the exposure to risk. Moreover, the information is too late to be of value to the deceased and often is too late to help others exposed to the same risks.

Another tool used in environmental epidemiology is analysis of mortality by cause and area. This can provide much interesting information. Regional variations in cancer mortality have been mapped in the United States, Canada, China, Japan, and many other nations. This has drawn attention to the existence of high-risk regions, where either environmental or occupational factors can be further investigated. An interesting example of regional variation is that of cardiovascular mortality in relation to drinking water quality; this has been observed in several countries. It remains uncertain whether the presence in hard water of certain salts has a protective effect, the absence of some factor from soft water should be incriminated, or whether the evidence has been spuriously inflated in importance by the use of inappropriate statistical methods.

B. DEFINITION OF OCCUPATIONAL AND ENVIRONMENTAL EPIDEMIOLOGY

Epidemiology is the study of the distribution and determinants of disease in human populations. Occupational epidemiology involves exposures and diseases in the workplace, whereas environmental epidemiology concerns non-workplace settings. Possible goals for an occupational or environmental epidemiologic study include:

1. Data collection for setting occupational or environmental standards,
2. Description of mechanism of toxicity,
3. Determination of health consequences and exposure,
4. Estimation of individual risk and extent of problem in the general population,
5. Evaluation of dose-response relationship, and
6. Recommendations for corrective action to eliminate or control exposure.

C. BASIC EPIDEMIOLOGIC MEASURES

Surveillance of toxic hazards requires quantitative assessments of both absolute and relative risk.

1. Absolute Risk

The first distinction made is between a ratio and a proportion. Ratios of measured quantities can often be used as risk indices but are frequently not very informative. A true proportion, in which the denominator contains the numerator, is often more useful. These proportions are frequently called "rates," although time may not explicitly enter the proportion. For example, the infant mortality rate is described as the number of infant deaths in the first 28 days of life divided by the total number of live births. This rate may be determined over any suitable interval of time.

Infant Mortality Rate (IMR) = Infant deaths/total live births.

Other basic descriptive epidemiologic measures are prevalence and incidence. Prevalence is a measure of existing cases in a defined population at some time. It is defined as:

Prevalence = Number of existing cases/size of the population.

In contrast, the incidence rate is a measure of new cases that arise in a population during a defined interval. The incidence rate is:

Incidence = Number of new cases/population at risk.

The incidence rate is an estimate of a true rate of change. Its precision, in part, depends on the width of the time interval (and other factors).

There is an exact mathematical relationship between the incidence rate, the prevalence rate, and the survival of subjects with the condition. However, when the incidence rate and survival remain constant for a sufficiently long period of time, the prevalence of any condition is directly proportional to the incidence:

Prevalence = Incidence × average duration of disease.

2. Relative Risk

Epidemiologists are constantly attempting to estimate the increased risk that exposure to a toxic substance in the environment imparts to an individual. One common and useful measure of increased risk is the "relative risk" (or risk ratio or rate ratio), which is available from cohort studies. Relative risk is defined as the rate of an exposed group over the disease rate of a suitable reference or control group:

Relative risk = Risk in exposed subjects / risk in unexposed subjects
             = (number of events among exposed / number exposed) / (number of events among unexposed / number unexposed).

If the relative risk is greater than 1.0, the risk of an event is greater in the exposed group. Relative risks as point estimates alone are seldom useful. Some estimate of their variability in the data or population being studied is essential. This is most commonly done by providing confidence limits for the estimated relative risk. Because of natural variability, confidence limits which overlap 1.0 do not provide evidence of increased (or decreased) risk.

3. Relative Odds

If a random sample of the population (e.g., cohort study) is not available, the relative risk can still be estimated under certain restrictions.

Table 3.1. Frequencies of Exposure among Cases and Controls in a Retrospective Study.

	Cases	Controls	Total
Exposed	a	b	a + b
Not exposed	c	d	c + d
Total	a + c	b + d	Total
Odds ratio = ad/bc			

Often, the odds ratio (Table 3.1) from a case-control study, calculated from summary data, accurately approximates the time relative risk.

4. Attributable Risk

The attributable risk (AR) is the proportion of events that can be attributed to the exposure in question. It is a useful concept when events can be caused by more than one factor. It is defined as:

AR = Number exposed with event/number exposed - number unexposed with event / number unexposed

AR = [a/(a+ c) — b/(b +d)/1 — b(b + d)].

5. Adjusted Rates

Invariably, it is necessary to account for the effects of confounding variables when comparing event rates. The process of accomplishing this is termed "adjustment." Unadjusted, or crude, rates can be compared reliably only if the composition of the comparison groups with respect to influential factors is similar. When this is not the case, adjustment is necessary.

Standardization is a common method in which the rates of two or more populations are adjusted to correspond with a standard distribution. The method of the standardized mortality ratio (SMR) is most frequently used. This adjustment technique may be used whether or not the rates refer to mortality. To generalize the concept, standardized event ratios (SERs) will be used. Basically, the SER is the rate in an exposed group compared with the rate that would be expected from the standard population. Mathematically,

Standardized mortality ratio = Observed rate/expected rate.

The expected rate or expected number of cases is obtained from the "average rate" operating on the standard population. Unfortunately, SMRs may not be directly comparable to one another, because adjustment is performed separately for each exposed group with its age distribution as the standard. In other words, two or more SMRs are not necessarily mutually standardized.

6. Multivariate Regression

To correct deficiencies in standardization, and to adjust on more than one confounding factor at a time, multiple regression techniques are often used. The most common of these for epidemiologic applications is logistic regression. In the dichotomous outcome case (diseased versus non-diseased), the outcome, coded as a 0 vs. 1, is modeled by a set of predictor variables, x, using the equation:

$$\text{Prob[outcome} = 1] = 1/(1 + e^{-Bx}),$$

Where B is a vector of parameter estimates, each of which is the logarithm of the odds ratio for that exposure factor. When the predictor variables are also dichotomous, the odds ratios can be interpreted directly as the odds of outcome given that characteristic divided by the odds of outcome without the characteristic. When the predictor variables are continuously distributed, the odds ratio is interpreted per unit change in the predictor variable. Thus, the technique is applicable when the predictor variables are not necessarily themselves categorical. Logistic regression methods are also applicable, with modification, when the design of a study incorporates matching and when outcomes have more than two ordinal levels.

D. INTERPRETATION OF EPIDEMIOLOGIC STUDIES

Because of the imperfect association between deterministic causes of disease (such as exposure to a toxin) and the ultimate development of a disease, epidemiologists have developed the concept of a "web of causation." This represents the interaction of factors that contribute to the occurrence of the disease. Although developed primarily for chronic diseases, it is a concept relevant to hazards from acute exposures as well.

The weight of the total amount of available information should be used in establishing an association between an exposure and a health outcome. The following causality criteria need to be considered:

1. **Strength**: a strong association between the suspected risk factor and the observed health outcome (e.g., high relative risk or odds ratio).
2. **Consistency**: the association holds up in different settings and among different groups.
3. **Specificity**: the specific exposure factor and specific health outcome are closely associated.
4. **Temporality**: the cause or exposure predates the health effect.
5. **Dose-response relationship**: as exposure intensifies, the severity of the health outcome is increased.
6. **Plausibility**: the association makes biologic sense.
7. **Coherence**: the association is consistent with what is known of the natural history and biology of the disease.
8. **Experimental evidence**: experimental studies support the hypothesis explaining the association.
9. **Analogy**: other examples with similar risk factors and health outcomes exist in the medical literature.

Strength of association is important because strong effects are less likely to be the result of epidemiologic confounding or bias. The variability in bias, which can enter epidemiologic studies, is often about the same magnitude as the effects being examined. While bias and confounding can produce large effects, it is more likely that strong associations are due to an underlying causality.

Evidence of true causality is also increased when results of independent studies are qualitatively and quantitatively similar. This consistency can be expected whether the causality or link is a strong one or a weak one. Biologic plausibility is an important component of proof of cause. It is important that a biologic mechanism exists that produces the observed effect from a toxic exposure. This evidence may rely on data gathered in species other than humans.

It seems self-evident that a causal exposure should proceed the onset of symptoms or disease. However, there is often ambiguity about the precise time of exposure, and long latent periods may further confuse the issues. Also, long latent periods may provide an opportunity for other factors to influence the onset of disease. Finally, dose-response association is important but difficult to demonstrate epidemiologically. In the laboratory, dose-response relationships can usually be shown for causal factors. However, the natural variability in human populations and the imprecision of epidemiologic studies may not allow a clear evidence of dose response.

E. EPIDEMIOLOGIC STUDY DESIGNS

Observational studies can be constructed in a variety of ways (Table 3.2). The common factor is the fact that the investigator did not control the exposure of subjects to any particular treatment. However, the sampling, data collection, and analyses are all carefully planned, leading to several broad categories of design.

1. Case Series

The simplest, oldest, and causally weakest type of epidemiologic study is the case series or case report. When causal factors are extremely large compared with the bias of case selection and with the natural person-to-person variability in outcomes, case reports may convey very useful information about the hazards of toxic exposures. However, most often case reports generate hypotheses that must be tested and strengthened by more valid types of studies.

Case reports are most useful when outcomes are extremely rare and/or when there is detailed knowledge about mechanisms of disease. For example, the Centers for Disease Control was able to alert physicians to the appearance of acquired immunodeficiency syndrome because of a few cases of **Pneumocystis carnii** pneumonia in New York City, which was previously an uncommon event.

In general, case series cannot be relied on to yield convincing causal evidence. When events can be attributed plausibly to several factors, case reports can potentially mislead. For example, isolating the causative "exposure" in suspected cancer clusters may be impossible or misleading if the cluster really represents random variation.

Table 3.2. Study Designs In Environmental Epidemiology That Use The Individual As The Unit Of Analysis. (Source: WHO, 1991).

STUDY DESIGN	Population	Exposure	Health Effect	Confounders	Problems	Advantages
Descriptive	Community or various subpopulations	Records of past measurements	Mortality and morbidity statistics; case registries; other reports	Difficult to sort out	Difficult to establish exposure-effect relationships	Cheap; useful to formulate hypotheses
Cross-sectional study	Communities or special groups; exposed vs. non-exposed	Current	Current	Usually easy to measure	Current exposure may be irrelevant to current disease	Can be done quickly; can use large populations; can estimate prevalence
Prospective cohort study	Community or special groups; exposed vs. non-exposed	Defined at outset of study (can change during study)	To be determined during study	Usually easy to measure	Expensive; time consuming; exposure categories can change; high dropout rate possible	Can estimate incidence and relative risk; can study many diseases in one study; can describe associations that suggest cause-effect relationships
Historical cohort study	Special groups, e.g., workers, patients, insured persons	Records of past measurements	Records of past or current diagnosis	Often difficult to measure because of retrospective nature; depends on quality of previously obtained data	Need to rely on records that may not be accurate	Less expensive and quicker than prospective study; can be used to study exposures that no longer exist
Case-control study	Usually small groups; diseases (cases) vs. non-diseases (controls)	Occurred in past; determined by records, or interview	Known at start of study	Possible to eliminate by matching for them	Difficult to generalize due to small study groups; some incorporate biases	Relatively cheap and quick; useful for studying rare diseases
Experimental (intervention study)	Community or special groups	Controlled/ known already	To be measured during study	Can be controlled by randomization of subjects	Expensive; ethical considerations; study subjects' compliance required	Well-accepted results; strong evidence for causality or efficacy of intervention

2. Cohort Studies

A cohort study is a design in which a population or sample of subjects at risk of disease is followed through time to ascertain which individuals develop the outcome of interest. The design may be implemented in real time (**prospectively**) or may be reconstructed from existing records (**retrospective**). This design closely resembles a true experiment in which the investigator controls exposure or treatment. In fact, clinical trials are a type of cohort study in which exposure (treatment) is controlled by the investigator. The cohort design allows estimation of both absolute risk and relative risk due to prognostic factors. However, it relies upon the outcome being relatively common. For example, a cohort study would be inefficient and unfeasible in a general population experiencing only a few events per thousand person-years of follow-up. Such a study might be useful in a high-risk population (e.g., industrially exposed workers). When cohort studies are performed prospectively, they have the advantage that many factors can be accurately determined on each subject at baseline. This can greatly limit selection bias. However, this design presupposes having a well-framed etiologic hypothesis when the study is started, i.e., it is not an exploratory tool.

When an epidemiologist can identify a group of people who were exposed to a toxic agent, a **cohort** study can be considered. With this study design, rates of diseases in a population exposed to a toxic agent are compared with rates in a demographically similar, but unexposed group. The disease rates for the unexposed population can be national or state averages for the entire population from which the exposed subjects are drawn, or they can be based on data collected from a population unexposed to the agent of interest. The association between exposure and disease in these studies is commonly expressed as the **relative risk** (the risk of disease in the exposed cohort divided by the risk in the unexposed cohort) for a particular toxic agent or dose level of a toxic agent. The criteria for exposure in a cohort study can be broad or narrow, depending on how accurately exposures or doses can be quantified, and the degree to which one desires the results to be generalizable. A cohort study can be restricted to a highly exposed group in order to maximize the chances of detecting an exposure - disease relation or it can include a large group with a wide range of exposures in order to produce results that are more generalizable or data that can be examined for exposure-response or dose-response relations with statistical models. There is no limit to the number of diseases that can be assessed in a cohort study, as long as the problem of multiple comparisons is addressed. The cohort design is useful for studying a toxic agent that is suspected to cause more than one disease. Cohort studies are also useful for studying the acute effects of environmental exposures that may not be severe enough to be recorded by disease surveillance systems.

Examples of cohort studies in environmental epidemiology include the study of cancer incidence in persons exposed to dioxins and other chemicals from an explosion at a chemical plant is Seveso, Italy, and studies of thyroid disease in children exposed to fallout from atmospheric tests of nuclear weapons at the Nevada Test site in the United States. Cohort studies in environmental epidemiology are usually retrospective or historical - that is, the cohort is defined after the exposure has occurred. Prospective cohort studies are rare, primarily because health agencies limit environmental exposures that are suspected to cause disease. However, when they can be done, prospective cohort studies can be quite effective.

3. Cross-Sectional Design

The cross-sectional design is also called a survey or prevalence design. It is based on random sampling of a population at a single point in time. Study subjects are characterized with regard to present, and perhaps past factors, and a determination of outcome status is made in each.

This design is most useful for studying chronic diseases of relatively high frequencies. When the sampling is properly done, cross-sectional studies are useful for characterizing the population under study, although the prevalence of outcomes can be determined, the cross-sectional study cannot estimate incidence, because it does not observe the transition from non-disease to disease status. Furthermore, certain factors may be seen to associate with prevalent cases, but the temporal and causal order of such associations cannot be determined from this study design.

4. Case-Control Designs

Case-control or **case-comparison** designs are primarily retrospective studies that compare previous exposure in subjects with disease to one or more groups of subjects without disease. The investigator plans and controls the selection of cases and non cases, but not the exposure. Cases may be prevalent or incident, case-control studies are extensively dealt with in many sources.

Because of the type of sampling employed, i.e., the cases are selected specifically because they have the outcome of interest; these designs allow estimation of the relative odds of exposure in cases and controls, but not absolute risk. In circumstances where the outcome is rare, the case-control design may be the only feasible one. These designs are further limited because information is obtained after the manifestation of disease, and cases and controls are often selected from different populations. Thus, this design is sometimes not suitable for exploring the consequences of an environmental exposure. Because these studies are inherently retrospective, they can be influenced by recall and other biases that arise from review of possibly incomplete documents.

Matching of cases and controls on one or more factors is often done to reduce the effects of confounders. For example, if age is related to outcome, controls may be selected to approximate within some interval the age of each case. In fact, matching induces confounding of a type, and its effects must be taken into account in the analysis. When there are too many confounders to make matching practical, an acceptable strategy is to match on only a few of the strongest confounders. Additional examples of matching factors are gender, race, ethnic background, and other socio-demographic characteristics. This approach compares a group of case subjects who have a disease with a group of control subjects who do not have the disease. Subjects in both groups are evaluated for exposure to one or more toxic agents, and the association between exposure or dose and disease is estimated with a statistic called the **odds ratio**, which, under appropriate conditions, approximates the relative risk.

Case-control studies are particularly useful for studying rare diseases such as cancer. Because exposures are assessed after the occurrence of disease, they must be measured carefully to avoid bias due to differing measurement protocols for cases and controls. Studies comparing exposures to electromagnetic fields in children with cancer to those in control groups are examples of case-control studies.

5. Other Study Designs

Numerous other designs have been employed in epidemiologic and surveillance studies. Such designs are often useful for taking advantage of specific exposure and outcome situations in a population.

a. Nested Case-control studies

Case-control studies can be nested within a cohort being followed for other purposes. In this setting, cases and controls are selected from the same defined population. Matching can also be employed.

b. Ecologic Studies

Ecologic studies have groups rather than individuals as the unit of analysis. Often the grouping variable is a geopolitical boundary (e.g., state, county, or country) and the outcome is average disease rate. Invariably, the results of such studies, which take advantage of existing databases, are intended to refer to individuals. There are potential fallacies in these types of inferences, and such studies are probably only reliable for hypothesis generation.

A study that assigns a single measure of exposure to a group of subjects is termed an ecologic study. Geopolitical boundaries are commonly used to define exposures in ecologic studies. In the United States, researchers choose counties, cities, or census tracts to define the boundaries for exposed and unexposed areas, and then compare disease rates for the populations within these boundaries.

Data from an ecologic study must be interpreted with caution, because persons within geographic units are usually not exposed to the same degree. Ecologic studies may include persons who have immigrated after the exposure occurred, and exclude persons who were exposed but emigrated before diseases were enumerated. Furthermore, environmental exposures are rarely homogeneous within geopolitical boundaries. Elevated disease rates produced by exposure to a toxic agent in a small section of a geographic area can therefore be diluted by many unexposed and unaffected subjects - an example of misclassification bias. The confounding effects of variables other than the exposure of interest can lead to inaccurate estimates of the toxicity of environmental agents. Some of these confounding effects can be controlled for by such methods as stratifying disease rates by specific time periods and by accounting for latent periods between the onset of exposure and the time of diagnosis or death.

c. Cluster Studies

Cluster studies examine outcome frequencies in groups defined by space, time, family, or other clustering. Special methods of analysis may be required to account for or detect non independence of outcomes.

One of the most common problems environmental epidemiologists encounter is determining whether reported cases of disease in an area are more numerous than would be expected by chance alone, and if so, whether there is an environmental exposure responsible for the "cluster." Determining whether a cluster is a statistically significant elevation in incidence or prevalence can be done using a fairly logical sequence of analyses, as outlined below. Whether a cluster is related to an environmental exposure is, however, far more difficult to determine.

The first and most important step in investigating a cluster is to learn as much as possible about how the cluster was discovered and whether possible causes of the cluster have been identified. Invariably, the news of a disease cluster in a community causes public concern, and members of the public can become quite angry with those who are thought to be responsible for its cause as well as with government officials and scientists who are perceived to work too slowly, to be insensitive to community concerns, or to be covering up the cause of the cluster.

Listening to those who are concerned about the cluster will help researchers design their investigation so that it will produce results that are relevant to the public's questions. Discussions of research goals will also inform the public about the limitations of epidemiologic analysis. In addition, these discussions help identify the exposure(s) thought to be responsible for the cluster - information that is extremely important for evaluating causal relations if the cluster is real. This information can also be used to address the problem with methods of risk assessment if there is not a statistically significant elevation in the incidence or prevalence of disease.

The second step in a cluster investigation is to determine whether the reported cluster represents a true increase in the usual occurrence of one or more diseases. Clusters can occur at random in space or in time, and there are statistical techniques for determining whether reported disease rates are significantly higher than rates expected by chance alone. Recently, software has been developed to make a variety of these techniques accessible to epidemiologists. The rapid advances in software development for geographic information systems should favorably influence the design of even better cluster analysis software in the future. Remember, however, that all techniques depend on reliable data for disease rates, which should be collected and verified for both the alleged cluster and for comparison groups before they are analyzed.

A statistically significant cluster of disease does not, by itself, confirm a proposed exposure - disease relation. Nor does the absence of a cluster mean the suspected source of exposure poses no health risk. If statistical analyses suggest a true increase in disease and if there are exposures that have been proposed as possible causes, then investigators can determine the feasibility of a cohort or case-control study.

In situations in which there is a statistically significant cluster but no hypothesized cause, a careful search for possible causes is necessary before planning an epidemiologic study. The search should involve a review of all agents known to cause the disease and possible sources of such agents, as well as the consideration of agents to which diseased subjects were exposed but which have not previously been associated with the disease. If there is no evidence for a disease cluster, then the previously described techniques of risk assessment can be used to estimate health risks.

Although the outlined procedure seems pretty straightforward, conducting a cluster investigation can be quite frustrating. This is particularly true for investigations of cancer, because exposure data for the pre-latent period are frequently unavailable and there are many lifestyle and dietary factors that could confound the effects of environmental exposures. Cluster investigations of acute diseases (called outbreak or epidemic investigations) are central to the practice of public health and have revealed the causes of many diseases. Clusters of chronic diseases with poorly understood etiologies also deserve the attention of epidemiologists, as they present opportunities for new discoveries. Clusters of diseases with known etiologies are less worthwhile to pursue.

6. Mapping Exposures And Diseases

Exposures and disease rates for geopolitically defined areas can also be mapped. In the past, important theories on the relation between the environment, insect vectors, and infectious diseases were based on such maps. To date, this type of analysis has failed to uncover new exposure-disease relations for cancer and other chronic diseases. Studies of mapped disease rates have mainly confirmed associations already known to exist, such as the relation between lung cancer and asbestos exposure in shipyards located in coastal counties of the United States, and between solar radiation and skin cancer in the southern United States.

Improvements in computer technology have eased the mapping of multiple data sets for environmental monitoring results, geologic factors, and disease rates. These **geographic information systems (GIS)** may be useful in graphically relating the distribution of toxic agents in the environment to the location of specific populations and in selecting remedial options for the cleanup of environmental contaminants that are most likely to reduce health risks. Whether such systems will improve current analytical approaches in environmental epidemiology remains unclear, however.

Mapped disease rates and ecologic studies have both been of limited use for the same reason: When geopolitical boundaries define exposures, persons with diseases caused by toxic exposures are mixed with those who have no exposure or disease and with those who have diseases caused by ubiquitous exposures, such as smoking. Furthermore, geopolitical boundaries are not very useful for evaluating dose-response (or exposure-disease) relations.

The distance between a suspected source of exposure and the place of residence at the time of diagnosis or death is commonly used in mapping, cohort, and case-control studies. Distance may not correlate with intensity of exposure, and place of residence at the time of diagnosis may not reflect earlier exposures at other residences. Results from studies with such crude measures of exposure must be confirmed with more detailed estimates of exposure or dose if they are to be accepted as evidence for causal relations.

In spite of these limitations, members of the public and practitioners of public health are seemingly infatuated with the distribution of diseases around potential sources of environmental exposure. If geographic information systems are used to construct maps of exposures and diseases for purposes of discussion and hypothesis generation, then they can provide useful information. Knowledge that disease rates in the community of interest are not ten times higher than the average for other areas can be helpful, as can the confirmation of a suspected increase in disease incidence or prevalence for a particular area. To evaluate causal relations, however, epidemiologists must employ other designs such as cohort and case-control studies with data for exposures or doses that are more accurate than those used in mapping studies.

7. Other Analytical Techniques

A number of other methods have been used to analyze exposure - disease relations. Exposure measurements such as concentrations of air pollutants can be related to disease rates with linear regression models. If disease rates are low, then Poisson regression models may be used.

Many types of environmental measurements have natural temporal patterns that vary diurnally, weekly, and seasonally. These effects can confound the exposure of interest if they are not accounted for. Seasonal weather cycles and the seasonal patterns of viral diseases, for instance, can confound the effects of air pollutants, which may also vary seasonally. **Time series** analysis is a popular method for making such adjustments, and has been used extensively in studies of air pollution and disease.

The effects of environmental agents on humans can also be assessed with studies of animals in contaminated environments. Studies in the fields of ecotoxicology and wildlife toxicology use designs similar to those of epidemiology. The results from such studies may be more relevant than laboratory studies, as animals are exposed to agents under environmental conditions that are more similar to those of humans.

It has been suggested that these animal studies can be designed as **sentinel** systems for identifying new health hazards to humans and other species and for generating data for risk assessment. A sentinel species must have a measurable response to the agent in question, have a territory or home range that overlaps the area for which there is concern about exposure to humans, be easily captured, and have a sufficient population size and density to permit enumeration. Candidates for sentinel species include food animals, pets, fish, and other wildlife.

To date, animal sentinel systems have been used rarely, and there appears to be no effort to implement them. The reason is due, in part, to their cost and the effort required to document normal rates of disease for sentinel species and to standardize an ongoing data collection program. The use of animal sampling for dose estimates, however, will continue to be popular for particular environmental exposures.

F. SAMPLE SIZE FOR EPIDEMIOLOGIC STUDIES

There are few decisions in the study more important than the choice of sample size. Study requirements for a certain number of cases and controls influence the economic feasibility of the study, the strength of the epidemiologic effect that can be detected, and the chances that valid conclusions will be reached. Four quantities are relevant to the assessment of sample size; the study designer must choose the first three, and the mathematical formulation yields the fourth:

1. **Type I error**: the chance that random variation will yield spurious evidence of risk associated with exposure when no such risk exists.
2. **Power**: the chance that a true risk associated with exposure will be detected. Note that a negative conclusion places a premium on this quantity; assertions that there is no effect require a study with a high chance of finding an effect if there is one.
3. **Relative risk**: a measure of the strength of the smallest risk associated with exposure that is considered "worth" detecting: the study is not justified if the true risk is smaller, and the study is obligatory if the true risk is at least as large. Using P_r, to

denote the chance of exposure among cases and P_n to denote the same chance among controls, standard epidemiologic theory indicates that the relative risk R is estimated by $P_r (1 — P_n)/P_n (1 — P_r)$.

4. C, the number of matched case-control sets (e.g., one case and two controls), needed to detect a true relative risk of R with given type I error and power. For this example with one case and two controls in each set, the study requires 3C subjects.

The relevant calculations can take into account matching which is justified only if matching factors have a very strong impact on the medical outcome, stratification (e.g., separate consideration of subjects in groups of similar age) and "dose" trend (e.g., possible increasing frequency of outcomes for those with longer exposure). In addition, assuming that those who cannot participate in the study or cannot be traced are similar to participants may not be correct. Because of losses and dropouts, inflation of the sample size is usually needed so that the desired number of subjects can actually be analyzed.

G. MAJOR METHODOLOGICAL ISSUES IN AN EPIDEMIOLOGIC STUDY

1. Precision

Precision is the reduction of random error as indicated by the variance of a measurement and associated confidence interval.

2. Validity

Validity is the reduction of systematic error (or systematic bias) as indicated by comparing what the study estimated and what it is intended to estimate.

3. Comparability and bias

A serious threat to the validity of any epidemiologic study is the possibility that the selection of study subjects or data collected is biased. In epidemiology, "bias" does not imply a prejudice or prejudgment on the part of the study investigators. Rather, "bias" generally refers to systematic or nonrandom errors, that is, errors due to factors other than sampling variability that prevent the true value of a disease rate or exposure status from being obtained. The introduction of bias renders study groups non-comparable in some important way that will distort study findings.

To understand how a study can become biased, it is useful to recall the degree to which the laboratory scientists strive to achieve comparability between exposed and unexposed animals in their experiments. This is accomplished by such means as using a single strain of test organism, random assignment of each study animal to an exposure group, maintaining uniform environmental and dietary conditions during the course of the study, and using a consistent protocol for examination. The examination for disease outcomes is performed with the investigator "blinded" to the subject's previous exposure history. Failure to achieve any of these major comparability elements can bias a study, and its conclusions must be regarded cautiously.

In epidemiologic research, using observational methods, an equivalent degree of comparability as that achieved in an experimental study cannot be achieved. The goal of the epidemiologist is to select from an existing population of exposed and non-exposed groups that are fundamentally comparable and from which equivalent data can be obtained. It is important to recognize that bias can be introduced in numerous ways, some of which cannot be known or controlled by the investigator. The following discussion provides examples of major types of biases that can occur in epidemiologic studies.

4. Biases

Bias can occur in virtually every aspect of epidemiologic research. However, the following examples illustrate only those biases that can arise:

a. In the process used to specify or select study participants (**selection bias**),
b. In the process of collecting data on study participants (**observation or information bias**),
c. Due to the existence of factors that are associated with both the exposure and the disease (**bias**).

Some types of bias can only occur in a particular study design, while others must be considered as a possibility with any design.

Non-response bias - Some portion of those who are selected or identified as study subjects cannot or will not participate in the study. Bias can occur when this group of non-respondents differs systematically from respondents with respect to exposure or disease status. For example, non-respondents may have more serious health problems. To minimize this bias, considerable effort must be expended to achieve a high participation rate (90% or better) or at least to obtain a sample of non-respondents to determine whether or how they may differ with regard to the risk of disease or exposure status.

Lost-to-follow-up-bias - A similar type of bias can occur when study participants are "lost to follow-up" in cohort studies. Those who are "lost" may differ in their disease status, thus removing from the study individuals with more serious health problems. Significant efforts must be made in cohort studies to minimize the proportion of individuals who cannot be located.

Detection bias - This bias refers to the situation in which a disease (such as a brain tumor) is more frequently diagnosed and ascertained in a particular population (such as an occupational group) than in the general population. This may result from better access to medical care or better diagnostic services. If the general population rates are used as a basis for comparison, it will appear that members of the particular population are at increased risk of the disease. In reality, they are at increased risk only of being diagnosed with the disease. Widespread publicity about some agent may prompt exposed persons to seek medical examination, again increasing the possibility of detection among members of that group.

Healthy worker effect - Overall the working population is healthier than the general population. Less healthy people are less likely to become or remain employed; thus employment serves as a selective factor. In occupational studies therefore a clear possibility of bias arises if the general population is used as the basis for obtaining expected disease rates as is often done in retrospective cohort studies. The use of general population rates can create the false appearance that employment in an industry actually affords protection against mortality or suggest that there is no excess mortality. This effect is more evident for some diseases than others. For example, in contrast to some chronic diseases, it does not appear that overall cancer mortality is typically lower than expected in occupational cohorts when compared with the general population. Cardiovascular disease on the other hand is typically found to be lower in an occupational cohort than would be expected based, on general population rates.

Incidence-prevalence bias - Newly diagnosed ("**incident**") cases of disease may differ in certain characteristics from all existing ("**prevalent**") cases of the disease. Studies that use prevalent cases are more likely to include longer duration cases and exclude both rapidly fatal and readily cured cases. Consequently, prevalence studies are more likely to yield information relating to disease duration rather than disease development.

Observation and measurement bias - Numerous biases involve non-comparable data or data collection procedures. For example, exposure data obtained from interviews will not be comparable to data obtained from environmental measurements.

Observation bias can also arise when interviews are used to obtain health outcome data. If the interviewer knows a subject's disease status as well as the hypothesis under study, the interviewer may subconsciously probe harder concerning past exposures. Furthermore, a subject who has been advised of a study's purpose may attempt to provide responses that are perceived as "favorable" or "helpful" to the interviewer. Thus, when possible, interviews are frequently conducted in a "double-blind" fashion where neither the interviewer nor the subject is aware of the specific hypothesis under investigation.

In follow-up studies, disease diagnosis may be influenced by the physician's knowledge of a subject's exposure history. This bias, which applies mainly to cohort studies, will tend to increase the association between exposure and disease.

Recall bias - A person who has developed a particular disease may be better motivated and better able to recall previous exposures compared with control subjects. The mother of a child born with a malformation may recall more completely (or perhaps exaggerate) exposures experienced during pregnancy compared with the mother of a healthy child. This is a serious potential bias in case-control studies.

Misclassification bias - This does not refer to random misclassification of some small proportion of the study population but to systematic misclassification of disease or exposure status. This could happen if, for example, the job title "electrician" is used to identify subjects occupationally exposed to electric and magnetic fields (EMF) and a large portion of these electricians work only on dead circuits, where EMF exposure is low. On the contrary, some other workers, who are identified as "non-electricians," might be exposed to EMF.

Berksonian bias - This bias, first described by Berkson in 1946, can arise when controls are selected from hospitals (usually the same hospitals from which the cases have been selected). Hospitalized controls are generally not representative of the overall population with respect to certain characteristics, such as smoking, alcohol, or coffee consumption. In order to detect and prevent Berksonian bias, multiple controls are suggested. Therefore, some case-control studies have used both hospital and neighborhood controls at the same time to detect this bias.

Confounding bias - Confounding bias occurs when there is a third variable that is not of interest to the study but is related to the exposure and is a cause of the disease under study. A study of lung cancer, for example, will find a significant association between alcohol consumption and the development of lung cancer. In such a study smoking would be considered a confounding variable since it is associated both with alcohol consumption and lung cancer. If the effect of smoking is removed in the study (by design strategies such as matching or analytic techniques such as stratification or adjustment), the association between drinking and lung cancer might not remain.

Most epidemiologic studies attempt to control at least several well-established confounding variables such as age, sex, race, and socioeconomic class. Other variables may be examined in a particular study; however, not all potentially confounding variables can be examined. Thus some degree of confounding bias is probably present in all data.

Given the difficulty in recognizing and controlling all potential sources of bias, no study should be considered completely free of bias. For example, rarely does a study attain 100% follow-up of subjects. Critics can always attribute study findings to some form of bias since there are indeed so many potential sources. However, in practice, it is difficult to actually demonstrate that some bias may fully explain or even materially affect the findings of a study. Strict adherence to established procedures and standards can reduce many, but not all, possibilities for bias. In many well-reported studies, the authors frequently discuss the possible sources of bias in their study and attempt to show, through logic and/or data, that their findings are not likely to be due to some bias. But there still remains the possibility that some unknown bias is operating.

II. STEPS IN CONDUCTING A DISEASE OUTBREAK INVESTIGATION

An investigation is an examination for the purpose of finding out about something. It differs from surveillance because when doing an investigation one assumes that a problem already exists. Moreover, an investigation may use information from an established data collection system, but it goes farther and gathers new information. Analysis, on the other hand, involves the study of a problem by breaking it down into its constituent parts. In carrying out an investigation, therefore, an epidemiologist must have some idea as to what analysis will ultimately be necessary.

Exactly what must be found out depends in part on what is already known. The classic epidemiological triad of host, agent, and environment first mentioned in the discussion of **determinants**, is a useful framework for thinking about epidemics. The epidemiologist often knows about the host as to signs and symptoms of an illness, or health event, and the number of people in the epidemic. This holds true for epidemics of infection, acute noninfectious problems, such as unexplained deaths in a hospital, and chronic disease problems, as illustrated by the occurrence of endometrial cancer and estrogen use.

When the investigation is complete, however, we must know about the host and have information on a wide range of risk factors for the health problem. In addition, we need detailed information about the agent to which the host is exposed and the environment of the exposure. Ultimately, we require effective control measures. This requires that the epidemiologist know how the agent is transmitted and, if possible, its portal of entry.

Epidemiological investigations meet both public service and scientific needs. If, for example, a community faces a health problem that is likely to continue to spread and about which the approach to control is uncertain, then the epidemiologist has an important role. Epidemics of viral infections that occur in presumably immunized young people, as has been the case of measles epidemics on college campuses, illustrate this problem. Moreover, public concern may also require the epidemiologist to provide assurance that no epidemic exists and none is threatening. Concern about transmission of AIDS by exposure to medical waste in public places is one such example, even though this environmental problem is not a real hazard for transmitting disease.

Scientific need is a second important reason for an epidemiologist to do a detailed field investigation. This kind of investigation recently led to the discovery of Lyme disease and Legionnaire's disease. Field investigation also identified the causal association between vinyl chloride exposure and angiosarcoma of the liver, as it was for oral contraceptive use and hepatocellular adenoma, and a wide range of other health conditions.

A. PREPARING FOR AN INVESTIGATION

Preparation for an epidemiological field investigation has three general elements:

1. Notification of essential people and organizations,
2. Identification of materials needed for the investigation, and
3. Travel planning.

The notification process will have begun before the epidemiologist departs for the field. However, initial reports require confirmation. In addition, the date and place of investigation and also its purpose needs the concurrence of supervisors, health officials where the investigation is being done, and other officials whose regions may include that area. Failure to notify these individuals can bring the investigation to a halt, limit access to people who have essential information, or lead to a withdrawal of support personnel needed to complete the investigation.

Before going to the field, materials must be assembled to help with the investigation. Depending on the nature of the problem, the epidemiologist may want reprints of scientific articles. In addition, other items may be useful. Among them are the following:

1. Copies of sample questionnaires,
2. Paper for line lists or the coding of data,

3. A hand-held calculator,
4. A portable computer,
5. A camera,
6. Containers for laboratory specimens,
7. Pocket references on microbial, physical, or chemical agents, and
8. Means for accessing the Internet.

B. BASIC STEPS OF AN INVESTIGATION

The following ten steps are essential considerations in every epidemiological investigation (Table 3.3). Practicing epidemiologists return more to this list than to any other.

Table 3.3. Steps in an Epidemiological Investigation.

1.	Determine the existence of an epidemic
2.	Confirm the diagnosis
3.	Define and count the cases
4.	Orient the data in terms of time, place, and person
5.	Determine who is at risk of having the health problem
6.	Develop and test an explanatory hypothesis
7.	Compare the hypothesis with the proven facts
8.	Plan a more systematic study
9.	Prepare a written report
10.	Propose measures for control and prevention

1. Ensure the existence of an epidemic. The first important decision is to decide if an epidemic exists. A preliminary count of people with similar symptoms is often the first criterion for this decision. Laboratory confirmation may be absent. It may even be inappropriate because of the urgent need to begin an investigation.

2. Confirm the diagnosis. The epidemiologist needs to know the diagnosis of the health problem being addressed. The number of cases is sometimes too great to do a history and physical examination on every person. Collection of laboratory specimens must then follow quickly, although decisions about epidemic control are often made before laboratory confirmation is available. Using this preliminary information, the epidemiologist must formulate a case definition of the health problem. The symptoms for the case definition are written down, as are the essential physical signs. Measurements of levels of severity of the health problem, or disease, must be determined. Confirming each reported case may not be possible, and laboratory specimens may be obtained on only 15 to 20 percent of the cases. In some large epidemics, a sample of cases gave the essential information about the agent, the host, the method of transmission, the portal of entry, and the environment of the disease. This proved to be the only way to deal with one epidemic in 1985, when **Salmonella** contaminated milk processed in Illinois and involved more than 200,000 individuals. Epidemiologists set up control measures more quickly using this approach than by an exhaustive detection of every ill individual.

3. Estimate the number of cases. Case finding often begins with a single report or a small cluster of cases. Initially, the epidemiologist casts a wide net, using a preliminary case definition that is sensitive and excludes as few true cases as possible. After making a preliminary estimate, the epidemiologist must make a key judgment. Should all cases be studied or is the epidemic so large that investigating a sample will lead to a decision more quickly? If only a sample is selected, then only the most severe cases should be studied because they are the ones of most value. Outlying observations deserve special attention because explaining their relationship to the epidemic is often the key to understanding its mode of spread.

Given a workable definition, the epidemiologist must count the cases and collect data about them. Once the ill persons are identified, the characteristics of the illness from beginning to the present and the demographic characteristics of each individual need to be determined. Next, data on the places where the ill people live, work, and have traveled to, and the possible exposures that might lead to health impairment all must be documented. Among the questions the epidemiologist may want to answer are the following:

a. What signs and symptoms are the most important?
b. Are any of them pathognomonic?
c. What is the laboratory test most likely to confirm the diagnosis?
d. Can both the exposure to the presumed source and the severity of the illness be characterized at different levels?
e. What must be done to identify the people with these problems should long-term follow-up be necessary?
f. Are there any in apparent or sub-clinical cases?
g. What role do they play in determining the future size of this epidemic or the susceptibility of the people in this community?

4. Orient the data as to time, place, and person. Data on each case must include the date of onset of the illness, the place where the person lives and/or became ill, and the characteristics of each individual, including age, sex, and occupation. A simple histogram, often called "the epidemic curve," shows the relationship between the occurrence of cases and their time of onset. The spatial relationships of cases are often shown best on a spot map. Maps, for instance, help show that the cases occurred in proximity to a body of water, a sewage treatment plant, or its outflow. Characterizing individuals by age, sex, and other relevant attributes permits the epidemiologist to estimate rates of occurrence and compare them with other appropriate community groups.

5. Determine who is at risk of having the health problem. The epidemiologist will calculate rates at which a health problem, or disease, occurs using the number of the population at risk as the denominator, while the number of those individuals with the problem form the numerator. If the original reports of an illness come from a state surveillance system, then the first estimations of rates may be based on a state's population. If the epidemic occurs only in school-age children from a particular school, however, the population at risk may be only the children who attend that school. Those not ill must be characterized by the same attributes as those who are ill, that is, age, sex, grade in school, or classroom.

6. Develop an explanatory hypothesis. During a field investigation comparing the rates of occurrence among those at greatest risk with other groups helps the epidemiologist develop hypotheses to explain the cause and transmission of a health problem. Besides examining rates, other approaches to developing hypotheses of cause include further, more-detailed interviews with ill individuals or with local health officials and residents, careful examination of outlying cases, or describing the epidemic in more detail. Depending on the extent of the epidemiologist's field library, reference to current and historical literature can stimulate new hypotheses.

7. Compare the hypothesis with the established facts. The hypothesis that explains the epidemic must be consistent with all the facts the epidemiologist knows. If the hypothesis is not so, then it must be reexamined. It should do more than just strengthen speculation explaining the cases at the peak of the epidemic. The epidemiologist may need to repeat the interview of case subjects, reassess medical records, gather additional laboratory specimens, and repeat calculations.

8. Plan a more systematic study. When the initial field investigations and preliminary calculations are complete, the investigator may need to conduct one or more case control studies. The data for such studies may be in hand, but more often additional information will be needed. It may be collected by either interviewing subjects in more detail, or surveying the population. Sometimes, a serological survey or extensive sampling of the environment for chemical or biological agents will generate new facts. Sometimes a visual record helps, requiring extensive photography or video taping of a work process. If there is a food-borne infection, a detailed food history is necessary. If a water-borne infection is suspected, a food and liquid intake history stimulates additional causal associations. For example, a water-borne epidemic may be discovered by knowing the number of glasses of water drunk by each person, thereby permitting the epidemiologist to estimate a dose-response relationship. An occupational illness might be determined by a specific machine that each worker used and the number of hours that each one used.

9. Prepare a written report. Preparing a written document is an essential step in any epidemiological investigation. An epidemic report need not be a publishable paper. However, it should be a benchmark in the conduct of an investigation, just as a hospital discharge summary is for patient care or a thesis is for the advancement of a scholar. The epidemic report is an essential public health document, and it may be the basis for action by health officials who may close a restaurant or face a major industry's attorneys in court. For the public, it may provide information for those concerned about the epidemic, its spread, and the likelihood that others will be involved. A report may have scientific epidemiological importance in documenting the discovery of a new agent, a new route of transmission, or a new and imaginative approach to epidemiological investigation. Moreover, many investigative reports are useful in teaching.

10. Propose measures for control and prevention. The ultimate purpose of an epidemiological investigation is to control a health problem in a community. The epidemiologist is part of the team that develops the approach to control and prevention.

The establishment of a surveillance system for the population at risk is an important element in ensuring the effectiveness of the control program. This is an essential element of an epidemiologist's responsibility in fulfilling a public need and carrying out a scientific study.

III. EXAMPLE OF ENVIRONMENTAL EPIDEMIOLOGY STUDY

Often recognized as the founder of epidemiology, John Snow conducted what is regarded today as a classic study of the transmission of cholera in London in the mid-1800s. The case illustrates many of the principles of a valid environmental epidemiologic study.

As pointed out by Monson, several factors make Snow's study a model of environmental epidemiology:

1. Snow recognized an association between exposure and disease - that is, between the source of the drinking-water supply and the incidence of cholera;
2. He formulated a hypothesis - that fecal contamination of drinking water was the specific agent of transmission of the disease;
3. He collected information to substantiate his hypothesis - in sub-districts where the drinking water was supplied by only one company, the association was stronger;
4. He recognized that there could be an alternative explanation for the association - that social class or place of residence might influence transmission of the disease;
5. He applied a method to minimize the effects of the alternative explanation - he compared cholera rates within a single district or neighborhood, rather than between neighborhoods, on the basis of their water supply;
6. He effectively minimized the collection of biased or false information - since most residents were not aware of the name of the company that supplied their water, he applied a chemical test to make this determination in a positive manner.

These criteria have withstood the test of time. In fact, investigators today assess the associations between environmental agents and disease based on the design of environmental epidemiologic studies that incorporate many of the principles established by John Snow.

IV. MAJOR CHALLENGES IN ENVIRONMENTAL EPIDEMIOLOGY

A. EXPOSURE ASSESSMENT

Valid environmental monitoring measurements and accurate estimates of exposures are essential. Exposure to physical agents such as noise or vibration may be transitory. In some cases assessment personnel do not yet fully understand which parameters are indicative of exposure. Nor do they know if the average or peak exposures are important.

The importance of movement and interactions is exemplified by the fact that physical and chemical contaminants can be readily altered. Exposures Assessment from airborne particulate exposures requires identifying:

1. What the contaminant is,
2. Its physical form (amorphous, crystalline, discrete particulate, or fibrous),
3. Particle size distribution, and
4. Physicochemical surface properties.

5. Factors that can contribute to indoor air quality are:

a. Family eating habits,
b. Type of cooking facilities,
c. Personal hobbies and recreational activities,
d. Pesticide applications within the home and garden, and
e. Nature of domestic water supply.

Contaminants released into the air during showering, bathing, and cooking may become sources of exposure through inhalation. Table 3.4 illustrates the hierarchy of exposure data or surrogates, ranging from quantified measurements of individual exposures to simply knowing the person's residence or place of employment.

Table 3.4. Hierarchy of Exposure Data or Surrogates. (Source: Moeller, 1997).

Types of data	Approximation to actual exposure
Quantified personal measurements Quantified area or ambient measurements in vicinity of residence or other sites of activity Quantified surrogates of exposure (e.g., estimates of drinking water and food consumption) Residence or employment in proximity to site of source of exposure Residence or employment in general geographic area (e.g., county) of site of source of exposure	Best ↑↓ Poorest

B. HEALTH ENDPOINTS

The selection of the health endpoints to be evaluated is a second major challenge in the design and implementation of an environmental epidemiologic study. Before, there was a determination of the chemical and physical agent in question that was causing an increase in mortality or hospital admissions (morbidity) among exposed populations. Then the potential increase in the incidence of cancer became the primary important health indicator.

Today, environmental and public health officials are concerned about the impacts of environmental agents on the quality of life. They are insisting that a variety of possible pathological conditions: biochemical, physiological, and neurological dysfunctions be considered (including effects on respiratory and cardiovascular, central nervous, and musculoskeletal systems, as well as behavioral, hematopoietic, growth, and reproductive effects).

Assessment of any of these endpoints requires some standardized measure of effects. Indicators that have been developed for measuring behavioral effects of noxious environmental agents fall into two broad categories: measures of psychological and psychophysiological functioning, and measures of mental state and behavior.

The range of indicators of exposure to various environmental agents has been expanded to include biologic markers (Figure 3.1). They are divided into 3 groups and defined as any cellular or molecular indicator of **toxic exposure**, **adverse health effect**, or **susceptibility**.

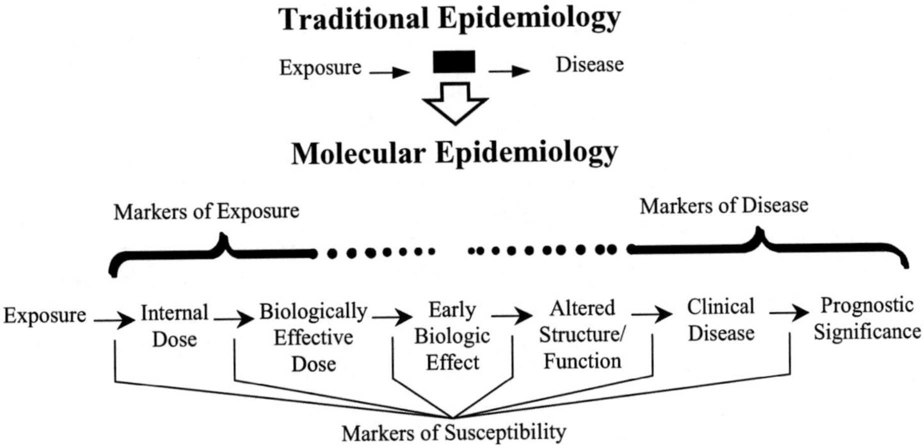

Figure 3.1. Evolution of the Detailed Continuum for Molecular Epidemiologic Research. (Source: Schulte, 1993).

V. MOLECULAR EPIDEMIOLOGY

A. CAPABILITIES OF MOLECULAR EPIDEMIOLOGY

1. Delineation of a Continuum of Events between Exposure and Disease

A rich level of detail can supplement previous categorical models that linked exposure and disease. The concept of a continuum of events between exposure and disease provides the opportunity to insure that epidemiologic research has a biologic basis for hypotheses and provides the analyses to test these ideas. New opportunities for classical and hybrid epidemiologic study designs can be applied to this continuum.

2. Identification of Exposures to Smaller Amounts of Xenobiotics and Enhanced Dose Reconstruction

The powerful tools of molecular biology, analytical chemistry, and related disciplines now allow exposure determinations on the order of 1 part in 10^{18} or 10^{21}. This ability to identify small amounts of a xenobiotic makes more active consideration of "background" levels of target xenobiotics in nominally nonexposed subjects important when designing studies and assessing covariates and confounding factors.

A key capability of molecular epidemiology is assessing past exposures and reconstructing doses received from past exposures by using biologic measurements on samples taken from small groups of subject. This procedure is termed "biologic dosimetry." Biologic dosimetry can complement traditional methods of dose reconstruction by using personal dosimeters to measure ambient exposure, by estimating body burdens through sampling fat, urine, or other materials, or by detecting adducts, gene mutations, chromosome aberrations, or other relevant markers.

3. Identification of Events Earlier in the Natural History

When a continuum or part of a continuum between an exposure and a disease is identified and understood, it is possible to focus on preclinical rather than clinical events. Thus, asymptomatic individuals who are at increased risk of manifesting clinical disease can be identified. Some examples of indicators include the decrease in CD4 lymphocytes in HIV-infected persons, expression of p300 in bladder cells in people at risk of bladder cancer, elevated levels of lipoprotein Lp(a) in persons at risk for cardiovascular disease, and various sperm parameters in individuals at risk of reduced fertility.

The ability to identify prodromal events expands the pool of potential cases for epidemiologic studies. It permits studies of interventions that can have impact on the group being studied as well as on the individuals to whom the results can be generalized.

4. Reduction of Misclassification of Variables

Misclassification of exposure and disease variables is a major weakness of epidemiologic studies. Better classification of exposure than that achieved using historical characteristics and measurements may be accomplished by assessing markers of internal and biologically effective doses. More homogeneous disease groupings can be defined using markers of effect such as specific mutations indicative of exposure (mutational spectra). The validity and precision of point estimates may be increased as misclassifications are reduced.

5. Indication of Mechanisms

Delineating a continuum of events between exposure and disease provides opportunities for insight into the mechanism of action. Much epidemiologic research has been based on theorization about mechanisms, or at least some prior speculation that exposure and outcome are related. Molecular epidemiologic approaches facilitate testing the association between mechanistic events in a defined continuum. Knowledge of the mechanism can guide future research and intervention applications.

6. Accounting for Variability and Effect Modification

Perhaps one of the greatest contributions of molecular epidemiology is the ability to discern the role of host factors, particularly genetic factors, in accounting for variation in response. Why similarly exposed people do not get the same diseases is a target question for molecular epidemiology. In most disease systems, susceptibility markers are being identified and evaluated. These markers can be incorporated into epidemiologic models as effect modifiers.

7. Enhanced Individual and Group Risk Assessments

The use of epidemiologic data to provide individual and group risk assessments is well established. For example, individual risk functions have played a strong role in cardiovascular disease research and control, in pulmonary and occupational medicine, in infectious disease control, and in genetic epidemiology and counseling. Molecular epidemiology can enhance individual and group risk assessments by providing more person-specific information, allowing extrapolation of risk from one group to another, from animal species to humans, and from groups to individual.

The "parallelogram approach" used in genetic toxicology is a model for animal-to-human extrapolation. A marker appropriate to both species (animal and human) that can be related to exposure-disease relationships in the animal can serve as the basis for predicting effects in exposed humans. Similarly, extrapolation from group to group, group to individual, or individual to group follows the same general model (see examples in Figures 3.2 and 3.3). Identification of a detailed continuum of events between an exposure and disease, coupled with covariates of the event variables in multivariate models, permits the calculation of individual risk functions.

Molecular markers can heighten the specificity of these functions and allow reduced confidence intervals around estimates. Not only is it now possible to say that a middle-aged man with heart disease and a cholesterol level above 240 mg/dl will have a one-in-five chance of dying from a heart attack within 10 years, it may soon be possible to indicate which man that will be. Some readers may view the term "molecular epidemiology" as an oxymoron.

Epidemiology is the study of health effects in groups of people. "Molecular" and "cellular" indicate assessment of the individual at the component level. Epidemiology relies on observation and inference of associations between variables. Molecular and cellular sciences use experimental proof of cause and effect. Despite these different scopes, scales, and approaches, molecular sciences and epidemiology are compatible, if not inevitably linked.

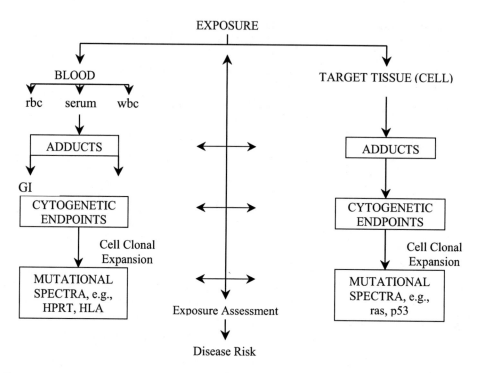

<u>Figure 3.2.</u> Exposure Assessment Paradigm for Linking Carcinogen-Macromolecular Adducts, Cytogenetic Aberrations and Mutational Spectra. GI, gastrointestinal tract. (Source: Schulte, 1993).

There is a historical basis for such a link, as well as a conceptual and epistemological framework for epidemiologic research that incorporates biologic measurements of human processes. In a sense, molecular epidemiology is a signpost that flags the need to incorporate an understanding of biologic phenomena at the physiologic, cellular, and molecular levels into epidemiologic research (Figure 3.4). Epidemiologists long have used biologic markers (e.g., antibody titers, serum lipids, blood lead). However, in the past when high "exposures" and single outcomes were more prevalent and frequent, epidemiologists argued that knowledge of associations was more useful than understanding the mechanisms, since prevention through control of exposures was often feasible even in the absence of understanding cellular processes. Previous success in public health led to the identification of the major single or primary cause of diseases.

Today, exposures are often smaller and mixed. Understanding mechanisms could be more important in determining appropriate intervention strategies. The health conditions of interest today are multicausal; to investigate them requires a wide array of disciplines. If molecular epidemiology has characteristics of a field or speciality, they are its hybrid interdisciplinary qualities. This new specialty requires attention to new organizational and educational structures and adherence to principles and practices derived from both its molecular biology and epidemiology roots.

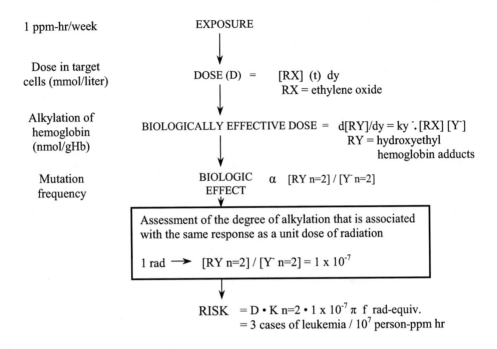

Figure 3.3. Example of Risk Assessment of Workers Exposed to Ethylene Oxide at a Swedish Plant. (Source: Schulte, 1993).

Molecular epidemiology is not a fundamental departure from the past, but an evolutionary step. The goal of molecular epidemiology should be to supplement and integrate, not to replace, existing methods. Molecular epidemiology is also a heuristic term used to describe an enhanced capability of epidemiology to understand disease in terms of the interaction of environment and heredity. Although this practice too has been part of the epidemiologic tradition, it generally has been confined to the specialty area of "genetic epidemiology."

Researchers easily can become arrogant in the face of the potential that molecular epidemiology offers. Believing that merely making molecular measurements leads to enhanced understanding of biologic phenomena is tempting. However, this is not always true and can be misleading, because such a reductionist approach fails to pay attention to the social and cultural characteristics of human populations and to the impact that this type of research has at the population level. Ultimately, research at both the "micro" and the "macro" level is necessary.

B. STRENGTHS AND LIMITATIONS OF OBSERVATIONAL EPIDEMIOLOGY

Epidemiology is the study of the distribution and determinants of health-related states and events in populations and the application of the results of this study to control health problems.

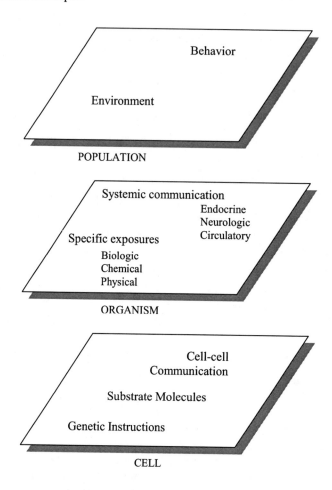

Figure 3.4. Component Levels of Molecular Epidemiologic Research: The Example of Cancer. (Source: Schulte, 1993).

The focus of epidemiology is the group rather than the individual; understanding is gained through inferences drawn from observations within and among groups. Causation is inferred rather than proved. The strengths and weaknesses of epidemiology derive from the field's primary goal: identification and control of the causes of human diseases. The strength of epidemiology is that it does not require extrapolation from other species or laboratory experiments. The weakness of the field stems from ethical constraints imposed on human experimentation and, thus, the requirement to study human disease in its natural state. The epidemiologic study of "free living" humans is more problematic than the study of controlled animals. Factors such as history, geography, social characteristics, and status are exceedingly powerful predictors of the health of human populations. Whereas laboratory animals are usually genetically homogeneous and live in controlled conditions, humans are genetically heterogeneous and live in diverse conditions. In short, because of the subject, all major methods of epidemiology (except for clinical trials) are essentially observational and nonexperimental. Drawing inferences about causation from observational studies is considerably more difficult than drawing them from experiments that use random samples and controls.

Much of epidemiology has been essentially ecologic. Often an individual is assigned the characteristics of a group; categorical descriptors are used to assess risk factors and health status. These descriptors range from dichotomous characterizations (exposed or not; diseased or not) to more quantitative representations of categories (high, medium, or low exposure). Analytic epidemiology uses measurements made on each subject or applies some specific criterion to classify subjects. In many instances, these measurements are surrogates, for example, measures of ambient air exposure for dose or measures of symptoms in lieu of underlying disease. In general, in epidemiology the group is the unit of comparison.

The epidemiologic approach has been highly successful and is the cornerstone of public health. From John Snow's assessment and control of the cholera epidemic in London to the understanding of the role of environmental factors in cancer and cardiovascular disease, epidemiology has contributed to finding causes and remedies. Despite these contributions, epidemiology has been limited by its fundamental conceptual and technical characteristics. Ecologic characterization of variables has hindered the epidemiologic approach in addressing the interdependence of multiple agents and variations in susceptibility that lead to disease. Epidemiology is also limited in its ability to classify individuals into exposure categories (misclassification), to identify mechanisms of action, and to detect disease at a time in its natural history when intervention in the study population or in other preclinical populations would be most effective.

Emerging abilities to assess exposure and disease at the cellular and molecular levels are promising supplements to traditional epidemiology. Instead of characterizing groups solely by geographic location, job title, or questionnaire-derived history, it is possible to measure dose by collecting biologic specimens and assessing xenobiotic interactions with biologic sites and molecules. At the other end of the spectrum, instead of making comparisons of cases of frank disease with controls, it will be possible to make assessments based on preclinical events such as abnormal DNA content or oncogene alteration, once these end points are established as predictive of clinical disease. Additionally, molecular methods make it possible to distinguish subtypes of clinical disease that have potentially different etiologies.

A long-observed weakness of epidemiology is its limited ability to address host factors that contribute to variable responses. Why similarly exposed people do not all acquire the same disease is a difficult question. Certainly, gross categories of host factors, such as age, race, and sex, are controlled routinely in epidemiologic studies. However, genetic factors generally have been considered to a lesser extent than environmental factors. Evaluation of gene-environment interactions has been minimal. "In the past epidemiologists tended to favor a 'black box' approach to their work: they have measured inputs from external agents and from susceptibility factors and disease outcomes; but they have not been concerned with explaining how the two come to be related".

Molecular epidemiology is not just a term that describes adding new techniques to epidemiology. Rather, it represents an opportunity to use new resolving powers to develop theories of disease causation that acknowledge complex interactions involved in the health-disease process. Considering disease at the molecular level without confronting the other events, such as genetic differences and competing biochemical processes, that occur at the molecular level is not sufficient. The question addressed in this volume is how to integrate these molecular biologic capabilities-measurements made in individuals-into a science that uses comparisons of groups to find causes of disease and opportunities for health protection.

C. USE OF BIOLOGICAL MARKERS IN EPIDEMIOLOGIC RESEARCH

1. Events in the Continuum between Exposure and Disease

A functional definition of molecular epidemiology is the use of biologic markers or biologic measurements in epidemiologic research. Biologic markers (or biomarkers) generally include biochemical, molecular, genetic, immunologic, or physiologic signals of events in biologic systems. The events represented can be depicted as parts of a continuum between a causal initiating event (sometimes an exposure to a xenobiotic substance) and resultant disease. By definition, a continuum is a whole, no part of which can be distinguished from neighboring parts except by arbitrary divisions.

The proposed continuum between exposure and disease is shown in Figure 3.5. Between **exposure (E)** in the environment and the development of **clinical disease (CD)**, four generic component classes of biologic markers have been identified: the **internal dose (ID)**, the **biologically effective dose (BED)**, **early biologic effects (EBE)**, and **altered structure and function (ASF)**. Clinical disease can be represented not only by biologic markers for the current disease but also by markers for **prognostic significance (PS)**. Each marker represents an event in the continuum. The relationships among the markers are influenced by various factors (such as genetic or other host characteristics) that reflect susceptibility to any of the events in the continuum. These indicators for susceptibility also can be represented by markers.

Definition of all the marker events has been elaborated elsewhere but is summarized briefly here. The continuum between cigarette smoking and lung cancer serves as illustration. **ID** is the amount of a xenobiotic substance or its metabolites found in a biologic medium (e.g., serum cotinine as an indicator of nicotine). The **BED** is the amount of that xenobiotic material that interacts with critical sub-cellular, cellular, and tissue targets, or with an established surrogate tissue (e.g., DNA adducts in peripheral lymphocytes). The **BED** represents the integration of exposure and effect modification by the host. A marker **EBE** (e.g., sister chromatid exchange) represents an event correlated with, and possibly predictive of, health impairment. Altered structure or function (e.g., abnormal sputum cytology) and DNA hyperploidy are precursor biologic changes that are more closely related to the development of disease. Markers of **CD** (e.g., tumor-associated antigen) and of **PS** (e.g., tumor markers such as CA-125) show the presence or future development of disease, respectively. Markers of susceptibility are indicators of increased (or decreased) risk for any component in the continuum [e.g., extensive debrisoquine metabolizers are at 4-to 6-fold increased risk for lung cancer.

2. Interdisciplinary Nature of Molecular Epidemiology

Molecular epidemiologic studies require interdisciplinary collaboration between population and field scientists (such as epidemiologists, statisticians, industrial hygienists, exposure assessors, and clinicians) and laboratory scientists from disciplines such as molecular biology, genetics, immunology, biochemistry, pathology, and clinical and analytical chemistry. Interdisciplinary collaboration is not new to epidemiology, but the level and extent of diversity of disciplines that molecular epidemiology will require is unprecedented.

Collaboration requires attention to the underlying assumptions, paradigms, and languages of various disciplines as well as to issues of the institutional context of research. Every discipline uses assumptions and paradigms to approach a research question. Often these conventions are so fundamental and integrated that investigators may not be conscious of them and, hence, rarely recognize them or make them explicit when interacting with members of other disciplines. Problems in collaborative research can occur when these fundamentals are not shared. Epidemiologists generally speak in terms of groups and risks to groups. Laboratory scientists tend to focus on individuals or components of an individual. Different disciplines may use common terms in very different ways. Words such as "sensitivity," "small," "valid," "normal," "bias," and "epidemiology" may have different meanings in various disciplines. Too often, the differences may be subtle, for example, understanding of the term "sensitivity." To the laboratory scientist, it refers to the extent to which an assay is capable of detecting a particular marker at some concentration. To an epidemiologist, the same word means the extent to which people with a marker respond positively on a test.

Critical in these types of studies are the need for specialists in study design and for subject selection, exposure assessment, and marker assay development to be integrated in all aspects of the work. The amount of data generated is generally much greater than in a classic epidemiologic study because, in addition to questionnaires and recorded data common to both, data are accumulated from biologic specimen analysis. For example, a study of 30 mortuary science students that assessed cytogenetic effects and DNA repair caused by formaldehyde exposure required 1800 slides and generated more than 3600 data points. Some of these data came from questionnaires and some from biologic measurements.

Molecular epidemiology also requires paying attention to the collection, handling, and storage of biologic specimens. Specimens must be stored to be usable for analyses not yet developed in addition to currently known analyses. The actual collection of biologic specimens also may require attention to timing, so specimens are collected when the influence of factors such as therapeutic treatments will be minimal. For example, a study of the role of oncogenes and colon cancer will be more informative if specimens are collected before DNA-altering chemotherapy or radiation is administered. Other new issues also arise, such as how to address the difficulty of obtaining biologic specimens from controls. For example, in a case-control study of colon cancer, how can usable colon specimens be obtained from controls?

Use of markers of susceptibility also may have a great impact on the organization and conduct of molecular epidemiologic research. Biologic monitoring data derived from molecular epidemiologic studies are likely to be sought by a diversity of societal groups ranging from insurers and employers to potential mates. The possibility that individual markers can predict future characteristics and outcomes makes them a target of interest. The use of susceptibility markers will be required increasingly in molecular epidemiological studies that assess exposure or effects at the DNA level, since effect modification or confounding caused by inherited or other non-study factors can influence associations under study. The analysis of biologic marker data may create new obligations for researchers that were not present in traditional epidemiology. What is the responsibility for follow-up of "abnormal" results, how will individuals with these results be treated, and what will be done if other pathologic conditions are observed?

The use of biologic markers of effect that permit focus on and detection of pre-clinical and extremely early disease also raises questions about the true preventability and treatability of these conditions. At present, insufficient information is available to determine whether particular levels of a certain biologic marker reflect normal ranges of that marker in a person over time or whether they reflect early stages of a preventable disease. Researchers currently face this challenge.

Finally, from an organizational viewpoint, epidemiologists may potentially be polarized into two worlds: one of molecular epidemiologists who emphasize the molecular and genetic causes of disease and the other of social epidemiologists who stress the role of social, psychological, and economic factors in health. Neither approach alone will satisfactorily address the health issues of the current era. History has shown that complete reliance on reductionist approaches is antithetical to public health, yet failure to use the powerful tools available also will not safeguard public health. A synthesis of the two approaches is needed that can address the entire scope of health issues.

3. Design Considerations in Molecular Epidemiology

a. Introduction

Molecular epidemiology does not differ in purpose from epidemiology in general, that is, the study of the distribution and determinants of health-related states and events in populations, and the application of this study to the control of health problems. Further, molecular epidemiologic studies generally are based on classic epidemiologic designs. What makes molecular epidemiology distinctive is its ability to look inside the "black box" of the exposure-disease continuum. In the process, it may reduce misclassification of exposure, provide insight into underlying mechanisms, identify gene-gene and gene-environment interactions, and provide information when intervention is potentially more effective.

b. Biomarker Categories

Designing studies that incorporate biomarkers requires understanding where along the continuum of exposure to disease a biomarker is located. To determine this location and to develop more effective communication about biomarkers in general, it has been necessary to develop a new vocabulary. The continuum between exposure and disease is presented in Figure 3.5.

One way to conceptualize marker categories is to consider exposure (E), internal dose (ID), or biologically effective dose (BED) in one category as markers of exposure and altered structure and function (ASF), clinical disease (CD), and prognostic significance (PS) as markers of effect. Early biologic effects (EBE) are ambiguous markers used prior to study and may be regarded as markers of exposure or markers of effect.

Generally, a study may test if an exposure (E) is related to a marker (M):

$E \longrightarrow M_E$ (e.g., paths 1, 7, 8, 9)

If a marker (M) is related to a disease (D):

$M_D \longrightarrow D$ (e.g., paths 20,21)

Or if exposures and their markers are related to diseases and their markers:

$E \text{ or } M_E \longrightarrow M_D \text{ or } D$ (e.g., 9, 10, 16, 17)

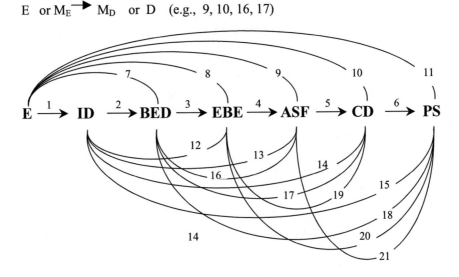

Figure 3.5. A Continuum of Markers between Exposure and Disease. [**E**, Exposure; **ID**, internal dose; **BED**, biologically effective dose; **EBE**, early biological effects; **ASF**, altered structure and function; **CD**, clinical disease; **PS**, prognostic significance. Numbers refer to studies presented in Table 3.5.]. (Source: Schulte, 1993).

These models are however, admittedly simplistic because they imply a single necessary and sufficient antecedent cause and subsequent effect, and a single mechanistic pathway. In most instances, particularly in chronic diseases, causation is multiple and potentially interactive. Despite its limitations, the continuum of exogenous exposure and resultant disease is a useful way to conceptualize molecular epidemiologic investigations.

Table 3.5. Potential Studies of Biological Marker Relationship[a] in the Continuum between an Exposure and Disease. (Source: Schulte, 1993).

Relationship to be studied[b]			Capability
1. E	↔	ID	Validation of exposure marker
2. ID	↔	BED	Assessment of dose
3. BED	↔	EBE	Association of dose and effect
4. EBE	↔	ASF	Determination of pathogenicity of an effect
5. ASF	↔	CD	Validation of pre-clinical marker
6. CD	↔	PS	Validation of prognostic marker
7. E	↔	BED	Validation of exposure marker
8. E	↔	EBE	Association of exposure with an effect marker
9. E	↔	ASF	Association of exposure with a pathogenic effect
10. E	↔	CD	Association of exposure with disease
11. E	↔	PS	Association of exposure with severity of disease
12. ID	↔	EBE	Association of dose and effect
13. ID	↔	ASF	Association of dose and pre-clinical effect
14. ID	↔	CD	Association of dose and disease
15. ID	↔	PS	Association of dose and severity of disease
16. BED	↔	ASF	Best indicator of association of dose and pre-clinical effect
17. BED	↔	CD	Association of dose and disease; indicator of risk
18. BED	↔	PS	Association of dose with severity of disease
19. EBE	↔	CD	Validation of marker of effect regarding disease
20. EBE	↔	PS	Validation of marker of effect of severity of disease
21. ASF	↔	PS	Validation of pre-clinical marker with severity of disease
22.			Repeat of studies 1-21 with marker of susceptibility as effect modifier

[a] The causal relationship between any two markers is generally from left to right, but the bi-directional arrow indicates that the relationship can be studied prospectively or retrospectively. Numbers correspond to paths in Figure 3.5.
[b] E, Exposure; ID, internal dose; BED, biologically effective dose; EBE, early biological effect ; ASF, altered structure/function; CD, clinical disease; PS, prognostic significance.

c. Using Biomarkers in Epidemiologic Research

Biomarkers may be used to enhance the assessment of the standard types of risk factors evaluated in epidemiologic investigations, for example, exogenous exposure, demographics, and genetic susceptibility. In addition, biomarkers may be used to evaluate disease status by defining more homogeneous case groups.

However, a series of new relationships can be evaluated when studying a series of biomarkers that represent the continuum of exposure to disease, that is, the associations between all that precedes a marker in the continuum and all that follows it (Table 3.5). Exploring these associations may provide a better description of disease progression and its determinants, and ultimately may result in improved primary, secondary, and tertiary prevention strategies and application. However, the ultimate significance of biomarkers that represent any point in the continuum up to disease itself can be assessed only by determining the association of these markers with disease.

VI. CASE STUDIES

A. FLUORIDE IN DRINKING WATER AND DENTAL CARIES

One of the earliest case-control studies was the determination of an association between fluoride in drinking water and the condition of the teeth of those who consumed the water. This occurred after observing reports of mottled enamel on the teeth of people who drank water from certain sources. The U.S. Public Health Service in the late 1920s began a series of epidemiologic studies to try to identify the cause of the problem.

Investigators discovered a noted difference depending on which spring served as the source of drinking water. Analyses of the water in the various springs showed a marked difference in fluoride concentration. Studies showed that children who lived in areas where mottled teeth were endemic had less tooth decay than those who lived where mottled teeth were nonexistent.

B. CIGARETTES AND LUNG CANCER

The determination of the definitive association between cigarette smoking and lung cancer is a classic example of the useful application of environmental epidemiology.

It is also an example of how the personal choices of individuals can have an extremely detrimental effect on their health and the difficulty in implementing effective control measures, even when a relationship has been thoroughly demonstrated.

In the middle to late 1940s, physicians in several of the industrialized countries of the world, including the United States and the United Kingdom, noted an increasing number of diagnoses of men with lung cancer. A decade earlier such cancer had been a medical curiosity. Although cigarette smoking was immediately suspected as a cause, obviously the presumption had to be confirmed. Two types of studies were undertaken, case-control studies in which persons with and without lung cancer were asked about past habits, including smoking, and cohort studies in which smokers and nonsmokers were followed and the rates of development of a variety of diseases, including lung cancer, were measured.

One of the leading epidemiologists who conducted such studies was Richard Doll, working first with A. Bradford Hill and later with Richard Feto. On the basis of an initial case-control study, Doll and Hill in 1930 concluded that "smoking" is a factor, and an important factor, in the production of carcinoma of the lung." They admitted, however, that they had no evidence about the nature of the carcinogen. As a result of a subsequent series of longer-term cohort studies, Doll and Peto in 1976 concluded that the death rate from lung cancer in smokers was ten tines the rate in nonsmokers.

This and related research by other investigators led to an increasing awareness of a definite association between cigarette smoking and lung cancer and the conclusion by public health officials, that cigarette smoking was a cause of lung cancer. In 1964, as a result of such concerns, the Surgeon General issued a report on Smoking and Health and antismoking campaigns were developed, including the banning in this country of cigarette commercials on television.

One of the principal actions that caused a noticeable reduction in cigarette smoking in the US was publication of epidemiologic study results that showed that nonsmokers were affected by secondhand smoke.

C. Ionizing Radiation And Cancer

After the discovery of X-rays in 1895, reports of radiation injuries including the subsequent development of cancers began to appear in published literature. It was soon recognized that ionizing radiation had harmful health effects and that standards were needed for the control of related exposures. The evidence was followed several decades later by the observation of the development of bone sarcoma in a number of young women who ingested radium while painting watch dials.

Shortly after detonation of the 2 atomic bombs in Japan near the end of WWII, researchers saw that these events though tragic, offered an opportunity to quantify the relationship between exposures to ionizing radiation and health effects. The dominant effects of ionizing radiation among the Japanese survivors were solid tumors - cancers of lungs, breast, thyroid, etc.

D. Electric And Magnetic Fields And Leukemia

A case-control study of leukemia was conducted among children living in the Denver area. The investigators concluded that the relative cancer risk for children living near high-current power lines is double that for children living elsewhere. But, based on measurements of the magnetic fields no statistically significant correlation was found between exposures and childhood cancer.

Subsequent reviews of several of the studies of the health effects of electric and magnetic fields revealed a number of methodological deficiencies. In nearly all instances, no quantitative assessment of power-frequency field exposures was made, that is, most of the estimates of exposure were based on surrogate measures. In many studies, the sample populations were small, thus the observed increases in cancer could have been due either to chance or to some unidentified factor.

VII. BIBLIOGRAPHY

Buffler, P.A. (1995). Uses of Epidemiology in Environmental Medicine. In Brooks, S.M., Gochfeld, M., Herzstein, J., Jackson, R.J. & Schenker, M.B. (Eds). Environmental Medicine (pp.46-62). St. Louis, MO: Mosby

Doll, R., & A. Bradford H. (1930, September 30). Smoking and Carcinoma of the Lung— Preliminary Report. British Medical Journal 2, 739-748.

Doll R., & Peto R. (1981) The Causes of Cancer. New York: Oxford University Press.

Doll, R., & Richard P. (1976, December 25). Mortality in Relation to Smoking: 20 Years' Observations on Male British Doctors. British Medical Journal 2, 1525-36.

English, O. (1992). Geographical Epidemiology and Ecological Studies. In Elliott, P., Guzick, J., English, D., Stern, R. (Eds). Geographical and Environmental Epidemiology: Methods for Small-Area Studies (pp. 3-13). New York, NY: Oxford University Press.

Fraumeni, I.F. Jr, Hoover R.N. (1985, March 14). Current Views of Epidemiological Methods. Federal Register, 58-64.

Goldsmith, J.R. (1986). Environmental Epidemiology: Epidemiological Investigation of Community Health Problems. Boca Raton, FL: CRC Press.

Griffith, J. & Aldrich, T.E. (1993). Epidemiology: The Environmental Influence. In Aldrich, T.E., Griffith, J. & Cooke, C. (Eds). Environmental Epidemiology and Risk Assessment (pp.13-26).

Hill, A.B. (1965). The Environment and Disease: Association or Causation? Proceedings of the Royal Society of Medicine 3, 259-300.

Last, J.M. (1998). Public Health and Human Ecology 2nd Edition (pp. 153-203). Stamford, CT: Appleton and Lange.

McLaughlin, J.K. & Brookmeyer, R. (1994). Epidemiology and Biostatistics. In McCunney, R.J. A Practical Approach to Occupational and Environmental Medicine, 2nd Edition (pp.346-357). Boston, MA: Little Brown and Company.

Moeller, D.W. (1997). Environmental Health (pp. 33-51). Cambridge, MA: Harvard University Press.

Monson, R. (1990). Occupational Epidemiology 2nd Edition. Boca Raton, FL.: CRC Press.

NRC. (1991). Environmental Epidemiology—Public Health and Hazardous Wastes. National Research Council. Washington, D.C.: National Academy Press.

Osorio, A.M. (1999). Principles of Occupational and Environmental Epidemiology. In Bowler, R.M & Cone, J.E. (Eds), Occupational Medicine Secrets (pp. 1-6). Philadelphia, PA: Hanley & Belfus, INC.

Piantadosi, S. (1992). Epidemiology and Principles of Surveillance Regarding Toxic Hazards in the Environment. In Sullivan, J.B. & Krieger, G.R. (Eds). Hazardous Materials Toxicology Clinical Principles of Environmental Health (pp. 61-64). Baltimore, MD: Williams & Wilkins.

Ruttenber, A.J. (1995). Environmental Epidemiology: Assessing Health Risks from Toxic Agents in the Environment. In Blumenthal, D.S. & Ruttenber, J. (Eds). Introduction to Environmental Health (pp. 321-362). New York, NY: Springer Publishing Company.

Schulte, P.A. (1993). A Conceptual and Historical Framework for Molecular Epidemiology. In Molecular Epidemiology: Principles and Practices (pp. 3-36). Academic Press, Inc.

Snow, J. (1965). On the Mode of Communication of Cholera 2nd Edition. Churchill, London. Reproduced in Snow on Cholera. Commonwealth Fund, New York, 1936. Reprinted by Hafner, New York.

Surgeon General. (1989, March 24). Executive Summary, The Surgeon General's 1989 Report on Reducing the Health Consequences of Smoking: 25 Years of Progress. Morbidity and Mortality Weekly Report 38, No. 5-2, 8.

Terracini, B. (1992). Environmental Epidemiology: A Historical Perspective.

Trichopoulos, D. (1994, August). Risk of Lung Cancer from Passive Smoking. Principles and Practice of Oncology: PPO Updates 8, No. 8, 1-8.

Tyler, C.W. & Last J.M. (1998). Epidemiology. In Wallace, R.B. (Ed). Maxcy-Rosenau-Last Public Health & Preventive Medicine (pp. 5-33). Stamford, CT: Appleton & Lange.

USPHS. (1964). Smoking and Health: Report. Surgeon General's Advisory Committee on Smoking and Health, Publication No. 1103, Washington, D.C.: U.S. Public Health Service.

Wertheimc N., & Leeper, E. (1979). Electrical Wiring Configurations and Childhood Cancer. American Journal of Epidemiology 109, 273-284.

WHO. (1991). Investigating Environmental Disease Outbreaks: A Training Manual. WHO Document WHO/PEP/91.35. Geneva: WHO.

WHO. (1983). Guidelines on Studies in Environmental Epidemiology. Environmental Criteria 27.

Yassi, A., Kjellstrom, T., Kok, T.D., & Guidotti, T.L. (2001). Basic Environmental Health (pp. 107-113). New York, NY: Oxford University Press.

CHAPTER

4

DISEASE

I. <u>INTRODUCTION</u>

A disease is any pathologic process having a characteristic set of signs and symptoms which are detrimental to the well-being of the individual and are the consequence of external factors, including exposure to physical or chemical agents, poor nutrition, and social or cultural behaviors.

Polluted air and water, excessive levels of noise, sunshine, nuclear weapons fall-out, overcrowded slums, toxic waste dumps, inadequate or overly adequate diet, stress, food contaminants, medical x-rays, drugs, cigarettes, unsafe working conditions - these comprise but a partial listing of the many environmental factors which, through their adverse impact on human health, can be regarded as causative agents of environmental disease. In recent years public concern about rising levels of pollution and environmental degradation has increasingly focused on the question of whether such trends may be influencing disease rates, particularly ailments such as heart disease, cancer, and stroke. If such a connection exists, as virtually all authorities agree it does, then society's response should be clear that most environmentally induced diseases, unlike those caused by bacteria or other pathogens, are difficult to cure but theoretically simple to prevent - remove the adverse environmental influence and the ailment will disappear. In other words, by preventing the discharge of poisons into our air, water, and food, by avoiding exposure to radiation, by refusing to fill our lungs with cigarette smoke or our stomachs with synthetic food colorings, we can protect our health far more effectively and cheaply than we can by desperately searching for an often nonexistent cure after our bodies succumb to a malignancy or degeneration of vital organs or when our children are born deformed.

II. <u>ENVIRONMENTAL DISEASE</u>

Environmental health threats are mostly the traditional problems long since solved in the developed countries, such as a lack of potable water, sanitation, adequate housing and protection from mosquitoes and other insect and animal disease vectors. The occurrence of diseases induced by environmental health threats varies geographically and with the economic status of each country. In the developed countries, pollution control, changes in technology, and environmental laws and regulations have substantially reduced human exposures to toxic agents over the past 30 years. On the other hand, new environmental problems have emerged as urban areas continue to expand. Transboundary air quality in many regions of the United States and Europe continues to deteriorate from the combined impact of increasing automobile traffic in contiguous urban areas. Furthermore, there is good evidence that air pollution levels in many North American and European cities, although within regulatory limits, will increase the risk for death from cardiovascular and chronic pulmonary diseases.

Many developed countries are experiencing problems with fresh water availability that stem from high rates of consumption without regard for the capacity of regional hydrologic cycles to maintain these rates. Fossil fuel use and generation of ozone-depleting gases in developed countries have contributed to the climate change, the greenhouse effect and stratospheric ozone depletion to a degree far in excess of the per capita average for the planet. Reduced availability of fresh water, the greenhouse effect, and ozone depletion each have important indirect effects on public health.

Common environmental diseases in the developed world are lung cancer from radon and its decay products, skin cancer from solar radiation, unintentional injuries from automobiles, intentional injuries from weapons, and allergic reactions to natural and synthetic compounds. Since the 1980s, large outbreaks of gastrointestinal illness from poorly treated drinking water have begun to occur more frequently in developed countries - due in part to the scarcity of clean drinking water sources for large populations and increased dependence on complex treatment strategies for water of marginal quality.

In the Third World many environmentally based diseases - both **infectious** and **noninfectious** - are endemic. Although diseases from environmental chemicals account for only a small portion of total morbidity and mortality in these countries, exposures to toxic agents are far higher than in Europe, North America, and in most areas of the former Soviet Union. Furthermore, urban centers in Third World countries are now experiencing the same health risks from air and water pollution as cities in heavily industrialized nations. Recently, Third World governmental agencies have expressed more interest in reducing the health risks from industrial and agricultural chemicals, and scientists from other nations are beginning to assist in such efforts. Without opportunities for economic improvement, however, long-term success will not be realized. Countries that are emerging from Third World status (Taiwan, for example) have environmental problems common to both industrialized and Third World countries. Circumstances are similar for the East European and the other former Communist Bloc nations. These countries have air pollution levels that are among the highest in the world because the push for rapid economic growth has outpaced the use of appropriate pollution control technology and environmental planning. There are similar problems with surface and ground water pollution. To some extent rapidly developing countries have conquered the Third World problems of sewage disposal and fresh water distribution and their environmental diseases now have longer latent periods than those for infectious diseases.

The People's Republic of China has one of the world's largest gross national products and is one of the largest generators of the greenhouse gas but, because it also has the world's largest population, its per capita gross national product is similar to small Third World countries. Because of extensive foreign investment in China, the level of industrial development and standard of living is rapidly expanding. As a result, air pollution from industry and coal burning (not automobiles) is the greatest environmental health problem.

Workers and the general public in all countries, regardless of their levels of development, are at risk for diseases caused by industrial accidents. The health effects from such accidents can vary widely, as evidenced by the explosions at chemical plants in Bhopal, India and by the Chernobyl nuclear reactor accident in Ukraine.

Just as the risks from environmental exposures are strongly correlated with the development status of countries, they also are related to the socio-economic status of individuals and communities. The poor are almost always afforded less protection from environmental risks than the rich, whether the risks are from factories, hazardous waste sites, urban atmospheres, contaminated drinking water, or indoor environments. This is true in cities, suburbs, and rural areas as well as in the workplace, regardless of the development status of a country. Minority races and ethnic groups that have been discriminated against economically are also at increased risk for the toxic effects of environmental exposures. Just as Third World countries find it difficult to devote scarce resources to environmental health, under most economic systems the poor and minorities are also faced with prioritizing their resources. Food, housing, and the health of children are deemed more important than protection from the more abstract risks posed by environmental agents.

Although some would argue that minority groups are not consciously placed at risk from environmental hazards, there is evidence that this has happened. Exposure to such risk is highest in communities with the least political power, and this lack of power is associated with either lower economic status or minority racial status, or both. Many feel that change will depend on a greatly heightened awareness of this issue. Recently in the United States, groups have begun to organize around the issue of environmental racism and make demands for environmental justice. It may be just as difficult to improve the environmental quality and reduce risks from environmental agents for the poor without first improving their opportunities for economic equity as it will be for Third World countries to focus on environmental health without first improving economically. On the other hand, substantial improvements in the environments of humans could be made in tandem with efforts to correct economic and racial inequities. We believe that all too often scientists working in the field of environmental health become mesmerized by the technical issues of environmental problems and lose sight of the important social aspects.

III. PATHOPHYSIOLOGY OF ENVIRONMENTAL DISEASE

The effects of toxic agents in the environment include known diseases as well as biologic effects that are not associated with recognized diseases or that may represent the early changes that precede disease. Such effects may be acute or chronic. Acute effects quickly follow exposure to precipitating agents; the pathology of these diseases commonly involves sudden changes in structure or function, which are usually transient but may be irreversible. Often, these changes are readily apparent and the responsible agents are easily identified.

Chronic effects last for long time periods, are often caused by multiple exposures, and may be irreversible. They also may follow a latent period between exposure and the first appearance of disease. For this reason, it may be difficult to identify the agents responsible for chronic toxicity.

Toxic effects can have both **acute** and **chronic** phases. For instance, gastrointestinal and neurologic disturbances occur early in the course of mercury vapor poisoning and may be followed by chronic, irreversible pulmonary fibrosis.

A. HEMATOPOIETIC AND IMMUNE SYSTEMS

Toxic agents in the bloodstream can damage developing and mature blood cells and induce illness by activating the immune system. Benzene interferes with the production of red and white blood cells and causes **aplastic anemia**, a disease of the bone marrow that can be irreversible. A high dose of ionizing radiation also causes transient depression of blood cell production and raises the risk for severe infections and hemorrhage. In mature red blood cells, lead inhibits enzymes and alters cell metabolism, thereby impairing heme synthesis and shortening red blood cell lifespan. Both effects contribute to anemia in victims of lead poisoning.

The immune system effectively eliminates molecules that are toxic to the host and destroys tumor cells. It comprises the bone marrow and thymus, where lymphocytes are produced and differentiate, and the lymph nodes, spleen, and lymphoid tissue of the mucosa, where lymphocytes concentrate. Damage to the immune system from toxic agents can result in **immunopotentiation**, characterized by allergic and hypersensitivity reactions, **immunosuppression**, which results in increased susceptibility to infection and cancer, or **autoimmunity**, the stimulation of an immune response to tissue of the host precipitated by **xenobiotic** agents (biologically active molecules that originate from outside the body).

There are two major types of immune response: **cell-mediated**, which involves sensitized T-lymphocytes, and **humoral**, which is implemented by antibodies in the cell-free portions of the blood. Xenobiotic agents commonly stimulate allergic reactions, which can be grouped into six categories, these involve antigen-antibody responses that induce production of immunoglobulin E (IgE) and the release of histamine and other compounds which produce vasodilation, urticaria, and edema. Such responses usually occur in the organs where antigens from the environment are introduced: the gastrointestinal tract for antigens in food, the circulatory system for those that reach the bloodstream, and the respiratory system for inhaled antigens. **Asthma**, **seasonal rhinitis**, and **atopic dermatitis** (eczema) are examples of immediate hypersensitivity reactions to environmental substances. Asthma is induced by bioaerosols in the environment and by many different industrial chemicals such as isocyanates, formaldehyde, metals, and metal salts.

Cytotoxic *(***Type II***)* reactions are antibody-mediated responses that ultimately destroy antigen-carrying bacteria and viruses. Antibodies produced in response to an antigen may also react with cell membrane proteins in the host organism, resulting in damage to tissues such as blood cells, platelets, the glomeruli of the kidneys, and the delicate vasculature of the lung.

Arthus *(***Type III***)* reactions deposit antigen - antibody complex in different tissues, thereby obstructing fluid transport and producing localized tissue damage. Common sites for deposition are blood vessels skin, joints, and renal glomeruli. The acute phase of **Hypersensitivity pneumonitis**, an important environmental and occupational lung disease, involves the deposition of antigen - antibody complexes in the interstitial tissue of the lungs following exposure to a variety of organic and inorganic dusts. Heavy metals such as gold and mercury also elicit Type III responses, resulting in membranous glomerulonephritis.

In **delayed hypersensitivity** *(***Type IV***)* reactions, antigens in the skin elicit responses from T lymphocytes. As in immediate hypersensitivity reactions, delayed hypersensitivity reactions follow a previous exposure - or **sensitization** - to a chemical or a toxin (a complex chemical molecule produced by an organism). Compared with immediate hypersensitivity, the response time for delayed hypersensitivity is longer. An example of delayed hypersensitivity is contact dermatitis - an allergic response to organic chemicals or heavy metals in natural and manufactured substances - as evidenced by the rash and urticaria from poison ivy and by nickel dermatitis.

Type V or **stimulatory hypersensitivity** reactions and **innate hypersensitivity** are additional types of allergic reactions. The former occurs when antibodies react with cell surface receptors and disrupt cell function. In the latter, excessive release of immune system components that are not associated with acquired immune responses can lead to conditions such as the adult respiratory distress syndrome.

Chemicals and biologic agents can induce other acute changes in the immune system, which can be detected as altered ratios of different types of white blood cells. Inflammation - the reaction of vascularized tissue to local damage - involves both the circulatory and immune systems and is caused by a variety of environmental agents including bacteria, viruses, chemical irritants, and both ionizing and non-ionizing radiation. Inflammatory responses can destroy, dilute, or isolate toxic agents and are also involved in hypersensitivity reactions. Acute inflammation is characterized by the build-up of fluid and plasma proteins and a local increase in the concentration of neutrophils, lymphocytes, and macrophages. Acute inflammation can resolve completely, lead to scarring or abscess formation, or progress to chronic inflammation. The features of chronic inflammation include increased concentrations of a variety of different types of white blood cells, proliferation of fibroblasts resulting in fibrosis, and tissue destruction. Exposures to silica and beryllium induce chronic granulomatous inflammation - characterized by clusters of macrophages, fibroblasts, and neutrophils (called **granulomas***)* that are usually surrounded by lymphocytes.

Immunosuppression from exposure to environmental agents is not well understood, and most evidence comes from animal studies. Polychlorinated biphenyls, dibenzodioxins, certain pesticides, and metals have been shown to depress the immune response in animals; similar effects, however, have not been convincingly demonstrated in humans.

Disorders of immunity sometimes present with complex clinical features that may not signal a pathophysiology that is readily traced to the immune system. The toxic oil syndrome - caused by rapeseed oil that was denatured with aniline for industrial use, but was marketed as cooking oil in Spanish villages in 1981 - began with pulmonary signs and symptoms, which were followed by eosinophilia and a gastrointestinal syndrome. Some of the exposed persons then developed myalgia and muscle atrophy, skin thickening reminiscent of scleroderma, pulmonary hypertension, and vasculitis - features more consistent with an immune system disorder than those noted at the onset of disease. The causative agent in the rapeseed oil and the pathophysiology of this disease have yet to be specified. Another progressive, multisystem disease with features of immune system damage is the eosinophilia - myalgia syndrome, which occurred as an epidemic in the United States in 1989. This syndrome followed use of the amino acid food supplement L-tryptophan and presented with flu-like symptoms, myalgias, shortness of breath, pulmonary interstitial infiltrates, fatigue, and skin rash. Some patients later developed scleroderma-like skin thickening and rheumatoid symptoms. Other features included pulmonary hypertension, neuropathy, myocarditis, and cardiac arrhythmias. Many of these signs and symptoms are similar to those of the toxic oil syndrome. The cause of this syndrome has been narrowed to one or more contaminants of L-tryptophan and has been linked to changes in the bioengineering process used to produce L-tryptophan from bacteria.

B. NERVOUS SYSTEM

Neurotoxins cause damage in both central and peripheral neurons. Not all tissues are equally vulnerable. The blood - brain barrier, for instance, restricts access to the brain for polar chemical compounds. It is maintained by tight junctions between the endothelial cells - junctions that are present throughout the nervous system. To enter the brain and other nerve tissue, molecules usually must pass through the membranes of endothelial cells, rather than between them as in other tissues. In children, the tight junctions are poorly developed and they are more susceptible than adults to central nervous system damage from certain chemicals.

The exact location of neuronal damage determines the clinical effects produced by neurotoxins. The physical and chemical properties of neurotoxins help determine where they are distributed, and thus where damage can occur. Neurotoxins compromise sensory, motor, and integrative functions. Loss or distortion of sensation may follow damage to either peripheral or central neurons, as exemplified by peripheral sensory loss in lower extremities following arsenic poisoning and visual field constriction and tremor caused by central nervous system damage from organic mercury.

Damage to motor function is characterized by weakness and paralysis and is produced by exposure to such chemicals as triethyl tin and hexachlorophene. Integrative functions of the central nervous system include coordination of sensation and movement, symbolic reasoning, and emotional responses. Organic solvents, including ethanol, commonly affect the integration of sensory and motor function. Inorganic lead and both the inorganic and organic forms of mercury can affect all the three processes.

Neurotoxins produce both acute and chronic damage, which may be reversible or permanent. Acute irreversible central nervous system disease is caused by destruction of cells in the brain and spinal column following exposure to chemical neurotoxins, or from the bacteria and viruses that cause encephalitis and meningitis. Chronic exposure to high concentrations of manganese and acute exposure to 1,2,4,6-methylphenyl-tetrahydropyridine (MPTP) - a contaminant of an analog of the synthetic narcotic meperidine - have produced irreversible parkinsonism by destroying cells in the substantia nigra in manganese miners and narcotics abusers respectively. It is possible that chronic exposures to many chemicals in the environment are under-recognized as causes of neurologic disease. Cell death does not always lead to irreversible neurologic disease - the remaining healthy cells can alter their function and compensate for neurons that are destroyed or damaged. Neurons can also develop tolerance to the effects of toxic agents. Damage to the central nervous system can also reversibly alter consciousness, as evidenced by the transient intoxication produced by many organic solvents. Recovery from such exposures usually occurs when the exposure stops. A reversible form of parkinsonism following environmental exposures to CO has been observed.

A number of chronic neurologic diseases have been associated with environmental exposures. Aluminum has been hypothesized to cause Alzheimer's disease, but concentrations of this metal in tissue samples could result from but not cause Alzheimer's disease, or be due to aluminum in the chemicals used to stain brain tissue. Multiple sclerosis (a disease with pathology in both central and peripheral neurons) has occurred in clusters that suggest a viral etiology, but little evidence has been developed to support this theory. Poliomyelitis is a well-known acute infection produced by a virus found in sewage-contaminated water. This infection may permanently damage peripheral nerves. Aggressive environmental monitoring for the polio virus has been suggested for Third World countries, where this disease is still a public health problem.

Toxic agents can damage both the heart and blood vessels. Disruption of the coordinated signals in the neuronal conducting system is the most common and dangerous effect produced by toxic agents in the heart. Such damage results in **arrhythmias**, which may lead to **cardiac arrest**. Many different chemicals and drugs - nonhalogenated and halogenated industrial solvents, hydrogen sulfide, directly induce arrhythmias. Gases such as NO can produce the same effect indirectly by displacing oxygen in the lung and producing anoxia in heart tissue.

Cardiac function can also be compromised by agents that induce structural damage to heart muscle *(***cardiomyopathy***)*, which acutely or chronically disrupts the contraction of heart muscle, leading to reduced pumping ability *(***congestive heart failure***)*, as well as to depressed circulation of blood to the entire body *(***shock***)*. Cobalt has been linked to cardiomyopathy in beer drinkers who consumed beer that contained this element as a foam stabilizer.

Hypertensive cardiac disease results from an increase in the rate and strength of cardiac contractility and from the constriction of peripheral vasculature. Chronic exposure to lead has been linked to hypertension in a number of studies. Although cadmium may elevate blood pressure and cause renal damage, it has not been shown to cause hypertension in exposed workers. Some natural constituents of foods such as glycyrrhizin in licorice also induce hypertension.

Exposures to industrial chemicals have also been associated with coronary artery disease, although the mechanisms for such damage are still not clear. For example, workers exposed to carbon disulfide during the production of rayon have been shown to have increased mortality from arteriosclerotic heart disease. Cadmium and CO are chemicals that may damage the endothelium of blood vessels and produce atherosclerosis - deposits of lipids and fibrous tissue that can occlude the vessels and cause anoxic damage to cardiac muscle leading to **myocardial infarction**.

Coronary arteries can be occluded by acute vasospastic constriction caused by chemicals such as nicotine, cocaine, and nitrates. Studies of workers exposed to nitroglycerin, ethylene glycol dinitrate, and other aliphatic nitrates used in the manufacture of explosives and pharmaceuticals have identified increased risks for coronary vasospasm, myocardial infarction, angina, and arrhythmias on the withdrawal of exposure to these vasoactive compounds. Chronic exposure to arsenic-contaminated well water has been linked to atherosclerosis and peripheral vascular disease (blackfoot disease) in Taiwan.

Chemicals and ionizing radiation produce hemorrhage at sites throughout the body by damaging the lining of blood vessels or by disrupting the complex biochemical system responsible for blood clotting. The yellow fever virus produces gastrointestinal hemorrhage by damaging blood vessels that supply the mucosa. Hypersensitivity reactions can acutely damage the smooth muscle lining of blood vessels and produce hemorrhage. Toxic agents also disrupt the vascular membranes that maintain the blood-brain barrier and thereby enter the brain.

C. DIGESTIVE SYSTEM

Environmental exposures to viruses, bacteria, and parasites commonly cause acute damage to the digestive system. These infections usually inflame the mucosa and result in localized fluid loss. Vomiting and failure to replace fluid by oral intake may lead to generalized fluid loss, dehydration, and, if not treated, cardiac arrest. Infants and children in Third World countries frequently die as a result of this series of events. Gastrointestinal parasites compete with their human hosts for nutrients, induce chronic inflammation and diarrhea, and may physically obstruct the intestinal tract.

The liver is an important site for metabolizing chemicals and may produce metabolites that are more toxic than their parent compounds. Acute and chronic **hepatitis** may follow exposure to many organic chemicals, including carbon tetrachloride, **aflatoxins** (organic toxins produced by a species of the fungus **Aspergilus flavus** that contaminates grains and nuts), and viruses. Hepatitis A is caused by exposure to feces-contaminated water, shellfish, and other contaminated food. Hepatitis B, Hepatitis C, and non-A, non-B Hepatitis are primarily transmitted by blood and body secretions, though several epidemics of non-A, non-B Hepatitis have been linked to contaminated water.

In the early stages of disease, the liver accumulates lipids. Such **fatty change** follows excessive exposure to many different chemicals, including ethanol and carbon tetrachloride. Liver necrosis may follow. Chronic exposure to toxic agents can lead to **cirrhosis** - a serious stage of liver damage, characterized by disrupted liver architecture and proliferating fibrous tissue. Cirrhosis can follow exposures to both chemical and biologic agents. Chemicals can also acutely damage the liver by altering or obstructing blood flow and producing hemorrhage and necrosis. Some drugs cause bile to accumulate in the liver, which can damage hepatocytes.

D. RESPIRATORY SYSTEM

The chemical, physical, and biological properties of toxic agents, such as pH, solubility, reactivity, fibrogenicity, and immunogenicity determine the extent to which they damage the respiratory system. The physiologic status of the respiratory system and unique metabolic conditions also modify toxicity. Substances in air, particularly in enclosed spaces, may produce acute damage by: (1) **asphyxiation** (the displacement of oxygen by other gases, resulting in death by a combination of cardiac and respiratory processes); (2) alteration of respiratory enzyme function; (3) irritation or necrosis of lung tissue; (4) constriction or obstruction of airways; (5) production of **pulmonary edema** (accumulation of fluid in the airways); (6) hemorrhage or inflammation of vascular tissue; and (7) allergic responses.

Pneumonia is another example of an acute disease that can follow exposure to bacteria, viruses, parasites, or aspirated chemicals such as petroleum products. It is characterized by inflammation and fluid secretion in the small airways and, in severe cases, cardio-respiratory failure that may be fatal.

Damage in the upper airways produces throat inflammation, dry cough, and hoarseness. In the middle airways, irritant and reactive chemicals cause inflammation, constriction of bronchi and bronchioles, bronchospasm, and asthma-like responses by a non-allergic mechanism. **Asthma** is an allergic response to chemicals and toxins that involves antibody production, airway constriction, and mucous plugging of bronchioles.

In the lower airways, toxic agents produce pulmonary edema, bronchiolar obstruction, and fibrosis. **Emphysema**, a disease most commonly caused by cigarette smoking, has also been associated with air pollution. Its pathogenesis involves the disruption of the network of elastic fibers surrounding the alveoli, producing extensive enlargement of lower airways.

Diffuse alveolar damage with edema and hemorrhage is produced by toxic agents in the epithelium of the lower airways. Alveolar damage can be caused by reactive chemicals such as oxygen in high concentrations, ammonia, and cadmium and by bacteria, viruses, and ionizing radiation. This disorder can be acute or chronic, depending on the intensity and duration of exposure. In chronic alveolar damage, the respiratory epithelium and adjoining tissue are replaced by fibrous tissue. Acute pulmonary edema produced by chemicals such as mercury vapor, chlorine, or phosgene can be fatal.

Hypersensitivity pneumonitis is a group of diseases induced by organic toxins and some reactive chemicals. This term encompasses the true allergic responses as well as pathologic effects not associated with antibody production. Farmer's lung disease is the classic form of hypersensitivity pneumonitis. Acute hypersensitivity pneumonitis usually resolves, but can be fatal. Prolonged responses can result in chronic disease as well as damage that are less severe and not clinically evident.

Pneumoconiosis comprises a group of chronic pulmonary diseases caused by inhaled inorganic dusts. The term has also been used to describe chronic pulmonary disease associated with other agents. The damage is produced by particles less than 5 μm in diameter that deposit in the terminal bronchioles and alveoli. The pathology of these diseases is characterized by local or diffuse fibrosis; their severity depends on the intensity and duration of exposure. Common environmental pneumoconioses are asbestosis and silicosis.

E. EXCRETORY SYSTEM

The kidneys excrete metabolic wastes and exogenous chemicals, regulate the concentrations of salt in body fluids, and help control blood pressure. The pathophysiology of toxic exposure to the kidney is best understood by regarding the organ as a collection of **nephrons**. Each nephron comprises three important structures: (1) the glomerulus, which serves as a blood filtration unit; (2) the arterioles that carry blood to and from the glomerulus; and (3) the collecting tubule, which receives the material filtered from the glomerulus, exchanges chemical compounds, ions, and water with surrounding renal tissue, and collects the liquid wastes that are released as urine through the ureters and bladder.

The kidneys are perfused by the circulatory system and are vulnerable to blood-borne chemical and infectious agents. The capillary walls of the glomerulus can be damaged by many different chemicals, resulting in reduced filtration and release of proteins and other large molecules to the urine. Heavy metals and organic chemicals usually damage the collecting tubules near the glomerulus by inducing vasoconstriction.

Some chemicals selectively damage the epithelium of the collecting tubules, causing toxic nephropathy. These chemicals include carbon tetrachloride, ethylene glycol (antifreeze), mercuric chloride, and phosphorus. Toxic nephropathy may also result from idiosyncratic reactions to drugs and from antibiotics administered to infants.

F. SKIN AND SENSORY ORGANS

The skin is a common site of deposition and intake for toxic agents in water, air, and soil. Reactive chemicals produce inflammation (contact dermatitis) and necrosis (chemical bums) in the epidermal, dermal, and subcutaneous layers of the skin. Parasites, bacteria, and viruses also produce inflammation, irritation, and necrosis. In addition, acute and chronic damage can be caused by nonionizing radiation from the sun, microwaves, and lasers. Such radiation can cause burns and destroy collagen in the connective tissue below the dermal layer. All forms of ionizing radiation except alpha particles, which cannot penetrate the skin's epidermal layer, cause erythema, irritation, and necrosis.

Some chemicals may discolor the skin and skin diseases may be part of a systemic reaction, such as pink disease (acrodynia) in small children poisoned by inorganic and organic forms of mercury, and argyria, which is caused by exposure to silver. **Chloracne,** an acneiform skin disease with comedones, hyperpigmentation, and yellow cysts, follows local or systemic exposure to polyhalogenated organic compounds, including chlorinated naphthalenes, PCBs, chlorinated dibenzofurans, and 2,3,7,8-tetra-chloro-p-dioxin (TCDD).

Environmental exposures to the eye involve four regions: the cornea, the anterior chamber, which contains the lens, the retina, and the optic nerve. The most common serious environmental eye injury is scarring of the cornea by chemicals, physical trauma, or electromagnetic radiation. Acute reversible contraction of the iris is a sign of toxicity from organophosphate insecticides and other chemicals that inhibit the metabolism of the neurotransmitter acetylcholine. Methanol damages the optic nerve in humans and monkeys by interfering with folic acid dependent pathways that metabolize methanol to carbon dioxide, resulting in the accumulation of toxic concentrations of formic acid.

Cataracts can be induced by most forms of electromagnetic energy, including heat, microwaves, and X-rays, and by chemicals such as 2,4-dinitrophenol and naphthalene. Lasers and other sources of intense light can also scar the retina. Conjunctivitis is caused by a variety of chemicals, bacteria, and viruses.

The external ear, comprising the external auditory meatus, the ear canal, and the tympanic membrane (ear drum), is the site of entry for chemicals, biologic agents, and the build up of air pressure. Infection and inflammation are the most common damages, but are usually not related to air or water pollution. The middle ear houses the delicate bones that transmit sound to the sensory cells in the inner ear. Most damage to the inner ear occurs in the sensory cells from noise and infection, though the auditory nerve can also be damaged by chemicals, including antibiotics.   An increased air pressure differential between the inner and outer ear can rupture the tympanic membrane and damage structures of the middle ear. Persons who survive lightning strikes often have damage to structures in the external, middle, and inner ear.

G. CANCER

No other environmentally related disease has received as much attention as cancer. Cancer is the malignant variety of **neoplasia** - the process of uncontrolled and undifferentiated cell growth. It results from damage to chromosomal DNA and from the failure of the immune system to destroy malignant cells - a process called **immune surveillance**. The term **malignant** refers to both the appearance and the behavior of neoplastic cells. Compared with cells of benign neoplasms, malignant cells have enlarged nuclei, divide more frequently, and infiltrate surrounding tissues.

Genotoxic agents can induce cancer in the developing fetus by inducing mutations in DNA, and breaks and sister chromatid exchange in chromosomes. For instance, exposure to ionizing radiation in utero has been associated with induction of acute lymphocytic leukemia. Wilm's tumor of the kidney, neuroblastoma, and primary carcinoma of the liver are other cancers induced prenatally. The etiology of these tumors has not been well established, though inherited genetic damage and in utero exposure to environmental agents, such as ionizing radiation, have been suggested.

Some cancers respond to medical treatment, but many are ultimately fatal, causing death by damaging crucial organs or physiologic processes. Cancer cells can also separate from the original tumor mass or neoplasm and **metastasize** to other locations through the circulatory or lymphatic systems. At these distant sites they form new implants of the tumor.

Cancers are classified according to the type of cells from which they arise: **carcinoma** for epithelial cells, **adenocarcinoma** for secretory epithelium, **germ cell cancer** for reproductive tissue, **sarcoma** for tissue of mesenchymal origin (connective tissue and bone), **lymphoma** for lymphatic tissue, and **leukemia** for hemopoietic tissue in the bone marrow. The etiology of many cancers is unknown. Based on results from animal studies, it is now presumed that cancer is caused or promoted by many different factors, including viral infection, diet, and physical and chemical agents.

Initiators (genotoxic agents) are carcinogens that produce mutations in DNA at different functional sites on chromosomes. They are thought to operate by activating oncogenes, interfering with the functions of tumor suppressor genes, and through mechanisms that have yet to be identified. **Promoters** (epigenetic agents) are carcinogens that stimulate cell division - thereby increasing the probability that a mutation will survive and proliferate. Some promoters are thought to stimulate tumor growth by deleting gap junctions between cells, thereby disrupting communication between them. Others, such as TCDD, act through a specific receptor molecule. Recently, a number of additional processes have been recognized to play important roles in the development of cancer. Tumor suppressor genes have been identified and shown to regulate division of cancer cells, repair of damaged DNA, and stimulation of apoptosis - the process of cell death that plays an important role in removing cells with damaged genomes and structural defects. Mutations in DNA repair genes have also been linked to hereditary cancers.

Because not all exposures to carcinogens result in cancer, the effects of carcinogens are best described as stochastic or probabilistic processes. Some exposures produce no damage, whereas others cause damage that is either repaired or results in cell death. The probability of developing cancer, however, increases with the magnitude and duration of exposure to a carcinogen.

Cancers do not appear immediately after the initial damage to cellular DNA. In humans it usually takes many years for a cancer to be recognized, though some have short **latent periods** ranging from a few months (leukemia induced by **in utero** exposure to ionizing radiation) to a few years (leukemia in adults exposed to ionizing radiation and hepatic angiosarcoma from vinyl chloride exposure). Factors such as age at tumor initiation and dose (cumulative dose as well as dose rate) of a carcinogen influence the length of the latent period.

H. ADVERSE REPRODUCTIVE OUTCOMES AND INFERTILITY

Environmental agents affect reproduction by damaging the gametes of one or both parents, the somatic (non-reproductive) tissues of the fetus, or by altering the fertility of one or both parents. Diseases of the mother may also be deleterious to the fetus. Genetic damage includes gains or losses of complete chromosomes, additions, rearrangements or deletions of sections of chromosomes, and mutations. Such damage can be caused by a variety of environmental agents. It is currently thought that most genetic damage is repaired by biochemical processes in the nucleus. Ova and zygotes with mutations that have not been repaired are also at risk for failing to implant in the uterus or for being spontaneously aborted following implantation. The extent of genetically induced damage in the fetus is determined by the particular enzyme systems and other physiologic processes that are under the control of the damaged DNA and the degree to which the altered DNA code is actually expressed.

Approximately 30% of implanted ova result in spontaneous abortions, with most occurring during the first trimester. Usually, the products of conception consist of the placenta only, or the placenta and a severely deformed and nonviable fetus. In most cases a logical explanation cannot be given for why a pregnancy results in miscarriage. Exposures to environmental agents have been suggested as possible causes, but these have been hard to prove.

A number of physiologic changes in pregnancy enhance the toxicity of chemicals to the fetus. Transport of digested food in the small intestine is delayed, thereby enhancing the uptake of toxic compounds. In the maternal lung, tidal volume is decreased and residual lung volume is increased, leading to increased absorption of volatile and soluble compounds.

Pregnancy also increases total body water and fat and decreases both the protein concentration in plasma and the total plasma volume. Expanding the volume of extracellular fluid (exhibited as maternal edema) can increase the distribution of chemicals throughout the mother, and enhance transport through the placenta. The placenta has enzymes for transforming toxic chemicals. It also permits transport of non-polar compounds and blocks passage of charged molecules. Toxic chemicals can also be concentrated in amniotic fluid; from there they can penetrate the developing skin and digestive tract of the fetus.

Teratogens are agents that cause fetal abnormalities or birth defects without damaging the DNA of the fetus. They stop or retard cell replication and cause cell death. The time at which a teratogen begins to exert its effects on the fetus has a strong influence on the type of damage that results. Toxic effects can occur in the embryo before implantation, during organogenesis in the implanted embryo, and in the fetal and perinatal phases of development. The critical period for teratogenicity is from the third to the ninth week of gestation (Figure 4.1).

Birth defects are classified by structure and function, and are divided into major defects, which cause severe medical or cosmetic consequences, and minor defects, which are less significant. Examples of environmental teratogenicity include:

1. **Fetal rubella syndrome**, which causes eye, heart, and hearing abnormalities as well as mental retardation;
2. **Methyl mercury poisoning** or **Minamata disease**, which causes growth deficiency, microcephaly and neurologic damage;
3. **Fetal iodine deficiency**, which leads to mental retardation (cretinism) and neurologic damage to the eyes and ears;
4. **Hypothermia** - from maternal fever and, reportedly, from exposure in saunas and hot tubs - which can retard fetal growth and neurologic development;
5. **Maternal malnutrition, caloric restriction**, and **protein deficiency**, which lead to growth retardation, thyroid deficiencies, and delayed maturation of the central nervous system in the fetus;
6. **Vitamin A** and **folic acid deficiencies**, which cause malformations, growth retardation, and embryonic death; and
7. **Maternal exposure to high doses of vitamin A** during pregnancy, which produces major fetal abnormalities.

Toxic agents impair fertility by causing mutations in sperm and ova, which often lead to cell death. Other causes of infertility from toxic exposures include damage to reproductive processes under the control of the endocrine system - spermatogenesis and ejaculation in men and oogenesis, ovulation, fertilization, and implantation in women.

Environmental agents that cause infertility include heat, which decreases sperm count and motility; metals such as lead, arsenic, and mercury; pesticides such as dibromochloropropane (DBCP) and Kepone® (chlordecone), the fumigant ethylene dibromide (EDB), and solvents. Most cases of infertility linked to these agents have occurred in workers who were exposed to comparatively high concentrations - not in the general public.

I. ENDOCRINE SYSTEM

Little is known about the effects of environmental agents on the endocrine system of humans. Compounds such as chlorinated hydrocarbons (DDT, chlordecone, PCBs, dioxins, and atrazine) and polycyclic aromatic hydrocarbons affect estrogen production and metabolism. These "xenoestrogens" have been shown to disrupt endocrine system development in a variety of wildlife species and laboratory animals.

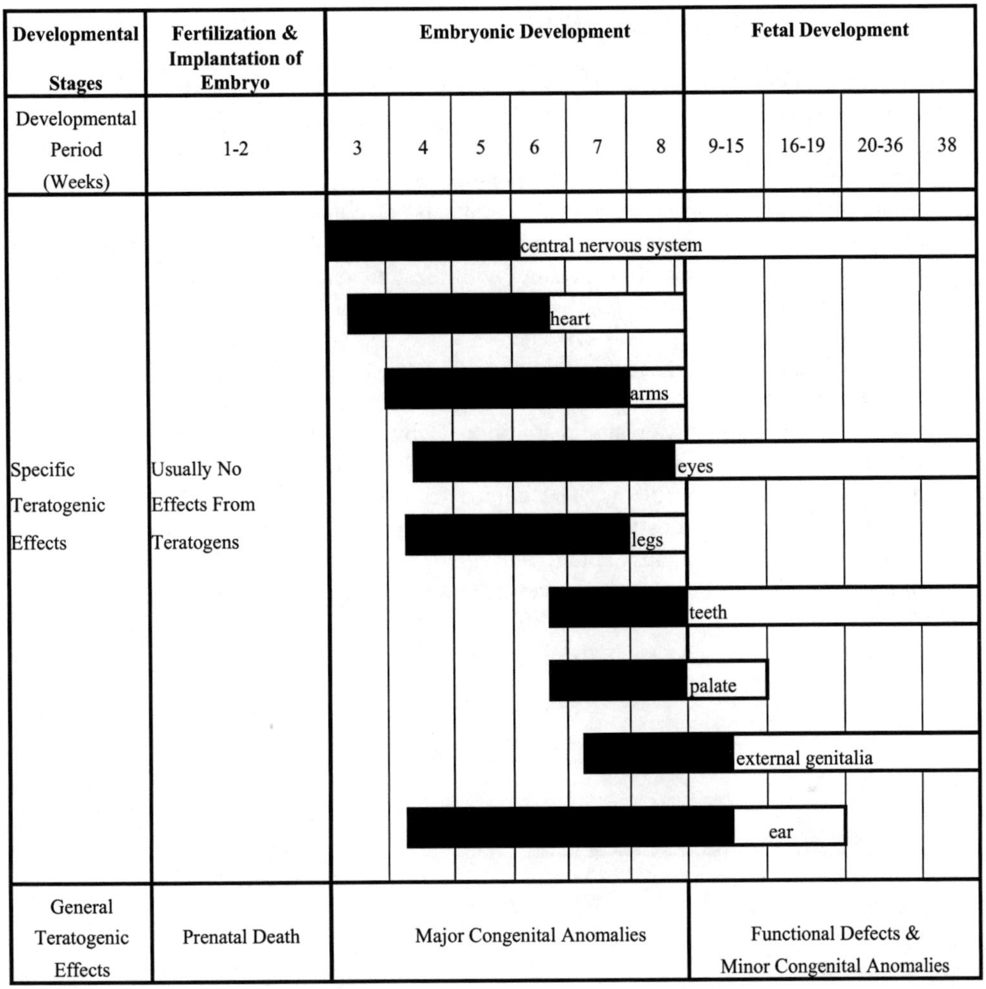

Developmental Stages	Fertilization & Implantation of Embryo	Embryonic Development						Fetal Development			
Developmental Period (Weeks)	1-2	3	4	5	6	7	8	9-15	16-19	20-36	38
Specific Teratogenic Effects	Usually No Effects From Teratogens	central nervous system									
			heart								
				arms							
				eyes							
				legs							
						teeth					
						palate					
								external genitalia			
				ear							
General Teratogenic Effects	Prenatal Death	Major Congenital Anomalies						Functional Defects & Minor Congenital Anomalies			

Note: Dark portions of the bars= periods during which the developing embryo or fetus is highly sensitive to teratogens.

Figure 4.1. Critical Periods of Development for Human Organs and Organ Systems. (Source: Ruttenber and Kimbrough, 1995).

Because estrogens and progestins play important roles in the development of breast cancer, some have theorized that xenoestrogens may be responsible for the steady increases in breast cancer in the United States. Recent epidemiologic evidence is contradictory on this point for DDT and PCBs. So far, there is no evidence that the effects of xenoestrogens noted in animals are found in exposed humans, but such effects would be difficult to evaluate in epidemiologic studies.

J. MULTIPLE CHEMICAL SENSITIVITIES

After seeing patients with a variety of complaints relating to exposure to one or more chemicals and not being able to explain these findings, allergists and occupational physicians began using the term **multiple chemical sensitivities (MCS)** to describe disorders characterized by recurrent symptoms in multiple organ systems that follow exposure to many different unrelated chemicals at concentrations lower than those usually associated with disease. Although disorders of the immune system may explain some complaints, many are not consistent with these mechanisms. Some believe that the majority of complaints have psychological origins and others postulate interactions between the immune and nervous systems.

The consistent appearance of patients with complaints more compatible with MCS than with other diagnoses has made it difficult for the medical community to disregard this complex problem. Physicians in traditional clinical specialties as well as the less-traditional clinical ecologists and environmental physicians diagnose and treat patients with MCS and related problems. The clinical ecologists have developed a variety of definitions, theories, diagnostic strategies, and treatments that rely on abnormalities in the immune system to help explain and treat MCS and other "environmental" or "ecologic" illnesses. Many argue, however, that their theories have not been adequately tested, and recent data suggest that MCS are more closely related to psychological symptoms than to immune system dysfunction.

IV. SPECIFIC DISEASES

A. DISEASES OF THE LUNG AND PLEURA

1. Asthma

Occupational asthma is defined as a disease characterized by variable airflow obstruction and/or airway hyper-responsiveness due to agents in the working environment. These agents can give rise to asthma through immunologic and non-immunologic mechanisms.

Many agents found in the workplace have been implicated in causing asthma (Table 4.1). Although many of these agents have been confirmed by specific challenge studies, others have been less well studied. Such a list serves a useful function in alerting health professionals that their patients may be suffering from occupational asthma if they were exposed to one of these agents. Because the list is steadily growing, the absence of previous reports of association should not rule out the possibility of occupational asthma if diagnostic evidence is strong.

The overall prevalence of occupational asthma is unknown. In the United States, the 1978 Social Security Disability Survey showed that 7.7% of the participants identified asthma as a personal medical condition and 1.2% attributed it to workplace exposure. In Japan, it has been estimated that 15% of all asthma in men is due to occupational exposure. In both Quebec and British Columbia in Canada, occupational asthma has become the most prevalent occupational lung disease, exceeding asbestosis and silicosis

Table 4.1. Agents That Cause Occupational Asthma. (Source: Chan-Yeung, 1994).

Asthma-Inducing agents	Common sources of exposure

Animal-Derived Material
  Dander
  Excreta
  Secretions
  Serum
	Animal poultry and insect work, veterinary medicine, fishing and fish processing, laboratory work

Plant-derived material
  Carmine
  Castor beans
  Coffee beans (green)
  Colophony
  Flour
  Grain
  Psyllium
  Tamarind seed
  Tea
  Tobacco
  Vegetable gums
  Wood Dusts
    (i.e., western red cedar,
    mahogany, oak, California
    redwood)
	Natural oil manufacturing, food processing, textile manufacturing, grain handling, tobacco processing, printing, sawmill and furniture work, carpentry, electronics soldering

Enzymes
  Alcalase
  Bacillus subtilis-derived enzyme
  Bromelain
  Pancreatic extracts
  Papain
  Trypsin (hog)
	Food processing, detergent industry, pharmaceutical industry

Drugs
  Amprolium hydrochloride
  Cimetidine
  Penicillins
  Phenylglycine acid chloride
  Piperazine
  Spiramycin
  Sulfonamide
  Tetracycline
	Pharmaceutical industry

Metal fumes and salts
  Chromium
  Cobalt
  Nickel
  Platinum salts
  Welding flux
	Chemical industries, metal refining, metal plating, metal grinding, welding

in the number of compensation claims submitted in 1986. In general prevalence of occupational asthma depends largely on the industrial agent, the degree of exposure, and the host susceptibility factor. Some agents are more potent sensitizers compared with others.

2. Byssinosis and Other Textile Dust-Related Lung Diseases

For nearly three hundred years, work in the textile industry has been recognized as an occupational hazard. In the early 18th century, Ramazzini described a peculiar form of asthma among those who card flax and hemp. The "foul and poisonous dust" that he observed "makes the workmen cough incessantly and by degrees brings on asthmatic troubles." That such symptoms did in fact occur in the early textile industry has been illustrated by Bouhuys in his physiologic studies at Philipsburg Manor (a restoration project of life in the early Dutch colonies in North Tarrytown, New York). In a primitive workshop where raw flax fiber was processed, this study documented objective lung function changes characteristic of those seen in modem textile workers.

The term **byssinosis** derives from a Greek and a Latin (byssus) root first applied to the description of illnesses of textile workers by the Belgian public health physician Achille Adrien Proust in the late 19th century. Although numerous authors throughout the 19th and early 20th centuries in both Britain and Europe described the respiratory manifestations of work-related illness in textile mills with increasing frequency, the disease remained essentially unrecognized in the United States until recently. Preliminary studies in the early 1960s under the direction of Richard Schilling indicated that despite pronouncements to the contrary by both industry and government, characteristic **byssinosis** did occur in this country.

From this modest beginning, through the efforts of epidemiologic and clinical investigations, the United States not only recognizes the important prevalence of this illness among its textile workers, but has, as a result of these findings, developed some of the most stringent environmental standards in the world. Additionally, these cotton dust standards are coupled with medical surveillance within the industry. Such an approach has the promise of reducing the prevalence of **byssinosis** in the United States, although residual disease in older and retired workers remains a serious problem. Moreover, shifts in the textile industry to other centers throughout the world and particularly to developing countries have recently confirmed that with inadequate control, **byssinosis** is and will continue to be a major occupational illness of international concern.

Natural fibers have been defined as cells or groups of cells with lengths much greater than their widths, Fibers are common in the vegetable world, particularly among plants structured with cellulose (e.g., cotton, wood, straw); however, only a limited number of these natural fibers can be used for textile products based on their physical properties (e.g., length, strength, pliability, elasticity). The use of these vegetable fibers for the manufacture of textiles dates back to the 3rd millennium BC. Cotton was processed in India, flax in Egypt, and silk in China. The manufacture of these textiles, however, remained relatively limited, and the processes for converting them to yarn and fabric were primitive until the Industrial Revolution, at which time the cleaning and spinning of textiles became automated and developed on a large scale.

3. Irritant Bronchitis

The past 20 years have been marked by an increasing awareness of the potential for exposure to occupational pollutants, including nonspecific irritants, to cause chronic bronchitis and chronic airflow limitation. This section focuses on the association between occupational exposures and chronic bronchitis, as well as the association among occupational exposures, bronchitis, and the development of respiratory impairment.

Chronic bronchitis is a common symptom affecting up to 15% of the general population depending on how risk factors, methods of data collection, and case definitions are defined. Prevalence rates for occupational bronchitis range from zero for a nonsmoker to as high as 60% for a smoker with industrial exposure. When compared with lesser-exposed or non-exposed controls, the occupationally exposed cohorts generally have higher rates of bronchitis.

a. Occupational Bronchitis

Chronic airflow obstruction (chronic obstructive pulmonary disease) frequently is thought to be the result of three overlapping disease processes: chronic bronchitis, emphysema, and asthma. Chronic bronchitis is defined by the nature and duration of cough, but it can be associated with both airflow obstruction and abnormalities in gas exchange. Asthma is more difficult to define, but it frequently is characterized as reversible airflow obstruction. Bronchitic symptoms are common in patients with asthma who, in addition to having symptoms of breathlessness, wheezing, and chest tightness, often report a chronic productive cough. Emphysema, defined as an abnormal permanent enlargement of airspaces, often is seen in the setting of both productive cough and wheezing. Physiologically, all three conditions are associated with airflow obstruction, frequently with a reversible component to a greater (e.g., asthma) or lesser extent (e.g., chronic bronchitis and emphysema).

b. Chronic Bronchitis

Chronic bronchitic symptoms result from mucus hypersecretion, which is associated with histologic abnormalities of the large and small bronchi and bronchioles. These changes are most notable for the hypertrophy and hyperplasia of the submucosal glands. Mucus-secreting goblet cells, which are normally limited to the larger airways, may greatly increase in size and number and can extend all the way to the bronchiole. The Reid Index, a measure of the ratio of the size of the goblet cells relative to the thickness of the bronchial walls (measured from the inside of the cartilage plates to the lumen), normally is 0.3 mm and, in chronic bronchitis, increases to 0.6 mm. Additional changes include bronchial wall edema and the presence of inflammatory cells, especially with concurrent bacterial infection.

The result of these changes is mucus hypersecretion and impairment of the mucociliary defense mechanism that helps clear pollutants and secretions from the lower respiratory tract. The natural history of chronic bronchitis depends on multiple factors such as the extent of mucus hypersecretion and deterioration of host defense mechanisms, presence of infection, and continued presence of irritant exposures such as cigarette smoke or other inhaled irritants. Chronic inflammation can result in bronchial wall ulceration. The process of bronchial wall ulceration, destruction, and repair may result in destruction and narrowing of small airways due to scarring as well as loss of elastic support. The effect of the processes of chronic inflammation and repair, coupled with mucus obstructing the small airways, can result in chronic airflow obstruction.

c. Emphysema

Emphysema is defined as the enlargement of airspaces accompanied by destruction of alveolar walls. Although considered a pathologic diagnosis based on lung morphology, clinical signs can be used to suggest a diagnosis of emphysema. Key signs include hyperinflation on chest radiographs, increased total lung capacity, reduced FEV, reduced DLCO, and of increasing importance, the presence of avascular spaces on computed tomographic (CT) scans of the lung.

Emphysema is categorized microscopically into multiple types based on the distribution of airspace enlargement and destruction. Major categories include centriacinar, focal, centrilobular, panacinar, and distal acinar emphysema. Of particular importance to those exposed to environmental and occupational agents are focal and centrilobular emphysema. Focal emphysematous changes are commonly distributed throughout the lung. This type of emphysema is associated with exposure to dusts such as coal dust. Centrilobular emphysema, commonly found in the upper lobes, is most often associated with cigarette smoking and perhaps with chronic irritant exposure.

d. Effect of Inhaled Pollutant on the Genesis of Chronic Bronchitis and Abnormalities of Ventilatory Function

The development of chronic airflow limitation with the attendant adverse effects on ventilatory function and gas exchange are the focus of two theories known as the **British hypothesis** and **Dutch hypothesis**.

The British hypothesis suggests that chronic mucus hypersecretion results in the development of chronic airflow obstruction. Although there is a close association between airflow obstruction and mucus hypersecretion, there are adequate data to suggest that mucus hypersecretion is not an independent risk factor for airflow obstruction. Nonetheless, mucus hypersecretion and airflow obstruction are both related to chronic irritant exposure (e.g., cigarette smoking). Chronic irritant exposures also are likely to have multiple loci of adverse effects, including secreting cells (mucus hypersecretion), lung walls (airflow obstruction), and lung parenchyma (interstitial fibrosis, emphysema, or both).

Other pollutants that have a substantial contribution to the prevalence of bronchitic symptoms and other pulmonary manifestations are the following: 1) cigarette smoke, 2) asbestos, 3) silica, 4) coal dust, 5) organic dusts, 6) cotton and other vegetable dusts, 7) welding fumes, 8) exposures associated with firefighting, 9) irritant gases (sulfur dioxide, nitrogen dioxide and ozone), 10) synthetic vitreous fibers.

4. Acute Inhalational Injury

a. Introduction

The events in Bhopal, India, dramatically illustrate the potential consequences of acute exposure to toxic inhalants. In the workplace, toxic inhalants have been reported to cause a variety of clinical problems ranging from mild irritation of the upper airways to noncardiogenic pulmonary edema (adult respiratory distress syndrome [ARDS]) and death. Exposure to toxic inhalants present problems in clinical management for the following reasons:
1. Exposures occur at infrequent, unpredictable intervals,
2. Exposures may involve large numbers of individuals,
3. The exact toxic agent may not be known to the patient or physician,
4. There is a broad range of acute clinical symptoms with a varying time of onset, and
5. The chronic effects of acute exposures have not been clearly characterized.

Despite these problems, knowledge of the basic principles underlying these acute parenchymal responses allows the clinician to respond appropriately. Although many agents, such as asphyxiants (e.g., carbon monoxide and hydrogen cyanide), metal fumes (e.g.. cadmium), and immunologically active inhalants (e.g., red cedar dust, animal dander, and grain dust) are potent mediators of acute lung injury, the section touches on some of the agents that are capable of causing toxic pneumonitis. Importantly, many of the exposures that can result in acute toxic airway and parenchymal injury also may result in subacute and chronic abnormalities that can dramatically alter lung function. The subacute and chronic effects of acute inhalational injury are poorly understood. However, delayed effects from acute high-dose exposures regularly occur in the clinical setting.

b. Major Causes of Inhalation Injury

(1) Irritant Gases

Irritant gases that are major causes of inhalational injury are the following: 1) ammonia (NH_3), 2) chlorine, 3) hydrogen chloride, 4) oxides of nitrogen, 5) ozone, 6) phosgene, and 7) sulfur dioxide.

(2) Metals

The metals associated with inhalational injury are the following: 1) cadmium, 2) mercury, 3) metal fumes (metal oxides such as zinc, copper, and magnesium), and 3) smoke.

5. Hypersensitivity Pneumonitis

Hypersensitivity pneumonitis, also known as extrinsic allergic alveolitis, constitutes a spectrum of granulomatous, interstitial, and alveolar-filling lung diseases that result from repeated inhalation of and sensitization to a wide variety of organic dusts and low-molecular-weight chemical antigens. The illness is characterized by granulomatous pneumonitis, with potential reversibility if antigen exposure is terminated. Continued antigen exposure may lead to chronic interstitial fibrosis. No single historical feature or laboratory test is diagnostic of hypersensitivity pneumonitis. Rather, diagnosis relies on a strong index of suspicion and a constellation of clinical findings.

6. Beryllium And Hard Metal-Related Disease

Both Beryllium and Cobalt are relatively light metals that have the potential to cause pulmonary toxicity through host responses that appear to involve immunologically mediated sensitization rather than overburdening of clearance mechanisms. Aluminum, cadmium, and titanium are other metals that appear to have such potential. Although much more is understood of host responses to inhaled beryllium than to inhaled cobalt, the diseases that result from chronic occupational exposure to these metals (chronic beryllium disease and hard metal-related disease, respectively) remain intriguing models of pulmonary toxicity about which there are many unanswered questions.

Two different types of pulmonary disease can result from the inhalation of Beryllium fumes or dust, or both. Short-term, high-intensity exposure can cause acute lung injury that is clinically and pathologically indistinguishable from toxic pneumonitis caused by the inhalation of other chemically irritating materials. Repeated exposure to lower concentrations of Beryllium in workplace air over months to years can lead to the development of a chronic granulomatous disease that is similar to sarcoidosis. Acute toxic pneumonitis due to Beryllium is now rare, at least in developed countries, because the primary production industry is aware of the metal's toxic potential and has taken steps to prevent massive exposures. However, many thousands of workers in the United States and elsewhere remain at risk for the development of chronic Beryllium disease because of relatively low-intensity exposures in industries involved in the fabrication and machining of beryllium-containing alloys. Non-occupational environmental exposures to Beryllium also have been reported to lead to chronic Beryllium disease.

7. Asbestosis And Asbestos-Related Pleural Disease

Asbestos, also known as asbestiform minerals, is a term applied to a group of minerals that are naturally occurring, often magnesium-containing fibrous hydrated silicates. Six fibrous silicates are commonly referred to as asbestos, including the three most common commercial forms: chrysotile, or white asbestos; amosite, or brown asbestos; and crocidolite, or blue asbestos. Although there is some evidence that the biologic potency differs among the various fibers, from the point of view of the clinician, it should be recognized that the three main commercial types have been associated with all of the major malignant and nonmalignant asbestos-related conditions.

The range of health effects from asbestos exposure is protean, including both pulmonary and non-pulmonary malignant and nonmalignant conditions. This section focuses on two major nonmalignant pulmonary sequelae: asbestosis and asbestos-induced pleural disease. Although these two types of outcomes - pleural and parenchymal - have distinct pathologic manifestations, it is helpful to consider them together, both because it is often difficult to distinguish their clinical effects and because although they can occur in isolation, they are commonly present in the same individual because both are dose-dependent outcomes of the same asbestos exposure.

8. Silicosis

Silicosis was first reported by the ancient Greeks and is apparently as old as human history. The prevalence of this illness peaked in the last half of the 19th century and the early part of this century, when mechanized industry was developing and the relationship between dust exposure and disease was less well understood. Yet, even today in developed countries, sporadic outbreaks of silicosis occur when workers are consistently exposed to silica particles of respirable size (0.5 to 5.0 μm in diameter) at levels exceeding those recognized to be safe.

Classic silicosis encompasses a continuum of severity ranging from simple silicosis (presenting as pulmonary fibrosis with or without symptoms) to progressive massive fibrosis (severely disabling restrictive lung disease). These features usually develop slowly and frequently require the person to work a lifetime to develop. However, in a small percentage of workers, the radiographic features of simple silicosis and then progressive massive fibrosis develop in less than 10 years. Because these features develop relatively quickly, workers with these findings are described as having accelerated silicosis. Development of these radiographic features so soon after beginning exposure to silica means that progression of disease and severe respiratory impairment is very likely to occur.

9. Coal Workers' Pneumoconiosis And Other Coal-Related Lung Disease

The growth in coal mining is virtually coincident with the Industrial Revolution. Although shallow mining of coal seam outcrops is reported to have occurred since the 9th century, the 18th century brought increased demand for coal as well as the technology to pursue the mining of seams well below the earth's surface. By the early 1800s coal mining had become an important industry in the United States. Employment in coal mining peaked about 100 years later in 1923, when over 800,000 coal miners were working. From that point, although production and consumption of coal continued to increase, mechanization progressively reduced the size of the workforce. In 1990, a total of 126,642 coal miners were at work in the United States, of whom almost half were employed on surface operations. The majority of coal production is still based in the eastern Appalachian coal fields. However, western states account for an increasing proportion of coal output.

In Europe, recognition of the adverse health consequences of coal mining followed the marked increase in the population of miners. Ramazzini cites Wedel, who in 1672 wrote of miner's asthma, but was probably referring to hard rock miners. According to Kerr, the term was first applied to coal miners in 1822. Laennec described the black pigment in the lungs of coal miners as melanosis in 1806 and, by 1819, clearly differentiated the condition from malignant melanoma. Several years later, the term miners' black lung was used to describe the disease in Scotland. In 1919, silicosis became a certifiable disease in the United Kingdom, and British miners with coal workers' pneumoconiosis (CWP) became eligible for certain benefits. Based on studies of British coal miners, CWP was differentiated from silicosis in the early 1940s.

10. Other Pnemoconiosis

The fibrogenic potential of mineral dust is dependent on various physical and chemical properties of the dust, the dose retained in the lung, and specific physiologic and immunologic characteristics of the individual. Silicon dioxide (SiO_2) as free silica is the most common naturally occurring fibrogenic dust. Silicates are silicon dioxide combined with various cautions. The crystalline structure of silicates can vary from a platy occurrence or habit, such as mica, to a very fibrous habit, such as with crocidolite and amosite asbestos. Specific silicate ore sources such as talc can exist in a very pure deposit or can contain minor concentrations of free silica or intergrowths of other minerals such as the amphibole tremolite. Proper mineralogic analysis of samples of an ore body taken from different locations, and ongoing analysis of environmental samples from the mine, mill, and secondary and end users are crucial in the recognition, evaluation, and control of potential pulmonary health risks. The Material Safety Data Sheets may not provide enough information to adequately characterize the physical and chemical properties of a specific silicate or potential contaminant minerals.

Specific elements that cause pneumoconiosis are the following: 1) aluminum, 2) antimony, 3) barium, 4) graphite, 5) iron, 6) kaolin, 7) synthetic vitreous fibers, 8) mica, mixed dusts, 9) oil shale, 10) polyvinylchloride, 11) talc, 12) vermiculite, 13) tin, and 14) zeolite.

B. Environmental Carcinogens

1. Introduction

A carcinogen is defined as any agent, mixture, or exposure circumstances that produces cancer. The U.S. Department of Health and Human Services (DHHS) National Toxicology Program uses specific criteria for identifying human carcinogens in the Report on Carcinogens, which is published every 2 years.

Agents, substances, mixtures, or exposure circumstances known to be "human carcinogens" are defined as those for which there is sufficient evidence from studies in humans to indicate as causal relationship between exposure and human cancer.

Human studies can include traditional cancer epidemiology studies, data from clinical studies, and/or data derived from the study of tissues from humans exposed to the substance in question. This may be useful for evaluating whether a relevant cancer mechanism is operating in people.

Agents, substances, mixtures, or exposure circumstances "reasonably anticipated to be human carcinogens" are those for which there is limited evidence of carcinogenicity in humans and/or sufficient evidence of carcinogenicity in experimental animals.

An environmental carcinogen can be defined as any agent, mixture, or exposure circumstance that is present in a person's environment and that has been shown to cause cancer in humans or experimental animals. Cancer attacks the most basic unit of life, the cell. It is a group of many different diseases that have the common characteristic of uncontrolled cellular growth. Many types of cells make up the human body. These cells normally grow and divide to replace old cells as a natural function to keep the body healthy. However, this process can malfunction, causing cells to divide when new cells are not needed and to multiply without control. This leads to the formation of a tumor.

Tumors can be benign or malignant. Benign tumors are not cancer and are rarely a threat to life. In most cases they can be removed and do not return. Malignant tumors are cancer and cause the destruction of healthy tissue. The cells from a cancer tumor can also "metastasize" by circulating in the body's blood stream or lymphatic system, forming new tumors in other parts of the body.

Most cancers are named for the type of cell or the organ in which they begin. When tumor cells spread, the new tumors have the same kinds of abnormal cells and the same name as the primary tumor. For example, if lung cancer spreads to the brain, the cancer cells in the brain are lung cancer cells. The disease is called metastic lung cancer and not brain cancer.

Most cancer researchers believe that a significant fraction of all cancer cases may be associated with the environment in which we live and work. In this context, the "environment" is defined as anything that interacts with humans, including life-style choices, such as what we eat, drink, and smoke, and aspects of sexual behavior: natural and medical radiation, including exposure to the sun; workplace exposures; drugs; socioeconomic factors affecting exposures and susceptibility; and substances in air, water, and soil.

We rarely know what environmental factors and conditions are responsible for the onset and development of cancers. However, in some cases we have some understanding, especially for cancers related to certain occupational exposures, the use of specific drags or cancer chemotherapeutic agents, and certain life-styles (e.g., smoking). Many scientists knowledgeable in these areas firmly believe that much of the cancer associated with the environment may be avoided.

2. Identification of Environmental Carcinogens

The United States government, industry, academia and other research organizations have studied various substances to identify those that might cause cancer. Information on specific chemicals or occupational exposures is usually published in the scientific literature or in publicly available reports. Information from studies in both humans and animals is used to evaluate whether agents are possible human carcinogens. The strongest evidence for establishing a relationship between exposure to any given chemical and cancer in humans comes from cancer epidemiology studies.

Scientists evaluate groups of people who have been exposed to certain agents and then compare the cancer incidence, or number of people who have developed cancer, to another group of people who have not been exposed to that agent. These studies of human exposure and cancer must consider the latency period (time from exposure to the development of cancer) for cancer development, because the exposure to the carcinogen often occurs many years (sometimes 20 to 30 years or more) before the first sign of cancer appears. In addition, other life-style factors, such as smoking, must be taken into account to ensure the cancers observed are not due to factors other than the exposure to the agent of concern.

The most common method for identifying substances as potential human carcinogens is the long-term animal bioassay. This type of study is designed to provide accurate information about the level and duration of exposure to the agent of concern and any interactions of the agent with other factors in the experimental animal's environment. In these studies, the agent is administered to one or, usually, two laboratory rodent species at different doses and for different time periods, with the experimental conditions carefully chosen to maximize the likelihood of identifying any carcinogenic effects.

It is not possible from animal studies alone to predict absolutely which agents or exposure circumstances will be carcinogenic in humans; however, all known human carcinogens that have been studied adequately also produce cancers in laboratory animals.

Experimental carcinogenesis research is based on the scientific assumption that chemicals causing cancer in animals will have similar effects in humans. The adverse responses of laboratory animals to chemicals (of which cancer is only one) do not always strictly correspond to the effects observed in humans exposed to the same agent; however, laboratory animals remain the best tool for detecting potential human health hazards of all kinds, including cancer.

3. The Effects of Environmental Carcinogens

According to the **American Cancer Society**, environmental causes of cancer probably account for more than half of all cancer cases. The number of new cases of cancer in the United States is going up each year. Information from the **National Cancer Institute** indicates that people of all ages get cancer, but nearly all types of cancer are more common in middle-aged and elderly people than in young people.

Skin cancer is the most common type of cancer for both men and women. The next most common type is prostate cancer in men, and breast cancer in women. Lung cancer is the leading cause of death from cancer for both men and women in the United States.

4. Sources of Environmental Carcinogens

There are three major sources of exposure to environmental carcinogens:

a. Workplace

Exposure to agents such as chemicals, metals, dusts, etc. can increase one's risk of cancer. A number of these agents found in the workplace are known human carcinogens (e.g., arsenic, asbestos. benzene, benzidine, vinyl chloride), and others are considered anticipated carcinogens (e.g.. carbon tetrachloride, chloroform, DDT, formaldehyde, glass wool). These may act alone or together with other carcinogens, such as tobacco smoke. For example, inhaling asbestos fibers increases the risk of lung cancer, and this risk is especially high for asbestos workers who smoke. It is especially important to follow safe work practices to avoid or minimize exposure to carcinogenic agents in the workplace.

b. Radiation

Only high-frequency radiation, such as ionizing radiation and ultraviolet radiation, have been proved to be human carcinogens. Sources of ionizing radiation exposure include radon in indoor air, radiation from rocks and soil, outer-space, sun, x-rays, and nuclear medicine exams. Exposure to high doses of ionizing radiation has been shown to cause cancer in atomic bomb survivors, uranium miners, and individuals who have received radiotherapy in the treatment of diseases. Ionizing radiation can cause cancer in virtually any part of the body but is especially associated with leukemia and thyroid cancer.

It is important to note that the x-rays used for diagnosis by your doctor or dentist expose you to very little radiation and the benefits of this very minor exposure outweigh any risk.

Repeated exposure to solar ultraviolet radiation has been shown to cause skin cancer (cutaneous malignant melanoma). Exposure to ultraviolet radiation from sunlamps or sunbeds has also been shown to cause cutaneous malignant melanoma. The data for these cancer studies indicate that there is a relationship between the length of time of exposure and the formation of cancer. The effects were especially pronounced in individuals under 30 years of age and those who experienced sunburn. It is important for people to protect themselves from the harmful effects of ultraviolet radiation by using protective clothing, such as a hat and long sleeves, and by using a sunscreen.

c. Lifestyle

Choices individuals make in their lifestyle may expose them to carcinogens in their living environment.

One of the most evident "lifestyle environmental carcinogens" is **tobacco**. Tobacco smoking has been determined to cause cancer of the lung, urinary bladder, renal pelvis, oral cavity, pharynx, larynx, esophagus, lip, and pancreas in humans. Smoking accounts for more than 85% of all lung cancer deaths. Smoking cessation is associated with a decreased risk of developing cancer. Using smokeless tobacco products has been determined to cause cancers of the oral cavity.

Cancers of the oral cavity have been associated with the use of chewing tobacco as well as snuff, which are the two main forms of smokeless tobacco used in the United States. Tumors often arise at the site of placement of the tobacco.

Exposure to environmental tobacco smoke (ETS) is associated with an increase in lung cancer in nonsmokers. Evidence for an increased cancer risk from ETS is from studies examining nonsmoking spouses living with individuals who smoke cigarettes, exposures of nonsmokers to ETS in occupational settings, and childhood exposure to ETS from smoking parents. Many studies have demonstrated increased risks of about 20% for developing lung cancer following prolonged exposure to ETS, with some studies suggesting higher risks with higher exposures. Exposure to ETS from spousal smoking or exposure in an occupational setting appears most strongly related to increased risk of developing cancer.

Another lifestyle choice associated with increased risk for cancer is consumption of **alcoholic beverages**. Studies have shown that consumption of alcoholic beverages can lead to cancers of the mouth, pharynx, larynx, and esophagus. These studies are in a variety of human populations and are notable for their consistency in reporting the presence of moderate to strong associations, which increase with increasing consumption of alcoholic beverages for these four cancer sites. Studies indicate that the risk is highest among smokers and at the highest levels of consumption (i.e., more than three drinks per day).

A third example of how lifestyle can be associated with increased risk for cancer comes from **dietary** studies. These studies indicate a link between high-fat diets and cancer of the breast, colon, uterus, and prostate. Being seriously overweight has also been linked to increases in these same cancers. Researchers have reported that you reduce your cancer risk by maintaining a well- balanced diet that includes ample amounts of high-fiber foods that are also high in vitamins and minerals and by reducing the amount of fatty foods in the diet.

5. Avoidance of Environmental Carcinogens

The more information made available by research into what environmental factors cause cancer, the better one will be able to determine the most effective ways to avoid or minimize exposure. Many environmental carcinogens can be avoided. For those that cannot be avoided, either because of job, life-style, or other factors, it is helpful to be aware of what these environmental carcinogens are and to take steps to protect oneself and minimize the exposure.

The risk - the probability of developing cancer - depends on many things, including the intensity, route, and duration of exposure to environmental carcinogens. Individuals may respond differently to similar exposures, depending on host factors such as age, sex, nutritional status, overall health, and inherited characteristics.

Some researchers believe that the cancer risk is directly proportional to exposure and that reduction of exposure by any means will decrease the incidence of cancer.

This is the basis of current regulatory policies that aim to lower human exposure to environmental carcinogens and thereby improve public health.

C. Environmental Endocrine Disruptors

1. Definition of Endocrine Disruptors

An endocrine disruptor is a chemical, or mixture of chemicals, that alters the normal functioning of the hormones within the body. Because hormones play such an essential role in controlling biological processes, especially during development of the reproductive and nervous systems, concern has risen that endocrine disruptors present in the environment could have profound effects on humans and wildlife exposed to such substances.

Although many pharmacologic agents are intentionally designed to modulate the endocrine system to induce some desired biological response (e.g., birth control pills to prevent pregnancy, thyroid hormone supplements for hypothyroid patients, estrogen therapy to prevent bone loss in postmenopausal women, antiestrogen therapy for women at risk for breast cancer, antiandrogen therapy for men with prostate cancer), the concern with environmental endocrine disruptors is that the exposures can be covert (contaminants in our food or water) and widespread [due to the environmental persistence of some endocrine-disrupting chemicals (EDCs)], and can occur during life stages that are known to be particularly vulnerable to alterations in endocrine function.

The public health importance of the issue of endocrine disruption is evident from the publications of a number of conferences and workshops over the past few years. Further stimulus resulted from the 1996 publication of "Our Stolen Future" in the lay press. Various perspectives and views on the scientific issues can be found in scientific publications and in a number of internet sites. In 1998, the International Programme on Chemical Safety (IPCS) of the World Health Organization provided a definition of endocrine disruptors as "exogenous substances that alter function(s) of the endocrine system and consequently cause adverse health effects in an intact organism, or its progeny, or (sub) populations."

2. **Other Terms Used to Describe Such Chemicals**

A number of synonyms have been used to describe substances that can interact with the endocrine system, including endocrine active chemicals (EACs), endocrine modulators, and hormonally active agents (HAAs). This last term was used by the **National Academy of Sciences** in their comprehensive review of the scientific literature, because it was felt that the term "endocrine disruptor" was "fraught with emotional overtones and was tantamount to a prejudgment of the problem" and that HAA was a more neutral, mechanistically based definition.

Others have recommended the use of the adjective "potential" endocrine disruptor, or modulator, when a chemical has been shown to have the ability to interact with the endocrine system in some fashion, but there has not yet been a clear demonstration of cause and effect in an intact organism.

3. **Endocrine Disruption as an Environmental Concern**

Support for endocrine disruption as an environmental issue comes from four basic areas:

In vitro experiments demonstrating that a chemical can either bind to a hormone receptor, activate hormonally responsive genes, or block the effect of a hormone on expression of a hormonally responsive gene.

In vivo experiments in which exposure to a chemical during some phase of the life cycle produces alterations in either function or morphology that are consistent with either over- or underactivity of a particular hormone.

Status and trends studies demonstrating that some biological end point or disease with an endocrine basis (e.g., breast cancer, prostate cancer, hypospadias) has been increasing during the modern era of synthetic chemistry (essentially since the 1940s).

Epidemiological studies in wildlife or humans demonstrating a cause-and-effect relationship between a chemical with a known endocrine action and a particular adverse health outcome.

By far, the last area provides the strongest scientific evidence for concern, particularly with supporting evidence from laboratory studies in experimental animals. While intriguing, evidence from status and trends studies can only suggest an environmental etiology. Thus, indications of increased incidences of certain hormonally mediated cancers (e.g., breast, testicular, and prostate), hormonally mediated birth defects (e.g., cryptorchidism, hypospadias), or deficits in reproductive function (e.g., diminished semen quality, endometriosis) overtime in certain geographic areas, while causes for concern, must be viewed with caution as to causation.

In such instances, it is critical that confounding influences such as the increase in lifespan, altered life-styles, dietary habits, increased diagnostic capability, improved reporting systems, and other exposures be adequately evaluated in the search for risk factors. Studies indicating that a chemical can act like a hormone in an *in vitro* system indicate only that the potential exists to cause biological effects via that mode of action in a whole organism.

4. Exposure to Endocrine Disruptors

Endocrine-disrupting chemicals encompass a variety of compounds, including natural and synthetic hormones, natural plant constituents, pesticides, monomers and additives used in the plastics industry, detergent components and breakdown products, and persistent environmental pollutants. For humans, the principal source of exposures of adults to nonpharmaceutical chemicals is via food, due to the biomagnification of certain persistent organochlorine pesticides such as DDT and industrial chemicals such as the polychlorinated biphenyls (PCBs); drinking water is a potential secondary source. Food with residues of fungicides or herbicides with endocrine-disrupting potential represents another significant possibility for exposure. Certain plants, such as soya beans, contain high amounts of phytoestrogens (natural constituents that have estrogenic properties when consumed by animals) and therefore soy-containing food products are a source of exposure to naturally occurring chemicals capable of altering the function of the endocrine system.

Exposures could also occur through leaching from plastics in medical devices (e.g., dialysis therapy and phthalates in the tubing), various plastics used in consumer goods, or food packaging materials that contain labile endocrine-disrupting chemicals. Included in this class are the phthalates, which are diester derivatives of phthalic acid used to make certain plastics more flexible. Of particular concern is the potential for exposure of young children through chewing of phthalate-containing toys. Finally, because many endocrine-disrupting chemicals are lipid soluble, trans-generational transfer can occur via lactation to infants. For wildlife, the aquatic environment provides the greatest opportunity for exposure, and top predators such as fish-eating birds often have the highest body burdens. In certain rivers, evidence of exposure to estrogenic substances (i.e., vittelogenin induction in male fish) has been traced to release of sewage effluent containing active components of birth control pills as a result of excretion by women.

5. Biological Effects of Endocrine Disruptors

Overall, the best evidence of endocrine disruption is found in wildlife living in polluted environments such as the Great Lakes (e.g., reproductive failures and malformations in fish and birds), the Baltic (decreased immune function in seals), and in Florida, Lake Apopka (altered reproductive development in alligators following a chemical spill from a pesticide-manufacturing plant in the early 1980's).

For human health, two principal adverse health outcomes are generally accepted as being caused by endocrine disruption. The first outcome is that of cancers of the uterus (adenocarcinomas) and other reproductive tract anomalies present in women whose mothers received diethylstilbestrol (DES) during pregnancy in an attempt to prevent miscarriage. DES is a potent synthetic estrogen and this therapy was used in the 1950s and 1960s before the effects were detected in the clinical setting. The other outcome of concern is that of neurological disorders in offspring of women exposed to PCBs and related co-pollutants during pregnancy. In this later instance, the mode of action is currently unknown.

A number of other adverse health outcomes (e.g., breast cancer, testes cancer, decreased semen quality) have been attributed to endocrine disruption, but for these there has been no clear association with particular exposures. In laboratory animal studies, clearer pictures of the impact of endocrine-disrupting chemicals are evident.

6. Identification of Endocrine Disruptors

The ultimate way an endocrine disruptor is identified is by inducing in a whole organism a biological response that is known to be controlled by a hormonal system (e.g., acceleration of the rate of transit through puberty in a female exposed to endogenous estrogen).

Traditionally, bioassays such as the uterotrophic assay (which measures an increase in uterine weight in response to an estrogen) and the Hershberger assay (which measures the potential of a chemical to block the supportive effect of androgens on male sex accessory glands) have been used to detect chemicals that interact with the female and male sex hormones. More recently, cellular-based assays have been developed, these assays can indicate the potential of a chemical to act as a hormone (either through endogenous responses such as cell proliferation by estrogen-sensitive cells, or through expression of specific hormone-sensitive reporter genes engineered into cells). Finally, other studies examine the ability of a chemical to bind to the receptor pocket normally used by the endogenous hormone. Because many events can intervene between the binding to a receptor and a biological event, the strength of the evidence that a chemical can be an endocrine disruptor is stronger when in vivo assays for hormonal activity are employed.

In 1996, the U.S. Congress mandated that the U.S. Environmental Protection Agency (EPA) develop and implement a screening program to identify a wide variety of chemicals that could interfere with the function of estrogen, or other hormones as deemed appropriate. The U.S. EPA convened an advisory committee (the Endocrine Disruptor Screening and Testing Advisory Committee, or EDSTAC) to help implement this mandate. The EDSTAC recommended a battery of assays to screen initially for a chemical's potential to affect the function of estrogen, androgen, or thyroid hormones. Depending on results of the screening program, chemicals would enter a testing phase in which multigeneration studies would be conducted in fish, birds, and/or mammals.

These batteries of biological tests are currently being developed and validated for widespread use, and it is anticipated that potentially several thousands of chemicals, including pesticides, pesticidal inert ingredients, and drinking water contaminants, will be evaluated for endocrine activity as the EPA mandate becomes implemented.

7. <u>Significance of Endocrine Disruptors as an Environmental Issue</u>

The general scientific consensus is that, with few exceptions, we simply do not know the extent to which endocrine-disrupting substances present in the general environment are producing any adverse effects in humans. We do know that the normal functioning of the endocrine system is critical for developing and reproduction, and we do know that certain chemicals found in the environment are capable of altering the actions or hormones in at least some test systems. We also know that in certain ecologic situations, where there has been persistent and cumulative contamination by endocrine-disrupting chemicals, that certain species have experienced severe population-level impacts.

What we do not know is whether these chemicals are present in the general human environment at sufficiently high levels, and whether humans come into contact with them in sufficient quantity and during the critical exposure periods, to cause adverse health outcomes. Considerable resources are being devoted to answering these questions in the United States, Canada, the European Union, and Japan. Indeed, the amount of cooperation and coordination in addressing the research needs is unprecedented. One product of this effort is a compilation of an international inventory of research on endocrine disruptors, this is accessible via the internet (http://www.epa/gov/endocrine) and contains nearly 800 individual research projects. Such coordination and focusing of resources is expected to clarify the level of concern over the next few years.

D. PERSISTENT ENVIRONMENTAL CONTAMINANTS

1. <u>Halogenated Dioxins/Furans</u>

a. Definition of Halogenated Dioxins and Furans

Dioxins and furans are related compounds characterized by a similar backbone that varies in the number and position of halogen atom substitutions, as shown in the figure below. Although there are many forms of these compounds, the best known is 2,3,7,8-tetrachlorodibenzo-p-dioxin (TCDD). TCDD is the most potent of this class of chemicals, and as a result the biological activities of the other dioxins and furans are often described relative to that of TCDD. Only a small subset of the total dioxins and furans, however, are thought to induce health effects through the same mechanism of TCDD.

b. Dioxins/Furans and the Environment

Halogenated dioxins and furans are not thought to be naturally occurring, rather they are formed as by-products of various industrial and combustion processes. Potential sources of release to the environment include chlorination processes such as paper bleaching, manufacture of chlorinated organic chemicals, including some pesticides; and combustion of fossil fuels and municipal and hazardous waste. Chlorinated dioxins and furans can also be present in cigarette smoke. Once these compounds are released into the environment they are resistant to being degraded, and thus they tend to be persistent. They are generally hydrophobic and for this reason they can bio-accumulate in the fatty tissues of animals that have ingested contaminated vegetation, soil, or water. The diet, primarily in meat and dairy products, is thought to be the major pathway for chronic low-level exposure in humans.

c. Exposure to Dioxins/Furans and Primary Health Effects

TCDD is noted for the wide array of physiological systems affected. A hallmark symptom of high TCDD exposure in humans is chloracne, a severe skin disease characterized by acne-like lesions. Chloracne has been associated with body burdens of TCDD ranging from 18 to 2357 ng/kg body weight. Erythematous or red skin rashes, discoloration, and excessive body hair have also been reported to occur in people following exposure to high concentrations of TCDD. Mild and reversible alterations in the ability of the liver to metabolize hemoglobin, lipids, sugar, and protein have been reported to occur in people following exposure to high concentrations of TCDD. Other effects have been less consistently reported in people. It is not clear whether TCDD can induce adverse reproductive or developmental effects in humans and the carcinogenicity data for TCDD have provided mixed results, with varying interpretations.

The International Agency for Research on Cancer concluded that TCDD can cause cancer in humans and the U.S. Environmental Protection Agency (EPA) classifies TCDD as a possible human carcinogen. TCDD dosing has been shown to induce adverse effects in many target organs in animal toxicity studies, including a wasting syndrome, thymic atrophy and other immunological effects, and effects on reproduction and development. It should be noted that there is considerable variability in species sensitivity to the effects of TCDD, therefore for many end points the applicability to exposed humans remains unclear.

2. Polychlorinated Biphenyls

a. Definition of Polychlorinated Biphenyls

The polychlorinated biphenyls (PCBs) are a group of 209 different compounds, referred to as congeners, characterized by a similar chemical backbone that varies in the number and position of chlorine atoms. In most cases, PCBs are described based on the toxicity of several PCB mixtures that have been commercially available. These mixtures, called arochlors, are unique mixtures identified by a number indicating the number of carbon atoms per molecule and percentage of chlorine in the mixture. For example, the U.S. EPA has reviewed the toxicity data for the development of human health risk values for arochlors 1016,1248, and 1254.

b. PCBs and the Environment

PCBs are not known to be naturally occurring. They once were manufactured extensively for use as electrical insulators in transformers and capacitors. Although no longer used in these products, PCBs can be released into the environment by leaking from old electrical equipment that still contains PCBs. These compounds can also be generated during the combustion of municipal and industrial waste. Due to their hydrophobic nature, PCBs are resistant to degradation in the environment, where they associate with organic matter in sediment. Similarly to dioxins and furans, PCBs bio-accumulate in the adipose tissues of animals that have ingested contaminated vegetation, soil, or water and in the diet, primarily in meat and dairy products. This is thought to be the major pathway for chronic low level exposure in humans.

c. Primary Health Effects of Exposure to PCBs

Acute exposures to PCBs have been associated with a variety of symptoms in exposed people. These include skin irritation, acne and rashes, neurological effects such as general weakness and numbness, respiratory irritation following exposure by the inhalation route, altered immune function, and liver damage.

Toxicity studies in animals have shown a similar array of effects following acute exposures. In chronic animal exposure studies, PCB treatment administered orally resulted in effects on the liver, stomach, and thyroid gland and decreased reproductive ability. The human evidence is inconclusive regarding the ability of PCBs to cause cancer, but animal studies have reported increased tumor incidence in PCB-treated animals. Based on these data, the U.S. EPA classifies PCBs as probable human carcinogens and the International Agency for Research on Cancer has determined that PCBs may reasonably be anticipated to be human carcinogens.

3. Mercury

a. Introduction

Each year, anywhere from 2700 to 6000 tons of mercury is released into the environment from natural sources, and another 2000 to 3000 tons is contributed by human activities. Three forms of mercury exist, each having different physical and chemical properties, routes of exposure, and health effects.

The first is metallic mercury, or mercury in its elemental form. It appears shiny and silver and is a liquid at room temperature. Mercury vapor is released from the metal in this state. The second form is a group of inorganic mercury compounds, or mercury salts. These are formed when mercury combines with other elements such as oxygen, sulfur, or chlorine. Most exist as powders or crystals. The third form is organic mercury, which is created when mercury combines with carbon-based molecules. The most common organic mercury compound is methyl mercury.

b. Exposure to Inorganic (Metallic and Inorganic) Mercury

Broken thermometers, shattered fluorescent tubes, or damaged electrical switches can expose people to metallic mercury through inhalation of the vapors. Breathing mercury vapors is a concern in closed areas, because 80% of inhaled mercury vapor is absorbed directly into the bloodstream. Swallowing metallic mercury is not as much of a health concern, because the stomach or intestines absorb less than 0.01% of the dose. Dermal contact with the metal can cause rashes.

c. Exposure to Methylmercury

Microorganisms in the water can convert metallic mercury into methylmercury. Methylmercury bioaccumulates, and can be present in significant concentrations in the tissues of organisms near the tops of food chains-shark, swordfish, and large tuna being several examples. Cooking does not appreciably reduce the methylmercury concentration in food. Methylmercury causes fetal methylmercury poisoning, and can be passed in breast milk. Children and fetuses are the most sensitive to exposure.

d. Effects of Mercury Exposure

Mercury impacts the nervous system. Remember the Mad Hatter in Alice in Wonderland? "Mad as a hatter!" is a saying describing milliners who had developed mercury poisoning from their exposure to mercurious nitrate, once used in the manufacture of hats. A variety of symptoms are possible for exposure to the various forms of mercury, and depend on degree of exposure.

Short-term exposure to metallic mercury vapor can irritate and damage the tissue lining the mouth and lungs, causing a burning sensation and tightness of breath. Paresthesia, a numbness and tingling sensation around the fingers, toes, and lips, is usually an early nervous system manifestation of exposure. The next progressive symptom is characterized by a difficulty walking and talking, followed by a constriction of visual fields, and finally tunnel vision and loss of hearing. People may demonstrate nervousness, irritability, shyness, an inability to concentrate, and memory loss. Severe exposures can lead to tremors or jerks. Kidney damage can occur, especially after exposure to toxic concentrations. Coma or death is the end to this progression.

e. Measurement of Exposure to Mercury

Mercury levels in the body can be measured in blood, urine, or hair samples. Breast milk can also be tested for mercury concentrations. Urine samples can indicate exposure to metallic mercury vapor and to inorganic forms of mercury, whereas whole blood and scalp hair mercury concentrations correlate to methylmercury exposure.

f. Health Risk from Mercury in Dental Fillings

Metallic mercury is often present in dental amalgam, which is used in fillings. Although U.S. government evaluations conclude there is no health threat posed to the general population from dental amalgam, there is currently an investigation on the health risks for sensitive populations and the possibility of subtle immune or behavioral effects.

4. Pesticides

a. Definition and Categories of Pesticides

The USEPA defines pesticide as any substance or mixture of substances intended for preventing, destroying, repelling, or mitigating any pest.

There are five broad categories:

The first category is **insecticides**, containing the organochlorine, anticholinesterase, pyrethroid, and botanical insecticides.
The second category is **herbicides,** encompassing the chlorophenoxy compounds and bipyridyl derivatives.
The third category is **fungicides**, grouping hexachlorobenzene, pentachlorophenol, phthalimides, and dithiocarbamates.
The fourth category is **fumigants,** including phosphine and ethylene dibromide / dibromochloropropane.
The final and fifth category is the **rodenticides**, including the zinc phosphide, fluoroacetic acid and derivatives, alpha-naphthyl thiourea (ANTU), and anticoagulants.

b. History of the Use of Pesticides

Pesticides are in use in agriculture, home gardens and lawns, in homes, and in some public places such as parks or airplanes. The most likely population to be exposed to potentially unsafe levels is the occupationally exposed, such as farm-workers or workers in a pesticide manufacturing plant. Exposure can occur by dermal, oral, or inhalation routes. In extreme situations, poisonings can occur. Residues of pesticides have been found on food, such as produce.

5. DDT (P, P' - Dichlorodiphenyltrichloroethane)

a. DDT as Pollutant of Concern in the United States

DDT was recognized to have insecticide properties in the late 1930s and was used extensively in the United States until its ban in 1972. Since that time, levels of DDT in the environment in many parts of the United States have decreased; however, DDT is still used in other parts of the world and atmospheric deposition of DDT represents a source of current contamination. In addition, DDT undergoes a gradual breakdown in the environment to DDE. Therefore contaminated sites can still have significant levels of both DDT and DDE arising from prior pesticide use. Because of its continued international use and environmental persistence, exposure to DDT and DDE can result from consumption of contaminated fish, crops grown in contaminated soil, or imported crops that were sprayed with DDE. Lactational transfer is a pathway for exposure of infants.

b. Ban of DDT

In 1962, Rachel Carson published "Silent Spring," warning the world about the widespread use (or more appropriately, misuse) of pesticides. Subsequently, DDT was shown to interfere with the shell-making capability (reproduction) of avian wildlife, causing a dramatic decrease in the population of many birds, including the American bald eagle. As a result, DDT was banned for use in the United States.

c. Health Effects Associated with DDT and DDE

Similarly to other persistent chlorinated pollutants, DDT has been associated with liver and neurological effects.   The evidence for carcinogenicity is mixed in human epidemiology studies, but based on positive results in animal studies, the U.S. EPA has classified DDE as a probable human carcinogen. A primary effect of concern is the potential adverse reproductive effects of DDT and DDE. Although the human evidence for adverse effects are not conclusive, a variety of adverse effects have been reported in animal toxicology studies.

d. Sport Fish and Possible Health Risk

Many persistent environmental pollutants can bio-accumulate in wildlife that are exposed to contaminated environments.   Based on the recognition that human exposures to pollutants can be significant from eating fish, the U.S. EPA and many state agencies establish fish consumption advisories. Advisories have been established for many bodies of water and are based on levels of pollutants such as mercury, PCBs, dioxins, chlordane, and DDT, among others. Fish consumption advisories are available though the U.S. EPA databases or from state health or environmental agencies.

Although the potential for adverse effects of eating highly contaminated fish is clearly recognized, the trade-off between risk from low levels of these pollutants and the health risk from substituting fish with less healthy dietary alternatives is uncertain and is an area of active research. Current work focuses on development of methods to assess these comparative risks.

E. ASBESTOS AS AN ENVIRONMENTAL HAZARD

1. Definition of Asbestos

Asbestos is a naturally occurring rock that has marketable mineral properties. This rock is being strip mined from the ground in various countries. Canada, South Africa, Russia, China, and Brazil have been able to market this mineral in large quantities to Third-World countries over the past few years. The increase in export of asbestos to Third-World countries was partially the result of a major decline of asbestos products shipped into the United States. This was known as the "ban and phaseout period," which started in the mid- 1970s.

2. Different Types of Asbestos

There are six different mineral types of asbestos. The three most common types are chrysotile, amosite, and crocidolite. The three remaining types of asbestos ate anthophyllite, tremolite, and actinolite.

Chrysotile asbestos has always been the most common type of asbestos used. This mineral is commonly known as the "white" asbestos and has the physical characteristic of flexible silky fibers. It belongs to the serpentine group, with which it is easily associated because of its snake-like, long, curly fibers.

Amosite asbestos is the next most common type of asbestos used. This mineral is commonly known as the "brown" asbestos and has the physical characteristic of brittle fibers. This mineral belongs to the amphibole group, and many people remember this group because they associate the shape of amosite fibers with needles or straight pins.

Crocidolite asbestos is not commonly used but it is known in the European countries. This mineral is commonly known as the "blue" asbestos and has characteristics similar to amosite asbestos.

Anthophyillite, tremolite, and actinolite asbestos minerals are rarely used. These three types of asbestos are confusing because the mineral types can either be in an asbestos fibrous form or non-fibrous form. In fact, the mining industry was able to convince the Occupational Safety and Health Administration (OSHA), which regulates asbestos, to no longer regulate the nonfibrous forms.

3. Use of Asbestos

Asbestos has some interesting physical properties. It is chemically resistant, especially to acids. It does not readily burn. It is a poor conductor of electricity. It is a good heat insulator and because of its fibrous nature, it provides good flexibility, wear, and friction properties.

4. Products that Contain Asbestos

Asbestos has been used in over 3000 building materials. Some of these products are still commercially available today in the United States. Since the signing of the North American Free Trade Agreement, other products containing asbestos have been entering the United States. Existing structures containing asbestos products are single-family dwellings and public, commercial, and industrial facilities. Asbestos can be present on the exterior or interior of boilers and duct systems and in materials used to cover steam pipes and water pipes. Asbestos can be present in cementitious siding, roofing shingles, and ceiling and wall panels; all forms of ceiling tiles; asphalts, adhesives, and felt roof materials; and wallboard or sheetrock and mud joint compound.

It also may be a component of sprayed-on or trowelled-on surface materials on walls or ceilings as decorative coatings for sound-proofing, or for fireproofing metal beams or decking. Asbestos can be present in floor tiles and sheet vinyl floor coverings. Water pipes made of asbestos are used to transport drinking water. Most people associate asbestos with brake pads and clutch plates. Asbestos was so readily available and commonly used that asbestos has even been used in bunsen burners, fume hoods, blankets, gloves, fire-fighting suits, cement-leveling compounds, and packings and gaskets. Asbestos has even been used in certain paints and to repair museum artifacts.

5. Asbestos in the Facility

Before conducting a renovation or demolition activity at a facility it is important to determine whether asbestos-containing materials are present and will be disturbed. In most states, the only individual who can take samples of suspect material is an accredited asbestos inspector. This individual will take representative samples of various suspect materials and submit the samples to a laboratory for analysis. In return, the laboratory will subject the suspect materials to an analytical method used to determine the presence or absence of asbestos. The two most commonly used methods to determine if a sample contains asbestos are the polarized light microscopy (PLM) method and the transmission electron microscopy (TEM) method.

The PLM method is the least expensive method used to determine the presence of asbestos. The method uses an oil dispersion staining process. The lab analyst will subject the suspect material to various dyes and look for certain physical properties. Remember the colors white, brown, and blue? After the lab analyst determines what type of asbestos is present, the next step is to determine the quantity or amount of asbestos present in the sample. This determination is important because existing asbestos regulations define asbestos materials as containing greater than 1% asbestos. The TEM method uses an electron microscope to determine the presence or absence of asbestos. This method can be expensive but is preferred for suspect materials that have a lot of binding materials, which can mask the presence of asbestos fibers when using the standard PLM method. It is recommended that the TEM method be used on complicated materials such as floor tiles, plaster, and roofing products.

6. Exposure to Asbestos

Inhalation is the primary route of exposure. Individuals inhale asbestos fibers when the asbestos materials are disturbed and fibers become airborne. An individual can also ingest asbestos when asbestos-containing materials are swallowed. This exposure can result from renovation or demolition activities. Exposure can also occur when asbestos materials have deteriorated from natural aging. Asbestos-containing materials (ACM) are divided into two categories: friable and nonfriable.

Friable ACM is defined as containing greater than 1% asbestos, which, when dry, can be crumbled with normal hand pressure. Materials such as fireproofing and pipe insulation are examples of friable asbestos.

Nonfriable ACM is defined as containing greater than 1% asbestos, which, when dry, cannot be crumbled with normal hand pressure. Materials such as floor tiles or cementitious shingles are examples of nonfriable asbestos. It is important to remember that even nonfriable asbestos products can become friable if mechanical forces are exerted on the products. Asbestos materials in either condition are considered regulated and come under the requirements of various government agencies.

7. Diseases Associated With Exposure

There are several diseases associated with exposure to asbestos fibers. The diseases associated with asbestos are based on the amount(s) of exposure and the length(s) of exposure. The period of time it takes to develop or show signs of an asbestos-related disease is referred to as the "latency period." The latency period for asbestos-related diseases can range from 10 to 40 years. This is something to keep in mind if children have been exposed to an unknown amount of asbestos fibers.

Asbestosis is the result of scarring of the lungs. This scarring is the result of the body being unable to naturally remove asbestos fibers. It is a progressive disease that leads to shortness of breath and a dry cough. In the more advanced stages, an individual can develop clubbing of the fingers and cardiac distress. There is no effective treatment or cure for this disease.

Lung cancer is responsible for the largest number of deaths associated with asbestos exposures. When an individual develops lung cancer, the person may notice a change in breathing and develop a cough. As the cancer progresses, the individual will notice shortness of breath, possibly chest pains, weight loss, and hemoptysis. There is also a "synergistic" effect associated with exposure to asbestos that dramatically increases the odds of contracting an asbestos-related disease. Studies have shown that smoking and being exposed to asbestos fibers will have a synergistic effect on an individual.

Mesothelioma is a rare form of cancer that occurs in the lining of the lungs of the chest and other pleural surfaces, such as the pericardium and the peritoneum. This disease is almost exclusively associated with asbestos exposure. The good news about this disease is that it is rare. The bad news about this disease is that it is always fatal, and by the time the physician diagnoses the disease, the individual has only a few months to a few years to live.

Pleural diseases have also been known to develop from asbestos exposure. The exposure to asbestos results in the thickening or scarring of the pleural tissues. The disease is usually not fatal but is an indicator of asbestos exposure. Examples of asbestos-related pleural diseases include pleural plaques, pleural effusions, and diffuse pleural thickening.

Other cancers, such as **laryngeal, kidney**, and **gastrointestinal cancers**, have been associated with ingestion of asbestos fibers. These cancers are rare and are usually associated with heavy exposure to asbestos fibers.

Asbestos warts have been shown to develop in individuals who have had asbestos fibers enter the skin tissue, usually on their hands or arms. Individuals have not been known to develop cancer from this type of asbestos exposure.

8. Medical Tests Used To Measure Asbestos Exposure

When an individual has been exposed to an unknown amount of asbestos fibers, it is often after asbestos has been accidentally disturbed. Considering the amount of exposure, the length of exposure, the latency period, and possibly a synergistic effect, it is prudent to consult a medical physician.

A physician will usually recommend that a base-line medical screen be conducted. This would include at least a medical questionnaire, physical examination, chest x-ray, and a pulmonary function test. It is important to remember that this base-line information can be used to detect pre-existing conditions or early signs of lung disease but it cannot tell you if the latest asbestos exposure has caused an asbestos-related illness. Only time can answer this question, along with more extensive evaluation and possibly invasive testing.

9. Precautions To Be Taken Before Disturbing Asbestos

First, determine if any asbestos materials are present. An asbestos survey is usually conducted by an individual who is an accredited inspector. Asbestos that has been identified and is in good condition should be left alone and properly managed. Second, if the asbestos will be disturbed during a renovation or demolition activity, or if the asbestos has already been damaged from previous events, then it will need to be removed by individuals properly trained or accredited by the appropriate state agency to prevent exposure.

10. Asbestos and its Removal

Accredited individuals who remove friable or regulated asbestos should have the necessary training and experience to address asbestos removal. This is not an activity for the novice. Workers and supervisors who remove friable asbestos will wear protective clothing and respirators approved to protect them from asbestos exposures. The location where the asbestos will be removed is isolated from the public and enclosed with a rigid containment. This is to ensure that asbestos fibers do not escape the work area. The asbestos will be continuously wetted down to minimize the concentration of airborne asbestos fibers. The adequately wet asbestos will be collected, placed in leak-tight containers, and properly labeled for disposal at an approved landfill.

After the asbestos has been removed and the area is properly cleaned, an accredited asbestos air monitor will usually conduct a thorough visual inspection of the workplace and take ambient air samples. If the workplace passes visual inspection and the ambient air samples contain asbestos concentrations below the allowable limit set by the appropriate state agency, then the area is acceptable for general occupancy.

11. Action To Take If Asbestos Has Been Disturbed

If asbestos has been accidentally disturbed, immediately isolate the area. Turn off or modify the heating and air-conditioning system to prevent further distribution of asbestos fibers to the area. After the area is secure, contact your local or state environmental protection agency for further assistance.

F. EMERGING DISEASES

1. Introduction

Infectious diseases continue to be the foremost cause of death worldwide. The Centers for Disease Control and Prevention (CDC) reported a 58 percent rise in deaths from infectious diseases since 1980. Although AIDS has been responsible for most of the increase, deaths from other infectious diseases have risen dramatically and according to some studies by as much as 22 percent.

Despite scientific progress and the development of sanitary methods, infectious diseases still cause human suffering and misery, deplete already scarce resources, impede social and economic development and is a contributory factor to global instability. Recent outbreaks underscore the potential and unrelenting danger that these new and emerging diseases bring. The main emerging diseases in the United States are 1) **Cryptosporidium**, 2) **AIDS**, 3) **Escherichia coli**, 4) **Hanta Virus**, 5) **Lyme Disease**, and 6) **Group A Strep.**

2. <u>Emerging Diseases Worldwide</u>

These and other infectious diseases have potential worldwide significance (Figure 4.2). As an example, the possibility of **Dengue fever** reaching the United States is very real. Until 1995, Dengue fever had been isolated in Costa Rica's coastal mountain regions along the Pacific shore. But rising temperatures permitted the mosquitoes responsible for Dengue fever, to break the coastal mountain barriers and invade the rest of the country. By September, the epidemic had infected 140,000 people and claimed the lives of 4,000. Dengue fever, a debilitating tropical disease transmitted by mosquitoes, is re-emerging with such force that it has now reached epidemic proportions in Central America and is bearing down on the United States. Each year 35-60 million people worldwide contract Dengue fever.

The **Ebola virus** grabbed global attention with a flurry of news articles and films as one of the deadliest viruses known, killing nearly 90 percent of those infected. There is no treatment or vaccine. Ebola and other hemorrhagic fever viruses typically start suddenly with malaise, fever, and flu-like symptoms which are often followed with rashes and bleeding along with kidney and liver failure as these organs and other body parts dissolve into mush.

According to the Pan American Health Organization, **Chagas** is the most important parasitic illness in Latin America causing over 40,000 deaths each year. The protozoan disease is transmitted by a beetle known as the kissing bug (**Rhodnius prolixus**) which thrives in dark houses with cracked floors and walls and comes out at night to feed on blood sucked from the face of the human host. The inoculated Trypanosome parasite invades the stomach, heart, and muscles of the human host to produce disabling fatigue, energy loss, and often death.

In the 1990s, epidemic **cholera** reappeared in the Americas after being absent for nearly a century; from 1991 through June of 1994 more than one million cases and nearly 10,000 deaths were reported.

In 1994 an extended period of monsoon season in northern India followed by 3 months of extremely hot weather (100^0F) drove rats into the cities, causing pneumonic plague from **Yersinia pestis** in Surat. The subsequent panic claimed the lives of many people and cost India $2 billion.

Malaria is the world's largest widespread mosquito-borne illness and is potentially the worst threat to humans in the future. Global warming provides an environment for mosquitoes to multiply, migrate, and increase their metabolism, forcing them to feed (bite) more often. Socioeconomic development combined with programs to eradicate malaria have reduced endemic areas, but malaria has seen an increase in many parts of the world despite continued efforts to eradicate it. More than 100 million clinical cases occur annually and more than 1 million people, mostly children, die each year in tropical Africa. Malaria has reemerged as a major international infectious disease with nearly half a billion people worldwide developing the disease each year. Deaths are mainly due to drug resistant strain of malaria. Malaria has also begun to reappear in the United States, and is now re-emerging at a geometric rate in South America.

The World Health Organization (WHO) reported that efforts to control tuberculosis have failed and that drug resistant strains of **Mycobacterium tuberculosis** are rising.

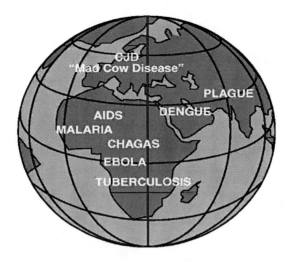

Figure 4.2. Emerging Diseases Worldwide. (Source: Moore, 1999).

Tuberculosis is considered one of the worlds leading infectious diseases and kills over 3 million worldwide each year with many more becoming ill.

3. Definition of an Emerging Infectious Disease

New infections are emerging, and old ones are expanding their geographical range faster than we can deploy resources to stop the organisms responsible. International travel and commerce are increasing, and technology is rapidly changing the conditions that increase the risk of exposure to infectious agents. The spectrum of infectious disease is changing quickly in conjunction with dramatic societal and environmental changes. Worldwide, explosive population growth in developing nations, with expanding poverty and urban migration is contributing to proliferation of both new and old infectious diseases. Once expected to be eliminated as a public health problem, infectious diseases remain the leading cause of death and disability-adjusted life years (DALYs). Some of these diseases may be new to the human species. Others may simply have never been seen in North America before. The term "emerging infectious diseases" is now being applied to this phenomenon, and awareness of these emerging diseases has reached international levels. The term "emerging infectious diseases" refers to diseases of infectious origin whose incidence in humans has either increased within the past two decades or threatens to increase in the near future.

Emerging infectious diseases, often with unknown long-term public health impact, continue to be identified. Table 4.2 lists major diseases or etiologic agents identified just within the last 20 years. New agents are regularly added to the list, particularly with the availability of nucleic acid amplification techniques for detecting and identifying otherwise non-cultivable microorganisms. In many cases, diseases became better recognized or defined (e.g., Legionnaires' disease, Lyme disease, human ehrlichiosis).

Others are completely new. A previously unknown and deadly disease, acquired immunodeficiency syndrome (AIDS), originated from uncertain sources in one part of the world and spread globally at a speed that would have been unthinkable in earlier times.

4. Factors Responsible for the Emergence of Infectious Disease

Factors responsible for the emergence of infectious disease are the following: a. **ecological changes**; b. **human demographic changes**; c. **travel and commerce**; d. **technology and industry (globalization)**; e. **microbial adaptation** and **change (resistance)**; and f. **breakdown of public health measures**.

a. Ecological Changes

(1) Agriculture

Ecological changes are often present when outbreaks of formerly unrecognized diseases occur. These diseases are usually introduced from animal hosts when people are placed in close contact with a host where the disease organism is present. People may expand into an area where the animal host thrives, the animal host may expand into human living areas. Lyme Disease is an example of an ecological change, where the effects of deforestation have increased the population of deer and deer tick, the vector of Lyme Disease. The movement of people into these areas has placed a larger population closer to the vector.

(2) Climate

The earth's climate is becoming a significant factor in facilitating the spread of infectious diseases. According to the World Health Organization (WHO), the temperature of the planet will increase by as much 8 degrees Fahrenheit by the year 2030. This will profoundly affect human health. Global warming enlarges the territories of disease carrying insects and according to the WHO will increase the at-risk population by 620 million by the year 2050. In addition, extreme weather patterns, as a result of natural fluctuations in the atmosphere or man-made changes (i.e., global warming) have routinely been followed by outbreaks of disease (El Niño, Vibrio, Hanta Virus).

b. Human Demographic Changes

Population movements and upheavals caused by migration or war are often responsible for disease emergence. Increased population density in urban areas- migration in hopes of a better, more comfortable lifestyle- has surpassed basic services, including clean water supplies, sanitary conditions such as sewage disposal and adequate housing.

Public health measures in overcrowded cities are often strained or unavailable to large groups of the urban impoverished living in inner city slums or in shanty-towns on the periphery, thereby increasing the opportunity for emerging infections such as HIV, cholera, and dengue.

Table 4.2. Major New and Re-emerging Etiologic Agents of Infectious Diseases and the Reason for their Emergence. (Source: Moore, 1999).

VIRAL

Viral Diseases that have been identified since 1973*

1977 Ebola, Marburg
Origin undetermined (importation of monkeys associated with outbreaks in these primates in Europe and the United States).
1980 HTLV Influenza (pandemic)
Pig-duck agriculture thought to contribute to reassortment of avian and mammalian influenza viruses.
1983 HIV
Transmission by intimate contact as in sexual transmission, contaminated hypodermic needles, transfusions, organ transplants. Contributing conditions that spread the disease include war or civil conflict, urban decay, migration to cities, and travel.
1989 Hepatitis C
Transmission in infected blood such as by transfusions, contaminated hypodermic needles, and sexual transmission.
1993 Hantaviruses
Increased contact with rodent hosts because of ecological or environmental changes.

Viral Diseases that have re-emerged

Argentine, Bolivian hemorragic fever
Agricultural changes that promote growth of rodents.
Bovine spongiform encephalopathy (cattle)
Alterations in the rendering of meat products.
Dengue, dengue hemorrhagic fever
Travel, transportation, urbanization, and migration.
Lassa fever
Conditions such as urbanization that favor rodent host, increasing exposure (usually in homes).
Rift Valley fever
Irrigation dam building, agriculture: possibly change in virulence.
Yellow fever
Conditions favoring mosquito vector (in "new" areas).

BACTERIAL

Bacterial Diseases that have been identified since 1973*

1977 Legionella disease
Cooling and plumbing systems that allow the organism to grow in biofilms that form on water
1982 Hemolytic uremic syndrome (Escherichia coli – 0157:H7)
Modern food processing on a large scale permitting contamination through meat storage tanks and unsterile plumbing.
1982 Lyme borreliosis (Borrelia burgdorferi)
Close contact between homeowners encroaching on forested areas and the mice and deer (a secondary reservoir host) that maintain the tick vector for Borrelia.
1983 Helicobacter pylori
Newly recognized as agent involved with gastric ulcers, probably widespread before recognition.
1987 Toxic shock syndrome (Staphylococcus aureus)
Ultra-absorbency tampons.
1992 Cholera (type 0139)
Likely introduced from Asia to South America by ship, with spread made possible by reduced water chlorination; Strain (type 0139) from Asia newly spread by travel (similarly to past introductions of classic cholera).

Bacterial Diseases that have re-emerged

Tuberculosis
Breakdown in Public Health measures such as reduction in prevention programs, inadequate sanitation, homelessness, AIDS.
Streptococcus, group A (invasive necrotizing)
Unknown, may be increased use of NAIDS.

PARASITES

Parasitic Diseases that have been identified since 1973*

1976 Cryptosporidium, other waterborne pathogens
Contaminated surface water, lack of proper filtration methods.

Parasitic Diseases that have re-emerged

Malaria (in "new" areas)
Spread of mosquito vectors, worldwide travel or migration, "Airport" malaria.
Schistosomiasis
Agriculture, dam building, deforestation, flood/drought, famine, climate changes.

---

*Compiled by CDC staff. Dates of discovery are assigned on the basis of the year the isolation or identification of etiologic agents was reported.

Table 4.2. Continued.

c. Travel and Commerce

Increased economic growth into national and international boundaries has led to increased travel, contributing to the notion of "diseases without boundaries." The incubation period for infectious diseases can range from a period of hours up to weeks. As a consequence, the potential to spread diseases from one country or continent to another is possible within a matter of hours. The following four diseases are often spread through travel and commerce: 1) **Bubonic Plague**, 2) **Smallpox**, 3) **Aedes aegypti**, 4) **Vibrio cholerae**.

d. Technology and Industrialization (Globalization)

Globalization is defined as the process of denationalization of markets, laws, and politics in the sense of interlacing peoples and individuals for the sake of the common good. Globalization is influencing public health in three ways:

1. First, the diseases are moving rapidly around the globe because of technology and economic interdependence which has increased international travel and the international nature of food processing and handling
2. The funding of public health programs has been reduced because of increased competition in the global market and increased pressures to cut expenditures.
3. Public health programs have become international through WHO and health-related nongovernmental organizations.

These successes have contributed to a population crisis, producing overcrowding, inadequate sanitation, and overstretched public health infrastructures.

e. Microbial Adaptation and Change (Resistance)

Antibiotic-resistant bacteria are emerging from the environment in response to the wide distribution of anti-microbials. Selection for antibiotic-resistant bacteria, and drug-resistant parasites have become common, generated by the wide and often unsuitable use of anti-microbial drugs.

There is growing concern that bacterial pathogens are developing a resistance to antibiotics as a result of patients not completing the prescribed course of treatment or the inappropriate and over prescribing of common antibiotics by physicians. The use of unsupervised prophylactic tetracycline administration to 100,000 pilgrims en route to Mecca from Indonesia is thought to have been significantly responsible for the fact that 50% of cholera strains in that country are now tetracycline resistant. It took fifteen years for widespread penicillin resistance to be reported to **N. gonorrhoea**. Many hospitals consider Vancomycin and Rocephin their "big guns" in the disease war. A recent report by the CDC found that Vancomycin resistance measured at 0.3% in 1986, rose to 7.9% across several facilities in 1994. Antibiotics have no effect on viruses, and vaccines are often ineffective against bacterial infections.

f. Breakdown of Public Health Measures

During the eighteenth and nineteenth centuries advancements in public health vastly improved the overall health of the populace, particularly in urban settings. Vector control, chlorination of water, pasteurization of milk, immunization, and proper sewage disposal are classical public health and sanitation measures that have successfully minimized the spread of infectious diseases in humans.

Well-understood and recognized diseases such as cholera are rapidly increasing because once active public health measures have lapsed. This apparent retrogression is apparent in both developing countries and inner cities of the industrialized world. One such example is the rapidly expanding cholera outbreak in South America which has been the result of reductions in chlorine levels used to treat the water supplies. Cholera follows the fecal oral route of transmission and is frequently promoted by the lack of reliable water supplies.

5. Specific Emerging Diseases

a. Viruses

The viruses with the greatest potential for emergence in the near future include: **hantaan (hantavirus)**, **dengue**, **influenza**, **ebola** and **HIV**.

(1) Hantavirus

Hantavirus outbreak was first called "Navajo Flu" by the media. CDC personnel trapped and tested rodents from the first suspected area, they found the deer mouse, **Peromyscus maniculatis** as the primary reservoir in New Mexico.

The hantaviruses that emerged in the Four Corners region of the United States were determined to be the cause of an acute respiratory disease now termed hantavirus pulmonary syndrome (HPS). Initial symptoms of the American version (HPS) were flu-like and manifested as fever, chills, headache, muscular aches and pains. With time the lungs fill with fluids causing severe respiratory distress for which there is no specific treatment. The virus is spread to humans from contact with rodents. The most common route of transmission to humans is by aerosolized mouse droppings containing the virus particles, although there is evidence that bites may also transmit the disease.

It is now established that hantaviruses can be carried by at least 16 various rodent species including rats, mice, and voles. Investigations have linked virus exposure to such activities as heavy farm work, threshing, sleeping on the ground, and military exercises.

(2) Dengue Fever

There are in excess of tens of million cases of dengue fever annually, with several hundred thousand cases of the more severe dengue hemorrhagic fever (DHF). There are four antigenically distinct viral serotypes. There is no cross-protective immunity with any of the viruses, so that it is possible for a person to acquire multiple dengue infections. Dengue is primarily an urban tropical disease with severe flu-like symptoms that causes high fevers, frontal headache, severe body aches and pains, nausea and vomiting. When the fever eases, patients start to develop "leaky capillary syndrome" in which the blood vessels leak and untreated patients will go into shock and die. The greatest emerging health menace from dengue/DHF has been in Central and South America. Complacency in mosquito control programs has allowed *Aedes aegypti* to return with a vengeance and it is a competent vector for dengue viruses.

(3) Influenza

Types A and B are responsible for the epidemics of respiratory influenza. Type C produces very mild symptoms or none at all. Influenza is normally characterized by a fever (100 °F to 103 °F); respiratory symptoms, that include cough, sore throat, stuffy nose; muscle aches and pain; and extreme fatigue. There are about 20,000 deaths annually in the United States with the majority of serious illness and death occurring in the aged, very young, and debilitated. To this date, there have been more than 30 pandemics of influenza with three occurring within the last 80 years. The **Spanish Flu** (1918-19) caused an estimated 500,000 deaths in the United States and 20 million deaths worldwide.

(4) Ebola

Ebola and Marburg viruses belong to a family of viruses called Filoviridae. Their extreme pathogenicity combined with the lack of effective vaccines or antiviral drugs classify them as biosafety level four agents.

Ebola fever typically starts suddenly 4 to 16 days after infection with malaise, fever and flu-like symptoms, which can be followed by rashes, bleeding and kidney and liver failure. Generalized bleeding occurs with massive internal hemorrhaging of the internal organs, with bleeding into the gastrointestinal tract, from the skin, and even from injection sites as the clotting ability of the blood is diminished. The death of the patient usually occurs from shock within 7 to 16 days and is accompanied by extreme blood loss.

Infections from Ebola virus were first reported in 1976 when two outbreaks occurred at the same time but in different locations and with different subtypes of the Ebola virus: Sudan and Congo. The total number of cases in these two outbreaks was 550 with 340 deaths. The case fatality rate from the Congo subtype Ebola virus was 90 percent and case fatality rate for the Sudan subtype was 50 percent.

(5) AIDS/HIV

The AIDS virus belongs to a special group of viruses known as retroviruses and is referred to as human immunodeficiency virus (HIV). The AIDS virus almost exclusively focuses on the white blood cells since the helper T cells have CD4 molecules on the surface to which the AIDS virus binds. The viral genetic information is then able to enter the cell and is transferred to the nucleus. HIV is transmitted most commonly by sexual contact with an infected partner and can enter the body through the vaginal lining, vulva, penis, rectum or mouth. Since the virus appears in the blood and many body fluids, it can be transmitted by infected blood as through contaminated needles. HIV has been transmitted to fetuses during pregnancy and birth. Many people remain asymptomatic for months or years after acquiring the infection.

Symptoms may emerge that include prolonged enlargement of lymph nodes, energy and weight loss, recurrent sweating and fevers, skin rashes, or flaky skin, yeast infections, and pelvic inflammatory disease. The disease will often advance to a stage referred to as AIDS or acquired immunodeficiency syndrome. Opportunistic infections produce a myriad of debilitating symptoms from respiratory distress, severe headaches, extreme fatigue, nausea, vomiting, to wasting and coma. A joint surveillance effort by UNAIDS and WHO now estimates that over 30 million people are living with HIV infection at the end of 1997. This figure also includes over 1 million children under the age of fifteen. More than two-thirds of the total number of people in the world living with HIV are from sub-Saharan Africa (Figure 4.3).

b. Bacteria

(1) Escherichia coli

Gram negative, facultatively anaerobic, short straight rods that characteristically inhabit the intestines of humans and other animals and belong to the family Enterobacteriaceae. Members of the enterics cause gastroenteritis, mostly, but have also been implicated in urinary tract infections, wound infections, pneumonia, septicemia, and meningitis. The strains of **E. coli** capable of causing hemorrhagic colitis are referred to as Enterohemorrhagic **Escherichia coli** (EHEC). **Escherichia coli** 0157:H7 is pathogenic for humans and has characteristically produced bloody diarrhea with abdominal cramps; sometimes the infection causes nonbloody diarrhea with very few symptoms.

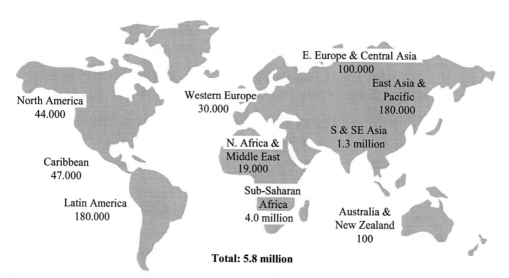

Total: 5.8 million

<u>Figure 4.3.</u> Distribution of HIV Infected Persons Globally for 1997. (Source: Moore, 1999).

Children under 5 years of age and the elderly, the infection may progress into a more severe and life-threatening form of the disease known as hemolytic uremic syndrome (HUS). In the United States, HUS is the leading cause of acute kidney failure in children.

The majority of infections with serotype O157:H7 have come from eating undercooked beef products, but many other sources of infection have been identified. In 1993 a foodborne outbreak of serotype O157:H7 was linked to the undercooked hamburgers eaten at a fast-food chain restaurant. The outbreak involved the infection of 700 persons from 4 different states with 51 of these persons developing HUS and four people dying from the syndrome.

(2) Lyme Disease

Lyme disease is caused by the spirochete **Borrelia burgdorferi**, a gram negative, slender, flexible bacteria that is helically coiled. The organism is anaerobic and fermentative in its energy metabolism and it is spread to humans by the bite of ticks of the genus Ixodes. Lyme disease was first reported in 1975 near Lyme, Connecticut, following a mysterious outbreak of arthritis. The early stages of Lyme disease are characterized by headache, fever, chills, swollen lymph glands, muscle and joint pain, and a characteristic skin rash (erythema migrans). Lyme disease rarely results in death but chronic Lyme disease can lead to permanent damage to joints or the nervous system. Prevention is best accomplished by avoiding tick-infested areas in the summer periods. Spraying with DEET on exposed skin surfaces other than the face will also be helpful.

(3) Streptococcus

Streptococci are gram positive cocci (spheres) arranged in chains or in pairs. The major pathogens are included in groups A and B, and their pathogenicity is associated with certain enzymes and surface proteins including hemolysins, erythrogenic toxins, and M-protein. Hemolysins are enzymes capable of breaking or lysing blood cells. The streptococci may produce a broad of array of enzymes including neuraminidases, hyaluronidases, streptokinases, ATPases, DNAses, and many others that participate in the destruction and invasion of human tissue.

The Group A Streptococci produce a variety of diseases that include strep throat, impetigo, and scarlet fever. The more severe of these invasions results in necrotizing fasciitis and / or streptococcal toxic shock syndrome. Streptococcal toxic-shock syndrome (strep TSS) is defined as any Group A streptococcal infection associated with the early onset of shock and organ failure. Beginning in the 1980s there has been a sudden elevation in the reporting of a highly invasive group A streptococci infection with or without necrotizing fasciitis associated with shock and organ failure. The mortality rate for streptococcal TSS is about 60 percent of the 2,000 to 3,000 cases reported per year. Annually, about 20 percent of the 500-1,500 patients who acquire Streptococcal fasciitis have died.

(4) Tuberculosis

Tuberculosis (TB) is a chronic infectious disease of the lower respiratory tract caused by **Mycobacterium tuberculosis**, a slender, acid-fast rod with cell walls containing high lipid levels. The slow growing bacilli are transmitted by aerosols from persons with active disease. Symptoms normally begin to develop at this stage from a cell mediated immunity that walls off the pathogen within multinucleated giant cells surrounded by lymphocytes and macrophages. Tuberculosis kills over 3 million people worldwide each year, and many more become ill from it. Tuberculosis was declared a U.S. public health emergency in 1992. WHO estimates that the 1990's will see 90 million new cases and 30 million deaths with annual rates in infection in developing countries exceeding 2 percent.

c. Parasites

(1) Cryptosporidium

Cryptosporidium is a single celled microscopic protozoan parasite that belongs to the Class Sporozoa. The resistant form of the parasite is called an oocyst which is characterized by an outer protective shell which protects the organism against environmental extremes such as heat, cold, dryness, and chemical insult. It is estimated that as few as 30 or even one oocyst(s) may cause infection when swallowed. Cryptosporidium is resistant to chlorine and difficult to filter thereby making it a serious threat to water supplies.

The ingested oocysts reach the upper small bowel where they excyst and produce four infectious sporozoites that attach to the surface epithelium of the digestive tract and reproduce, forming more oocysts and sporozoites. The symptoms are self-limiting, and include watery diarrhea, stomach cramps, nausea, and a slight fever. The immunocompromised are at increased risk from infection, and may develop serious and life-threatening illness from this organism. There have been five major outbreaks associated with public water supplies of Cryptosporidium gastroenteritis in the USA and seven in the UK since 1983. Contamination of drinking water by Cryptosporidium is a growing concern especially after the outbreak in Milwaukee in 1993 which affected some 400,000 people. Cryptosporidium is found in animal droppings and human feces, soil, drinking water and recreational water, food, hands, and surfaces contaminated by such wastes.

(2) Malaria

Malarial diseases are caused by protozoan parasites belonging to the genus Plasmodium. There are four species known to infest humans and they are: **P. falciparum, P. vivax, P. ovale,** and **P. malariae**. These parasites are transmitted from human to human by the bite of a female anophelene mosquito in which the parasite has gone through a complex development cycle.

A complex cycle takes place that involves the union of the gametocytes in the stomach of the mosquito and results in the development of slender, microscopic sporozoites that appear in the salivary glands, and are infective for humans. Inside the cell, the parasite form the classical signet ring stage and feed on the cells contents as they grow through the stages of trophozoites, and schizonts. The symptomology and pathogenesis of malaria infection is related to the parasite's stage of growth and the host's parasitemia. High parasitemias result in decreased hemoglobin and a lower oxygen carrying capacity. Untreated infections lead to splenomegaly (enlarged spleen) and particularly in falciparum to cerebral malaria and death. The World Health Organization (WHO) estimates that there are 300 to 500 million people worldwide infected with malaria. The majority of malarial transmission occurs in tropical and subtropical countries. The re-emergence of the disease is due to the following: 1) decreased spraying of homes with DDT, 2) drug resistant malaria, 3) global warming. There have been 76 cases of malaria reported from 1957 through 1994 including the three outbreaks occurring in the densely populated areas of New Jersey (1991), New York (1993) and Texas (1994).

d. Practical Approaches to Limiting the Emergence of Infectious Disease

The emergence of 29 new infectious diseases and re-emergence of many others are creating national and international crises. A Prevention Strategy Plan for the United States was developed with four major goals:
1. Promptly investigate and monitor emerging pathogens, the diseases they cause, and factors of emergence;
2. Integrate laboratory science and epidemiology to optimize public health practice;
3. Enhance communication of public health information about emerging diseases and ensure prompt implementation prevention strategies; and
4. Strengthen local, state, and federal public health infrastructures to support surveillance and implement prevention and control programs.

G. PSYCHOSOCIAL HAZARDS - HEALTH EFFECTS OF STRESS

The modern perception of stress is that it is a negative or adverse reaction. The evolutionary perspective is different, in that stress is considered to be an important mechanism to prepare the human organism for urgent action, both physically and mentally. The physiological characteristics of stress reaction include increases in heart rate, blood pressure, respiration, and blood transport to skeletal muscles and a simultaneous decrease in digestive activity. Increased production of stress hormones, such as epinephrine and cortisol, also play an important role in this reaction. All of these reactions prepare the individual for defensive actions - attack or flight. They thus improve the individual's chance of survival and can influence the success of a given species.

If an individual is continuously exposed to environmental stressors and has no adequate coping strategies, adverse health effects are a likely outcome. Cardiovascular diseases such as arterial hypertension and ischemic heart disease may be associated with stress. Other medical conditions such as peptic ulcer disease, bronchial asthma, and rheumatoid arthritis are influenced by psychological factors, although the prevalence of these diseases is less than that of cardiovascular diseases.

Attempts have been made to identify physiological stress indicators such as screening measurements (ratio of epinephrine to norepinephrine in urine or blood) and screening measurements of the ratio of potassium to sodium in urine or the levels of lipoproteins (cholesterol and triglyceride) in blood.

V. BIBLIOGRAPHY

Barnhart, S. (1994). Irritant Bronchitis. In Rosenstock, L. & Cullen, M. (Eds). Textbook of Clinical Occupational and Environmental Medicine (pp.224-232). Philadelphia, PA: W.B. Saunders Company.

Chan-Yeung, M. (1994). Asthma. In Rosenstock, L. & Cullen, M. (Eds). Textbook of Clinical Occupational and Environmental Medicine (pp.197-209). Philadelphia, PA: W.B. Saunders Company.

Dellinger, J.W. (2001). Asbestos as an Environmental Hazard. In Williams, L.K., Langley, R.L. (Eds) Environmental Health Secrets (pp. 197-200). Philadelphia, PA: Hanley & Belfus, Inc.

Frumkin, H. (1994). Occupational Cancers. In McCunney, R.J. (Ed). A Practical Approach to Occupational and Environmental Medicine 2nd Edition (pp.187-198). Boston, MA: Little, Brown and Company.

Greaves, I.A. (1994). Occupational Pulmonary Disease. In McCunney, R.J. (Ed). A Practical Approach to Occupational and Environmental Medicine 2nd Edition (pp.145-165). Boston, MA: Little, Brown and Company.

Jameson, C.W. (2001). Environmental Carcinogens. In Williams, L.K., Langley, R.L. (Eds). Environmental Health Secrets (pp. 106-109). Philadelphia, PA: Hanley & Belfus, Inc.

Kavlock, R.J. (2001). Environmental Endocrine Disruptors. In Williams, L.K., Langley, R.L. (Eds) Environmental Health Secrets (pp. 116-120). Philadelphia, PA: Hanley & Belfus, Inc.

McArleton, C., Maier, A., & Poirier, K.A. (2001). Persistent Environmental Contaminants. In Williams, L.K., Langley, R.L. (Eds) Environmental Health Secrets (pp. 121-126). Philadelphia, PA: Hanley & Belfus, Inc.

Moore, G.S. (1999). Living with the Earth: Concepts in Environmental Health Science (pp. 4.1 - 4.41 & 7.1 - 7.52). Boca Raton, FL: Lewis Publishers.

Nadakavukaren, A. (2000). Our Global Environment: A Health Perspective 5th Edition (pp.187-224). IL: Waveland Press, Inc.

Petsonk, E.L. & Attfield, M.D. (1994). Coal Workers' Pneumoconiosis and Other Coal-Related Lung Disease. In Rosenstock, L. & Cullen, M. (Eds). Textbook of Clinical Occupational and Environmental Medicine (pp.274-287). Philadelphia, PA: W.B. Saunders Company.

Rosenstock, L. (1994). Asbestosis and Asbestos-Related Pleural Disease. In Rosenstock, L. & Cullen, M. (Eds). Textbook of Clinical Occupational and Environmental Medicine (pp.254-274). Philadelphia, PA: W.B. Saunders Company.

Ruttenber, A.J. & Kimbrough, R.D. (1995). The Pathophysiology of Environmental Diseases. In Blumenthal, D.S. & Ruttenber, A.J. (Eds). Introduction to Environmental Health (pp.35-67). New York, NY: Springer Publishing Company.

Ruttenber, A.J. & Ragsdale, H.L. (1995). The Ecologic Basis of Health and Disease. In Blumenthal, D.S. & Ruttenber, A.J. (Eds). Introduction to Environmental Health (pp.3-33). New York, NY: Springer Publishing Company.

Schachter, E.N. (1994). Byssinosis and Other Textile Dust-Related Lung Diseases. In Rosenstock, L. & Cullen, M. (Eds). Textbook of Clinical Occupational and Environmental Medicine (pp.209-224). Philadelphia, PA: W.B. Saunders Company.

Schwartz, D.A. (1994). Acute Inhalational Injury. In Rosenstock, L. & Cullen, M. (Eds). Textbook of Clinical Occupational and Environmental Medicine (pp.232-254). Philadelphia, PA: W.B. Saunders Company.

Wakeman, M.A. & Lockey, J.E. (1994). Other Pneumoconioses. In Rosenstock, L. & Cullen, M. (Eds). Textbook of Clinical Occupational and Environmental Medicine (pp.287-296). Philadelphia, PA: W.B. Saunders Company.

CHAPTER

5

LAW

I. <u>INTRODUCTION</u>

The governmental system in a democratic society performs two distinct functions. It provides a foundation for debate on issues and a vehicle for the solution of problems. It also provides a service and regulatory function, since the individual in a complex society cannot provide for all of his or her needs. These needs include adequate police, fire, and health protection. For the society to operate properly, the individual or group must adhere to rules and regulations formulated and enforced by the elected government.

According to the U.S. Constitution and Amendments thereto, federal powers include the control of interstate and foreign commerce, conduct of foreign policy, and national defense. The federal government cannot levy direct taxes, other than income taxes, except in proportion to the population of the states, and they cannot abridge civil rights. The state is sovereign. The powers not delegated to the federal government or prohibited by the constitution are reserved for the states or the people. The state's powers include the administration of elections, the establishment and operation of local government, education, intrastate commerce, the creation of corporations, police force, and the promotion of health, safety, and welfare. Although the federal government cannot dictate organization and administration of programs, or the establishment of policy, it has gained some control via its use of funds. In order for a state to receive federal funds, it must adhere to certain requirements established by the federal government for the use of these funds. These requirements include preparation and submission of plans, approval of plans by a central federal agency, the establishment of necessary state agencies, provision for matching state funds, and the supervision and auditing of state programs by the appropriate federal agencies.

Public policy is a result of the interaction of groups and individuals. The formulated policy is not necessarily ideal for the public. Major pressure groups - including business, industry, agriculture, labor, medicine, and religion, try to influence the legislature to pass laws beneficial to their own self-interest. These groups also pressure administrative agencies to make or change decisions on policies that are not in the best interest of the public. These groups compete with each other for public support. They use sizable sums of money to influence opinions on legislation. Citizens groups properly educated and stimulated by trained professional public health workers could use the techniques of the pressure groups to establish public policy that would be beneficial to the citizens and would improve the environment.

The state is divided into local government, including counties, townships, villages, cities, and boroughs. Local government functions may include all the functions of the state government, such as the powers of taxation, establishment of budgets, licensing, and the administration of health, safety, and environmental programs. The local government is expected to deliver quality service and to protect the public. It should prevent the duplication of efforts, budgets, and facilities of the state government. The environmentalist must recognize that although concern for the environment is foremost in his or her mind, the county commissioners or township supervisors may be more concerned with other programs, such as road building, recreational facilities, police and fire service, etc. The environmentalist has to compete for budget monies with each of the other operating departments.

State and local governments obtain their funds for operation from taxes levied on sales, automobile licensing, gasoline, corporations, personal income, alcohol and tobacco, gross receipts, property, and establishment licensing. In many cases, tax rates become oppressive and yet income derived from taxes is inadequate to properly finance the necessary programs for the community. Then it becomes necessary for the federal government to supply funds; in this way, the federal government exercises control in some states even at the township level.

II. <u>THE MAKING OF A LAW</u>

The average time for an environmental law to be passed at the federal level may take several years. Every federal law starts as a bill and passes through a complex system of checks and balances in the Congress originally created by the framers of the constitution as a way of dispersing power and preventing tyrants from abusing that power. The bill is first introduced into the House, and if it is passed, it goes to the Senate. These bills are then forwarded by the leadership to a standing committee (subcommittee) for review and support. Nearly 90 percent of bills never make it through this process. Recommended bills are brought forward through hearings for comments and opinions. The committee then meets to mark up (discuss and amend) the bill and to vote on it. If the subcommittee and the parent committee in the Senate vote favorably for the bill, it is sent (reported) to the full chamber for debate and a vote. Before a bill is sent to the House, it goes first to the Rules committee where a time limit is set for debate and it also indicates whether floor amendments are allowed. This is not so in the Senate where riders are often attached to popular bills that may have no relationship to the original bill, but often are passed along with it, forcing the president to accept it or veto the entire bill.

If both the Senate and the House pass a bill with some differences (as is usually the case), then they go to a conference committee to resolve these differences. Should these differences be resolved, and the same version approved by both House and Senate, the bill moves forward to the President who may sign it into law or veto it. Although Congress may override a veto by a two-thirds majority vote in each chamber, it is very difficult to do so.

Virtually all of the environmental laws require some form of compliance that falls within one or more of the following areas:

1. Notification requirements
2. Discharge or waste controls
3. Process controls and pollution prevention
4. Product controls
5. Regulation of activities
6. Safe transportation requirements
7. Response and remediation requirements, and
8. Compensation requirements.

Notification requirements are meant to deal with any intended or accidental releases of pollutants or hazardous wastes that need to be immediately reported to local and state and/or federal authorities. Failure to do so can significantly impact the environment, endanger public health, and cause significant liability to the persons associated with the release. **Discharge or waste controls** are regulations designed to prevent or minimize the discharge, release, or disposal of wastes and pollutants into the environment. **Process controls and pollution prevention** are regulations that promote minimizing waste generation, reducing the quantities produced and released, and preventing the release or discharge of pollutants into the environment. **Product controls** can reduce the generation and disposal of solid waste by altering the design or packaging of a product, along with the process by which it may be produced. Some regulations promote the use of less hazardous materials and reduced packaging to achieve these goals. The **regulation of activities** that threaten the natural habitat, fragile ecosystems, and vital resources may be necessary to provide protection for resources, endangered species, or habitat. Some of those activities include mining, harvesting of lumber, oil refining, and construction. **Safe transportation requirements** recognize that accidents and spills along our highways occur at an enormous rate, and laws have been established to reduce the risks associated with the transport of hazardous materials. These laws provide for special packaging, labeling, placarding, operator training, and methods of response. **Response and remediation laws** have been promulgated that regulate the cleanup of pollutants and hazardous wastes released to the environment. Laws such as CERCLA have specific provisions for the payment of cleanup costs. These same laws provide for **compensation requirements** requiring responsible parties to pay for cleanup costs for damages done to the health or environment of the private sector. Compensation for damages done to public assets may be recovered by representatives of the "public interest."

III. ENVIRONMENTAL LAWS AS PART OF A SYSTEM

Environmental law is more than a collection of unrelated regulations, it is a system of statutes, regulations, executive orders, factual conclusions, case specific interpretations, and accepted environmental principles that have evolved into "Environmental Law." Understanding the unifying principles of this law system is both a challenge and the key to understanding its complexity. Environmental law is a system that uses all of the laws in our legal system to minimize, prevent, punish or remedy the consequences of actions that damage or threaten the environment and public health and safety. Environmental law encompasses all the environmental protections that originate from: United States Constitution and state constitutions;

1. Federal, state, and local statutes;
2. Regulations published by federal, state and local agencies;
3. Presidential executive orders;
4. Court decisions interpreting these laws and regulations; and
5. Common law.

The system of environmental law includes federal statutes, executive orders, state laws, tax laws, local and municipal laws, business and regulatory law, environmental law and judicial decisions, common law, and torts.

Federal statutes include such regulations as the Clean Air Act or Clean Water Act, that establish federal and state regulatory programs which allow states to enact and enforce laws that meet federal minimum standards and to achieve the regulatory objectives established by Congress. Most states have taken over regulatory programs as allowed under federal regulations, and are often more stringent than the federal counterpart. These states are subject to federal intervention only when they fail to enforce the regulations. **Executive orders** are issued by the president and require federal facilities to provide leadership in protecting the environment and to comply with federal statutes and policies regarding the protection of the environment. They were first used in 1970 and include more than 18 executive orders including such areas as federal compliance with Right-To-Know laws and pollution prevention requirements, to federal actions that address environmental justice in minority populations and low-income populations.

Tax laws are being used to create incentives for environmentally safe products and activities, and disincentives against environmentally detrimental products and activities. Among the approaches which have been adopted or seriously considered are recycling tax credits, taxes on use of virgin materials, taxes on hazardous waste generation and excise taxes on various products. Many state attorney generals use their business regulatory authorities to control environmental claims made for products. Full disclosure of environmental liabilities in statements and reports has been required by the Securities and Exchange Commission for some time. **Local and municipal laws** include zoning and noise control ordinances, nuisance laws, air emission requirements, landfill restrictions or closures, local emergency planning, and product recycling incentives. These are not trivial ordinances and regulations and must be incorporated into any compliance program. Such laws have been effectively used to control the operation and location of facilities. Court interpretations of these laws and regulations are dynamic and changing, and therefore, judicial decisions have important impacts on the manner in which environmental laws are applied. The environmental system of laws also incorporates **common law**, which is a body of rules and principles that pertain to the government and the security of persons and property. These basic rules were originally developed in England and were then brought to the American colonies. After the American Revolution, these basic rules were formally adopted and enforced by the states.

Civil suits, in which the plaintiff seeks to remedy a violation of his rights, are common law actions. Under common law, **"tort"** is a private wrong or wrongful act for which the injured party can bring forth a civil action. There is a general legal duty and responsibility to avoid causing harm to others, by acts of omission or commission. When a person's rights have been violated by acts of carelessness, the injured party may seek compensation or restitution by means of a lawsuit.

The 1990s have been called the era of "toxic torts" due to the filing of tens of thousands of lawsuits involving asbestos and toxic chemical litigation cases. The three most common types of torts encountered in environmental law include:

1. **Nuisance:** Generally, a person may use his land or personal property as he sees fit with the limitation that the owner use his property in a reasonable manner Whenever a

person uses his property to cause material injury or annoyance to his neighbor, his actions constitute a nuisance.

2. **Trespass:** An invasion of another's rights is the general definition of trespass. A more limiting definition of trespass is an injury to the person, property or rights of another immediately resulting from an unlawful act. Unlawful intent is not necessary to constitute trespass.

3. **Negligence:** This is the portion of the tort law that deals with acts not intended to inflict injury. A case becomes one of criminal law if an intent to inflict injury exists. The degree of care and caution that would be taken or used by an ordinary person in similar circumstances is defined as the standard of care required by law in negligence cases. A defendant is liable if his actions cause injury, and without those actions the end result would not have happened. This involves a natural and continuous sequence of actions, unbroken by intervention. Persons harmed by the careless and improper handling or disposal of hazardous wastes can file suit to recover damages for their losses even if there has been full compliance with all government regulations and permit conditions.

IV. <u>BACKGROUND</u>

Laws providing for protection of the environment date back to the late 1800s. However, modern U.S. environmental law had its birth with the enactment of the National Environmental Policy Act (**NEPA**) in 1969. This law declared that it was national policy to:

1. Encourage productive and enjoyable harmony between people and their environment and the biosphere and stimulate the health and welfare of man,
2. Promote efforts that will prevent or eliminate damage to the environment and biosphere and stimulate health and welfare of man, and
3. Enrich our understanding of ecological systems and natural resources important to the nation.

In enacting this legislation, Congress recognized the profound impact of human activities, particularly of population growth, high-density urbanization, industrial expansion, resource exploitation, and new and expanding technological advances - on the interrelation of all components of the natural environment.

The basic goal of the NEPA was to administer federal programs in the most environmentally sound manner, consistent with other national priorities. Through this act Congress made it mandatory that each federal agency prepare an environmental impact statement (EIS) if a proposed action is:

1. Federal
2. Qualifies as "major," and
3. Will have a significant effect on environment.

The primary purpose of the EIS is to disclose to the agency and the public, the environmental consequences of a proposed action, as well as the repercussions of the alternative courses of action. Projects or activities to which this act applies cover the construction of new facilities (bridges, highways, airports, hydroelectric and/or nuclear power plants), the dredging or channeling of a river or harbor, large-scale aerial spraying of pesticides, and disposal of munitions and other hazardous material. Included are not only projects undertaken directly by federal agencies but also those that are supported in whole or in part by federal contracts, grants, subsidies, loans, or other forms of funding assistance.

A significant initiative of the NEPA was the establishment of a Council on Environmental Quality (CEQ) within the Executive Office of the President. Responsibilities assigned to the CEQ included developing new environmental programs and policies, coordinating the wide array of federal environmental efforts, ensuring that officials responsible for federal activities take environmental considerations into account, and assisting the President in assessing and solving environmental problems. Among the duties of the CEQ was the preparation of an annual report on the quality of the environment.

Although the National Environmental Policy Act was far-reaching and all encompassing, it focused primarily on process rather than substance. Nonetheless, in many cases proposed projects were halted after initiation of the NEPA litigation. In other cases, federal agencies have refrained from taking controversial actions, to avoid the expense and delay of litigation. Undoubtedly some environmentally unjustifiable projects have either been abandoned or were never formally proposed because of the NEPA requirements. In addition, a host of projects have been modified to reduce their environmental impact. The unanswered question is whether the benefits thus attained are sufficient to justify the expense and delay created in instances when the project has ultimately proceeded.

Interestingly, the NEPA contains no requirements relative to how clean the air and water must be or to how much pollution can be discharged into the environment. To meet these needs, Congress has passed a wide range of laws that address air and water pollution, solid waste disposal, the purity of food and drinking water, and problems of the occupational environment. Many of the laws were passed prior to the NEPA.

V. ENVIRONMENTAL RULES AND REGULATIONS

A. COMPREHENSIVE ENVIRONMENTAL RESPONSE, COMPENSATION, AND LIABILITY ACT (CERCLA)

The Superfund program is dedicated to cleaning up hazardous waste sites and to protecting public health and the environment. Sources of hazardous wastes include operations that use hazardous wastes or create them as a by-product, illegal dumping, accidental releases, and other releases that threaten health and the environment.

The authority for the Superfund program is provided by the Comprehensive Environmental Response, Compensation, and Liability Act (CERCLA). The Superfund program is described, along with citations to statutes, regulations, and guidance, on the Superfund home page Internet site (http://www.epa.gov.superfund). This site also provides links to EPA regional offices and related federal, state, and other Internet web sites of interest.

Waste sites are discovered by local and state agencies, businesses, the U.S. Environmental Protection Agency (EPA), the U.S. Coast Guard, and citizens. Releases of hazardous substances (including oil spills) should be reported to the National Response Center hotline at 1-800-424-8802.

The EPA works closely with the Agency for Toxic Substances and Disease Registry (ATSDR), a federal environmental health agency created by CERCLA legislation, and with state health agencies in evaluating the impacts of hazardous waste sites on public health.

Superfund site impacts are real. Hundreds of drinking water wells across the country have been shut down due to contamination. Studies conducted by ATSDR show a variety of health effects associated with some Superfund sites, including birth defects, cardiac disorders, changes in pulmonary function, impacts on the immune system (the body's natural defense system against disease and sickness), infertility, and increases in chronic lymphicytic leukemia.

Physician information on pollution-related impacts that are thought to be associated with abandoned hazardous waste sites is of interest to the EPA, ATSDR, and state health agencies. Reports of health-related impacts should be reported to EPA regional or headquarters offices, ATSIDR (888-42ATSDR) and state health agencies. Reports of pollution-related illness can provide the basis for actions at a site.

The Superfund statute authorizes the United States, the states, and Indian tribes to act on behalf of the public as Natural Resource Trustees for natural resources under their respective trusteeship. An example of a trust responsibility is the responsibility for the protection of groundwater, which is generally a trust responsibility of the states. The EPA works with a variety of federal, state, and tribal partners in addressing sites. Although there are clearly interests relating to the protection of health, "trustee" agencies have "trust" responsibilities for "natural resources." Natural resources include, but are not limited to groundwater fisheries, and tribal hunting grounds. There is overlap between protection of health and the environment and protecting against impacts on natural resources. When environmental cleanups for health and the environment do not adequately address natural resources (as determined by the trustee agencies), trustee agencies can file a claim for natural resource damages.

B. EMERGENCY PLANNING AND COMMUNITY RIGHT-TO-KNOW ACT (EPCRA)

In 1984 and 1985, twin releases of cyanide gas into the environment, one in Bhopal, India and the other in Institute, West Virginia, demonstrated the need for enhanced preparedness and planning for chemical accidents.

In 1986, Congress passed the Superfund Amendments and Reauthorization Act, Title III of which comes the Emergency Planning and Community Right-to-Know Act (EPCRA). The Act requires facilities with hazardous substances, at specified quantities, to report the inventories to government authorities. With this information, emergency planners and responders may prepare for dealing with accidental chemical releases. The Act also provides for public access to data submitted by facilities. The Major Sections of EPCRA are shown in Table 5.1.

Table 5.1. Major Sections of EPCRA. (Source: Berman, 2001).

Subtitle A – Planning and Notification	Function
Section 301	Establishes State Emergency Response Commissioners (SERCs) and local emergency planning /committees (LEPCs).
Section 302	Requires Facilities with extremely hazardous substances (EHSs) at or above the listed threshold planning quantity (TPQ) to notify the SERC and LEPC; each facility is subject to EPCRA regulations.
Section 303	Requires (1) EHS facilities to provide the name of their emergency coordinator to the LEPC and (2) LEPCs to develop an emergency plan to address emergency responses to EHS facilities.
Section 304	Requires notification to the SERC, the LEPC, and in some cases the National Response Center (NRC) of releases of certain hazardous substances at or above their reportable quantity (RQ).
Subtitle B – Reporting Requirements	
Section 311	Requires updating of inventory information within 90 days of changes.
Section 312	Requires filing of a tier I or II report identifying the inventory and storage locations of EHSs and other hazardous substances above applicable thresholds.
Section 313	Requires filing of a Toxic Release Inventory (TRI) report identifying the amount of toxic chemicals released into the environment by specified sectors of industry.
Subtitle C – General Provisions	
Section 323	Provides for disclosure to health professionals, doctors, and nurses in the event of exposure to a hazardous substance or for preventative measures.
Section 324	Provides for public availability of all materials, with certain exceptions, submitted under EPCRA.
Section 329	Contains definitions for words used in the Act.

The universe of substances potentially regulated by EPCRA totals around 500,000 chemicals. These are substances for which the federal Occupational Safety and Health Administration (OSHA) requires a material safety data sheet (MSDS) under the Hazard Communication Standard.

Subsets of the universe include substances specifically listed by the federal Environmental Protection Agency (EPA). The three subsets are:

1. Extremely hazardous substances,
2. Toxic chemicals, and
3. Hazardous substances.

The composition of each subset list may be found in EPA regulations. Each year between January 1st and March 1st facilities must report inventories of substances subject to EPCRA for the previous calendar year. Substances that must be reported include (1) EHSs at the TPQ or 500 pounds, whichever is less, and (2) other hazardous substances for which OSHA requires an MSDS, at or above 10,000 pounds. The Tier II Emergency and Hazardous Chemical Inventory form is submitted to state and local authorities and the local fire department. This form provides information about the facility, the chemicals, and where and how the chemicals are located.

EPCRA Section 311 requires facility owners or operators to submit a material safety data sheet or a list of MSDSs for substances present at the facility. Because the Tier II report lists substances present during the previous calendar year, this section requires an update of inventories during the current calendar year. The notification can take the form of submission of an MSDS for each chemical, or a list of chemicals. The MSDSs or the list are sent to the SERC, LEPC and local fire department with jurisdiction over the facility. Due to the voluminous paper involved with MSDSs, the receiving agencies may prefer a list.

The Toxic Release Inventory, a report prepared by facilities, identifies toxic chemicals released into the environment during the previous calendar year. Only federal facilities and facilities from sectors of industry specified by EPA regulations are subject to this reporting requirement. In addition, facilities must manufacture, process, or otherwise use a listed toxic chemical in quantities exceeding the applicable threshold. A final requirement is that the facility must have two or more full-time employees. The TRI is submitted to the federal EPA and the SERC by July 1st of each year.

C. RESOURCE CONSERVATION AND RECOVERY ACT (RCRA)

RCRA ("rick-rah") is an acronym for the Resource Conservation and Recovery Act. Congress enacted RCRA in 1976 as an amendment to the Solid Waste Disposal Act of 1965 to address the growing amount of waste generated in the United States. The Act gave the Environmental Protection Agency (EPA) the authority to create regulations to implement and enforce RCRA to ensure the proper management and disposal of household, municipal, commercial, and industrial solid and hazardous waste.

RCRA focuses on active and future facilities and does not address abandoned or historical sites. The Act has been amended several times since 1976 and continues to evolve to meet the changing needs in waste management.

The major goals of the RCRA are the following:

1. To protect human health and the environment from the hazards posed by waste disposal,
2. To conserve energy and natural resources through waste recycling and recovery,
3. To reduce the amount of waste generated, including hazardous waste, and
4. To ensure that wastes are managed in a manner that is protective of human health and the environment.

According to the EPA regulations, a solid waste is mostly non-hazardous garbage from businesses and homes (e.g., coffee grounds, milk cartons), refuse (e.g., metal scrap), sludge from waste treatment plants and water supply treatment plants, non-hazardous industrial wastes, and other discarded materials from industrial, commercial, mining, agricultural, and community activities. In 1995, approximately 208 million tons of garbage was generated in the United States. By 2000, we are expected to produce over 220 million tons of garbage per year.

A hazardous waste is a waste with properties that make it dangerous or capable of having a harmful effect on human health or the environment. To cover this wide range, the EPA developed a system to identify specific substances known to be hazardous and established criteria for identifying other materials that may be hazardous. For example, a waste may be considered hazardous if it is ignitable (burns readily), corrosive (strong acid or base) or reactive (explosive). A waste may also be considered hazardous if it contains certain amounts of toxic chemicals.

The EPA has developed a list of over 500 specific hazardous wastes. The criteria for determining if a waste is hazardous and the lists of specific hazardous wastes can be found in Title 40, Part 261 of the hazardous waste regulations. These regulations are located on the Internet at http://www.epa.gov/epahome/cfr40.htm.

In 1995, about 279 million metric tons of hazardous waste was generated in the United States. An underground storage tank (UST) is a large metal or fiberglass container designed to be buried in the ground for storage of liquid chemicals such as gasoline. There are approximately 1.5 million UST's in the United States that contain hazardous substances or petroleum products not counting farm and heating-oil tanks. Nearly 25% are leaking or will leak in the future.

D. FEDERAL INSECTICIDE, FUNGICIDE, AND RODENTICIDE ACT

The term "**pesticide**" includes many kinds of ingredients used in products to prevent, destroy, repel, or mitigate insects, weeds, fungi, nematodes, rodents, and other pests. Pesticide products are also used as antimicrobial's, disinfectants, swimming pool chemicals, fumigants plant growth regulators, desiccants, defoliants, insect growth regulators and bio-pesticides (naturally occurring chemicals with pesticidal properties).

The basis for the EPA's pesticide regulation under FIFRA is pesticide registration. The EPA must register each pesticide (including imported pesticides) and its label before any person in any state may distribute or sell the pesticide to any person. According to the EPA's pesticide registration information internet site, pesticide registration is a scientific, legal and administrative process through which the EPA examines the ingredients of a pesticide; the particular site or crop on which it is to be used; the amount, frequency, and timing of use; and storage and disposal practices.

For each prospective pesticide product, manufacturers must develop extensive data for EPA review. Pesticide manufacturers are required to submit their proposed labeling, a statement of all claims to be made for the pesticide, complete directions for use, a confidential statement of the product's complete formula, and a description of all tests on which the manufacturer's claims are based.

Data provided by the manufacturers must be developed in tests done according to EPA guidelines. These tests must determine whether a pesticide has the potential to cause adverse effects on humans, wildlife, fish and plants, including endangered species and non-target organisms, as well as possible contamination of surface water or groundwater from leaching runoff, and spray drift. Potential human risks include short-term toxicity and long-term effects such as cancer and reproductive system disorders.

Before any pesticide can be legally applied to a food crop, the EPA must set a "**tolerance**." The tolerance is the maximum amount of pesticide residue that can remain on food. The EPA's current standard under the Food Quality Protection Act in setting any new pesticide tolerance, or in reassessing existing tolerances, is one of "**reasonable certainty of no harm**." In meeting this standard, the EPA must weigh carefully several factors concerning the pesticide. Factors used by EPA to determine "tolerance"are the following:

1. The aggregate, non-occupational exposure from the pesticide, i.e., through diet, from use of pesticides in and around the home, and from drinking water,
2. The cumulative effects from pesticides that produce similar effects on the human body (similar "modes of action"),
3. Whether there is increased susceptibility to infants and children, or other sensitive sub-populations, from exposure to the pesticide, or
4. Whether the pesticide produces an effect in humans similar to a naturally occurring estrogen or produces other endocrine-disruption effects.

The Food Quality Protection Act requires the EPA to reregister all pesticides originally registered before November 1, 1984, to make certain they meet current strict safety standards. The EPA's top priorities are pesticides registered for use on foods and animal feeds. The EPA also places high priority on registering "reduced risk" pesticides that are safer than any older pesticides currently on the market, those pesticides with public health benefits, as well as pesticides that are of particular economic importance.

The EPA can suspend and cancel the registration of any pesticide if it determines that continued availability and use would create unreasonable adverse impacts to human health, safety, and welfare, or cause unreasonable harm to the environment.

E. TOXIC SUBSTANCES CONTROL ACT (TSCA)

TSCA ("tosca") is the Toxic Substance Control Act. Originally enacted in 1976 and amended several times since. TSCA gives the Environmental Protection Agency (EPA) authority to regulate manufacturing, processing, distribution, use, and disposal of chemical substances when these activities may pose an unreasonable risk to health and the environment. TSCA is probably best known for its programs regulating:

1. Asbestos,
2. Polychlorinated biphenyls (PCBs),
3. Chlorofluorocarbons (CFCs), and more recently,
4. Lead-based paint.

TSCA Section 4 allows the EPA to require manufacturers, importers, and chemical processors to perform toxicological tests on chemical substances to determine whether they might pose such risks. From 1979 through 1997, approximately 550 chemicals were subject to testing actions through these test rules, consent agreements, and voluntary testing agreements. The EPA maintains an inventory (the TSCA Inventory) of these substances and their use.

Some of the TSCA programs are delegated to the states and Indian tribes because they are often the entities that implement the programs; these are key stakeholders throughout the development of most programs. Where states or tribes do not seek to become authorized for particular programs, they may be implemented and enforced at the federal level.

The EPA has various mechanisms to involve the public in TSCA as well as other initiatives. TSCA rulemakings often include stakeholder meetings early on in the development of initiatives, and rulemakings always provide for a public comment period and often include additional public meetings to explain proposed actions and further solicit comment.

F. CLEAN AIR ACT (CAA)

The average person breathes 13,000 liters of air each day. Clean air is critical for a healthy quality of life. Originally passed into law in 1970, the Clean Air Act provides the federal authority to preserve and protect the nation's air. The Clean Air Act Amendments of 1990 were designed to curb three major threats to the environment and to the health of millions of Americans: **acid rain**, **urban air pollution**, and **toxic air emissions**.

The overall goal of the Clean Air Act is to reduce the pollutants in our air by 56 billion pounds a year - 224 pounds for every man, woman, and child. The dramatic reduction of lead in the air is one of the most striking successes of the Clean Air Act:

1. Since 1970, emissions of a lead - pollutant known to cause learning disabilities in children - have dropped 98%.
2. Eliminating lead from gasoline has been the catalyst for this astounding accomplishment.
3. The United States began phasing out lead from gasoline in the 1970s, when the first generation of pollution control equipment was installed on cars and trucks, and completely eliminated lead in gasoline in the early 1990s.

For each requirement of the Clean Air Act, the law prescribes specific reporting or compliance mechanisms. The states share responsibility for enforcing the provisions of the Act, but the federal government is the "800-pound gorilla in the closet." States that do not submit plans to implement the NAAQS, for example, are subject to economic growth sanctions and road-building funding restrictions from the federal government. In addition the EPA can step in and issue a federal plan where a state or local government has failed to act. Furthermore, the 1990 amendments to the Act also greatly expanded a citizen's authority to take legal action to enforce Clean Air Act requirements. The Clean Air Act also includes extensive civil and criminal enforcement provisions.

G. CLEAN WATER ACT

The Federal Water Pollution Control Act Amendments, commonly called the Clean Water Act, were enacted on October 18,1972. This law, subsequent amendments, and implementing regulations constitute the national water-quality policy for the United States. The objective is to restore and maintain the chemical, physical, and biological integrity of the nation's water. Three national goals supported this objective:

1. Elimination of all pollutant discharges into navigable waters by 1985,
2. Achievement of fishable and swimmable waters wherever attainable by 1983, and
3. Prohibition of discharges of toxic pollutants in toxic amounts.

The Clean Water Act defines "pollutants" as dredged spoil, solid waste, incinerator residue, sewage-garbage, sewage-sludge, munitions, chemical wastes, biological materials, radioactive materials, heat, wrecked or discarded equipment, rock, sand, cellar dirt, and industrial, municipal, and agricultural waste discharged into water. "Toxic pollutants" are defined as including disease-causing agents that after discharge and on exposure or ingestion inhalation, or assimilation by any living thing either directly from the environment or indirectly by ingestion through the food chain - will cause death, disease, behavioral abnormalities, cancer, genetic mutations, physiological malfunctions, or physical deformities, in the exposed organism or its offspring.

The Clean Water Act requires States and Native American tribes, which are to be treated as States, to adopt water quality standards that protect human health. Water quality standards for any given water-body have three main components: the designated use of the water body, water-quality criteria to protect the use, and anti-degradation policy to maintain the water's quality. States and Tribes are to take into consideration the water's use and value for public water supplies; agricultural, industrial, and other uses; propagation of fish and wildlife; and recreational purposes and use.

States and Tribes are to adopt water-quality standards to protect human health. Narrative criteria most closely associated with public health may specify that no toxics can be discharged in toxic amounts. The numerical criteria may specify concentrations of chemical pollutants and pathogen indicators that cannot be exceeded in order to protect human health. The numerical criteria for chemical pollutants are to be based on human exposure through consumption of drinking water and fish/shellfish. The numerical criteria for pathogen indicators are to be based on human exposure through accidental ingestion of water while swimming.

H. SAFE DRINKING WATER ACT (SDWA)

SDWA was passed in 1974. The general objective was to ensure that public drinking-water supplies are free of potentially harmful materials and that they meet minimum national standards for protection of public health. The act includes regulations pertaining to the underground injection of liquid wastes. Under the SDWA, the EPA was authorized to established national drinking-water quality standards, including the specification of maximum contaminant levels (MCLs) for specific substances in water. The MCLs must be set at a level that allows no known or anticipated adverse health effects. Through passage of the1977 amendments to the SDWA, Congress recognized the finite nature of the nation's water supplies and the need to assess present and future supplies and demands. The SDWA was amended in 1986 and 1996 to specify additional contaminants to be regulated and acceptable treatment techniques for each such contaminant.

I. POLLUTION PREVENTION ACT (PPA)

Both the CAA and the CWA emphasize treatment or remediation, rather than prevention, of pollution. Recognizing this deficiency, Congress passed the PPA of 1990. This act established a national policy to assure that pollution is prevented or reduced at the source, recycled or treated in an environmentally safe manner, and disposed of or released into environment only as a last resort. It also created a clearinghouse to encourage the sharing and transfer of source reduction technology and provided financial assistance to states to promote pollution prevention.

J. RADIOACTIVE WASTES

For purposes of classification, radioactive wastes in the U.S. have been divided into two categories: **high level** and **low level**.

1. Nuclear Waste Policy Act (High-Level Waste)

Through the Nuclear Waste Policy Act of 1982 and the Nuclear Waste Policy Amendments Act of 1987, Congress took what it considered to be positive steps to solve the high-level waste disposal problem. The program initiated by these laws has three essential components:

a. The design and construction of a geologic repository for permanent disposal of spent fuel from nuclear power plants and other high-level waste;
b. The establishment of a monitored retrievable storage (MRS) facility for temporary storage and packaging of spent fuel prior to placement in a repository; and
c. The development of a transportation system for moving the waste from its source to the MRS facility and ultimately to the repository.

2. Low-Level Radioactive Waste Policy Amendments Act

For several decades there were only 3 low-level disposal facilities in U.S., located in Nevada, S. Carolina, and Washington. These states did not want to be "dumping ground" for wastes from other states. In an effort to alleviate this situation, Congress passed the Low-Level Radioactive Waste Policy Amendments Act of 1985. Each of these states, either individually or as part of a regional compact, was made responsible for the disposal of low-level radioactive wastes produced as a result of commercial or federally sponsored activities within its borders.

K. FEDERAL FOOD, DRUG, AND COSMETIC ACT (FDCA)

FDCA was enacted in 1938, to replace the Pure Food and Drug Act of 1906. The Act covers food for humans and animals, human and veterinary drugs, medical devices, and cosmetics. The FDCA was revised with the passage of the 1958 Food Additives Amendment, which required that the safety of substances classified as "food additives" be demonstrated prior to marketing. Any review of laws regulating food would be incomplete without mention of Delaney clause, which Congress added to the FDCA in 1958. Recognizing that cancer was a major and widely feared health problem, this clause stated that "no additive shall be deemed safe if it is found to induce cancer when ingested by man or animal."

L. ATOMIC ENERGY ACT (AEA)

The AEA of 1954 established the Atomic Energy Commission, which was later replaced by the Nuclear Regulatory Commission and the U.S. Department of Energy (DOE). Under this act, the USNRC is responsible for licensing transfer, manufacture, acquisition, possession, or use of any nuclear facility, and for regulating radioactive materials and their by-products. The USNRC is required by law to ensure that radioactive materials and related facilities are managed so as to protect the public health and the environment.

M. OTHER ENVIRONMENTAL LAWS

A number of other laws pertain to environmental protection, those concerning energy policy, flood plains and wetlands, and endangered species. In the 1970s, Congress passed several laws designed to encourage energy conservation. The Energy Policy and Conservation Act of 1975, for example, promoted disclosure of efficiency ratings of appliances. The Endangered Species Act of 1973 is designed to protect plant and animal resources from adverse effects of development.

VI. <u>FEDERAL AGENCIES INVOLVED IN ENVIRONMENTAL ISSUES</u>

A. <u>INTRODUCTION</u>

There really is no coordination, let alone integration, of federal environmental policy. The President's Council on Environmental Quality (CEQ), established under the National Environmental Policy Act of 1969, was once seen as a possible source of executive branch coordination. But rather than evolving into an integrating force, CEQ was largely disbanded in the Reagan administration.

Neither the Bush nor Clinton administrations attempted to rebuild an agency dedicated to and capable or coordinating the work of the myriad federal agencies whose activities significantly affect the environment. Hence, to understand the environmental work of federal agencies, one has to monitor each of a large number of agencies, including, but not limited to the following agencies or organizations:

Following is a list of federal agencies involved with the environment:

1. U.S. Environmental Protection Agency (EPA)
2. Several subagencies within the Department of Interior (notably U.S. Fish and Wildlife, U.S. Geological Survey, the Bureau of Land Management and the National Park Service)
3. Several subagencies in the Department of Agriculture (notably the U.S. Forest Service, the Natural Resource Conservation Service, and the Rural Utilities Service)
4. National Oceanic and Atmospheric Association (NOAA) in the Department of Commerce
5. The independent Federal Energy Regulatory Commission and Nuclear Regulatory Commission
6. Each branch of the Department of Defense, particularly the U.S. Army Corps of Engineers
7. Parts of the Department of Transportation, particularly the U.S. Coast Guard
8. National Aeronautics and Space Administration (NASA)

B. <u>USEPA (U.S. ENVIRONMENTAL PROTECTION AGENCY)</u>

The EPA was formed in 1970 to consolidate, centralize, and raise the visibility of many pollution control programs. For example, the National Air Pollution Control Administration was previously "buried" in the Department of Health, Education, and Welfare; the Federal Water Pollution Control Administration was "buried" within the Department of the Interior. As major new federal environmental programs were created in the 1970s and 1980s, such as the Superfund-program (1980), the EPA accumulated many, but not all, of the federal environmental responsibilities.

The original planners of the EPA gave some consideration to combining pollution control and natural resource management functions, but there was not felt to be adequate political capital to respond fully to President Nixon's original address to the CEQ in 1970, "Message on the Environment," which noted that "Federal institutions for dealing with the environment and natural resources have developed piecemeal over the years in response to specific needs, not all of which were originally perceived in the light of the concerns we recognize today. Many of their missions appear to overlap, and even to conflict.

The EPA does have the primary authority to set these standards. Typically, the federal environmental laws then allow states to adopt the federal standards or to set more stringent standards of their own. This ensures a degree of national uniformity in core pollution control standards.

C. FEMA (FEDERAL EMERGENCY MANAGEMENT AGENCY)

The disaster recovery work of the Federal Emergency Management Agency (FEMA) fits generally into two phases:

1. The immediate, post-disaster relief is carried out under authority that gives broad powers to take actions necessary to restore structures to pre-disaster conditions without having to conduct environmental assessments (see 42 United States Code, Section 5159)
2. The longer term hazard mitigation projects that FEMA funds do have to demonstrate compliance with environmental laws, including the National Environmental Policy Act, as well as related laws such as historic preservation requirements.

D. USDOI

The lead agency on federally listed threatened and endangered species is the U.S. Fish and Wildlife Service, in the Department of Interior.

The federal environmental laws for cleanup of spills, such as the Comprehensive Environmental Response, Compensation, and Recovery Act (CERCLA) and the Oil Pollution Act (OFA), provide for "natural resource trustees" who represent federal (and state) agency landowners and who may bring actions to recover damages to natural resources under their care.

E. USDOA

The Soil Conservation Service began as an agricultural erosion control agency in the New Deal era. It has grown into the Natural Resources Conservation Service and its work has evolved from farm-oriented conservation programs to broader multipurpose water resource engineering projects and habitat protection. Today its projects are sometimes indistinguishable from projects of the Army Corps of Engineers and the Bureau of Reclamation.

F. USDOC

Congress passed the Coastal Zone Management Act in 1972 to encourage environmental planning and management in and around coastal areas. The National Oceanic and Atmospheric Administration within the U.S. Department of Commerce, including the National Marine Fisheries Service, keep tabs on coastal zone development issues.

G. USDOF

The Corps was recognized as the nation's lead agency for construction of projects in waters of the United States with the 1824 Rivers and Harbors Act. It gained responsibility for permitting projects in navigable waters that might impair navigation in the 1899 Rivers and Harbors Act. When the 1972 Federal Water Pollution Control Act added a permitting requirement for all projects that affect waters of the United States, including wetlands (Section 404), the Corps was well established as the federal permitting agency in this area.

H. OTHER AGENCIES

There are many agencies. A complete list is almost unimaginable. Environmental issues by definition defy narrow categories. Still, in any list of federal environmental agencies, one should include the following:

1. **Federal Energy Regulatory Commission**, which in its role as licensor of hydroelectric facilities is centrally concerned with the environment in and around rivers.
2. The **National Aeronautics and Space Administration** conducts and provides a space platform for others to conduct a substantial amount of research on the environment, from space.
3. The **Nuclear Regulatory Commission** has wide-ranging regulatory jurisdiction over radioactive materials, another area full of environmental issues.
4. The **Department of Energy** has both regulatory and research programs that are very important to the nation's (and world's) environment.
5. The **Tennessee Valley Authority and other federal agencies** with broad regional mandates play important roles in the environment of their particular regions.
6. **United States-sponsored international organizations**, such as the World Bank, the International Monetary Fund, and the General Agreement on Tariffs and Trade, all have a significant effect on international environmental policy.
7. Policies of the **Department of Housing and Urban Development** and the **Department of Transportation** greatly affect growth and land use patterns, and these in turn are very important to the environment.

VII. STANDARDS

A. INTRODUCTION

Many organizations have developed guidelines, recommendations and standards for limiting exposures to a variety of occupational and environmental contaminants:

1. **Environmental Protection Agency**, through its ambient air quality standards, has established limits for airborne contaminants in the outdoor environment; it has also set standards for various contaminants in drinking water and in rivers and streams.
2. Standards for limiting exposures to contaminants in food have been developed by the **Food and Drug Administration.**
3. Guidelines for limiting exposures to chemical and physical stresses in the workplace have been developed by the **American Conference of Governmental Industrial Hygienists.**
4. Standards for the environmental and occupational exposures to ionizing radiation have been set by the **Environmental Protection Agency,** and the **Nuclear Regulatory Commission** and the **Occupational Safety and Health Administration** have promulgated regulations to assure that the standards will be met.
5. Guidelines for protection against non-ionizing radiation have been set out by the **International Radiation Protection association** and the **International Commission on Non-Ionizing Radiation Protection.**

Unfortunately, because of the multitude of organizations involved, there is no uniform methodology for dealing with the host of considerations that must be taken into account in the development of occupational and environmental standards. Such considerations include the approaches used to develop the standards, the underlying scientific bases, the associated goals for limiting the risks to the public and the environment and the application of the standards, once developed.

B. CURRENT APPROACHES

The basic goal of many environmental standards is to protect human health. The associated guidelines are generally referred to as primary standards. Sometimes other affected entities must be considered as well; those associated guidelines are called secondary standards. In the case of air pollution, the secondary standards are aimed at protecting agricultural crops and property, such as buildings and statues. In the case of drinking water, the secondary standards assure the aesthetic qualities of the product such as temperature, color, taste, and odor. Interestingly, secondary standards for many contaminants in air and water are more stringent than the primary standards.

One of the first requirements in the development of primary standards is to identify or define the exposed member who is to be protected. Is it an adult, a child, an infant or a fetus? Aware of this need, the International Commission on Radiological Protection in 1994 published age-dependent guidance for use in protecting members of the public. A specific consideration in the development of occupational exposure standards is the need to protect pregnant women.

Once these types of decisions have been made, the next step is to decide whether the standard should protect the maximally exposed or the most susceptible member of a given group. In the case of the general population it may be difficult to identify such an individual and determine his or her exposure. For this reason some organizations have recommended that standards be based on protecting an average member of the "critical group," that is, the group that because of its location or living habits will be most heavily exposed. This group may be real, in which case the living habits of the members are known or predictable, or the group may be hypothetical, in which case the habits may be assumed, based on observations of similar groups elsewhere. The dose to an individual within the critical group is then assumed to be that received by a typical member of the group. This approach has the advantage of ensuring not only that members of the public do not receive unacceptable doses but also that decisions on the acceptability of a given practice are not prejudiced by a small number of individuals with unusual habits.

Once the basic standards have been developed - for example by placing limits on the permissible doses to members of the public - derived or tertiary guides must be established for determining through monitoring programs whether the standards are being met. These guides may include limits on the intakes of individual contaminants by members of the exposed population, and/or limits on the concentrations of individual contaminants within various environmental media (air, water, food). Derived guides can also be developed on the basis of allowable releases of specific contaminants into the environment via the airborne or liquid pathway.

Refinements and specificity can be added by setting limits on the inhalation of contaminants based on the size of the airborne particles: lower limits may be specified for certain sizes within the respirable range. This is the approach used today for setting limits on airborne particles in the ambient environment. Where the health effects of a contaminant tend to depend on the short-term concentration (as is the case for ozone), it may be necessary to set limits on hourly concentrations rather than on cumulative intake.

In certain cases it is difficult, expensive, and/or time-consuming to quantify the presence of a specific contaminant in a given medium (say, viruses and other disease organisms in drinking water). To circumvent this problem, current standards for drinking water are based primarily on limits on the concentrations of coliform organisms, which serve as **surrogates**. Although not normally a source of disease, these organisms are frequently present in the human intestines, and their identification in drinking water is an indicator of the possible presence of fecal matter. In a similar manner, it is sometimes easier to assure containment as in a waste disposal facility, through requirements directed to features other than those in question. For example, one of the concerns of the Nuclear Regulatory Commission is that interacting water will leach radionuclides from wastes in a disposal facility. Rather than specifying limits on leachability, the USNRC sets specific requirements for the structural stability of the wastes, the assumption being that radionuclides in such wastes will not be readily leached.

In taking a closer look at setting targets for the control of air pollution, it is necessary to set standards. The word **standard** implies a set of laws or regulations that limit allowable emissions or that do not permit degradation (deterioration) of air quality beyond a certain limit. The word guidelines imply a set of recommended levels against which to compare air quality from one region to another over time.

Standards may take two forms: ambient air quality standards and emissions standards. **Ambient air quality** is the general quality of outdoor air in the region. Guidelines are usually for ambient air quality only. **Emissions standards** set the amount of pollution that is allowed to come from a particular source. Ambient air quality standards or guidelines are levels of general air quality in the region that the jurisdiction responsible cannot allow to be exceeded. Sometimes the penalty for this is withholding of funds from the national government or some administrative penalty. Ambient air quality is monitored in various places within the region; an **exceedance** occurs when the level of a particular pollutant is exceeded. The number of exceedance, the average levels of air pollution, and the peak levels during 1 hr may all be used as indicators in air quality standards or guidelines. Ambient air quality standards may include a **non-degradation policy**, which means that not only should air pollution not exceed certain levels but also it cannot be permitted, on average, to get worse over time even within the allowable levels.

As seen in figure 5.1., control at the source may be regulated by product standards, process standards, or emission standards.

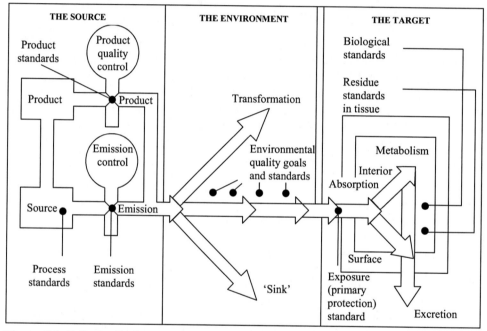

Figure 5.1. Pollutant Pathway Showing Possible Points At Which Standards May Be Set (Source: Yassi, 2001).

Product Standards If a substance does not have a known threshold level or has not been adequately tested, it may make sense to redesign the product to minimize the amount of the substance required, or search for a substitute. Governments can ban the use of a substance for specific purposes. Sweden, for example, banned the use of cadmium except in electroplating, pigments, and stabilizers for plastics (and soldering if the product does not come into contact with drinking water or food). Governments may also encourage the use of substitutes by imposing strict labeling requirements.

Process Standards If a pollutant enters the environment during a manufacturing process, governments can encourage the use of other processes for manufacture, through such measures as tax incentives or information exchange programs; legislation is another option. In Japan, for example, the outbreak of Minamata disease prompted the government to require the recycling of all water containing mercury and the replacement of mercury catalysts with other technology.

Emission Standards Emission limits on industrial discharges to air and water, and more recently to soil, have been in place for decades in many jurisdictions. These standards may be expressed in terms of the permissible concentration of a pollutant in units of air emitted or wastewater discharged by a source or in terms of a total load of pollutant per time, unit of production, or unit of energy or materials input. Emission or effluent standards may also be expressed in terms of danger to health or the environment, with a preferred method of control being specified. In this approach, the best available and economically feasible control technology is used.

Standards can also relate to operating practices, including maintenance measures to avoid spills, and measures to promote prompt cleanup, careful storage, and segregation of wastes. They may stipulate rules for cleaning and maintenance of equipment as well as training. Emergency measures may also be required. Many jurisdictions do, in fact, have regulations concerning the packaging, storage, handling, transportation, and disposal of toxic substances.

C. OCCUPATIONAL SAFETY AND HEALTH STANDARDS

Until 1970 there was almost total reliance on state and local governments and the forces of the market to improve working conditions related to occupational injuries, death, and disease. For more than 50 years state governments had attempted to inspect workplaces and to advise employers about hazards. Few of these programs, however, had adequate enforcement authority to compel abatement of dangerous conditions. In some states, no attempt was made by government to change workplace conditions, either by enforcement or by persuasion. Variations in state legislation resulted in comprehensive, strong regulation in some states (New York and Illinois) and nonexistent regulation in others (e.g., Mississippi). The doctrine of states rights and a tradition of state regulatory activity in the area of labor standards protected this status quo.

Another traditional approach was to trust market and private sector mechanisms to provide worker protection. Workers' compensation insurance carriers made some attempt to improve workplace safety for economic reasons. Many carriers provided consultative service to their clients and charged lower rates to large companies that were successful in reducing injuries. Then, as well as now, Insurance Companies' consultative resources are limited and are not available to all who may need them; while it may be possible to provide economic Incentives to large firms by basing their premium rates on accident experience, it is not possible to provide this same incentive to small firms, which have few employees to record a statistically significant accident experience. More importantly these economic incentives are inadequate where health problems are concerned because occupational diseases are not often diagnosed as workplace related. Occupational diseases often have complex origins; many years may elapse between exposure and the appearance of symptoms, making physicians and boards reluctant to attribute the symptoms to time spent with specific employers or to the exposure to particular working conditions.

A third approach evolved to cope with occupational safety and health problems; industry-based organizations filled the vacuum by producing guidelines for safe work practices for various types of industrial equipment and processes and for "acceptable" exposure limits to certain harmful substances. These "consensus standards" were adopted by the Occupational Safety and Health Administration (0SHA) in 1972 as federal standards.

Thus, a long series of private, voluntary efforts and a slowly evolving pattern of government initiatives [e.g., the Walsh-Healey Act (1936)], which authorized sanctions against federal contractors who violated standards) tested a variety of approaches to improving safety and health. These experiences served as the basis for broad federal legislation. As legislators had a record of approaches that had not worked, it became clear that voluntary-compliance approaches and consensus guidelines would have to be backed by a technically experienced federal enforcement staff and that inadequate state safety and health efforts would have to be reshaped to meet national standards of effectiveness. The economic realities of the marketplace had overwhelmed voluntary efforts, and the weak incentives of workers' compensation programs and of the states appeared unable to act effectively because of a need to compete among themselves for industry and jobs.

The Occupational Safety and Health Act was signed into law in 1970. It featured a strong standards-setting authority vested in the Secretary of Labor. The standards-setting process was open to labor, industry, and public inputs at all stages. The word "standard" connotes uniformity, consensus, and regulatory power. OSHA standards are an attempt, though the federal government's regulatory powers, to set a minimum level of protection for workers against specified hazards and to achieve that level through enforcement, education, and persuasion.

Sections 6 and 3(8) of the Occupational Safety and Health Act govern the standards-setting process. They contain three major schemes under which standards can be promulgated: (a) a short-lived authority for adoption of existing consensus standards, (b) development and promulgation of new or amended standards, and (c) promulgation of temporary emergency standards.

D. CONSENSUS STANDARDS

At the time the Occupational Safety and Health Act was passed, a large body of consensus standards was already in existence, developed as guidelines by such groups as the American National Standards Institute (ANSI), the National Fire Prevention Association (NFPA), and the American Conference of Governmental Industrial Hygienists (ACGIH). The standards represented industry's agreement on certain reasonable exposures, work practices, and equipment specifications. To establish as rapidly as possible a body of occupational safety and health rules already familiar to employers, Congress required adoption of these standards, but recognized that many were seriously out of date. The legislative history of the act emphasized that the standards would need to be constantly improved and replaced and that new standards were especially needed in the occupational health area.

Many of the consensus standards contained provisions that were irrelevant to safety and health (e.g., several pages of specifications for the wood to be used in ladders). The standards were adopted wholesale, however, without significant deletions, in the interest of speed. Competing priorities made it impossible to evaluate and amend the body of standards within the 2-year deadline allowed by Congress. Thus, OSHA began with initial standards derived from previous industry use, which had these key weaknesses. They were unduly complex and obsolete. One standard, for example, prohibited the use of ice in drinking water, a rule that dated from a time when ice was cut from contaminated rivers. Certain standards were only tangentially related to the safety or health of workers, e.g., the requirement for coat hooks in toilet stalls. The consensus standards were guidelines and not designed for enforcement and the adjudicatory process. Provisions that should have been advisory became inflexible law. Threshold limit values reflected industry consensus as to acceptable practice and were not necessarily designed for the greatest protection to workers and often lacked documentation.

By 1978 OSHA removed the most inappropriate of these rules from the books. At that time, 1110 standards provisions were proposed for deletion; after participation by labor and the business community, 927 were finally eliminated. Further improvements have included an updated fire protection standard.

E. PERMANENT STANDARDS

Section 6(b) of the act outlines the 9-step process for setting permanent safety or health standards:

1. **Decision to initiate standards development project:** The Secretary of Labor may begin the process on the basis of recommendations from the National Institute of Occupational Safety and Health or other governmental agencies, petitions of private parties, research findings from any source, accident and injury data, congressional input, or court decisions.
2. **Drafting the proposal:** Including economic and environmental impact statements to fulfill the requirements of the National Environmental Policy Act of 1969. Economic studies determine whether regulatory analysis will be required.
3. **Advisory committee:** An advisory committee may at the discretion of the Department of Labor be formed to provide help. The statute requires its composition and includes representatives of labor and industry, the safety and health professions, and recognized experts from government or the academic world.
4. **Revision and review:** By technical experts and attorneys. Where appropriate, review by other agencies also occurs.
5. Federal Register **publication of proposal:** The public is invited to comment.
6. **Informal hearings:** May be held to allow further public comment.
7. **Staff analysis of records:** Major issues requiring policy decisions are defined and presented to the assistant secretary. Alternate approaches, if appropriate, are presented.
8. **Final standard:** The staff develops a proposed final standard based on the record of rule making and submits the proposal for internal reviews.
9. **Final publication:** The completed final standard is published in its entirety in the Federal Register. A petition for review of the standard may be filed in a federal circuit court of appeals.

This process is only an outline. The length of time between steps may stretch for months or years. At times, proposals are abandoned after first hearings or public comment, and the decision to proceed with a rule making is reevaluated. If appropriate, an entirely new proposal may be developed.

F. TEMPORARY EMERGENCY STANDARDS

The Occupational Safety and Health Act requires that the Secretary of Labor "shall provide for an emergency temporary standard to take immediate effect upon publication in the Federal Register if employees are exposed to grave danger from exposure to substances or agents determined to be toxic or physically harmful or from new hazards." These standards are promulgated without the extensive Public participation characteristic of permanent standards. The act requires that they be replaced with a permanent standard within 6 months. Emergency temporary standards may be used as a "proposed standard" in the permanent standards proceedings. This provision of the act has been chilled because of unfavorable court decision and is currently rarely used.

G. CONTENTS OF OSHA STANDARDS

OSHA standards are written to control risks even if exposure continues throughout a person's working life. The effectiveness of the technology available for controlling exposures and the characteristics of the hazard in the particular workplace determine how compliance with the standard will be achieved. The standards are variable in several areas. The technical content necessarily differs according to the hazard being regulated, although it is possible to group related problems in a single standard. A specification approach or a performance approach may be employed, or the two approaches may be combined.

Specification standards tell precisely what protection an employer must provide. This approach has been used most often in developing safety standards. The advantage of specification standards is that they tell the employer exactly what must be provided to "be in compliance." The disadvantage of the specification standards is that they tend to be inflexible and may restrict an employer's efforts to provide equivalent protection using alternative - and sometimes more satisfactory - methods. In certain instances, employers may be granted a variance by OSHA.

The trend in OSHA regulation is toward performance standards that set exposures but leave the means of compliance largely to the decision of the employer. This greater degree of flexibility allows the employer to consider alternative methods and equipment and choose those most suited to the particular technology. Performance standards, however, do not give the employer carte blanche to substitute less effective means of protection (such as personal protective equipment) for engineering controls of dangerous emissions or other hazards.

Health standards are generally addressed by way of the performance, rather than the specification, approach. While many large corporations prefer performance standards in both the safety and health areas, it is advantageous, at least for small employers, to have an acceptable "specific" method of compliance included in the appendix of a performance standard.

H. Threshold Limit Values (TLVs), Permissible Exposure Limits (PELs), and Action Levels

Older occupational health standards (still used in developing countries) were based on **threshold limit values** (TLVs) developed by the ACGIH. In this system, maximum exposures were usually set based on the level of a contaminant known to produce acute effects, allowing some margin for safety and considering what was readily achievable by employers. Unfortunately, such limits do not protect against long-term chronic or subclinical effects on the body, such as changes in blood chemistry, liver function, or the reaction time of the central nervous system. In addition, these values were derived mainly for healthy, young adult, white males, not for the diverse makeup of working populations. In addition these TLVs were not designed to address the problem of irreversible health problems such as cancer.

Permissible exposure limits (PELs) are used in OSHA health standards. The lead standard, for example, contains a PEL of 50 mg of lead per cubic meter of air, averaged over an 8-hour period. PELs are based on consideration of the health effects of hazardous substances.

I. Medical Removal Protection

Medical removal protection (MRP) is a protective, preventive health mechanism complementing the medical surveillance portion of some OSHA standards. The lead standard, for example, calls for temporary removal for medical purposes of any worker having an elevated blood lead level. During the period of removal, the employer must maintain the worker's earnings, seniority, and other employment rights and benefits as though the worker had not been removed.

Medical removal protection is essential; without it, the major cost of health hazards falls directly on the worker and the worker's family in the event of illness, death, or lost wages. Without a requirement for the protection of workers' wages and job rights, removal could easily take the form of transfer to a lower-paying job, temporary layoff, or termination. A worker who participates in the medical surveillance program might risk losing his or her livelihood. The alternative has sometimes been to resist participation and thereby lose the protection that surveillance offers.

An interesting leveraging effect of MRP is its role as an economic incentive for employers to comply with the OSHA standards. For example, employers who do not comply with the lead standard will have a greater number of removals and thus will have higher labor costs over a long period, while employers who invest in the control technology will experience savings from lowered removal costs.

J. Compliance

To comply with the PELs, employers first conduct an industrial hygiene survey, including environmental sampling. This process identifies contaminants, their sources, and the severity of exposure. The employer then devises methods to reduce exposure to permissible levels. Methods commonly employed by industrial hygienists to control exposures fall into three basic categories: engineering controls, work practice controls (including administrative controls), and personal protective equipment.

Engineering controls employ mechanical means or process redesign to reduce exposure. The contaminant may be eliminated, contained, diverted, diluted, or collected at the source. Examples of this type of control include process isolation or enclosure, such as is used in uranium fuel processing. Employee isolation or machine and process enclosure are also used to protect workers from excessive fumes or noise. Closed material-handling systems, product substitution, and exhaust ventilation are also commonly employed.

Work practice controls rely on employees to perform certain activities in a carefully specified manner so that exposures are reduced or eliminated, For example, employers may instruct workers to keep lids on containers, to clean up spills immediately, or to observe specific, required hygiene practices. Such work practices are often required to complement engineering controls. This is particularly true if cases where engineering controls cannot provide complete compliance with the standard. Noise hazards are often controlled by a Combination of engineering steps and work practices limiting the amount of time workers are exposed to excessive noise levels.

Personal protective equipment controls exposure by isolating the employee from the emission source. Respirators are a common type of personal protective equipment, used when protection from an inhaled contaminant is required. Personal protective equipment is used to supplement engineering controls and work practices. Often overlooked is the great importance of personal hygiene, which includes the use of protective clothing to provide barriers to the worker and the worker's family, the provision for shower facilities, and the cleaning of protective clothing so that contaminants are not transferred to others.

Engineering control is the best method for effective and reliable control of worker exposure to many substances. It acts at the source of the emission and eliminates or reduces employee exposure without reliance on self-protective action by the employee. Work practices also act on the source of the emission, but rely on employee behavior, which requires supervision, motivation, and education for effectiveness. While personal protective equipment provides a cheaper alternative to engineering controls, it does so at the expense of safety and reliability. The equipment does not eliminate the source of the exposure, often fails to provide the degree of protection required (or fails to provide it with certainty in all cases), and may create additional hazards by interfering with vision, hearing, and mobility. Feasibility is a mandated requirement by the statute.

Individual differences in employees also affect the acceptability of personal protective equipment. For example, some employees develop infections from some ear-protection devices and respirator face pieces, and some who have impaired breathing cannot safely or comfortably use respirators. Additionally, personal protective equipment is made in standard sizes and facial configurations that may not properly fit female workers and unusually large or small workers.

OSHA should progress from a reactive, priority-setting system to one with an information-based approach. Highest priority must be given to hazards that cause irreversible adverse health effects. Court decisions have required the agency to establish a "reasonably necessary" approach, i.e., determine the number of workers affected and the number protected by the new regulation. This has been translated into a risk assessment requirement. For example, OSHA's cancer policy could be modified to increase the speed with which the particular carcinogens are regulated, with priorities shaped according to the population of the workers exposed, current exposure levels, and the potency of a substance. Consideration should be given to the ways in which these substances are used in actual operations and to the likelihood of substantial accidental exposures.

These same criteria can be applied to other health hazards. In the safety standards area, a parallel process must occur, which should include guidance in the establishment of standards for reducing deaths due to inappropriately designed lockout procedures, for reducing musculoskeletal injuries, and for controlling the development of stress-related diseases associated with newer technologies. Development of so-called generic standards, e.g., hazard identification, reaches many workers in providing protection. These types of standards are difficult to promulgate because of the divergent industrial sectors and numerous employers coming under the regulation.

Critics of occupational safety and health standards encourage the use of theoretical economic models based on cost-benefit analysis. Common sense indicates that the numbers of workers exposed, the severity of hazards, and the technological feasibility must be considered in setting standards. These factors should be explicit in OSHA's priority-setting processes. Precise costs and benefits, however, cannot be measured.

The costs of standards compliance can be estimated with some precision. New equipment, engineering modifications, and work practices have readily measurable costs. Industry, however, sometimes overestimates these costs by several magnitudes in their testimony against standards: actual costs for vinyl chloride standards compliance turned out to be but a fraction of those indicated in public testimony. More recently, even with the thoroughly worked and reworked estimates of the costs to comply with the cotton dust standard, it appears that costs were overestimated by the government and industry both. OSHA has never had the authority to require facilities to open their financial books in preparing economic feasibility impact studies so must be content with voluntarily divulged economic data.

The benefits of regulation, however, are more difficult to calculate. One cannot count all accidents that were avoided as one can number the accidents and injuries that actually occurred. One cannot precisely identify the health benefits that will accrue in 10, 20, or 30 years from current reduced exposures to toxic substances or carcinogens. The data for prediction do not exist, and causality mechanisms in occupational disease are too complex to be defined with the same certainty as the costs of a new ventilating system.

The largest problem with cost-benefit analysis, however, is not lack of information-it is the impossibility of weighing lives spared against the dollar costs for prevention. Workers are coming to realize that hazardous-pay differentials are in fact based on a dangerously false assumption that lives can be valued and, in effect, "prorated" on a cash basis. Public debate over regulatory costs can begin to clarify this issue and to uncover the hidden social costs of failure to regulate out of deference to faulty labor market mechanisms. These hidden social costs include not only loss of life and health of workers, but also increased incidence of illness and death among families of workers exposed to some substances such as lead and asbestos, and disruption of family and community life due to death and disability of workers and to local environmental effects of industrial contaminants.

K. GLOBAL STANDARDS

Particularly important for NIOSH and OSHA is participation in international occupational health and safety forums to achieve full awareness of available research and enforcement experience, including those of the Commission of the European Communities, the International Labor Organization, the World Health Organization, and many foreign national governments. It is critical that the United States shares information internationally and encourages other nations to adopt effective health and safety standards. Without comparable standards in other countries, U.S. industries can choose to export hazardous processes such as asbestos milling or pesticide formulation. This is doubly unacceptable because it not only exposes foreign workers to hazardous conditions but would tend to export jobs along with the hazards. Indeed the failure to participate in the global efforts for health and safely standards could lead U.S. workers backward if U.S. occupational safety and health standards are considered to be a bar tier to free trade under trade agreements, e.g., the North American Free Trade Agreement (NAFTA).

Standards alone will not guarantee healthful, safe working conditions. An enforcement inspection to determine whether compliance exists is essential. Training and education of workers and employers is also necessary. Government cannot provide direct, constant enforcement of employee protection; this effort must be assisted by employer and employee participation.

Workers' rights to a safe and healthful workplace are facilitated in part by the existence of employer standards, by federal and state enforcement activities, but most of all by the workers' own knowledge and vigilance. The Occupational Safety and Health Act recognizes this fact. It reinforces the workers' rights, with guarantees against reprisals by employers, when workers file and obtain abatement of health and safety hazards. Whether improvements come from voluntary employer action, from direct enforcement, or from labor-management negotiations, health and safety standards are essential to define the necessary levels of protection and the acceptable means of attaining them.

VIII. BIBLIOGRAPHY

Berman, R. (2001). Emergency Planning and Community Right-to-Know Act. In Williams, L.K. & Langley, R.L. (Eds). Environmental Health Secrets (pp. 87-90), Philadelphia, PA: Hanley & Belfus.

Bingham, E. (1998). Occupational Safety and Health Standards. In Wallace, R.B. (Ed). Maxcy-Rosenau-Last Public Health and Preventive Medicine, 14th Edition (pp.719-722). Stamford, CT: Appleton & Lange.

Bunn, W.B. (2001). Environmental Medicine: The Regulatory Issues. In McCunney, R.J. (Ed). A Practical Approach to Occupational and Environmental Medicine, 2nd Edition (pp. 614-622). New York: Little, Brown and Company.

Burnette, J. (2001). Federal Insecticide, Fungicide, and Rodenticide Act. In Williams, L.K. & Langley, R.L. (Eds). Environmental Health Secrets (pp. 92-95), Philadelphia, PA: Hanley & Belfus.

Lisko, E.A. (2001). Occupational Medicine and The Law. In Bowler, R.M. & Cone, J.E. (Eds). Occupational Medicine Secrets (pp. 323-330), Philadelphia, PA: Hanley & Belfus.

Moeller, D.W. (1997). Environmental Health, Revised Edition (pp. 270-294). Cambridge, MA: Harvard University Press.

Moore, G.S. (1999). Living with the Earth Concepts in Environmental Health Science (13.1 – 13.27). Boca Raton, FL: Lewis Publishers.

Moore, S.H. (2001). Resource Conservation and Recovery Act. In Williams, L.K. & Langley, R.L. (Eds). Environmental Health Secrets (pp. 90-92), Philadelphia, PA: Hanley & Belfus.

Noonan, J. (2001). Clean Air Act. In Williams, L.K. & Langley, R.L. (Eds). Environmental Health Secrets (pp. 97-98), Philadelphia, PA: Hanley & Belfus.

Southerland, E. (2001). Clean Water Act. In Williams, L.K. & Langley, R.L. (Eds). Environmental Health Secrets (pp. 98-101), Philadelphia, PA: Hanley & Belfus.

Topping, D.A. (2001). Toxic Substances Control Act. In Williams, L.K. & Langley, R.L. (Eds). Environmental Health Secrets (pp. 95-97), Philadelphia, PA: Hanley & Belfus.

Whisnant, R. (2001). Federal Agencies Involved in Environmental Issues. In Williams, L.K. & Langley, R.L. (Eds). Environmental Health Secrets (pp.102-105), Philadelphia, PA: Hanley & Belfus.

Yassi, A., Kjellstrom, T., & Kok, T.D. (2001). Basic Environmental Health (pp. 150-159). New York, NY: Oxford University Press.

Yassi, A., Kjellstrom, T., & Kok, T.D. (2001). Basic Environmental Health (pp. 202-204). New York, NY: Oxford University Press.

Zaragoza, L.J., Jones, S.L., & Reed, L. (2001). Comprehensive Environmental Response, Compensation, and Liability Act. In Williams, L.K. & Langley, R.L. (Eds). Environmental Health Secrets (pp. 85-87), Philadelphia, PA: Hanley & Belfus.

SECTION

II

EXPOSURE PATHWAYS

CHAPTER

6

AIR QUALITY

I. INTRODUCTION

Air pollution is the result of emission into the air of hazardous substances at a rate that exceeds the capacity of natural processes in the atmosphere (e.g.. rain and wind) to convert, deposit, or dilute them. Microbiological air pollution is mainly a problem of indoor air.

Air pollution is a problem of obvious importance in many places that affects human, plant, and animal health. For example, there is good evidence that the health of about 1 billion urban dwellers is compromised daily because of high levels of ambient air sulfur dioxide concentrations. Air pollution affects health most clearly when compounds accumulate to relatively high concentrations, producing an adverse effect on the body, e.g., bronchoconstriction or other asthmatic symptoms. Recent studies have shown that even low levels of exposure to fine particles can produce illness and deaths in a community. Often, this effect is not visible against the greater number of cases of illness or deaths caused by other factors, such as hot weather. Air pollution can also affect the properties of materials (such as rubber), visibility, and the quality of life in general.

Although people have caused air pollution ever since they learned how to use fire, anthropogenic air pollution has increased rapidly since industrialization began. In addition to the common air pollutants, many volatile organic compounds, inorganic compounds, and trace metals are emitted into the atmosphere by human activities. Worldwide, almost 100 million tons of sulfur oxides (SO_x), 68 million tons of nitrogen oxides (NO_x), 57 million tons of suspended particulate matter (SPM), and 177 million tons of carbon monoxide (CO) were released into the atmosphere in 1990 as a result of human activities. The Organization for Economic Cooperation and Development (OECD) countries accounted for about 40% of the SO_x, 52% of the NO_x, 71%, of the CO, and _23%_ of the SPM. The reductions in some of the emissions noted in the figure were likely due to regulation, education, changes in technology, and a rise in fuel prices in OECD countries.

The accumulation of chemically active compounds in the atmosphere is greatly affected by land features and atmospheric movements, Valleys, nearby mountain ranges, and the lack of open space (parks, forests, wilderness areas, bodies of water) strongly increase the severity of air pollution in a locale. These features hold the air mass like a container and prevent dilution and mixing. Stagnant air masses may receive emissions for days on end. When conditions are right usually in the morning or when there is descent of air from higher altitudes, a special atmospheric condition is created that is called **an inversion**. In an inversion, the temperature rises with increasing altitude rather than falling, which is normally the case. An inversion layer is a mass of air with an inverted temperature gradient (warmer above, cooler below). The motion of air in an inversion layer is suppressed and it limits the mixing and dilution of air pollution. Inversions are very common, especially in valleys and coastlines. The worst episodes of air pollution usually occur when inversions stay in place for days on end and the atmosphere underneath receives air pollution day after day with no mixing or wind to dilute it.

Air pollution is a very complicated physical and chemical system. It can be thought of as gases and particles that are dissolved or suspended in air respectively. Many air pollutants interact with one another to produce their effects. The severity of air pollution changes with the season, with daylight, with industrial activity, with changes in traffic, with the prevailing winds, and with precipitation (rain or snow), among many relevant factors. The composition of air pollution, therefore, is not constant from day to day or even week to week, but tends to cycle. Average levels go up and down fairly consistently depending on the time of year, but the actual levels are highly variable from one day to the next.

People have been aware for centuries of the effects of airborne pollutants on human health. As is frequently the case, several major, acute episodes were required to demonstrate conclusively to policy makers and the public that air pollution could have significant effects on health. In 1930, for example, in Belgium's Meuse River valley, high concentrations of air pollutants held close to the ground by a thermal atmospheric inversion during a period of cold, damp weather led to the deaths of 60 people. The principle sources of pollution were industrial operations, including a zinc smelter, a sulfuric acid plant, and glass factories. Most of the deaths occurred among older people with a history of heart and lung disease. In 1948, in another river valley in Donora, Pennsylvania, about 20 people died as a result of air pollution from iron and steel plants, zinc smelting, and an acid plant. Again, cold, damp weather was accompanied by a thermal atmosphere inversion. In London in 1952, 4,000 people died as a result of domestic coal burning during similar meteorological conditions.

Concern is mounting over the effects of decades of environmentally blind industrial development in Eastern Europe and the former Soviet Union, which appears to have produced widespread threats to health and life from air pollution. Today the effects of air pollution on human health and on the global environment are widely recognized. Most industrialized nations have taken steps to prevent the occurrence of acute episodes and to limit the long-term, or chronic, health effects of airborne releases.

II. THE ATMOSPHERE

A. INTRODUCTION

Human beings are dependent on the atmosphere for survival. An average adult male takes in roughly 3 lbs (1.4 kg) of food, about 4.5 lbs (2.0 kg or 2 liters) of water per day, and roughly 32 lbs (14.5 kg) or about 140 ft^3 (12.2 m^3) of air per day. Man can survive for days without food and water, but only minutes without air. The air we breathe supplies the oxygen that is needed for metabolism. Since a large amount of air is needed to sustain life, the quality of the air must be guarded so that potentially toxic materials are not inhaled along with the needed oxygen.

Concentrations of materials in the atmosphere are commonly expressed in several different ways. The concentration of particles and gases can be expressed in terms of mass per unit volume of air, e.g., μg/m^3. The concentration of gases can also be given in terms of parts per million (ppm) or percent (%). Unlike water measurements where ppm and % are based on mass, ppm and % for air concentrations are based on volume. It is possible to convert gas concentrations between a mass per unit volume measure (μg/m^3) and a volume measure (ppm or %) by utilizing the ideal gas law which states that the volume occupied by a given number of moles of a gas is related directly to temperature (absolute) and inversely to pressure (absolute).

B. AIR COMPOSITION

The composition of clean dry (no water) air is shown in Table 6.1. Air in the atmosphere also contains water and the concentration of water in the atmosphere is variable and can range between a few tenths of 1% to 5 or 6%, depending on weather conditions. Air is never found that is truly clean. Products from natural and anthropogenic activities add many other substances to the air. Natural occurrences such as volcanic eruptions and forest fires add particles and gases to the atmosphere. The winds can entrain particles off the ground and vegetation decay adds gases to the air. For now, it is sufficient to realize that the atmosphere is the recipient of products of both natural and human sources. Conditions in the atmosphere will, therefore, govern the exposure of people, structures, animals, and vegetation, to all of these materials.

Table 6.1. Typical Composition of Clean Dry Air. (Source: Sutton, 1953 and Stoker & Seager, 1972).

Constituent	Volume %	ppm
Nitrogen	78.08	780,800
Oxygen	20.95	209,500
Argon	0.934	9,340
Carbon dioxide	0.033	330
Neon	0.0018	18
Helium	0.0005	5
Methane	0.0002	2
Krypton	0.0001	1
Xenon	0.00001	0.1

C. ATMOSPHERIC STRUCTURE

Conditions in the atmosphere are not constant with increasing altitude. The variation of the temperature of the atmosphere with altitude is shown on Figure 6.1. With the exception of the emissions from supersonic aircraft, the emissions to the atmosphere from human and natural processes take place in the troposphere. Most of the materials emitted into the troposphere remain there. The movement of air in the troposphere can profoundly change the concentration of these emitted materials that various receptors experience.

D. ATMOSPHERIC MOTION

1. Lapse Rate and Stability

The negative of the change of atmospheric temperature with altitude is called the **lapse rate**. If an imaginary parcel of air were lifted adiabatically (without exchange of heat with surrounding air) and as long as the parcel of air does not become saturated with water vapor (relative humidity reaching 100%), then the temperature of the parcel will decrease 9.86°C per kilometer increase in altitude. This is called the **dry adiabatic lapse rate**. The ability of materials emitted into the atmosphere to disperse is partially governed by how the actual change in temperature with altitude compares to the dry adiabatic lapse rate. Consider a parcel of air at ground level. Assume that the temperature of this parcel of air is 20°C. If that parcel of air is lifted adiabatically 1 km, its temperature would decrease to 20°C - 9.86°C= 10.14°C. If the actual temperature of the atmosphere at an altitude of one kilometer is greater than 10.14°C, the parcel of air being cooler and hence denser than the atmosphere would begin to sink. This condition is termed "stable". If the temperature of the atmosphere at 1 km is less than 10.14°C, the parcel of air being warmer and hence less dense than the atmosphere would continue rising. This condition is termed "unstable". If the temperature of the atmosphere at an altitude of 1 km is 10.14°C, then the parcel of air being at the same temperature and density as the surrounding air would not rise or sink. This condition is termed "neutral stability".

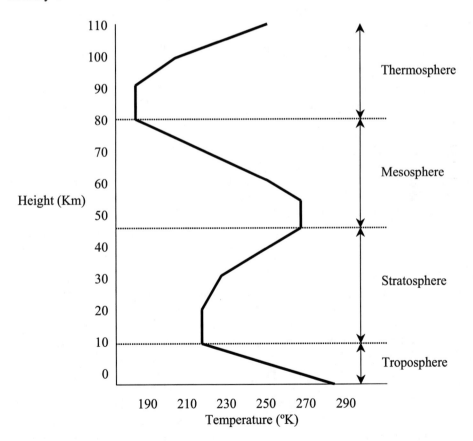

Figure 6.1. Temperature of the atmosphere as a function of altitude. (Source: Donn, 1965).

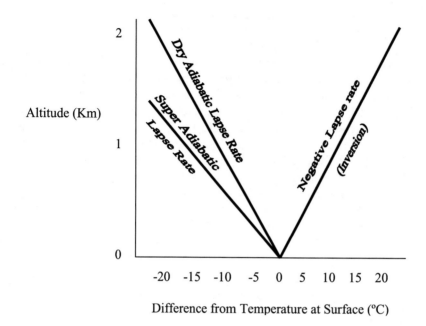

Figure 6.2. Air Temperature Lapse Rates. (Source: Rossano, 1969).

2. Dispersion

Two other terms are used to describe the actual change of temperature in the atmosphere with increasing altitude. If the temperature of the atmosphere decreases more than 9.86°C per km, then this lapse rate is termed, "**super adiabatic**." If the temperature of the atmosphere increases with increasing altitude, this condition is known as an "**inversion**." These two conditions are illustrated on Figure 6.2.

The actual lapse rate of the atmosphere and the presence of inversions can dramatically change the manner in which atmospheric emissions from a man-made or natural source are dispersed into the atmosphere. Several different atmospheric temperature profiles (solid line) along with the dry adiabatic lapse rate (dashed line) for comparison are shown on Figure 6.3.

The **plume** (trail of smoke) from a chimney is considerably different for each set of conditions. Conditions such as looping or lofting lead to rapid dispersal of the plume. Conditions such as fumigation or trapping lead to the plume being trapped near the ground with very limited dispersal. Therefore, the atmospheric conditions effect the manner in which air emissions are dispersed into the atmosphere, and hence the amount of the air emissions that reach ground based receptors (people included). There are three other factors which also effect the amount of an air emission that will reach a receptor: wind speed, amount or strength of the emission, and the spatial relationship between source and receptor (whether the receptor is upwind or downwind of the receptor).

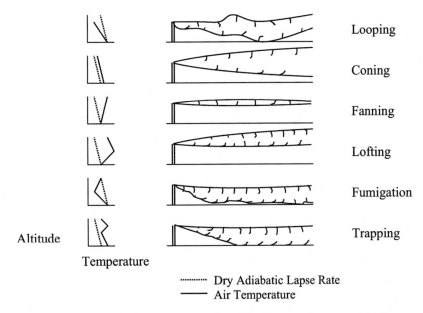

Looping

Coning

Fanning

Lofting

Fumigation

Altitude   Trapping

Temperature

·········· Dry Adiabatic Lapse Rate
——— Air Temperature

Figure 6.3. Plume Types and Air Temperature Profile. (Source: Rossano, 1969).

3. Macroscale Atmospheric Motion

The atmosphere is constantly in motion being driven in general by the movement of energy from the equator to the poles, a swirling results. Within the swirling motion are created large pools of air commonly referred to as "**air masses**". "An air mass is a large, horizontally homogeneous or uniform body of air within the atmosphere as a whole. Its uniformity is principally one of temperature and humidity". The passage of warm and cold fronts indicate the departure of one air mass and the arrival of another. Over North America, air masses generally move from west to east. There are northerly or southerly components to the movement of any air mass, but the average movement is west to east.

4. Microscale Atmospheric Motion

Superimposed on the macroscale atmospheric motion are smaller, microscale motions. These microscale motions can markedly effect air quality. Two of the microscale events that effect Chicago's air quality are the lake breeze and the urban heat island.

The lake breeze can cause the wind to reverse its direction predominantly along the western shore of Lake Michigan. The lake breeze is a result of the difference in temperature between lake water and land. (Land warms up and cools off more rapidly than water.) During the daytime in the summer the land will be warmer than the adjacent water. As a result the air over the land will be warmer and less dense than the air over the water. The result is that the denser air over the water pushes outward causing a breeze moving from the water to the land. The movement of the air is illustrated on Figure 6.4. The result is that air, and whatever contaminants it has picked up, are recirculated over a portion of the area.

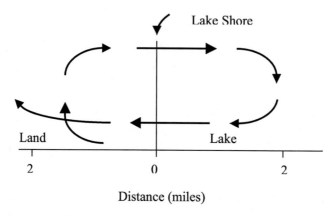

Distance (miles)

Figure 6.4. Lake Breeze. (Source: Lyons & Olsson, 1972).

The urban heat island is a nighttime event. Because the ground will cool faster than the air above it, nighttime inversions frequently occur. The urban area acts as a reservoir of heat. At night the release of the stored heat raises the altitude of the inversion in a kind of bubble as is illustrated on Figure 6.5. Contaminants released into the air inside the bubble remain trapped until the heat of the next day eliminates the inversion.

III. AIR POLLUTION

A. DEFINITION

Many attempts to define air pollution get into discussions of whether or not some chemical should be considered to be a pollutant or just a contaminant. A more general definition has been developed: "Air pollution means the presence of contaminants, such as dust, fumes, mist, odor, smoke or vapor, in quantities, of characteristics, and of duration such as to be injurious to human, plant or animal life or to property, or which unreasonably interferes with the comfortable enjoyment of life and property". Unfortunately, this definition of air pollution refers to **"outdoor atmosphere."**
This terminology probably stems from the division of responsibility for protection of environmental quality among Federal regulatory agencies.

The Environmental Protection Agency has been given responsibility for outdoor air quality while a portion of indoor air quality (occupational environments) is the responsibility of the Occupational Safety and Health Administration. Not all indoor environments are considered to be occupational and hence the air quality in non-occupational indoor environments is not officially regulated. Sources of air pollution are being identified in indoor environments and there is an exchange of pollutants between the outdoor and indoor environments. Therefore, the above definition of air pollution would be improved by replacing the phrase "outdoor atmosphere" with the phrase "air environment." Subsequent sections of this chapter will address outdoor and indoor air quality.

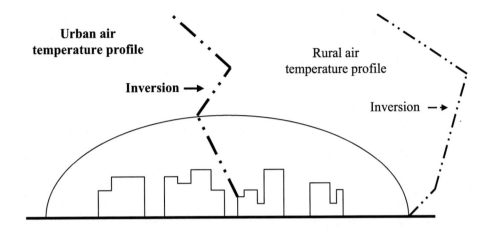

Figure 6.5. Idealized Urban Heat Island. (Source: Martin et al., 1967).

B. AIR POLLUTION EFFECTS

A variety of things can happen as a result of the addition of pollutants to the air. As the definition of air pollution indicated, air pollution can adversely effect human health and the health of other animals and vegetation; can soil, damage or accelerate the deterioration of materials; and can be esthetically unpleasant. Although a brief discussion of each of these kinds of effects will be presented here, more information on health effects of specific pollutants will be presented when individual pollutant are discussed.

The effects of air pollution on human health can be classified as infectious or noninfectious. Infections can be caused by microorganisms released into the air from a process such as sewage treatment or incineration of infectious wastes. These infections can then be transmitted among people. Noninfectious effects include all effects that are not initiated by release of an infectious organism into the air. Noninfectious effects can range from physiological changes of unknown significance to death. Diseases such as chronic bronchitis, emphysema and lung cancer are also associated with air pollution. It has also been suggested that air pollution increases susceptibility to respiratory diseases.

Air pollution has been linked to the death of livestock and vegetation. Another ecological impact can be the effect on lakes that have apparently been caused by acid rain. Material damage includes things such as soiling, deterioration of finish or material, deterioration of textiles, or accelerated weathering of monuments. Esthetic impacts may not cause illness or impacts on materials, but do interfere with enjoyment. Not being able to see the mountains from Los Angeles because of smog is an esthetic impact.

C. STANDARDS

There are several different kinds of regulations or standards that apply to air pollution. Furthermore, these standards have been established and enforced by different regulatory agencies.

Federal standards that relate to air pollution are:
1. National Ambient Air Quality Standards (NAAQS)
2. New Source Performance Standards (NSPS)
3. National Emission Standards for Hazardous Air Pollutants (NESHAP)
4. Threshold Limit Values (TLV) and Permissible Exposure Limits (PEL)
5. Prevention of Significant Deterioration (PSD)

The NAAQS, NSPS, and NESHAP are developed and enforced by the U.S. Environmental Protection Agency (EPA). TLVs are non-enforcible guidelines developed by the American Conference of Governmental Industrial Hygienists, and the Occupational Safety and Health Administration (OSHA) develops and enforces PELs. The purpose of each standard, the air environment where each standard applies, and the pollutants covered by each standard are usually different (although there is some overlap in pollutants regulated). A brief discussion of each type of standard is included below.

Federal standards do not govern all aspects of air pollution. Some authority is delegated to the States and the States are required to develop some standards and can choose to develop others. For example, Federal regulations require the States to develop a State Implementation Plan detailing how each state will meet the NAAQS. Each state then develops emission standards for air pollution sources (both new and existing) in the state. Although the states are required to develop such plans, the emission standards are developed by the states and no two state regulations need to be identical.

1. National Ambient Air Quality Standards (NAAQS)

The NAAQS apply to all outdoor air (except for occupational situations governed by PELs). The goal of all NAAQS is to specify the allowable concentration of pollutants in the ambient air, which will not adversely affect the public health (primary standard) or the public welfare (secondary standard). Pollutants presently governed by NAAQS are particles smaller than $10\mu m$ in size (PM_{10}) (formerly the standard was for total suspended particles (TSP), sulfur dioxide (SO_2), nitrogen dioxide (NO_2), carbon monoxide (CO), lead, (Pb), and ozone (O_3). There was a NAAQS for reactive hydrocarbons established in 1970, but the standard was eliminated in 1983.

2. New Source Performance Standards (NSPS)

NSPS, as the name indicates, applies to new sources of air pollution, not ones already in existence. The goal of NSPS is to limit emissions from a new air pollution source that cause or contribute to the endangerment of public health or welfare. Pollutants covered by NSPS are all the pollutants listed under NAAQS plus sulfuric acid mist (H_2SO_4), hydrogen sulfide (H_2S), fluorides (F) and (for certain sources) total reduced sulfur (S).

3. National Emission Standards for Hazardous Air Pollutants (NESHAP)

NESHAP is also an emission standard as was NSPS. NESHAP can apply to new and existing sources of air pollution. The goal of NESHAP is to control the emissions of pollutants for which there is no NAAQS and that may cause or contribute to an increase in mortality or an increase in serious irreversible or incapacitating reversible illness. NESHAPs have been established for vinyl chloride, asbestos, inorganic arsenic, beryllium, mercury, radionuclides, benzene, and coke oven emissions.

4. Threshold Limit Values (TLV) and Permissible Exposure Limits (PEL)

TLVs and PELs are air quality standards used in occupational settings. The goal of TLVs is to establish conditions under which it is believed that nearly all workers may be repeatedly exposed day after day without adverse effect. Because of wide variation in individual susceptibility, however, a small percentage of workers may experience discomfort from some substances at concentrations at or below the TLV; a smaller percentage may be affected more seriously by aggravation of a pre-existing condition or by development of an occupational illness. PELs are similar to TLVs, however, there is not complete correspondence in chemicals included or exposure levels between them. Hundreds of chemicals are covered by TLVs and PELs and the list is too long to include here.

5. Prevention of Significant Deterioration (PSD)

PSD is a different kind of air pollution standard. It does not directly specify a permissible concentration of a specific pollutant. The idea of PSD stems from concern about what could happen to areas where air is cleaner than present standards if sources of air contaminants were to be built there. The question raised is how much should air quality be allowed to deteriorate in areas where air is cleaner than the standards. The PSD regulations specify classifications of cleanness of the air and how much air quality will be allowed to deteriorate in such areas. Needless to say the concept is controversial. Its implementation is progressing.

D. AMBIENT AIR POLLUTANTS

As was mentioned when the NAAQs were discussed, seven air contaminants (now six) had been designated as air pollutants by EPA (PM_{10} [formerly TSP], SO_2 NO_2, CO, Pb, O_3 and HC). The major sources, typical concentrations, ambient standards, control techniques and health effects of each of these seven pollutants is presented below.

1. Ambient air Standards and Typical Pollutant Concentrations

The NAAQS are shown in Table 6.2. The standards for PM_{10}, SO_2, CO, O_3 and Pb are presently being reviewed and are subject to possible revision or as in the case of HC, elimination. All the NAAQS are required to be reviewed every five years so as to remain consistent with available knowledge of health effects. The concentrations of the various air pollutants can vary dramatically from place to place and time to time. Different cities have different combinations of natural and anthropogenic air pollution sources as well as differing meteorology, and hence have different air pollution problems. The most common way of presenting information on air quality is to present the values of the actual measurements made at specific monitoring stations.

Table 6.2. National Ambient Air Quality Standards (NAAQS) in the U.S. (Source: Williams, 2001).

POLLUTANT	PROMULGATION DATE	PRIMARY NAAQS	AVERAGING TIME	SECONDARY NAAQS
Ozone	7/18/97	0.08 ppm (157 µg/m^3)	8 hour	Same as primary
	3/9/93	0.12 ppm (235 µg/m^3)	1 hour	Same as primary
Nitrogen dioxide	10/8/96	0.053 ppm (100 µg/m^3)	Annual	Same as primary
Sulfur dioxide	5/22/96	0.03 ppm (80 µg/m^3)	Annual	None
	4/30/71	0.14 ppm (365 pg/m^3)	24 hour	None
	9/14/73	None	3 hour	0.5ppm (1300 µg/m^3)
Particular matter (PM $_{2.5}$)	7/18/97	15 µg/m^3	Annual	Same as primary
	7/18/97	65 µg/m^3	24hour	Same as primary
Particulate matter (PM $_{10}$)	7/18/97	150 µg/m^3	Annual	Same as primary
	7/1/87	50 µg/m^3	Annual	Same as primary
Particulate matter (TSP)	4/30/71	75 µg/ m^3	Annual	60 µg/ m^3
		260 µg/ m^3	24 hour	150 µg/ m^3
Carbon monoxide	8/1/94	9 ppm (10 mg/ m^3)	8 hour	None
		35 ppm (40 mg/ m^3)	1 hour	None
Lead	10/5/78	1.5 µg/ m^3	Maximum quarterly average	Same as primary

2. Control of Air Pollutant Emissions

There are two primary approaches toward reducing air pollution emissions from a process. The first approach is to change the process or raw material in such a way that fewer products are formed. Reduction of emissions through process modification is not always possible, or if possible may not be economically feasible because of the outdatedness of the process. The second approach is to attach pollution control equipment to the process. The process still produces the same amount of wastes, only the wastes are not permitted to escape in as large quantities. Note that the material captured by pollution control equipment must still be dealt with for disposal.

By far the most common approach to air emission control is the installation of emission control equipment. In general air pollution emissions can be classified as particle or gas. Pollution control equipment is therefore designed to capture either particles or gases. In Table 6.3 are listed several categories of particle collection devices, the principle of operation, and the size of particle collected with 90% efficiency. More detailed collection efficiency curves as a function of particle size for various control devices air shown on Figures 6.6 and 6.7. Control equipment for gaseous pollutants utilize one of four basic approaches: absorption, adsorption catalysis, or combustion. Absorption is a process whereby a gas is captured by a liquid. Devices operating on this basis are called scrubbers. Adsorption is a process in which a gas (or liquid) is captured by a solid. The solid adsorbent is frequently impregnated with another chemical to improve pollutant collection. Catalysis is a process where a catalyst (a material used to change the rate of chemical reaction but which is not consumed in the reaction) is used to convert a pollutant to a chemical form which is no longer considered to be a pollutant.

Table 6.3. Particle Collection Devices. (Source: American Chemical Society, 1969).

Control Device	Collection Mechanism	Particle Diameter (microns)[a]
Settling chamber	Gravity	50
Cyclone		
Large diameter	Centrifugal + Impaction	25
Small diameter	Centrifugal + Impaction	>5
Mechanical centrifugal rotor	Centrifugal + Impaction	>5
Scrubber		
Simple spray tower	Impaction + Direct Interception	25
Packed tower	Impaction + Direct Interception	5
Wet cyclone	Impaction + Direct Interception Centrifugal	5
Inertial-power driven	Impaction + Direct Interception Centrifugal	5
Self-induced spray	Impaction + Direct Interception	5
Venturi	Impaction + Direct Interception	<1
Filter		
High velocity impingement	Impaction + Direct Interception	10
Spun glass prefilters	Impaction + Direct Interception	5
Deep fiber bed	Impaction + Direct Interception Diffussion	1
High efficiency cellulose-asbestos or all glass Superfine fiber	Impaction + Direct Interception Diffussion	<1
Plastic fiber-superfine	Impaction + Direct Interception Diffussion + Electrostatic	0.1
Cellulose ester membrane	Impaction + Direct Interception Diffussion + Electrostatic	0.01
Bag or screen woven fabric	Impaction + Direct Interception Diffussion	<1
Reverse-jet felt	Impaction + Direct Interception Diffussion	<1
Electrostatic precipitators		
Single stage high voltage	Electrostatic	<1
Two stage low voltage	Electrostatic	<1

[a] Minimum particle size collected at approximately 90% efficiency under usual operating conditions.

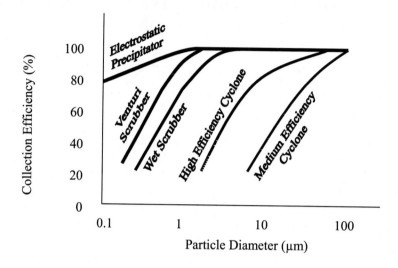

Figure 6.6. Collection Efficiency of Particle Collection Devices. (Source: Rossano, 1969).

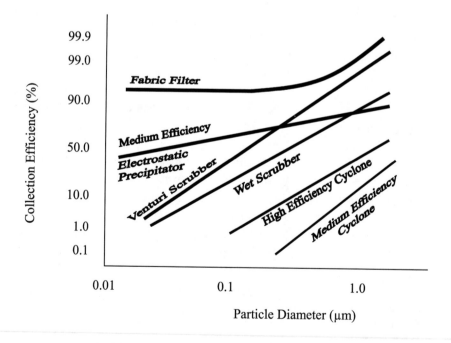

Figure 6.7 Particle Collection Device Efficiency for Particles Smaller Than 1 μm. (Source: Stern, 1977).

As an example, the catalytic converter of an automobile among other things aides in the conversion of CO to CO_2. Combustion is a process usually used in the control of HC emissions where the HC's are burned (reacted with O_2) in an attempt to form CO_2 and H_2O.

Of the six EPA-designated air pollutants PM_{10} and Pb emissions can be controlled by particle collection devices while CO, NOx and SO_2 emissions can be controlled by the kinds of gaseous pollutant control devices. Photochemical oxidants are not directly emitted into outdoor air and can not controlled by the control technology thus far presented. Photochemical oxidants are formed in the atmosphere by reactions among NO_x and HC in the presence of sunlight. Presently, control of photochemical oxidants can be achieved only by control of the precursors (NO_x and HC).

IV. AIR POLLUTION EFFECTS

A. CRITERIA POLLUTANTS

Criteria pollutants are ubiquitous outdoor air pollutants that can cause adverse health effects at current or historical outdoor (ambient) levels in the United States. Of the thousands of air pollutants, only a few meet this definition.

The current criteria pollutants are ozone (O_3), nitrogen dioxide (NO_2), sulfur dioxide (SO_2), particulate matter ($PM_{10 \text{ or } 2.5}$), carbon monoxide (CO), and lead (Pb).

B. REGULATION OF CRITERIA POLLUTANTS

The Clean Air Act (CAA) of the United States requires that the U.S. Environmental Protection Agency (EPA) must (a) identify these pollutants, (b) provide periodic compilations of scientific knowledge (criteria) about their effects on humans and the environment, and (c) set National Ambient Air Quality Standards (NAAQS) to protect public health and welfare from the adverse effects of these compounds in ambient air.

The EPA has designated reference and equivalent methods for sampling and analyzing the ambient air for criteria pollutants. There are a number of ways to express the amount of a pollutant in the atmosphere. Perhaps the most commonly used measure is concentration, which is the amount, or mass, of a substance in a given volume of air divided by that volume (e.g., mg/m^3, mol/m^3).

Often, however, quantities of gases are expressed as a volume mixing ratio, such as parts per million (ppm; the ratio of the concentration of a gas to the concentration of all the gaseous components in a given air volume). EPA is required under the CAA to provide an assessment of the latest criteria and reevaluate the NAAQS for these pollutants every 5 years.

1. Ozone

Ozone is a colorless gas composed of three atoms of oxygen. Ozone occurs both in the Earth's upper atmosphere and at ground level. The odor of ozone can be detected by some people, but the threshold varies widely. Ozone can be good or bad, depending on where it is found.   Ozone that occurs naturally in the Earth's upper atmosphere forms a protective layer that shields us from the sun's harmful ultraviolet rays.

This "good" O_3 is gradually being destroyed by man-made chemicals. In some areas where O_3 has been significantly depleted (such as the North and South poles), it is sometimes called an "ozone hole." In the Earth's lower atmosphere, O_3 is formed when hydrocarbons and nitrogen oxides emitted by cars, power plants, industrial boilers, refineries, chemical plants, and other sources react chemically to form O_3 in the presence of sunlight.   This "bad" O_3 occurs at ground level where it affects our environment and the health of some exposed people.

That depends on how sensitive you are and how much O_3 is in the air. Many people only have to worry about O_3 exposure when ground-level concentrations reach high levels.   Some people are affected by much lower O_3 levels.   During summer months, health warnings may be broadcast in some U.S. communities when the O_3 levels become unhealthy for sensitive people. Scientists have found that short-term exposures to O_3 can irritate the respiratory system, decrease lung function, cause lung inflammation, and provoke asthma, leading to increased visits to emergency departments and doctor's offices, and leading to more people being hospitalized for lung ailments.

Ozone also may aggravate other chronic lung diseases, such as emphysema and bronchitis, and could even reduce the immune system's defense against bacterial infections in the respiratory tract. Longer-term exposures to O_3 may cause permanent changes in the lung. Research is underway in an effort to understand the possible long-term effects of ozone exposure. Some people exposed to O_3 experience recognizable symptoms, including coughing, rapid or shallow breathing, and discomfort when breathing or general discomfort in the chest. Other people with asthma may experience increased wheezing or asthma attacks. Not all people will have symptoms, or the symptoms may disappear with continued exposure. Ozone can cause lung damage even if there are no symptoms.

In general, when ozone levels are elevated, your chances of being affected by ozone increase the longer you are active outdoors and the more strenuous the activity in which you engage. It is good advice to reduce your level of exertion, change the duration of exposure, or change the time of outdoor activities. Particularly sensitive individuals may want to stay indoors, especially in air- conditioned surroundings where ozone levels are generally much lower.

The information is provided in newspapers and on television and radio broadcasts in many communities with high ozone levels. With the help of state and local air agencies, the EPA developed a number of tools (e.g., the Air Quality Index) to provide people with information on local O_3 levels, their potential health effects, and suggested activities for reducing O_3 exposure. Ozone can affect all living things and even some nonliving materials such as natural rubber, synthetic elastomers, textile fibers, pigments, and dyes. Ozone also is the gaseous pollutant most injurious to agricultural crops, trees, and native vegetation.

2. Nitrogen Dioxide

Nitrogen makes up approximately 80% of our ambient air. Of the seven oxides of nitrogen that may be present in ambient air, two are generally found in the highest concentrations-nitric oxide (NO) and nitrogen dioxide (NO_2). Their interconvertibility in photochemical smog reactions has frequently resulted in their being grouped together under the designation NO_X. Combustion processes emit a variety of nitrogen compounds, but the most predominant compound is NO, which can be oxidized to NO_2 in ambient air. Of these NO_X compounds, NO_2 has the greatest potential impact on public health.

Key health effects of concern for NO_2 are respiratory illness in children, lung function effects in asthmatics, and the potential for alterations in lung host defenses and structure. Because homes with unvented gas combustion devices (principally gas stoves) have elevated levels of NO_2, they have been the subject of many epidemiologic studies. An analysis of homes with and without gas stoves showed that NO_2 was associated with an increased risk for lower respiratory symptoms and illness (such as shortness of breath, persistent wheeze, chronic cough, chronic phlegm, or bronchitis) in 5-to 12-year-old children. Despite uncertainties in these analyses, the general interpretation is that the respiratory effects in children are associated with repeated exposures over a longer period of time, rather than with an acute exposure.

Nitric oxide (NO) is a colorless and odorless gas. It is the primary form of NO_X resulting from the combustion process. However, in high temperature combustion nitrogen and oxygen can also combine to form NO_2. NO_2 is a reddish-orange brown gas with an unpleasant odor. It contributes to haze and a reduction of visibility. NO_X is also known to cause deterioration and fading of certain fabrics at concentrations between 0.6 and 2 ppm. Depending on concentration and extent of exposure plants may suffer leaf crop, lessions, and reduced crop yield. NO itself is not considered harmful to humans at concentrations found in the atmosphere, but NO_2 has been shown to cause inflammation in the lungs and bronchi in ranges from 0.062 to 0.109 ppm for a 24-hour mean concentration.

3. Sulfur Dioxide

Sulfur dioxide is the only gas-phase sulfur oxide compound that is found in ambient air in significant concentrations. It is detectable by taste and by its pungent irritating odor at high concentrations only (i.e., much higher than ambient concentrations); it is highly soluble in water and body fluids. Sulfur dioxide is formed by the combustion of fuels containing sulfur (mainly coal and oil); it also is produced by smelters, power plants, and cement factories. The highest levels of SO_2 are measured in the plumes near large industrial plants.

The effects of the oxides of sulfur on health are related to irritation of the respiratory system. Such injury may be temporary or permanent. The potentiation by particulate matter of toxic responses to sulfur dioxide (synergism) has been observed under conditions, which would promote the conversion of sulfur dioxide to sulfuric acid. The degree of potentiation is related to the concentration of particulate matter. A threefold to fourfold potentiation of the irritant response to sulfur dioxide is observed in the presence of particulate matter capable of oxidizing sulfur dioxide to sulfuric acid.

Sulfur dioxide can cause acute or chronic leaf injury to plants. Acute injury, produced by high concentrations for relatively short periods, usually results in injured tissue drying to an ivory color; it sometimes results in a darkening of the tissue to a reddish-brown. Chronic injury, which results from lower concentrations over a number of days or weeks, leads to pigmentation of leaf tissue, or leads to a gradual yellowing, or chlorosis, in which the chlorophyll-making mechanism is impeded. Both acute and chronic injury may be accompanied by the suppression of growth and yield. Corrosion rates are higher in urban and industrial atmospheres with relatively high levels of both particles and sulfur oxides than they are in rural and other areas of low pollution. Sulfur oxide pollution contributes to the damage of electrical equipment of all kinds. Building materials and textile fibers are also harmed by atmospheric sulfur oxides.

Sulfur dioxide is a public health problem because of its association with health effects in persons with cardiopulmonary disorders and its interactions with particles. The health effects of concern associated with SO_2 are increased morbidity and mortality, and the ability of short exposures (e.g., < 10 minutes) to affect asthmatics. Sulfur dioxide causes bronchoconstriction (airway narrowing). People with asthma are more sensitive to SO_2 than are typical healthy individuals. However, the sensitivity of asthmatics does not necessarily relate to the severity of their disease. Short-term exposure (minutes) of asthmatic individuals to SO_2 while they are exercising can affect the function of the lung and cause symptoms such as wheezing, chest tightness, or shortness of breath. Although these responses are typically self-limiting and may disappear without treatment in 30-60 minutes, a bronchodilator is sometimes necessary to relieve symptoms.

The association of SO_2 with mortality and various morbidity end points has been observed in epidemiologic studies. Increased mortality related to both respiratory and cardiovascular causes has been associated with SO_2. Sulfur dioxide levels also are associated with hospital admissions and emergency room visits for respiratory causes, including asthma. Some studies, however, show little or no association between SO_2 and mortality. Also, high levels of SO_2 are seldom present without high levels of particulate matter. In the United States, associations of mortality and morbidity with short-term PM levels generally have been stronger than associations with short-term SO_2 levels.

SO_2 can act alone to produce health effects but it also can produce effects when it combines with particulate matter in the air. Sulfur dioxide can coat the surfaces of very small particles and be carried deeper into the lungs where it can cause adverse effects. The effects of breathing SO_2 combined with high levels of PM for longer times may include respiratory illness, alterations in the defenses of the lung, and aggravation of preexisting respiratory disease. Responses to SO_2 also are exacerbated by breathing air with a low absolute humidity (either dry or cold), probably because drying of airway surface fluid leads to decreased removal of SO_2 in the upper airways.

SO_2 is a major precursor of acid rain and, along with NO_x, is associated with acidification of soils, lakes, and streams; accelerated corrosion of buildings and monuments; and reduced visibility. Sulfur dioxide is a major precursor of fine PM, which is also of significant health concern as well as a main pollutant that reduces visibility.

4. Particulate Matter (PM)

Particulate matter (PM) is the general term used to describe the mixture of solid particles and liquid droplets in ambient air. Some of these particles are large or dark enough, or are present in high enough concentrations, to be seen as soot or smoke.

Others are so small they can only he detected with an electron microscope. Particulate matter is classified by size. Particles greater than 2.5 μm in aerodynamic diameter are designated as "coarse" particles, whereas those less than 2.5 μm in aerodynamic diameter are classified as "fine" particles. Very small particles, those less than 0.1 μm in diameter, are classified as "ultrafine" particles. Atmospheric PM is composed of a complex mixture of organic and inorganic components that originate from many different stationary and mobile sources, as well as from natural sources. Fine particles ($PM_{\leq 2.5}$) result from fuel combustion by motor vehicles, power plants, and industrial facilities; as well as from residential fireplaces and woodstoves. Coarse particles ($PM_{>2.5}$) are formed by vehicles traveling on unpaved roads, volcanoes, and crushing and grinding operations; another source is windblown dust.

Although some particles are emitted directly by sources (such as smokestacks and motor vehicles), other particles are formed by complex reactions between gases (such as sulfur dioxide, nitrogen oxides, and volatile organic compounds) and other compounds in air to form fine particles. Ultrafine particles are formed by combustion sources such as gasoline and diesel engines. The chemical and physical composition by PM varies with location, weather, and time of year.

Particles entering the atmosphere differ in size and chemical properties. The effects of particles on health and welfare are directly related to their size and chemical composition. Particle pollutants enter the human body by way of the respiratory system, and, therefore, their most immediate effects are upon this system. The size of the particle determines the depth of penetration into the respiratory system. Particles over 5μm are generally stopped and deposited mainly in the nose and throat. Those that do penetrate deeper into the respiratory system into the air ducts (bronchi) are soon removed by ciliary action. Particles ranging in size from 0.5-5.0 μm in diameter can be deposited in the bronchi, with few reaching the air sacks (alveoli). Most particles deposited in the bronchioles are removed by the cilia within two hours. Particles less than 0.5 μm in diameter reach and may settle by the process of diffusion in the alveoli. The removal of particles from the alveoli is much less rapid and complete than from the larger passages. Some of the particles retained in the alveoli are absorbed into the blood.

High particle concentrations have been associated with increased mortality and bronchitis. The chemical nature of the particles may also result in an increased risk of cancer. Vegetation surfaces and growth rate may be adversely affected by particles. Particles also cause a wide range of damage to materials, including corrosion of metals, and electrical equipment, and soiling of textiles and buildings.

Inhalable PM can be deposited in the respiratory system and is associated with numerous health effects. Health effects of concern shown by epidemiologic studies to be associated with fine particles include increased hospital admissions and emergency room visits for heart and lung disease, increased respiratory symptoms and disease, decreased lung function, and even premature death, especially for the elderly (over 65 years of age). Exposure to PM also is associated with the aggravation of respiratory conditions such as asthma.

Groups that appear to be at greatest risk from the effects of PM include the elderly (persons over 65 years of age), individuals with cardiopulmonary disease (such as asthmatics), and children. Numerous studies are underway with humans and laboratory animals, with the goal being to understand the mechanisms of action of PM. Some of the possibilities implicate bioavailable transition metals in PM as mediating cardiopulmonary injury in healthy and compromised animal models (pulmonary vasculitis and hypertension). Critical PM components are now being identified, but it is unlikely that any single component of PM is responsible for all health effects. Potential differences in respiratory tract regional deposition, clearance, or retention of particles of varying size and composition may partially explain the increased sensitivity of the above-mentioned groups.

PM can act alone to produce health effects, but it also can produce effects by combining with other compounds, such as: SO_2, in the air. Such materials may become attached to the surfaces of very small particles and be carried deeper into the lungs where they can cause adverse effects. In addition to health problems, PM is the major cause of reduced visibility in many parts of the US. Airborne particles also can cause damage to paints and building materials. PM levels are decreasing, between 1988 and 1997, average PM_{10} concentrations decreased 26%. Short-term trends between 1996 and 1997 show a decrease of 1% in monitored PM_{10} concentration levels.

5. Carbon Monoxide (CO)

CO, a trace gas in the atmosphere, is produced by both natural processes and human activity. When fossil fuels are burned, two primary oxidized carbon gases are produced, carbon monoxide (CO) and carbon dioxide (CO_2). Both gases are important in the Earth's atmosphere; however, CO has greater potential impact on public health.

Carbon monoxide is a public health problem because it can affect the quality of life for sensitive people with heart disease and it is a leading cause of poisoning deaths worldwide. It is produced naturally within living organisms, and normal body functions utilize and control this endogenous CO. Inhalation of exogenous CO can overwhelm these normal functions and potentially endanger the exposed person. When inhaled, CO is readily absorbed from the lungs into the blood stream, where with hemoglobin (Hb) it forms a slowly reversible complex known as carboxyhemoglobin (COHb).

The presence of COHb in the blood decreases the oxygen-carrying capacity, potentially reducing the availability of oxygen to body tissues. Sufficient reduction in oxygen delivery, coupled with decreased blood flow because of an oxygen-deprived heart, will secondarily caused an impairment of cellular oxidative metabolism and greater loss of organ function, especially in the heart and brain. The toxic effect of high concentrations of CO (greater than 100 ppm) on the body is well known. Carbon monoxide is absorbed by the lungs and reacts with the hemoglobin of the blood. The absorption of CO is associated with a reduction in the oxygen-carrying capacity of blood. The affinity of hemoglobin for CO is over 200 times that for oxygen, indicating that carboxyhemoglobin (COHb) is a more stable compound than oxyhemoglobin. The higher the percentage of hemoglobin bound up in the form of carboxyhemoglobin, the more serious is the effect.

CO is impossible to detect by an exposed person because it is colorless, tasteless, and nonirritating. Electronic CO alarms have been developed for use in residences and some public buildings, but they will miss other possible exposures. The blood COHb level, which can be easily measured, represents a useful marker for predicting the potential health effects of total CO exposure. The amount of COHb formed depends on the CO concentration and duration of CO exposure, exercise (which increases the amount of air inhaled per unit time), the pulmonary diffusing capacity for CO, ambient pressure, health status, and specific metabolism of the exposed individual.

The level of COHb in the blood may be determined directly by blood analysis or indirectly by measuring gaseous CO in exhaled breath. The use of optical methods (e.g., CO oximetry) to measure COHb can provide useful information about mean levels in populations being studied or can aid in clinical diagnosis of CO poisoning. Gas chromatography is a better method for measuring low COHb levels (<5%).

Average levels for nonsmoking adults are < 1% COHb. Evaluation of human CO exposure situations indicates that occupational exposures in some workplaces and indoor exposures in buildings with faulty or unvented combustion appliances can exceed 100 ppm CO, often leading to COHb levels of 4-5% with 1-hour exposures and 10% or more with continued exposures for ≥ 8 hours. Carbon monoxide poisoning from such high exposure levels is not encountered by the general public exposed under outdoor (ambient) conditions.

More frequently, exposures to less than 25-50 ppm CO for an extended period of time occur among the general population in certain outdoor locations and situations associated with motor vehicle traffic. At the modest activity levels of most adults, resulting COHb levels typically remain below 2-3% for nonsmokers. Acute CO exposures, and resulting COHb levels, can be higher when a person is exposed to other combustion engine sources. Other sources may include riding behind high emitters (both on- and off-road vehicles) or riding in a vehicle with a defective exhaust system and using lawn mowers, weeders, tillers, or other garden equipment.

The CO concentration in tobacco smoke is very high -approximately 4.5% (45,000 ppm) - compared to typical exhaust from modern automobiles (7700 ppm). Levels of COHb in smokers average 4%, with a usual range of 3-8% for one- to two-pack-per-day smokers, reflecting absorption of CO from inhaled smoke. Levels as high as 15% COHb have been reported for chain smokers. Because smokers arc chronically exposed, they become adapted to higher COHb levels, as evidenced by increased red cell volumes or reduced plasma volumes. Carbon monoxide from tobacco smoke can be a significant exposure source for nonsmokers, especially in enclosed environments.

Health effects depend on the level and duration of exposure, the activity in which one is engaged, and his/her health status. For nonsmoking healthy individuals, low CO exposures producing <5% COHb will cause only small decrements in exercise performance, mostly affecting competing athletes rather that people engaged in everyday activities. At COHb levels >5%, small behavioral effects have been reported, including reductions in hand eye coordination (driving or tracking) and in attention or vigilance (detection of infrequent events).

Adverse effects have been observed in patients with diagnosed coronary artery disease (CAD) at 2-6% COHb. At these levels, individuals with angina pectoris are likely to experience a reduced capacity to exercise because of decreased time to onset of chest pain. Higher CO exposures, resulting in ≥ 6% COHb, can cause an increase in the number and complexity of exercise-related dysrhythmia (abnormal heart beat) in some people with CAD. Epidemiologic studies suggest that the effects of outdoor (ambient) CO exposure may increase the number of heart disease patients that seek medical treatment and hospitalization, but these studies are not conclusive.

The effects of exposure to low CO concentrations, resulting in COHb levels <5%, are far more subtle and considerably less threatening than those occurring in frank CO poisoning at mild (<10% COHb) and moderate (<20% COHb) levels. The effects of CO are generally more severe with higher COHb levels, including headache, dizziness, weakness, nausea, vomiting, confusion, disorientation, and visual disturbances. Breathing difficulty, increases in pulse and respiratory rates, and fainting are observed with continuous exposure. With extreme exposures, coma, convulsions, and cardiac arrest may occur. Although COHb levels can provide a general guide for clinical treatment, most physicians emphasize the poor relationship between COHb levels and clinical presentation of the poisoned patient.

Other people who may be sensitive to CO because of the effects of decreased oxygen delivery include fetuses; infants; pregnant women; the elderly; and patients with congestive heart failure, peripheral vascular or cerebrovascular disease, hematologic diseases such as anemias and obstructive lung diseases. Some people also may be at increased risk from exposure to CO because of medicinal or recreational drug use that affects the brain, from exposure to other pollutants (e.g., solvents) that increase endogenous production of CO, or from initial exposure to high altitude and CO. Unfortunately, little empirical evidence is available by which to specify health effects associated with ambient CO exposures in these probable risk groups.

One way is to avoid locations and times when vehicular traffic builds up, and to encourage vehicular inspection and maintenance to keep CO emissions low. Another way to avoid CO exposure, especially exposure to potentially dangerous levels, is to prevent high concentrations of CO from occurring in residences and other indoor environments. This can be accomplished by (a) not using tobacco products or unvented combustion sources (such as space heaters and cooking devices) indoors, and not misusing properly vented sources (e.g., using a gas oven/range for heating); (b) not allowing automobiles to idle in closed or open garages; (c) ensuring frequent inspection and routine maintenance of vented combustion appliances and fireplaces; and (d) installation of CO detectors or alarms.

6. Lead

Lead is a metal that has had many uses dating back to at least the Roman Empire. The fact that lead can be toxic has been known for centuries, although the amount of lead necessary to produce toxic effects has been the subject of debate. Lead affects multiple organs and systems of the body, but its effects on the nervous system, especially in the developing fetus and young child, have been of particular interest.

In man, lead primarily affects red blood cells, the central and peripheral nervous systems, soft tissues such as liver and kidney, and bone; the latter ultimately sequesters 95 percent of the body's lead burden. Significant biological indices of exposure to lead include microgram quantities of lead and of erythrocyte photoporphyrin (EP) per deciliter of blood ($\mu g/dl$). Adverse effects range from elevated EP and mild anemia at 20 to 40 μg Pb/dl - through gastrointestinal, renal, and hepatic pathologies - to severe neurobehavioral impairment at >80 to 120 μg Pb/dl, sometimes culminating at those levels in convulsions and abrupt death. Preschool children and developing fetuses are the populations at greatest risk.

Lead was considered a ubiquitous outdoor pollutant by the EPA primarily because of its use in gasoline. Tailpipe emissions of particles containing lead were widely dispersed in the atmosphere, becoming the predominant source of lead in outdoor (ambient) air. With the phase out of lead in gasoline, however, the importance of this source of lead exposure has declined in relation to other inhalation sources (such as dust from old leaded paint).

Lead has not been totally removed from gasoline. Many foreign countries continue to use leaded fuels. Lead also is released into the air from industrial processes, smelters, and incinerators. Besides inhaling lead-containing dust particles, however, lead exposure can come from ingestion of leaded paint and lead-contaminated food and herbal medicines, or drinking water contaminated by lead from soldered pipes. Lead also can be absorbed through the skin.

The most widely accepted indicator of lead exposure is the concentration of lead in whole blood. Although blood lead is not a perfect indicator of the body burden of lead, it is the best available measure of low-level exposure for risk assessment purposes, and it integrates exposure from all routes - inhalation, ingestion, and dermal.

The health effects of lead have been studied extensively, and recent health risk assessments have pointed to adverse health effects related to progressively lower levels of lead exposure. As consensus has grown on the adverse effects of lead exposure, especially on the hypertensive and developmental neurotoxic effects, efforts have shifted from further documentation of effects, to evaluating and reducing lead exposure.

Children are at greatest risk because of greater lead exposure, uptake, and sensitivity. Although the data base on lead health effects is massive and pertains to essentially every body system, health risk assessments of lead have tended to center on developmental neurotoxicity in children because of evidence indicating that such effects have among the lowest, if not the lowest, exposure-effect levels of any health effect of lead and because of the prima facie adverse nature of perturbations in the neurobehavioral development of children.

Numerous epidemiologic studies have been devoted to examining the relationship between measures of lead exposure (usually represented by blood lead level) and neurobehavioral development (often quantified as intelligence quotient). Collectively, these studies suggested that lead could affect neurobehavioral performance at low levels of exposure (i.e., below an average blood lead level of 30 µg/dl). The overall pattern of findings from more recent prospective epidemiologic studies points to an effect of lead on neurobehavioral development in children at blood lead levels around 10-15 µ g/dl and possibly lower.

The effects of lead on neurobehavioral development in children, although generally difficult to detect clinically in any given individual, are nonetheless significant in terms of population distributions and public health impacts. To illustrate, a shift of 4 points in the mean of a normal distribution of intelligence quotient scores would yield a 50% increase in the number of scores more than 1 standard deviation below the mean.

A number of federal agencies, including the Environmental Protection Agency, the Centers for Disease Control and Prevention, and the Department of Housing and Urban Development, are working with state and local agencies to take a variety of actions to educate the public and health care providers. Their goal is to reduce concentrations of, and exposures to, lead already in the environment (e.g., older homes with leaded paint, drinking water supplies).

A mathematical and statistical model has been developed for environmental risk assessment - the Integrated Exposure Uptake Biokinetic (IEUBK) Model for Lead. The IEUBK Model is designed to model exposure from lead in air, water, soil, dust, diet, and paint and other sources with pharmacokinetic modeling to predict blood lead levels in children 6 months to 7 years old. The IEUBK Model for lead in children can be used by health risk assessors to account more systematically for past exposures than can usually be done with a simple equation. By this means, it has been possible to refine regulatory or abatement efforts to address the specific sources that make the largest contributions to lead exposure on a population-by-population basis.

V. OTHER AIR POLLUTANTS

A. HAZARDOUS AIR POLLUTANTS

The EPA has designated a group of materials as "**hazardous air pollutants**" and has developed National Emission Standards for Hazardous Air Pollutants (NESHAP's) for each material. Although ambient air quality standards have not been developed for these materials, there are TLVs or PELs for most of these materials. NESHAPs are developed for materials which may cause or contribute to an increase in mortality or an increase in serious irreversible or incapacitating reversible illness. NESHAPs have been established for vinyl chloride, benzene, asbestos, inorganic arsenic, beryllium, mercury, and radionuclides.

B. VIABLE PARTICLES

Viable particles found in the air include pollen, spores, molds, fungi, bacteria, and viruses. The vast majority of the viable particles emanate from natural sources. There are no air pollution standards applicable to viable particles.

Research conducted at the University of Illinois at Chicago School of Public health has identified two anthropogenic sources of airborne viable particles, an activated sludge sewage treatment plant and a hospital incinerator. Although the sewage treatment plant was a source of viable particles, an epidemiological study of residents around the plant did not reveal a dose-response relation between exposure and self reported illness. In a study of bacterial emissions from a hospital incinerator, it has been found that burning of hospital waste possibly containing infectious agents does not necessarily sterilize the waste. Monitoring of stack gases at a hospital found an average bacterial concentration in the stack gas of 230 colonies/m^3 while simultaneous ambient air bacterial concentrations averaged 148 colonies/m^3. The bacteria collected were not identified so that it is as yet impossible to project the public health consequence of this finding.

C. HYDROCARBONS

Studies conducted thus far of the effects of ambient air concentrations of gaseous hydrocarbons have not demonstrated direct adverse effects from this class of pollution on human health. It has been demonstrated that ambient levels of photochemical oxidant, which do have adverse effects on health, are a direct function of gaseous hydrocarbon concentrations. Although an air quality standard was developed for hydrocarbons in order to take into account their contribution to the formation of hazardous photochemical oxidant, EPA feels that other regulations developed specifically to control oxidants (including reductions in hydrocarbon emissions) have made the hydrocarbon standard unnecessary.

VI. INDOOR AIR QUALITY

A. INTRODUCTION

Air pollution is not solely an outdoor concern. Outdoor air does come indoors. There are also indoor sources of pollutants. It is possible that indoor air quality can be quite different from outdoor air quality. Indoor air quality is a function of many variables including outdoor air quality, indoor pollutant sources, the pollutant, ventilation, and indoor decay of the pollutant. The air quality in the non-occupational environment can be a significant factor in overall pollutant exposure. These non-occupational indoor environments include places such as homes, schools, trains, stores, hospitals, restaurants, theaters, etc.

Generalizations can be made about how the indoor concentration of a pollutant compares with the outdoor concentration. Several of these generalizations are listed below. In all cases care must be taken to note words of phrases like "except' or "in the absence of" because the indoor-outdoor relationship can be markedly different under some circumstances.

B. COMMON POLLUTANTS

Sulfur Dioxide. The indoor concentration is roughly one-half the outdoor concentration.
Total Suspended Particulate Matter. The indoor concentration bears little relationship to the outdoor concentration. The size distribution and chemical composition of indoor particles is different from outdoor particles.
Carbon Monoxide. Over long averaging times and in the absence of indoor sources, indoor concentrations are about the same as outdoors. Indoor sources such as unvented or defective stoves, furnaces, and heaters as well as smoking can cause the indoor concentrations to be double or more the outdoor concentration.
Nitrogen Dioxide. If no indoor sources are present, the indoor concentration is about one-half the outdoor concentration. Indoor sources such as unvented stoves and heaters as well as smoking can cause the indoor concentration to be double or more the outdoor concentration.

Ozone. In the absence of indoor sources the concentration can be as little as one-fifth the outdoor concentration. Indoor sources such as electrostatic air cleaners and photocopying machines can cause the indoor concentration to be as high as 0.2 ppm.

Non-methane Hydrocarbons. The indoor concentration is typically 1.5 times the outdoor concentration because of many indoor sources.

Lead. There are no significant indoor sources and the indoor concentration is roughly two-thirds the outdoor concentration.

Formaldehyde. Urea formaldehyde resins have been used in a range of building products including urea-formaldehyde foam insulation, plywood, and particle board. It is unreacted formaldehyde that is given off by these products. Gas stoves have also been found to emit formaldehyde. Measurements made in two energy efficient homes showed the indoor formaldehyde concentration to be 5 to 10 times the outdoor concentration.

Radon. Radon-222 is an alpha decay product of radium-226 which naturally occurs in the earth's crust. Radium-226 is a component of building materials such as concrete, brick, and building stone. Measurements made in energy efficient homes have shown radon-222 levels to be 0.5 to 30 nC_i/m^3.

Smoking. Combustion of tobacco can be the source of numerous air pollutants. Data on the indoor concentration of these pollutants is not available, but emission factors for many of the chemicals are shown in Table 6.4.

C. BIOLOGICAL BUILDING CONTAMINANTS (BBCS)

BBCs are indoor contaminants that are either living organisms or substances originating from those organisms. Contaminant sources most often cited as creating health risks include **fungi** (molds), **bacterial endotoxins**, **arthropods** (house dust mites, cockroaches), and **fur-bearing animals**, domestic and otherwise.

Exposure occurs when these contaminants become aerosolized and are inhaled. These contaminants most commonly cause an allergic response in the respiratory tract. Symptoms can range from mild allergic rhinitis to a life-threatening asthmatic episode. From 10 to 20% of adults and children will respond to exposure to one or more of these allergens.

1. Atopic Individuals With Asthma

There is no question that indoor allergen exposure is a risk factor for frequency and severity of asthmatic attacks. And, although the data are not entirely clear, there is mounting evidence that exposure to allergens indoors plays a significant role in causation of the chronic asthmatic condition.

This is critical when considering that asthma is a serious disease and that prevalence of the chronic condition has increased more than 100% from 1987 to 1997. A 1998 survey of ninth graders in North Carolina found that 30% of participants had asthma symptoms in the year preceding the survey. National figures vary from 5 to 20% prevalence, depending on the source.

Fungi that grow indoors are saprophytic, meaning they are decay organisms. Fungi that grow indoors to form visible colonies are generally referred to as mold.

Table 6.4. Emission Factors for Mainstream and Sidestream Cigarette Smoke. (Source: Wadden & Scheff, 1982).

Properties	Mainstream Smoke	Sidestream Smoke
General Characteristics		
Duration of Smoke Production	20 sec	550 sec
Amount of Tobacco Burnt	347mg	411 mg
# of Particles Per Cigarette	1.05×10^{12}	3.5×10^{12}
Median Particle size	0.2 μm	0.15 μm
Particulate phase	(μg/cig)	μg/cig
Total Suspended Particulate Matter	36.2	25.8
Tar (Chloroform Extract)	<500-29.000	44100
Nicotine	100-2500	2.700-6750
Total Phenols	228	603
Pyrene	50-200	18-420
Benzo [A] pyrene	20-40	68-136
Naphthalene	2.8	40
Methylnaphthalene	2.2	60
Aniline	0.36	10.8
Nitrosonornicotine (NNN)	0.1-0.55	0.5-2.5
NNK[a]	0.08-0.22	0.8-2.2
Cadmium	0.13	0.45
Nickel	0.08	
Arsenic	0.012	
2-Naphthylamine	0.002-0.028	0.08
Hydrogen cyanide	74	
Polonium-210	0.029-0.044 pCi/cig	
Gases and Vapors	(μg/cig)	(μg/cig)
Water [b]	1.000-4.000	2.400-9.600
Carbon Monoxide	1.000-20.000	25.000-50.000
Carbon Dioxide	20.000-60.000	160000-480000
Acetaldehyde	18-1.400	40-3.100
Hydrogen cyanide	430	110
Methylchloride	650	1300
Acetone	100-600	250-1500
Ammonia	10-150	980-150000
Pyridine	9-93	90-930
Acrolein	25-140	55-300
Nitric Oxide	10-570	2300
Nitrogen dioxide	0.5-30	625
Formaldehyde	20-90	1300
Dimethylnitrosamine (DMN)	10-65	520-3380
Nitrosopyrolidine (NPy)	10-35	270-945

[a]   4- (N- methyl - N- nitrosamino) -1- (3 - pyridyl) -1-butanone (NNK).

[b]   3.5 mg of mainstream smoke water and 5.5 mg of sidestream smoke water in particulate phase; remainder in vapor phase.

Common genera that grow indoors include **Cladosporium**, **Aspergillus**, **Penicillium**, and **Alternaria**, among many others. Different genera can metabolize specific nutrient sources such as proteins, cellulose (wood or plant products), sugars, starches, and fats. There are always nutrient sources available indoors. The only thing that keeps fungi in check is indoor moisture control.

2. Production of Aerosols by Fungi

Fungal colonies can originate from a single vegetative cell or spore. In the presence of adequate moisture and nutrients, the vegetative or hyphal cells form a mass of growth, or mycelia. Reproductive cells, or spores, grow out of the mycelial mass. The microscopic spores are buoyant in air and are easily separated from the colony by air movement. The majority of aerosolized material is spores, but hyphae are likely to be airborne as well. Inhaled cells can result in allergy- mediated illness. Fungi may also produce mycotoxins, which may also be aerosolized. However, most illnesses due to mycotoxins are from ingestion.

When relative humidity indoors remains above 60 or 70% for more than a few hours a day, when a building surface is at or near the indoor dew point temperature, or when there is water intrusion by roof, window, or plumbing leaks, moisture can be adequate to cause fungal proliferation. Moisture that soaks into building materials is used by the fungi to solubilize nutrients in the material. Under ideal conditions a single spore can grow into a visible colony in 48 hours.

Warm air can hold more water vapor than can cold air. The temperature at which the air becomes saturated is the dew point. When a surface temperature is at or below the dew point temperature, water condenses on the surface, as it does on a glass of ice water. If the air temperature is at or below the dew point temperature, water vapor condenses into fog or rain. At a given temperature there is a maximum mass of water vapor the air can hold. Relative humidity is the percentage of water in the air that can exist in the air without the formation of condensate. If the RH is 100% the air is at dew point; if the RH is 50% the air is holding 50% of the mass of water vapor that could be held at that temperature. If the water vapor mass remains constant, RH will increase as the temperature drops, and will decrease as the temperature rises. High relative humidity and condensation on surfaces can occur as a result of heating, ventilating, and air conditioning (HVAC) system operation, occupant activities that generate water vapor, poor building insulation, or water intrusion that is not corrected.

Bathing, cooking, washing clothes, or any other activity that generates steam or adds water vapor to the air can create moisture problems indoors. Most of these activities should involve exhausting the moist air to the outdoors (e.g., clothes dryer vents, bathroom vents, range hoods).

3. HVAC System Operation

During the cooling season the air conditioning system must remove water vapor from the air that it cools. Water vapor removal occurs when chilled coolant runs through a heat exchange coil, which looks a lot like a radiator. Air is returned to the air-handling unit, where the blower and coil are located, and runs through the chilled coil. If the coil temperature is below the dew point temperature, as it should be, water will condense on the coil and drain out of the system. Removing water vapor from the air lowers relative humidity. If the system cools without removing water vapor, relative humidity will be increased indoors, which can result in fungal or other biological growth, particularly in hot, humid climates.

During cold weather, outdoor dew point temperatures are low. When outdoor air is heated to comfortable indoor temperatures, without the addition of significant amounts of water vapor (as by the use of humidifiers), relative humidity is reduced. Relative humidity levels below 30% (which are likely when outdoor temperatures are below freezing) will cause drying of the skin and mucous membranes, which can result in upper respiratory and eye irritation, and nose bleeds. Mechanical humidification of the air through the HVAC system is usually not recommended except in very cold climates, because of the risk of microbial contamination of the humidifier system.

4. Home and Office

Inexpensive temperature and humidity gauges (thermohygrometers) are available in hardware stores. Individuals should be aware that relative humidity changes hourly and the key is to look for trends. Generally if relative humidity stays above 70% for more than 4 or 5 consecutive hours per day there is likely to be trouble (mold growth).

If exterior walls and floors are not adequately insulated, their interior surfaces will be cold when the outdoor temperature is lower than the indoor temperature. If the walls are colder than the dew point temperature, water will condense on those walls, which can result in fungal growth. Other cold surfaces, such as chilled waterlines or air conditioning ducts that are poorly insulated, will have surface condensation as well. These types of problems, like many other indoor air problems, are most likely to occur in low income or poorly maintained housing.

Roof and plumbing leaks are probably the most common causes of biological contamination from water intrusions. Water can also move up through masonry floors by capillary motion. Water can then soak into carpet backing, creating excellent growth conditions for fungi.

5. Health Problems

Exposure to fungal and other antigens (bacterial or protozoan) indoors can cause Type III and Type IV reactions, such as hypersensitivity pneumonitis. This disease generally occurs after chronic exposure to relatively small antigenic particles that find their way into the lower reaches of the respiratory tract. Attack rates are generally low within the exposed population. The disease can be life threatening.

Only among immunocompromised individuals. Most fungi that grow indoors are saprophytic (decay organisms) rather than parasitic (infectious). Fungi that grow indoors are very ineffective infectious agents. **Aspergillus fumigatus** is a very common fungus that rarely causes infection in healthy individuals, even when massive exposure occurs, although severely immunocompromised individuals may develop an opportunistic respiratory infection.

Illness and disease caused by exposure to fungal toxins (mycotoxins) have been well documented over the years. Most of the reports involve livestock ingesting fungal-contaminated feed. Currently, however, there is only a suggestive causal link between mycotoxin exposure and illness and disease when fungal growth and exposure occur indoors.

In one study, pulmonary hemosiderosis (alveolar bleeding in the lungs) was reported in a significant number of infants in homes with high levels of toxigenic fungi, including Stachybotrys **chartarum (atra)**, compared to controls. Although this report raises concern about this type of exposure, there are questions about other exposures in these infants' environments and other fungi were found to be elevated significantly in their homes.

6. Environmental Sampling and Building Contamination

Usually, there is no need for environmental sampling. Most people know what fungal colonies look like, and will usually know if there are persistent moisture problems in the building. Because there are no exposure limits or guidelines for fungal exposures, the general recommendation is that there should be no fungal *growth* indoors. Visible fungal growth is a clear indicator that there is a moisture problem, and if the problem is widespread (more than a few colonies in the shower), there is an exposure risk for sensitized individuals.

The moisture problem causing the growth must be corrected in order to resolve the problem. If that has been done, simple cleaning should remove the growth from hard surfaces (tile and finished wood). Porous materials such as carpet and upholstered furniture may not be cleanable and may have to be discarded.

Remember that these contaminants are allergens. Fungal growth that is dead can still cause allergic illness if the cells become airborne and are inhaled.

Humans and contaminated water are the main sources of aerosolized bacteria in the indoor environment. Non-human-source organisms are most likely to cause illness when aerosols emanate from slime in humidifiers or from condensate collection pans in HVAC systems. There is suggestive evidence that exposure to low levels of endotoxin from gram-negative bacteria may correlate with building-related occupant complaints of respiratory and other nonspecific symptoms. High-dose endotoxin exposure, rarely encountered in the nonindustrial indoor environment, can cause acute and possibly chronic airway obstruction and possibly hypersensitivity pneumonitis.

D. BUILDING-RELATED ILLNESS

A building-related illness (BRI) is one that has an identifiable etiology that is associated with exposure in a building. Examples include allergy-induced illness (allergic rhinitis, asthma), carbon monoxide poisoning, and eye and upper respiratory irritation from formaldehyde exposure. For this designation to be made, there must be an identifiable (usually quantifiable) exposure and a tangible clinical outcome.

Sick building syndrome (SBS) is a phrase that was created in the 1980s to describe buildings in which the occupants complained of nonspecific symptoms, with generally unidentifiable etiology, that improved when they were away from the building. It is a fairly non-descriptive, if not misleading, term in that it implies that the buildings, rather than the people are sick, and that a building is either sick or it is not. In fact, if there are enough people in a building, you will be able to find some who have symptoms that they attribute to exposure in the building-that is, they have building-related complaints. In this light any building could be considered sick. A more descriptive phrase, and one that is used more now, is building-related occupant complaints (BROCs).

E. LEGIONELIA SP AS AN INDOOR BACTERIAL CONTAMINANT

Legionella is a ubiquitous bacterium with numerous environmental reservoirs indoor and out. It is the causal agent for Legionella pneumonia (Legionnaire's disease).

The organism becomes amplified indoors in warm stagnant water that contains significant organic slime. Exposure occurs when that water somehow becomes aerosolized and is inhaled.

Clusters of **Legionella** pneumonia are uncommon though not rare. A larger proportion of morbidity and mortality (legionellosis has a case fatality rate of approximately 15%) associated with the disease occurs in single or sporadic cases. Sporadic cases usually occur in immunocompromised individuals, whereas commonly encountered exposure does not affect healthy individuals with similar exposure.

Clusters of disease occur when large groups of susceptible individuals are exposed (as in a hospital setting) or when there is exposure to very high concentrations of the organism in the air.

Indoor hot water plumbing systems, whirlpool or hot tub spas, and evaporative cooling tower have been implicated in outbreaks. Nosocomial (originating in a hospital) infections result when large portions of the exposed population are immunocompromised. They are probably the most often reported outbreaks and typically result from exposure to aerosols from the plumbing system (specifically shower heads).

Sampling is not done in most cases. The incubation period is 5 to 6 days. Because disease can result from very short duration exposure, it would be necessary to monitor every environment that the individual visited during the incubation period. With a cluster of cases it is possible to use epidemiologic tools to determine probable exposure scenarios. The source(s) can then be analyzed, which is a process that typically involves sampling of the suspected water source.

F. INDOOR COMBUSTION POLLUTANTS

If the combustion process is 100% efficient (a rare event) the products of combustion are carbon dioxide (CO_2), water vapor, and oxides of nitrogen (NO_x,).

If the process is less efficient, then there are air contaminants such as combustion particulates ("smoke" when visible), unburned hydrodarbons, sulfur oxides, and carbon monoxide (CO). All of the contaminants can create health risks in the indoor environment, including those from efficient combustion. It is unlikely that carbon dioxide concentrations might reach levels that would be toxic (CO is a simple asphyxiant). Simple asphyxiants displace oxygen from the inspired air. Water vapor is not toxic, but if enough of it is generated it can condense on surfaces, which can result in fungal growth indoors.

When natural or liquid propane gas combustion processes are starved of oxygen, significant amounts of CO can be produced, enough to sicken or kill building occupants using unvented gas appliances. Oxygen sensors shut the gas unit down if there is insufficient oxygen to support efficient combustion. This innovation and home carbon monoxide sensors lessen the likelihood that there will be a catastrophic CO exposure event resulting from the use of gas appliances. It is still quite possible that low-dose CO exposure may have a significant health impact with sensor/detection systems in place and functional. They are not necessarily safe. There are still the products of combustion. Water vapor can create problems if the unvented units are used frequently or as a sole heat source, by creating a favorable environment for biological contaminants.

Pulmonary function deficits might result after indoor exposures. Numbers of studies have suggested that children living in homes with unvented gas appliances have more frequent upper respiratory infections, report more respiratory irritation, and are more likely to experience exacerbation of asthma symptoms.

A number of combustion pollutants are "intentionally" released indoors through use of kerosene space heaters, gas ranges, candles, tobacco, and incense. Many sources of combustion are unintentional: car exhaust (attached garages), back drafting fireplaces, back drafting combustion appliances (hot water heaters), and malfunctioning heating systems, among others.

The simple answer is, if you burn anything indoors it should be exhausted to the outdoors. If unvented appliances are used they should be used sparingly and never in a home with asthmatics or other susceptible occupants. Obviously burning a candle occasionally or using unvented gas logs for a few hours a week is not likely to endanger anyone. But it is simpler to recommend that combustion products should not be released indoors.

G. VENTILATION

Most of those buildings have heating, ventilating, and air conditioning systems that mechanically introduce outdoor air into the indoor environment. It is clear that in buildings, particularly crowded ones, with inadequate outdoor air ventilation, occupants are more likely to describe the air as stuffy or odorous. It is probable that inadequate outdoor air ventilation can increase the rate of building-related occupant complaints. What is much less clear still is whether a lack of outdoor air ventilation causes illness.

Outdoor air serves to dilute contaminants generated indoors. It is always preferable to remove the source (as in banning indoor smoking) rather than try to dilute the contaminants to a safe or desirable level. In most cases airborne allergen concentrations, for example, will not be significantly affected by increasing outdoor air ventilation.

There is one very important source of contaminants that cannot be removed from the indoor environment: people. People generate what we politely call **bioeffluents**. People generate odors and water vapor and the only practical means of dealing with that is to introduce outdoor air. Guidelines for ventilation rates are based on occupant density, supplying outdoor air at a specific rate per person.

Carbon Dioxide can be used to estimate outdoor air ventilation rates. A resting adult will expire about 30,000 parts per million CO_2. When CO_2 levels have stabilized in an occupied space, a concentration of 1000 ppm roughly approximates an outdoor air ventilation rate of 20 ft³/min per person. Carbon dioxide indoors may be at concentrations that are toxic (greater than 5000 ppm). Investigators measure CO_2 because it is an easy way to get a rough estimate of outdoor air ventilation rates.

H. ODORS

A medical dictionary defines an odor as "the volatile emanation that is perceived by the sense of smell." Odorants are the gases or compounds that produce the sense of smell (olfaction) when they are inhaled and deposited in the olfactory cleft of the nose.

When an odorant reaches one or more of the 5 million olfactory receptor cells in the nasal epithelium within the bridge of the nose, a signal is sent via the olfactory nerve to the olfactory cortex of the brain and an odor is detected. In addition to olfactory receptor cells, the nasal epithelium contains trigeminal (5th cranial nerve) nerve receptors, responsible for sensations such as irritation, tickling, burning, and cooling. These sensations often accompany olfaction. Chemical stimulation of the trigeminal nerves is referred to as chemesthesis, instead of the "common chemical sense," to emphasize that the trigeminal nerve is part of the somatic nervous system. In practice, olfaction and chemesthesis operate as a single perceptual system.

Information from the olfactory cortex is passed to an almond-shaped structure in the brain, the amyglada, sometimes called "the seat of emotion." This neuroanatomical connection is speculated to be one reason why odors seem to be associated with emotional-laden memories.

Humans can detect the odors of many pure substances at concentrations in air of parts per billion (ppb), near the analytical detection limits of modern analytical chemistry technique. Many environmental odorants are complex mixtures, and the understanding of human sensitivity to odorant mixtures is limited. Odorant mixtures in the field are often composed of gases and particulates.

Although there is active research on the "electronic nose" and prototypes have been deployed successfully, the current technology has not developed an analytical instrument that can accurately simulate the sensitivity of the human nose to environmental odorants under field conditions.

Airborne emissions from many operations are complex mixtures that contain gases and particles. Dust from industrial and agricultural sources may contain a high percentage of fine particulate (smaller than 5 μm in mass median diameter). Fine particulate is significant because it comes airborne easily, remains suspended for long time periods, may travel long distances, offers a large ratio of surface area to mass for adsorbing odorants, and is better able to penetrate and deposit in the deeper areas of the respiratory system.

The most reliable methods use odor panels-trained individuals or groups - exposed to creasing dilutions (increasing concentrations) of sample air until an odor can be detected. The number of dilutions of sample air required to reach the detection or irritation threshold is often used as a surrogate for intensity. A standardized, controlled, and statistical version of the panel method was developed by the food and fragrance industries and is reliable enough to have national standards. Although odor panels were developed for characterizing odors with positive characteristics (good smells), the technique is also applied to odors with aversive characteristics (bad smells). In addition to detecting odors, odor panelists have "calibrated noses" i.e., and the ability to compare and rank the odor to a reference odor using standard methods.

Odor panels typically measure and quantify the main parameters of odors:

1. **Concentration**: Detection and irritation threshold.
2. **Intensity**: The strength of an odor compared to a reference (usually butanol).
3. **Character**: Description of an odor using a standard vocabulary
4. **Hedonic tone**: A qualitative measurement of the degree of pleasantness or unpleasantness.

As the concentration of an odorant increases, the first level of importance is odor **detection level**, a level at which an odor can be differentiated from ambient air. Next, at the odor **recognition level**, a person begins to characterize the odor. At the **annoyance level**, a person may be annoyed by the odor but will show no physical reaction. At the odor **intolerance level**, an individual may show physical (somatic) symptoms. At the **perceived irritation level**, symptoms occur as a result of stimulation of nerve endings in the olfactory epithelium and other sections of the respiratory tract. **Somatic irritation**, **acute toxicity**, and **chronic toxicity** are in the realm of classical toxicology.

Model 1 - Irritant or other toxic effects occur at levels below the odor detection threshold. Some gases, such as carbon monoxide and arsine, have poor warning properties; odor perception will provide warning of serious acute impending toxicity.

Model 2 - Physical irritation or other toxicological effects occur at a level above, but within an order or magnitude of, the odor detection threshold. Many common industrial chemicals such as volatile organic compounds, formaldehyde, and hydrogen sulfide fall in this category.

Model 3 - Odor potency is far above the irritation or toxic level, but at levels that could stimulate the olfactory receptors or trigeminal receptors. In some people olfactory stimulation may trigger nontoxicological odor-related health effects. Factors such as hedonic tone, exposure history, beliefs about safety of the odor, and emotional status may be important factors in inducing or exacerbating health symptoms. These nontoxicological symptoms might trigger physiological stress and a cascade of other health effects.

Model 4 - The odorant is part of a mixture and one or more copollutants are responsible for the health symptoms; the odor is a marker for exposure. Confounding this model is that acquired conditioning may influence health effects from odors. In experimental studies people have been exposed to an odorant mix containing the odorant and some other compound that can cause a measurable response. After acquired conditioning, subsequent exposures to the odorant the co-pollutant will elicit the response.

In studying citizen telephone calls to a typical air pollution control district it was found that 70-80% of calls concerned environmental odors. The symptoms are acute in onset, self-limiting in duration, and difficult to validate with standard clinical tools. Symptoms most often include headache, nausea and mucous membrane irritation, and respiratory irritation.

Preexisting medical conditions - A wide variety of odors (flowers, perfume, cleaning products, and petroleum) are implicated as asthma triggers in some individuals. Another example of hypersensitivity is seen in "morning sickness" during pregnancy.

Preexisting psychological conditions - Some conditions, such as hypochondriasis might render some individuals more symptomatic in response to odor stimuli.

Odor aversion conditioning - A number of studies have documented conditioning responses after acute overexposure to irritant or other toxic chemicals such as pesticides. After the initial event, patients report they react to very low odor exposures. The phenomenon has many names, including acquired intolerance to pesticides, acquired intolerance to solvents, atypical posttraumatic stress disorder, behavioral sensitization, and odor-triggered panic attacks, among others.

I. INTENSIVE LIVESTOCK OPERATIONS

In modern agricultural meat and dairy production (swine, poultry, and cattle), large numbers of animals are raised or held inside confinement buildings under controlled environmental conditions. Intensive livestock operations (ILOs) are managed to grow the most meat for the least cost. The farmer manages every aspect of the production cycle, including diet, thermal control, and waste disposal.

Odorants from livestock operations come from four areas:

1. Dead animal management and disposal,
2. Confinement buildings and animal holding facilities,
3. Manure storage and treatment, and
4. Land application of treated liquids and sludge.

Although farmers attempt to reduce mortality, a large ILO may produce over 40,000 pounds of dead animals a year. The carcasses are disposed of by several methods, including commercial rendering, landfill, on-farm burial or incineration. Each of these methods can be significant odor sources if mismanaged.

Confinement buildings have a high odor potential due to high stocking density of animals and a large volume of feed and manure in storage. Many odorants are by-products of anaerobic microbial decomposition of organic material and manure. The easiest odor control method is to keep the building clean and remove accumulated organic materials before anaerobic decomposition begins.

Generally, increasing temperature and humidity will intensify odorant emissions because microbial activity generally increases when temperature rises. High ventilation rates in buildings are required to remove heat and moisture produced by animals. Large exhaust volumes will increase the emission rate from the building. In addition, higher amounts of dust seem to intensify odorants emissions.

Aerosols in poultry and livestock houses are primarily composed of dust from feed components and dried fecal material. Other materials may include dander (hair and skin cells, feathers), mold, pollen, and insect parts. Sources include the feed and the feed delivery systems, bedding, animal wastes, and animal shedding. Many volatile fatty acids or other volatile odorant compounds can be adsorbed to particles. Some of the components of ILO dust may contain constituents such as proteins and endotoxins, which can cause irritation or allergic response.

Manure is a combination of feces and urine. Feces are the end product of an animal's digestive system. Fecal material consists of water, enteric bacteria, and undigested and indigestible material in a slurry form. Urine, a liquid excreted by the kidneys, contains the many water-soluble nitrogenous and sulfurous wastes that are eliminated from the bloodstream. Swine manure is about 60% feces and 40% urine. A 1000-head swine finishing operation produces about 8,000 gallons of manure per day. Of course the amount of manure produced by a pig will vary depending on the age, weight, and life stage of the animal.

Most ILOs use anaerobic lagoons for wastewater treatment. Anaerobic lagoons are dynamic biological systems that use anaerobic (without oxygen) bacteria to digest pathogens and waste products. Well-managed lagoons emit few odors. However, improperly managed or agitated lagoons have the potential for releasing large amounts of odorants. Start-up lagoons will create odors until biological processes stabilize. A lagoon overloaded with a "slug" of waste will also release odors. Other conditions that destabilize the system, such as inadequate dilution of waste and inadequate treatment volume, can also cause odorants to be released. In some climates lagoons "turn over" on a seasonal basis due to thermal Inversions.

Eventually the anaerobic bacteria in a lagoon will digest pathogens and organic material to relatively low levels. Typically the upper layers from a lagoon will be removed and applied to fields at agronomic rates for fertilizer. The treated liquid may be sprayed or injected into fields. Spray application is aesthetically unattractive and may produce significant amounts of odor.

Several hundred different odorant compounds have been identified in the exhaust air from confinement buildings and manure.

There are four main chemical classes:

1. **Volatile fatty acids** - Acetic, butyric, isobutyric, propanoic, and caproic
2. **Indoles and phenols** - Indole, skatole, cresol, and 4-ethylphenol
3. **Volatile amines** - Putrescine, cadaverine, methylene, and ethylamine
4. **Ammonia**

Many studies have found a variety of acute health effects among people working in confinement buildings. Among the reported symptoms are cough, phlegm production, upper respiratory tract irritation (nose and throat), eye irritation, headaches, chest tightness, shortness of breath, wheezing, and muscle aches/pain. Long-term studies have shown an exposure-related response, with chronic cough and chronic phlegm production to be the most prevalent symptoms.

VII. BIBLIOGRAPHY

American Chemical Society. (1969). Cleaning our Environment. The Chemical Basis for Action. Washington, D.C.

Donn, W.L. (1965). Meteorology. McGraw-Hill.

Guidotti, T.L. (1994). The Environment and Health. In McCunney, R.J. A Practical Approach to Occupational and Environmental Medicine, 2nd Edition (pp. 605-613). Boston, MA: Little, Brown and Company.

Lyons, W.A., & C.E. Olsson. (1972). Mesoscale Air Pollution Transport in the Chicago Lake Breeeze, JAPCA, 22, pp. 876-881.

Martin, D.O., P.A. Humphrey & J.L. Dicke. (1967). Interstate Air Pollution Study Phase II Project Report: V. Meteorology and Topography. U.S. Department of Health, Education and Welfare.

McLellan, R.K. & McCunney, R.J. (1994). Indoor Air Pollution. In McCunney, R.J. A Practical Approach to Occupational and Environmental Medicine, 2nd Edition (pp. 633-650). Boston, MA: Little, Brown and Company.

Moeller, D. W. (1997). Air in the Home and Community. Environmental Health (pp.77-102). Cambridge, MA, and London, UK: Harvard University Press.

Moore, G. S. (1999). Air, Noise, and Radiation. Living with the Earth: Concepts in Environmental Health Sciences (pp.10.1 - 10.51). Boca Raton, FL: Lewis Publishers.

Nadakavukaren, A. (2000). Air Pollution. Our Global Environment: A Health Perspective, 5th Edition (pp.447-506). Prospective Heights, IL: Waveland Press, Inc.

Raub, J.A., McGrath, J.J., Davis, J.M., & Folinsbee, L.J. (2001). Criteria Pollutants. In Williams, L.K. & Langley, R.L. (Eds). Environmental Health Secrets (pp. 5-16), Philadelphia, PA: Hanley & Belfus.

Rossano, A.T., (Ed). (1969). Air Pollution Control: Guidebook for Management. Environmental Science Service Division, E.R.A. Inc, Stamford, CT.

Service, W. (2001). Indoor Air Quality. In L. Williams, & R. Langley (Eds.), Environmental Health Secrets (pp. 19-24). Philadelphia, PA: Hanley & Belfus, Inc.

Stern, A.C., (Ed). (1977). Air Pollution, Vol. IV Engineering Control of Air Pollution, 3rd. Edition, Academic Press.

Stoker, H. S., & Seager, S. L. (1972). Environmental Chemistry: Air and Water Pollution. Scott, Foresman and Company.

Sutton, O. G. (1953). Micrometeorology. McGraw-Hill.

Wadden, R.A., & Scheff, P.A. (1982). Indoor Air Pollution: Characterization, Prediction and Control. John Wiley and Sons, New York.

Watkins, A. M. (2001). Outdoor Pollution: Acid Rain. In L. Williams, & R. Langley (Eds.), Environmental Health Secrets (pp. 16-18). Philadelphia, PA: Hanley & Belfus, Inc.

Williams, L.K. (2001). Outdoor Pollution. Environmental Health Secrets (pp. 5-6), Philadelphia, PA: Hanley & Belfus.

Yassi, A., Kjellstrom, T., Kok, T.D. (2001). Basic Environmental Health (pp. 180-208). New York, NY: Oxford University Press.

Yassi, A., Kjellstrom, T., Kok, T.D. (2001). Basic Environmental Health (pp. 378-387). New York, NY: Oxford University Press.

CHAPTER

7

WATER QUALITY

I. <u>INTRODUCTION</u>

Water is the most abundant substance on Earth's surface. The oceans cover approximately 71 percent of the planet; glaciers and ice caps cover additional areas; and water is also found in lakes and streams, in soils and underground reservoirs, in the atmosphere, and in the bodies of all living organisms. Thus, water, in all its forms – ice, liquid water, and water vapor – is very familiar to us.

Compared with other substances, however, water has unique properties. Ice floats on liquid water; much energy is consumed when ice melts or when water evaporates; and water is an excellent solvent for many different kinds of substances. All these properties of water affect its role in the biosphere. The movement of water on Earth (the hydrologic cycle) is closely related to the energy changes that take place when water changes its form between solid, liquid, and vapor. The water can be a vehicle for spread of the pathogens and other environmental health hazards.

Water, a multiple use resource, has uses for: human consumption, agricultural production, electric power generation, navigation/transportation, industrial production, waste disposal, recreation, and aquatic life and wildlife.

Since there is a finite amount of water available for all of these uses, this chapter will discuss the following:
1. The hydrologic cycle and water resources,
2. Water pollution, receiving water and receptors,
3. Water parameters as a measure of water quality, biochemical oxygen demand, microorganisms, solids, temperature, plant nutrients, inorganic and organic chemicals, and
4. Treatment methods to improve water quality, municipal water and wastewater treatment.

II. <u>HYDROLOGIC CYCLE AND WATER RESOURCES</u>

Water moves through a hydrological cycle from the oceans to the atmosphere, from the atmosphere to the land, and from the land back to the oceans (Figure 7.1). Basically, solar energy evaporates water into the atmosphere from the oceans, lakes, rivers, soil, and plants (evapotranspiration). Then, it is cooled and precipitates as rain or snow onto the land and receiving bodies of water where by gravity it moves back to the oceans. It has been estimated that the maximum flow of fresh water resources that is available for human use each year in the world is about 38,000 cubic kilometers (10 quadrillion gallons).

In the United States, it has been estimated that the maximum flow of fresh water resources that is available for human use each day is 4.54 cubic kilometers (1200 billion gallons per day). Of this amount, only about 315 bdg (billion gallons per day) can realistically be developed as a sustained, dependable, water supply for human use. Of the water withdrawn for human use, about 9%, is used for domestic and commercial uses, 40% is used for irrigation, and 43% is used for industrial purposes (26% is for cooling electric power plants).

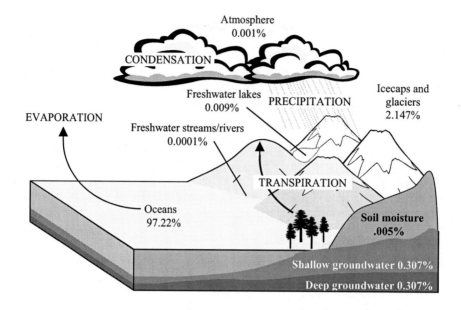

<u>Figure 7.1.</u> The Hydrological Cycle, and percentage of water in various earth compartments. (Source: Moore, 1999).

III. <u>HEALTH RISKS</u>

Historically, considerations of the effects on health of water contamination have focused on waterborne diseases, such as typhoid fever and cholera. Although today the most frequently reported waterborne disease in the United States is acute gastrointestinal illness (or gastroenteritis), this concern has expanded to include giardiasis and cryptosporidiosis. The latest data show that almost one million people in this country become sick each year from drinking contaminated water. Careful examination, however, shows that water can have effects on the health of a population far beyond those that result from its ingestion.

Although the transmission of infectious diseases by water has been virtually eliminated in the developed nations, concern is increasing about the health implications of a host of other contaminants, particularly toxic chemicals, that can be present in drinking-water supplies. Evaluation of the health effects of these newly recognized contaminants is complicated by the problems faced in essentially all other fields of environmental and occupational health, namely, the latency (time delay) in the appearance of effects and the lack of definitive data on dose-response relationships. In addition, the federal government has been slow to acknowledge the importance of drinking water to health; the first federal law directly addressing the subject, the Safe Drinking Water Act, was not passed by the U.S. Congress until December 1974.

Most diseases associated with water are caused by pathogens. These diseases are traditionally classified according to the nature of the pathogen. However, such a classification is not very useful for prevention. As explained in **Our Planet, Our Health** (WHO, 1992), a more useful way of classifying these diseases is according to the various aspects of the environment that human intervention can alter. The diseases are the following:

Waterborne Diseases These arise from the contamination of water by human or animal feces or urine infected by pathogenic viruses or bacteria, which are directly transmitted when the water is drunk or used in the preparation of food. Cholera, typhoid, and cryptosporidiosis are typical examples of Waterborne diseases (Table 7.1).

Water-Privation Diseases This category of diseases is affected more by the quantity of water rather than by quality. These diseases spread through direct contact with infected people or materials contaminated with the infectious agent. Infrequent washing and inadequate personal hygiene are the main factors in these types of diseases, such as certain types of diarrheal diseases, helminths, and skin and eye infections.

Water-Based Diseases In these diseases, water provides the habitat for intermediate host organisms in which some parasites pass part of their life cycle. These parasites are later the cause of disease in people as their infective larval forms in fresh water find their way back to humans, either by boring through wet skin or by being ingested with water plants, minute water crustacea, or raw or inadequately cooked fish. Schistosomiasis is an example of a water-based disease.

Water-Related Diseases Water may provide a habitat for insect vectors of water-related diseases. Mosquitoes breed in water and the adult mosquitoes may transmit parasite diseases, such as malaria, and virus infections, such as dengue, yellow fever, and Japanese encephalitis.

Water-Dispersed Infections The disease categories listed above are primarily problems in developing countries. A fifth category of diseases associated with water is emerging in developed countries-infections whose pathogens can proliferate in freshwater and enter the body through the respiratory tract. Some freshwater amoebae that are not usually pathogenic can proliferate in warm water, and if they enter the host in large numbers, they can invade the body along the olfactory tracts and cause fatal meningitis. These bacteria can be dispersed as aerosols from air-conditioning systems; an example of this type of disease is Legionella.

Projections regarding population growth have been made for the year 2000, and it is estimated that growth in the world alone will cause at least a doubling in the demand for water in nearly half of the countries of the world. Hardest hit will be those countries with low per capita water availability and high population growth (parts of Africa, South Asia, the Middle East, and Latin America).

Even though withdrawal of water already exceeds the dependable supply of 315 bgd, it is the consumption of water which is of greater concern. Consumption use means that the water is either lost to the atmosphere by evaporation and transpiration, or it becomes a part of some entity such that is cannot be retrieved to the water base. Although agriculture (irrigation) is the largest water consumer, future water consumption is estimated to remain well below what is available. However, uneven distribution of runoff in the United States causes some regions in the United States to experience either droughts or flooding.

Table 7.1. Waterborne Pathogens. (Source: Yassi, 2001).

Pathogen	Health Significance	Persistence in Water Supplies	Resistance to Chlorine	Relative Infective Dose	Important Animal Reservoir
BACTERIA					
Campylobacter jejuni, C. coli	High	Moderate	Low	Moderate	Yes
Pathogenic E. coli	High	Moderate	Low	High	Yes
Salmonella typhi	High	Moderate	Low	High	No
Other salmonellae	High	Long	Low	High	Yes
Shigella spp.	High	Short	Low	Moderate	No
Vtbrio choierae	High	Short	Low	High	No
Yersinia enterocolitica	High	Long	Low	High(?)	Yes
Pseudomonas aeruginosa	Moderate	May multiply	Moderate	High(?)	No
Aeromonas spp.	Moderate	May multiply	Low	High(?)	No
VIRUSES					
Adenoviruses	High	?	Moderate	Low	No
Enteroviruses	High	Long	Moderate	Low	No
Hepatitis A	High	?	Moderate	Low	No
Hepatitis E	High	?	?	Low	No
Norwalk virus	High	?	?	Moderate	No(?)
Rotavirus	High	?	?	Moderate	No(?)
Small round viruses	Moderate	?	?	Low (?)	No
PROTOZOA					
Entamoeba histolytica	High	Moderate	High	Low	No
Giardia intestinalis	High	Moderate	High	Low	Yes
Cryptosporidium parvum	High	Long	High	Low	Yes
HELMINTHS					
Dracuncuius medinensis	High	Moderate	Moderate	Low	Yes

Some methods suggested by scientists to reduce the likelihood of droughts and/or floods are:

1. Divert water from one region to another,
2. Create lake reservoirs by building dams,
3. Desalt seawater,
4. Tap and artificially recharge ground water supplies
5. Tow icebergs to regions short on water,
6. Control the precipitation patterns in the region,

7. Better pollution control,
8. Decrease evaporation losses in irrigation,
9. Encourage the reduction in population growth in areas with water problems,
10. Better design of industrial processes to decrease water use, and
11. Conservation of water.

Many of the above suggestions have inherent problems and impact on the environment and water quality. For instance, dams can have undesirable ecological and health effects because a large amount of land is permanently flooded. In addition to the loss of a large amount of land, the dams also can create a health problem in the still waters of the reservoir because the environment is ideal for the survival of snails and the transmission of a painful disease called schistosomiasis.

Another kind of impact can occur from water diversion projects where surface irrigation dissolves various salts as the waters flow over and through the ground. As this saline water is spread over the soil for irrigation, evaporation takes place and these soils can build up with salts and make the soil infertile. In addition, another problem associated with soil salinity, waterlogging, happens when irrigation water percolates downward, and the water table rises close to the soil surface as a result. Then, when too much water accumulates around plant roots, growth is inhibited.

Finally, the suggestion of tapping more ground water supplies as a solution to water supply problems has resulted in problems such as:

1. Depletion
2. Sinking or subsidence
3. Salinization
4. Contamination

Removing groundwater faster than it is recharged leads to groundwater depletion and subsidence. Groundwater can be naturally recharged as vegetation slows the runoff from a rain, and migrates through the soil to aquifers. Obviously, development of large urban areas and removal of vegetation leads to catchment deterioration, erosion and a decrease in water supply. Ground water can also be recharged artificially. When this is done, great care must be taken to prevent the groundwater from being contaminated. Coastal areas have a unique problem when groundwater is removed faster than it is replaced because saltwater intrusion occurs. This process happens when fresh groundwater is pumped from wells faster than it is replaced, and saline groundwater below the ocean bottom moves inland replacing the fresh groundwater area with unusable salt water. Other sources of groundwater contamination result from surface disposal of wastes, mine drainage, sanitary landfills, animal feedlot wastes, and agricultural pesticides and herbicides.

IV. <u>WATER POLLUTION, RECEIVING WATER AND RECEPTORS</u>

There is only a finite amount of water circulating through the hydrologic cycle. As water circulates through this cycle, its quality is continually changing, both by natural and man-made conditions. Receiving waters are affected naturally by the geophysical, hydrologic and meteorological characteristics of the drainage basin. Furthermore, precipitation picks up natural substances from the atmosphere such as gases, dust, microorganisms, pollen and other natural airborne particles. Once the precipitation contacts the land. It can pick up soil particles, vegetation, and microorganisms as the runoff moves to receiving waters, or it infiltrates into groundwater supplies.

Man-made changes in water quality (pollution) result from industrialization, urbanization, and agricultural practices. Basically, pollutants are discharged from point and non-point sources into the water environment. The amounts of these pollutants are best described as a mass/time rate, such as pounds/hour. Once the pollutants reach the receiving water, they are generally characterized by measuring their mass per unit volume (e.g., milligrams/liter) related to some averaging time of sample collection. Water quality models are used to predict the concentrations of pollutions in receiving waters. Finally, after the pollutant concentrations are determined in the receiving water, it is important to determine what the water is used for, and its impact on such receptors as human health, plants, materials, and aesthetics (Figure 7.2).

Water Models

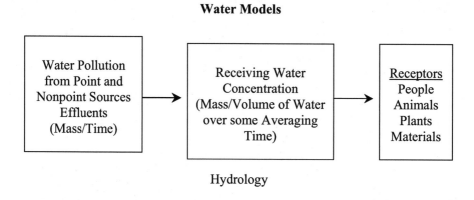

Figure 7.2. Water Pollution, Receiving Water and Receptors.

V. <u>WATER PARAMETERS AS A MEASURE OF WATER QUALITY</u>

In order to determine if a receiving water can be utilized for a specific use (e.g.,public drinking water supply or recreation), there are waterparameters such as biochemical oxygen demand (BOD)/dissolved oxygen (DO), microorganisms, solids, temperature, plant nutrients, inorganic and organic chemicals, and radioactive substances that can be measured to determine the quality of a water. By measuring these parameters, it can be determined whether a receiving water is acceptable for a water supply, a bathing beach, a fishing area, or any other use. Radioactive substances have been covered under the Solid Waste Management and Radiological Health chapters.

A. BIOCHEMICAL OXYGEN DEMAND (BOD)/DISSOLVED OXYGEN (DO)

Dissolved oxygen is a very important water quality parameter because the amount present determines whether desirable aquatic species such as trout will be present. Generally, if the DO of a receiving stream is decreasing appreciably, oxygen-demanding wastes such as sewage or certain industrial effluents are probably being carried into the water.

Basically, the following four processes determine the amount of oxygen in water: reaeration, photosynthesis, respiration, and the oxidation of biodegradable organic wastes. Reaeration is the process whereby oxygen enters the water from the atmosphere when the actual amount of oxygen in the water is less than the saturation value. The saturation value varies inversely with water temperature having an oxygen solubility of 14.7 mg/l at 0 ^{0}C and 7.4 mg/l at 30 ^{0}C. Reaeration from the atmosphere takes place at a rate which is proportional to the oxygen deficit.

The process of photosynthesis and respiration respectively increase and decrease the oxygen concentration in the water. Therefore, the processes of reaeration, photosynthesis and respiration result in a diurnal variation of DO.

The fourth process, which can impact appreciably on the amount of oxygen in water, is the oxidation of biodegradable organic wastes by bacteria as shown in the following equation:

$$\begin{array}{c} \text{Organic} \\ \text{Waste} \end{array} \xrightarrow[\text{oxygen consumption}]{\text{bacteria}} CO_2 + H_2O + \text{new bacteria}$$

If all the oxygen in the water is used up during the aerobic decomposition of the organic matter, the process will continue under anaerobic conditions with such undesirable reaction products as ammonia, methane and hydrogen sulfide. As long as the load of organic waste to a receiving water is not overwhelming, the processes of reaeration and deoxygenation from the decomposition of organic matter will simultaneously occur producing an oxygen sag phenomenon (Figure 7.3). The oxygen sag will occur some distance or time downstream from the point of discharge.

An important water quality parameter which gives the potential oxygen removal from an organic waste is called the biochemical oxygen demand (BOD). More specifically, BOD is the amount of oxygen required to stabilize (breakdown to inorganic forms) the decomposable organic matter present under aerobic conditions.

The rate of biochemical oxidation of organic matter is proportional to the remaining concentration of un-oxidized substance measured in terms of oxidizability. Therefore, the amount of organic matter remaining decreases exponentially with time. At time zero, the total oxygen requirement to oxidize the organic material is called the ultimate BOD. An equation describing this curve is as follows:

$$BOD_{remaining} = BOD_L \, e^{-kt}$$

Where k is a reaction-rate constant (days $^{-1}$), and t is time in days.

Dissolved oxygen (mg/L)

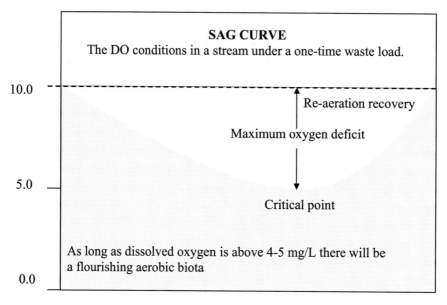

Time in days

Figure 7.3. Typical Sag Curve Resulting from the Deposit of High BOD Materials into a Receiving Body of Water. (Source: Moore, 1999).

The curve for BOD remaining versus time is depicted in Figure 7.4. Many times BOD data are reported as BOD utilized rather than BOD remaining. The BOD utilized curved is a mirror image of the BOD remaining curve, and is proportional to the amount of organic matter which has been oxidized (Figure 7.4). The equation for BOD utilized is as follows: $BOD_{utilized} = BOD_L (1-e^{-kt})$

In the laboratory, the BOD is determined by incubating a sample of some waste water for five days at 20°C. Once the amount of oxygen required by bacteria for the first five days of decomposition is determined, the ultimate BOD can be determined by using the equation for BOD utilized. The discussion of BOD to this point has only concerned the carbonaceous organic matter. An additional demand for oxygen in water results when nitrogenous organic matter is converted by a process of nitrification as shown in the following equation:

$$\text{Organic N} \xrightarrow[\text{Bacteria}]{O_2} NH_3 \xrightarrow[\text{Bacteria}]{O_2} NO_2 \xrightarrow[\text{Bacteria}]{O_2} NO_3$$

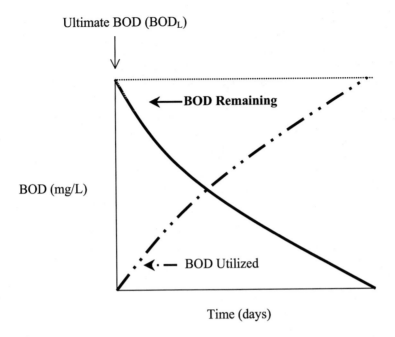

Figure 7.4. BOD as a Function of Time.

B. MICROORGANISMS

Another important parameter in determining water quality is microorganisms. The major concern with microorganisms is that there are many pathogenic bacteria, parasites, and viruses, which can cause outbreaks of waterborne diseases, such as typhoid, cholera, dysentery, and infectious hepatitis. Major sources of pathogenic organisms come from domestic sewage and animal wastes.

Since it is quite difficult to detect pathogenic microorganisms in a water supply, indicator organisms are used to determine if the water is full of pathogens. A good indicator organism is a non-pathogen that is found in large numbers in the excreta of humans and other warm-blooded animals. The assumption being made with indicator organisms is that their absence also means the absence of pathogens.

The two groups of organisms that are used most frequently to determine if the water is contaminated with sewage are the coliform and the enterococcus.

"The coliform group comprises all of the aerobic and facultative anaerobic gram-negative, non-spore-forming, rod-shaped bacteria that ferment lactose with gas formation within 48 hrs. at 35°C." Total coliform determinations are made to determine whether water can be used as a drinking water supply. Total coliforms are comprised of fecal coliforms such as **Escherichia coli**, which are found in the intestinal tracts of humans and warm-blooded animals, non-fecal vegetable coliform such as **Aerobacter sp.**, which are found in the soil and on plants, and intermediate-aerogenes-cloacal coliforms which are found in both fecal and non-fecal habitats. Fecal coliform determinations are generally made to determine whether a water source is acceptable for swimming.

The other group of nonpathogenic organisms that is commonly used as an indicator of fecal contamination is the fecal streptococci. Streptococci are more resistant than coliforms to chlorine and, as a consequence are considered to be a more sensitive test for swimming pools.

Once bacteria like fecal coliforms reach a receiving water, they tend to die-off at a constant rate according to Chick's law:

$$\frac{dN}{dT} = -kN$$

which can be integrated to:

$$N = N_0e^{-kt}$$

where: N = the residual number of bacteria after time t
N_0 = the initial number of bacteria
k = the die-off constant (day^{-1})

Coliforms are a group of bacteria that are normal inhabitants of the intestinal tract. They include **Escherichia coli** (or **E. coli***)* and various species of **Klebsiella, Enterobacter**, and **Citrobacter**. All but **E.coli** may also be present in the soil. A **colilert test** is the routine test used to determine if coliforms are absent or present in water. The presence of coliforms with the absence of **E. coli** (i.e., fecal coliforms) suggests that the naturally occurring bacteria from the soil possibly entered the water supply through runoff.

Coliform bacteria are rarely pathogenic, but there are a few exceptions. Certain strains of **E.coli** have been associated with gastrointestinal infections in adults (traveler's diarrhea, or Montezuma's revenge), urinary tract infections, and neonatal meningitis. **Klebsiella pneumoniae** has been associated with gastrointestinal infections, pneumonia, hospital-acquired urinary tract infections, and burn wound infections, and is seen as a secondary pathogen to other primary respiratory infections. **Enterobacter** has been associated with hospital-acquired urinary tract infections. **Citrobacter** has been associated with hospital-acquired urinary tract infections, superficial wound infections, osteomyelitis, neonatal meningitis, and gastroenteritis.

The **colilert test** first indicates either the presence or absence of total coliforms, then **E. coli** (a fecal coliform) may he identified. The presence of total coliforms and F. colt indicates that fecal contamination from human or animal waste has occurred and that contaminants such as pathogenic bacteria, protozoa, viruses, and helminths may be present in the water.

The principal bacterial pathogens associated with acute gastrointestinal illness (diarrhea, abdominal pain) from drinking contaminated water are **Aeromonas hydrophila**, **Campylobacter jejuni**, **E. coli** (specific strains), **Plesiomonas shigelloides**, various **Salmonella** species (e.g., **Salmonella typhi***)*, various **Shigella** species, **Vibrio cholerae**, and **Yersinia enterocolitica**.

The principal protozoa associated with acute gastrointestinal illness from drinking contaminated water are various **Cryptosporidium** species, **Entamoeba histolytica**, and **Giardia lamblia**.

The principal viruses associated with acute gastrointestinal illness from drinking contaminated water are **Astrovirus, Calicivirus, enteroviruses** (polio viruses, coxsackie viruses, and echo viruses), hepatitis A, hepatitis E, Norwalk and Norwalk-related viruses, Group A rotavirus, and Group B rotavirus,

The principal helminth associated with acute gastrointestinal illness from drinking contaminated water is **Dracunculus medinensis** (guinea worm).

There is a group of nuisance microorganisms collectively designated as iron bacteria, sulfur bacteria, and sulfate-reducing bacteria that may be found in drinking water. These bacteria are not pathogenic and are naturally found in soil. These nuisance bacteria are responsible for various transformations of iron, usually in the form of slime, and often cause a bad odor or taste in the water. Iron bacteria may cause plugging of wells and impart a reddish tinge to the water. Sulfur and sulfate-reducing bacteria may cause rusty water and corrosion of pipes.

C. SOLIDS

Solids impart a certain quality to water and impact directly on what uses are appropriate for a water source. Solids determination is important in both water and wastewater treatment processes. Total solids are defined as the matter that remains as residue upon evaporation and drying at 103°C. Solids can be broken up into dissolved and undissolved matter. The undissolved solids are referred to as suspended solids, and those solids that will settle out under quiescent conditions are called settleable solids.

The dissolved solids concentration in water has a bearing on its suitability for domestic use. Generally, water with a dissolved solids concentration of less than 250 mg/l is recommended for drinking water supplies because of possible physiological effects (laxative effect from sulfates, cardiovascular effect for people on low sodium diets), unpalatable mineral tastes, and higher costs because of the corrosion effect. Suspended solids cause turbidity in the water, and the settleable solids will blanket the benthos damaging invertebrate populations, destroying spawning beds, and increasing BOD demand. Finished drinking water supplies have to be low in turbidity because chlorine cannot properly disinfect turbid water.

D. TEMPERATURE

Heat from industrial and power plant cooling water can cause receiving water to increase in temperature with resulting deleterious environmental impacts. For instance, dissolved oxygen in water decreases with increasing temperature, and the metabolic rate of most aquatic organisms increases. Also, at highest water temperatures the rate of decomposition of wastes increases. The overall result is a decrease in the dissolved oxygen concentration.

Another deleterious impact of increased water temperature is a change in the predominant type of algae that will be present. As the water temperature increases, the algae population will shift from more desirable diatoms to green algae to the less desirable blue-green algae. Blue-green algae can cause taste and odor problems, and can even be toxic to some aquatic organisms.

Finally, water temperature increases can affect spawning of fish, and if the increase is rapid aquatic organisms can even be killed. Technology is presently available to protect receiving waters from thermal pollution.

E. PLANT NUTRIENTS

Plant nutrients such as nitrates and phosphates can speed up the aging of a lake through the production of algae blooms and excessive aquatic growths. This whole process of nutrient enrichment and its result is referred to as **eutrophication**. Sources of these nutrients come from natural and agricultural runoff from land, fertilizers, domestic sewage and industrial processes. In the past, detergents were a major source of phosphates.

The principle behind algae blooms and excessive aquatic growth is based on the work of Justus Liebig in 1840 and his '**Law of the Minimum**.' Since several nutrients are essential for algae growth, Liebig theorized that growth will be limited by the nutrient which is least available to the algae. If nutrients like nitrogen (nitrates) and phosphorus (phosphates) are readily available to the algae, blooms of algae can result because these important nutrients are no longer limiting.

One undesirable aspect of algae blooms is that dissolved oxygen levels in receiving waters will decline when the algae die. This process is made worse by a process of thermal stratification which takes place in lakes located in temperate zones. For example, in summer the warm surface water of a lake will float on top of colder water because the colder water is more dense than the warmer water (the maximum density of water is at $4°C$). As a consequence, dead algae sinking to the bottom of a thermally stratified lake will deplete oxygen in the bottom of lakes during the summer weather. This oxygen cannot be replenished until the fall overturn. If enough oxygen demanding wastes make their way to the bottom of a stratified lake, it is very possible for that portion of the lake to become anaerobic.

In addition to algal blooms and diminishing oxygen levels from plant nutrients, two health related effects have been attributed to the consumption of water containing high concentrations of nitrates (or nitrites): **methemoglobinemia** and the formation of nitrosamines which may have a carcinogenic potential. In methemoglobinemia, iron (Fe^{2+}) in the hemoglobin (oxygen carrier) of red blood cells becomes oxidized to (Fe^{3+}) and can no longer carry oxygen to tissues. Acute toxicity of nitrate occurs as a result of being reduced to nitrite in the stomach. Nitrite in the blood oxidizes the hemoglobin into methemoglobin. Since methamoglobin is not capable of carrying oxygen, anoxia and death may ensue. Methemoglobinemia is almost always seen in infants rather than adults because of the amount taken in per unit weight, the presence of nitrate-reducing bacteria in the upper gastrointestinal tract, the condition of the mucosa, and the greater ease of oxidation of fetal hemoglobin.

Blue-baby syndrome is another name for a condition observed in infants living in rural areas with groundwater or wells contaminated with high levels of nitrates and nitrites. Symptoms may include headache, dizziness, fatigue, lethargy, syncope, and dyspnea. In severe cases, arrhythmias, shock, convulsions or even death can occur. The lips and mucous membranes of the patients with nitrate/nitrite toxicity usually have more of a brownish than a bluish cast. It is a particular concern for infants because they have low levels of the detoxification enzyme methemoglobin reductase.

Contamination of groundwater and surface water will occur when animal waste is applied to land at rates above which soil and vegetation can absorb and utilize waste constituents.

The other nitrate related health hazard, that it may act as procarcinogen, is much more speculative. The following reactions are proposed in converting nitrates in water to nitrosamines (N-nitroso compounds): (a) reduction of nitrate to nitrite, (b) reaction of nitrite with secondary amines or amides in food or water to form N-nitroso compounds and (c) carcinogenic reactions of N-nitroso compounds.

F. INORGANIC AND ORGANIC CHEMICALS

Many inorganic and organic chemicals that are discharged into receiving waters degrade very slowly, bio-accumulate through the food chain, and are toxic to people, animals and aquatic organisms. For example, mercury can be discharged into aquatic systems around chlorine alkali - manufacturing plants and industrial processes involving the use of mercurial catalysts, and from the use of slimicides primarily in the paper-pulp industry and for the treatment of seeds.

The toxicity of mercury is dependent on its form. Mercury in the inorganic form is not very toxic and is precipitated out of the water into the bottom sediment as mercuric sulfide. However, it was eventually discovered that bacteria in the sediments can convert inorganic mercury into the highly toxic methylmercury. The Food and Drug Administration has established a guideline of 0.5 ppm for the maximum allowable concentration of mercury in fish for human consumption. Organic compounds that can bioaccumulate and remain for long periods of time in the bottom sediments include chlorinated pesticides, polychlorinated biphenyls (PCB's) and dioxins.

VI. MUNICIPAL WATER TREATMENT (DRINKING WATER)

A. INTRODUCTION

Drinking water from the tap may come from groundwater (Figure 7.5) or surface water. Large public water supply systems that serve well-populated cities and towns tend to rely on surface water resources, and smaller public water supply systems that serve smaller communities tend to use groundwater. Surface water resources include rivers, lakes, and reservoirs. Groundwater is pumped from private wells that are drilled into aquifers, geologic formations that contain water.

A public water supply is one that serves piped water to at least 25 persons or provides 15 service connections for at least 60 days per year. Water that does not come from a public water supply and serves one or only a few homes is called a private water supply.

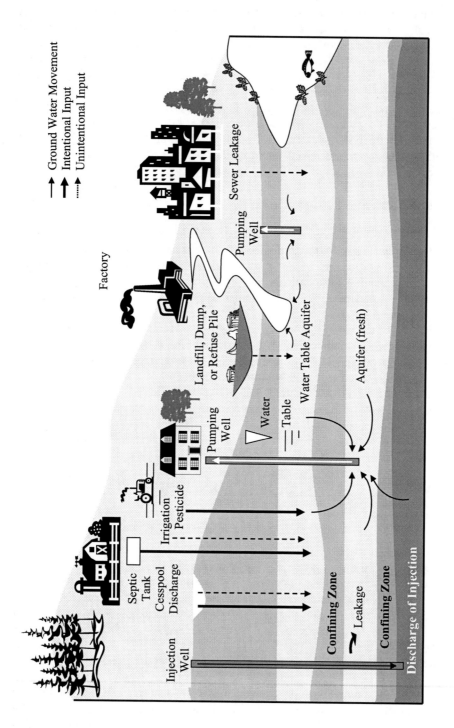

Figure 7.5. Sources of Ground Water. (Source: Nadakavukaren, 2000).

Tap water that meets United States Environmental Protection Agency (U.S. EPA) standards and state standards is considered safe to drink. However, some public water supplies do not meet all applicable standards. To find out if your public water supplier complies with federal and state standards, contact your local water supplier. The phone number should be on your water bill or in your local phone book. You can obtain information about U.S. EPA and state standards as well as about having your well tested by contacting your county or state health officials.

Gasoline contaminants have been detected throughout the United States in many water supplies that are close to a leaking underground gasoline storage tank. Because of their persistency and mobility in the environment, methyl tertiary butyl ether, ethylene dibromide (1,2-dibromoethane), 1,2-dichloroethane, 1,2-dichloropropane, diisopropyl ether, benzene, toluene, ethyl-benzene, and xylenes are some of the most commonly found gasoline constituents.

Methyl tertiary butyl ether, ethylene dibromide, 1,2-dichloroethane, and 1,2-dichloropropane have been reported to be associated with certain cancers in animals. Benzene has been associated with leukemia in humans. Diisopropyl ether and xylenes are thought to be associated with a decrease in body weight in animals. Toluene and ethylbenzene have been reported to be associated with liver and kidney toxicity in animals following ingestion.

It is common to find chemicals such as methyl ethyl ketone, acetone, and tetrahydrofuran in water supplies immediately after installing new water pipes. These chemicals are found in the glues that are used to seal joints in some water pipes. The concentrations of these chemicals are typically low and are below the recommended U.S. EPA and state standards. In time, with continued use of the water, the glue should harden and chemicals would not be expected to be released from the glue. In order to improve the taste and smell of your water, you may want to run the water for a few minutes to flush the chemicals out of the pipes.

Blue-green water may be an indicator of high copper and lead levels. If you have copper pipes, you may want to contact your county and state health officials for information about getting your water tested. Elevated copper and lead levels maybe found in drinking water where copper pipes are used because copper leaches from the pipes and lead leaches from the solder used to join the pipes together.

Drinking water with elevated copper levels has been associated with diarrhea, nausea, vomiting and anorexia in humans following short- and long-term exposure. More serious health effects have been reported in infants and children less than 1 year of age and in individual with liver disease, kidney disease, Wilson's disease, and glucose-6-phosphate dehydrogenase deficiency. The most serious health effects reported in the literature for these sensitive individuals include effects on the spleen, kidney, liver, and blood-forming cells.

Children and the developing fetus are particularly sensitive to lead. In most cases, overt symptoms are not observed in individuals who develop adverse health effects. Symptoms are usually not observed until blood lead levels exceed 35-50 μg/dl in children and 40-60 μg/dl in adults. The symptoms seen in children are often generalized and may include general fatigue, irritability, difficulty concentrating, tremors, headaches, abdominal pain, vomiting, weight loss, or constipation. The most critical effect identified in adults is increased blood pressure, which has been reported at blood lead levels of 7-34 μg/dl. Although overt symptoms may not appear until a blood level has reached 35 μg/dl in children, adverse health effects occur at lower blood lead levels. Even blood lead levels less than 5μg/dl have been associated with a decrease in intellectual quotient (IQ). No safe exposure is known to exist for lead.

Fluoride, chloride, total dissolved solids (sodium, potassium, calcium, magnesium, sulfate, bicarbonate, chloride, and organic matter), and hardness tend to increase in drinking water as one goes from the mountains to the coast.

Drinking water with fluoride levels at 2 mg/liter or greater has been associated with dental fluorosis, whereby white, brown, or black stains may be present along with pitting of the teeth. Daily consumption of water containing fluoride levels of 10mg/liter or more for 20 years or more may be associated with crippling skeletal fluorosis in humans.

Elevated levels of chloride and total dissolved solids in drinking water have been associated with an undesirable taste, corrosion of metal pipes, and decreased life-span of water heaters.

Arsenic levels in soil are sometimes elevated in areas where volcanoes were previously active. Depending on the conditions of the soil, the arsenic in the soil may leach into the groundwater, resulting in elevated arsenic levels. Drinking water with high levels of arsenic may be associated with the development of different cancers, including skin, lung, liver, bladder, and kidney cancers.

Radon is a soil gas. Radon gas levels in soil are sometimes elevated in areas where granite rock is present. Radon gas may be present in the soil following the decay of uranium found in granite rocks, which are usually found in mountainous areas- Radon gas can travel from the soil into water supplies. Radon gas is associated with lung cancer in humans when inhaled over a long period of time and may also be associated with stomach cancer following ingestion. Contact your county and state health officials for information about testing your water for radon.

Pesticides have been detected in many water supplies across the United States. Because of their persistency and mobility in the environments, chlorpyrifos, atrazine, simazine, chlordane, endrin, dieldrin, aldrin, dichlorodiphenyltrichloroethane / dichlorodiphenyldichloroethane (DDT/DDD) and dichlorodiphenyldichloroethylene (DDE) are sometimes found in drinking water. Chlordane, dieldrin, aldrin, DDT, DDD, and DDE have been associated with causing some cancers in animals. Endrin has been associated with causing liver toxicity and convulsions in animals. Atrazine and simazine have been associated with causing a decrease in body weight and cancer in animals. Chlorpyrifos has been associated with causing intestinal discomfort, changes in heart rate, and dizziness in humans. Pesticides from use on crops, nitrate and nitrite from fertilizers and animal waste, and microorganisms (fecal coliforms) from animal waste are sometimes found in water supplies located near farms.

Public water suppliers use a variety of treatment processes to remove contaminants from drinking water. The most commonly used processes include filtration of microorganisms and other contaminants, promoting sedimentation of contaminants, and disinfection using primarily chlorine, chloramines, or chlorine dioxide. Disinfection by-products can form when disinfectants react with organic matter that is in treated drinking water.

Some of the most commonly produced disinfection by-products are trihalomethanes (THMs) and haloacetic acids.

A series of studies with differing strengths and weaknesses support a small association between drinking higher levels of disinfection by-products and risk of bladder and rectal cancers.

Boiling your water with a rolling boil for 3 to 5 minutes should eliminate pathogenic microorganisms. In order to protect your health your water will need to be tested for fecal and total coliforms periodically to determine when it will be safe to use from the tap.

Private water supplies should be tested annually for nitrate, coliform, and fecal coliform bacteria to detect contamination problems early. If you suspect a problem, then your well water should be tested more frequently. Call your local and state health departments for information about having your water tested.

Typical water treatment plants are very good at removing suspended solids, taste, odor, color, and microorganisms, from raw water such that finished water is palatable and when consumed will not result in outbreaks of infectious disease. Basically, water treatment consists of such processes as coagulation, sedimentation, filtration and disinfection. As depicted in Figure 7.6 and 7.10, raw water passes into the water treatment plant to the intake basins where such things as fish and aquatic weeds are removed. From the intake basin water moves to chemical application basins where chlorine (disinfectant), alum (coagulant), and lime and/or caustic soda (corrosion control) are added. After the chemicals are added, the water moves to mixing basins where the chemicals are slowly mixed with wooden paddles and the coagulant forms a "floc." The "floc" is then removed in the settling basins. After the "floc" is removed, the water gets its final "polishing" in the sand and gravel filters, chlorine is added once more, and the finished water is distributed for consumption.

One health related concern with municipal water treatment is disinfection with chlorine. It has been shown that trihalomethanes are formed in drinking water that has been disinfected with chlorine. The overall health risk to gastrointestinal and urinary tract cancers from trihalomethanes still needs to be determined.

B. DRINKING WATER STANDARDS

As established, drinking standards include maximum contaminant levels (MCLs) for selected inorganic contaminants (such as arsenic, barium, cadmium, chromium, lead and mercury), volatile organic chemicals, and radioactive materials, as well as limits for turbidity and the presence of coliform organisms. Limits have also been specified for the amount of suspended solids (turbidity) in drinking water, both for aesthetics, and because efficacy of disinfection is related to the clarity of the water being treated.

To assure the limits specified in the 1ry standards are within the capabilities of current technologies, EPA has also identified treatment processes considered adequate for reducing concentration of individual regulated contaminants to acceptable levels. Some micro-organisms, cysts in particular, have a greater resistance to disinfection than coliform bacteria. These concerns assisted in passage of 1996 amendments to SDWA. Thus, analyses of drinking H2O supplies for contaminants (e.g., **Cryptosporidium**) are mandatory in many cases.

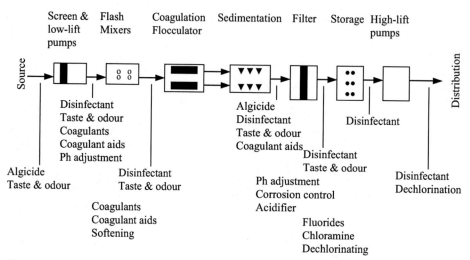

Screen &   Flash   Coagulation Sedimentation Filter   Storage High-lift
low-lift   Mixers   Flocculator   pumps
pumps

Figure 7.6. Diagram of a Water Treatment Process. (Source: Yassi, 2001).

C. WATER PURIFICATION

Preparing water for human consumption is a major industry. About 60,000 municipal water purification and distribution systems exist in U.S. The combined output of these systems is 40-50 billion gallons per day, or 160-200 gallons for each person in the U.S. The primary purposes of a water purification or treatment systems are to collect water from a source of supply, purify it for drinking if necessary, and distribute it to consumers. Capital investment in municipal water treatment facilities totals about $250 billion.

D. SLOW SAND FILTRATION

Raw water is passed slowly through sand bed 2-3 feet deep. Soon after a bed becomes operative, a biological growth develops on top of and within sand, removing and retaining particles from the raw water. This process removes most bacteria and disease organisms, including cysts of **Giardia lamblia**. Because excess turbidity in the raw water supply will rapidly plug the filter bed, preliminary settling is recommended. With proper care, slow sand filter beds can be operated 30-200 days before top layers of sand have to be scraped, cleaned or replaced.

E. RAPID SAND FILTRATION

First water is pumped or diverted from a river or stream into a raw storage basin. This provides a carryover or reserve in case the raw water supply becomes unfit for use for several days. Storage also removes color and reduces turbidity and bacteria. The initial step in the process is to add chemicals to the water to create a coagulant. Alum (Al2 $(SO_4)_3 \cdot 14H_2O$ is the chemical most commonly used in the US. A less commonly used chemical is ferric acid ($FeCl_3$).

Once the water has been rapidly mixed to assure proper coagulation, it is slowly and gently stirred to enable finely divided floc to agglomerate into larger particles that will rapidly settle. This process called flocculation, is accomplished by moving large paddles slowly through the water. Next, the water undergoes a period of quiescence. The settled floc or sludge is removed from the bottom of the settling tank and disposed off. Because settled water will still retain some traces of floc, it is passed through a bed of sand 2-3 feet deep. Sand filters become loaded with floc and must be cleaned by backwashing with purified water every 12-72 hours.

Once the clarified water is disinfected and fluoride has been added, it is sent to storage and is ready for distribution to consumers. Additional steps that can be taken in the purification of drinking water include procedures to remove hardness, iron and manganese, organic compounds, and tastes and odors.

F. ADDITIONAL STEPS IN THE PURIFICATION OF DRINKING WATER

Hardness - This is caused by the presence of calcium and magnesium. These chemicals do not pose any health effects to humans. One approach to removing calcium and magnesium is to install a water purification system (e.g., reverse osmosis unit) to purify the portion of the water used for cooking and drinking. The output of such units is small, but are readily available at a reasonable cost. Iron and Manganese are soluble in water only in the reduced chemical state.

Organic compounds, and tastes, and odors - the most common sources of bad tastes or odors in drinking water are hydrogen sulfide and algae growths, and byproducts resulting from reactions of chlorine with various chemicals in the water. Although not needed to make drinking water safe, (assuming that the public supply meets federal, state, and local drinking-water standards), certain devices can improve the quality of drinking water.

G. DEVICES USED TO IMPROVE THE QUALITY OF DRINKING WATER

1. **Particulate filters** that remove suspended materials from water.
2. **Chemical adsorbers** (such as activated carbon or charcoal) that removes chlorine, tastes and odors, and some organic compounds such as pesticides.
3. **Reverse osmosis units** that remove hardness, chemicals such as nitrates, and some organic chemicals.
4. **Water softeners** (e.g. ion exchange units) that remove hardness.
5. **Distillation units** that remove some organic and inorganic chemicals (such as calcium, magnesium, and nitrates).

VII. MUNICIPAL WASTEWATER TREATMENT

The main items of federal legislation pertaining to the control of water pollution comprise the original Federal Water Pollution Control Act passed in 1956, amendments to this act passed in 1972 and 1977, and the Water Quality Act of 1987.

With the passage of the Water Quality Act of 1987, primary attention was directed to the control of nonpoint sources of waste. The EPA was directed to promulgate regulations requiring municipal and industrial stormwater discharges to obtain permits to release such wastes to U.S. waters. A variety of methods is available for measuring the quantities of contaminants in a liquid waste.

One indicator is the concentration of suspended solids. Another is the amount of nutrients in the waste. Still another is the amount of chlorine required to oxidize the organic matter in the waste. The acidity or alkalinity of the waste may also be used as an indicator of its "strength," or polluting potential. In general, methods for treating liquid wastes, particularly domestic sewage, are designed primarily to stabilize or oxidize the organic matter therein, through biological processes. Fish cannot live in a stream that does not contain sufficient DO. Its concentration in a stream is expressed in mg of O_2 / l of H_2O.

A. TREATMENT OF MUNICIPAL SEWAGE

Three stages of treatment can be applied to municipal sewage: **primary**, **secondary** and **tertiary**.

1. **Primary treatment** consists of holding the wastes undisturbed in a tank for a sufficient period of time to permit the solids within the waste to settle and be removed.
2. **Secondary treatment** is the use of a biological process to oxidize the nutrients in the waste.
3. **Tertiary treatment** involves a variety of processes tailored to the intended uses of the finished product.

One of the more common tertiary or advanced methods of treating liquid wastes is very similar to the coagulation, settling, and filtration processes used in treating surface waters to make them acceptable for drinking.

Primary treatment consists in simply holding sewage in a large tank to permit the removal of solids by sedimentation. Grease and light solids that float are removed from the settling tank by a scraper and are pumped along with the settled solids to a large closed tank called a digester, where they are held for anaerobic digestion.

After primary treatment (settling), sewage can be subjected to secondary or biological treatment. In most cases this is accomplished by use of a trickling filter, the activated sludge process, or a waste stabilization pond. The trickling filter is one of the most common forms of secondary treatment.

The term treatment is a misnomer, since the system does not filter the sewage. Rather, a trickling filter consists of a large tank, roughly 6 feet deep, filled with stones 2-4 inches in diameter over which sewage is intermittently trickled or sprayed from a distributor. When the bacterial growth on the stones becomes too thick and heavy, it sloughs off and is carried away in the liquid effluent leaving the bottom of the filter bed. The activated sludge process is another form of aerobic secondary treatment for municipal sewage.

Sewage is sent into a large open tank, where it is held for several hours and its oxygen content maintained by means of aerators (air diffusers) or mechanical agitators (paddles or brushes). Used in other countries for many years, waste stabilization ponds were largely ignored in the United States until the 1950's. Since then, more and more have been built, particularly in the South. Waste stabilization ponds can be used singly or in series. They can be designed to receive either raw sewage or sewage that has undergone primary treatment. Most methods used in the tertiary treatment of sewage are modeled on those used in the purification of drinking water: a coagulant is added, a floc is formed and settled, the liquid is passed through a sand filter, and a disinfectant is added.

B. TREATMENT OF INDUSTRIAL WASTES

Early wastewater treatment systems were based on the traditional methods for treating municipal sewage, that is, they were designed to stabilize the organic matter in the waste. Later it was recognized that nutrients such as N & P also had to be removed. Today treatment systems are designed to remove toxic chemicals as well. Such approaches include physical and chemical, as well as biological processes, and they can be applied either singly or in combination.

1. Physical Processes:

a. **Remove suspended solids**. These processes can range from simply holding the wastes undisturbed in a tank to permit the solids to settle, to passing the wastes through filters to remove the solids, to centrifuging to separate the solids from the liquid wastes.

b. **Remove suspended oils, greases, and emulsified organics**. Aeration of the wastes causes such materials to float to the surface, where they can be removed by skimming devices.

c. **Remove dissolved materials such as organic and inorganic chemicals**. One way of removing organic and inorganic chemicals is to pass the wastes through beds of activated carbon that physically adsorb and remove these materials.

d. **Recover acids, such as nitric and hydrofluoric, from stainless steel pickling liquor, and pulping liquor from organic mixes**. One such process is electrodialysis, which employs a membrane filter coupled with an electric charge.

2. Chemical processes:

a. **Addition of acids** to neutralize wastes that are alkaline, or addition of bases to neutralize wastes that are acid. Frequently, this results in the production of precipitates that settle and can be removed from the wastes.

b. **Addition of chemicals** to liquid wastes to coagulate and precipitate suspended solids. This process is very similar to the tertiary or advanced systems applied to the effluents from municipal sewage treatment plants.

c. **Use of ion-exchange resins** to exchange innocuous chemicals for the contaminants in the wastes.

d. **Use of oxidants** such as chlorine, ozone, hydrogen, peroxide, and ultraviolet light to convert volatile and nonvolatile organic contaminants into nontoxic compounds.

3. Biological processes:

a. **Predigestion** of brewery, winery, and meat packing wastes in a tank under anaerobic conditions as an initial step in their treatment. Frequently, this is done at elevated temperatures to accelerate the process.

b. **Oxidation** of certain types of industrial wastes under aerobic conditions similar to those applied in the treatment of domestic sewage. Trickling filters and oxidation ponds are used, as well as the activated sludge process. Under normal circumstances, industrial wastes containing compounds such as formaldehyde, phenols, and pickle factory residues would be disruptive to the biological organisms present in municipal (sewage) treatment systems.

Another method used for the disposal of certain types of liquid chemical wastes is **deep well injection.** This technique, often applied without prior treatment of the wastes, involves injecting them into a deep underground formation using a specially designed well. According to EPA regulations, operators of injection wells must be able to show that hazardous concentrations of the waste will not migrate from the injection zone for a period of 10,000 years. Because of the intermittent flow rate of nonpoint sources and the difficulties in designing facilities to treat them, primary efforts to control such releases are being directed to reducing the volumes and improving the quality of such wastes, whether agricultural or human in origin.

One practice that has proved especially useful in reducing the presence of pollutants in agricultural runoff is the **optimization of pesticide application** rates and timing. The presence of contaminants in urban runoff can be reduced by providing convenient disposal sites for used oil and household hazardous waste; collecting leaves and yard trimmings on a frequent basis; and using vacuum equipment for street cleaning.

C. Land Disposal of Treated Wastewater

When pit privies were in common use, human excreta were disposed of primarily into the soil. The same approach is used by those who are served today by septic tanks. This procedure changed with the development of municipal sewage collection and treatment systems and the widespread use of chlorine as a disinfectant (beginning early in the twentieth century).

In recent years it has again been recognized that land disposal of treated wastewater offers many advantages. Such an approach:

1. Returns nutrients to the soil where they can be used for agriculture and forests; the nutrients can also support aquaculture.
2. Reclaims and / or preserves open spaces an existing wetlands and allows the development of new wetlands-parks, golf courses, and recreational areas irrigated with wastewater enhance human activities; wetlands receiving such wastes provide habitats for wildlife.
3. Creates an ideal environment in which natural biological, physical, and chemical processes can stabilize the wastes; wetlands serve as nutrient sinks and buffering zones to protect streams and other areas.

4. Provides a ready means for recharging groundwater sources.
5. Frequently results in economies in wastewater treatment, thus saving funds for application to other problems. Experience has shown that a properly developed land disposal system can be operated for 20 or more years.

Concerns related to the use of wastewater extend beyond disease organisms to include the possible presence in such water of trace metals, organics, and pesticides. In all cases, it is important not only to examine the purity of the treated wastewater under consideration for disposal, but also to develop detailed knowledge on industrial facilities that may discharge toxic materials into the treatment system. EPA estimates that the liquid waste treatment plants in the United States produce almost 8 million tons of sludge /yr.

One control method used to improve water quality by reducing the BOD, solids and nitrate and phosphate loads to receiving waters is treatment. Wastewater treatment plants are designed tertiary (advanced) treatment. Primary treatment plants remove approximately 35-40% of the BOD and 60% of the suspended solids by the physical process of sedimentation.

Secondary treatment can be added to a primary treatment plant through the design of an activated-sludge or trickling filter system. In Figure 7.7, a flow diagram depicts an activated-sludge process. After the effluent goes through primary treatment (screen, grit chamber, primary settling, Figure 7.8, it is brought into an aeration tank which is seeded with a sludge containing high concentrations of bacteria. The bacteria decompose the organic matter under aerobic conditions. After about six hours of aeration and bacterial digestion of the organic matter, the effluent passes on to a secondary settling tank where the bacterial masses are removed by sedimentation.

After sedimentation, some of the bacteria (sludge) is recycled back to the aeration tank to keep the digestion process going, and the remainder of the sludge from the secondary settling tank and the sludge from the primary settling tank is removed for processing and disposal. The combination of primary and secondary treatment will remove about 90% of the BOD and 90% of the suspended solids.

Another secondary treatment process is the trickling filter. After primary settling, the effluent will be sprinkled over a circular bed of rocks which are covered with a layer of slime teaming with bacteria. The bacteria digest the organic matter in the same fashion as the activated-sludge process. However, the trickling filter process is not quite as efficient in removing BOD and solids when compared to activated-sludge.

After secondary treatment, the effluent is generally passed through a chlorine contact chamber before it goes into the receiving water. The purpose for chlorinating the effluent is to kill off the pathogens before they get out into the environment. However, some scientists feel chlorinated effluents pose a greater environmental/health impact through the formation of chlorinated hydrocarbons.

Sludge which has been collected from the primary and secondary settling tanks is sent to anaerobic digestive tanks where it is converted into methane gas and carbon dioxide. The remaining solids are now stabilized, dried in drying beds or vacuum drums and disposed in landfills, incinerated or used for fertilizer.

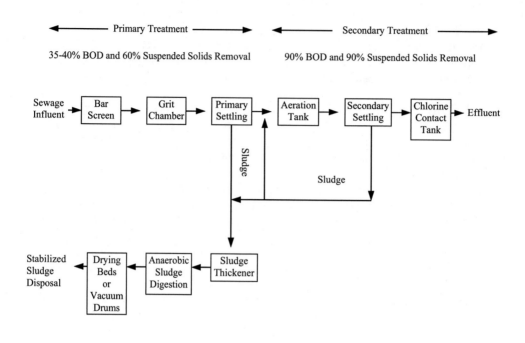

Figure 7.7. Flow Diagram of an Activated – Sludge Wastewater Treatment Plant. (Source: Masters, 1974).

Although secondary treatment does an adequate job in removing BOD and solids, it does a poor job of removing nutrients. As a consequence, some treatment plants have added tertiary or advanced treatment processes for the removal of nitrates and phosphates. Such processes as ammonia stripping and bacterial nitrification and denitrification can remove nitrogen from wastewater. Phosphorus can be removed by coagulation with lime and precipitated out. Other wastewater pollutants can be removed by such advanced processes as reverse osmosis, distillation, electrodialysis, carbon absorption and ion exchange. However, the costs of construction and operation of many of these advanced processes can be staggering.

VIII. STORMWATER RUNOFF

A. INTRODUCTION

When we have a rainfall event, several things can happen to the precipitation. Some infiltrates into the soil surface, some is taken up by plants, some is evaporated into the atmosphere, and some runs off of the land surface and impervious areas of stormwater runoff.

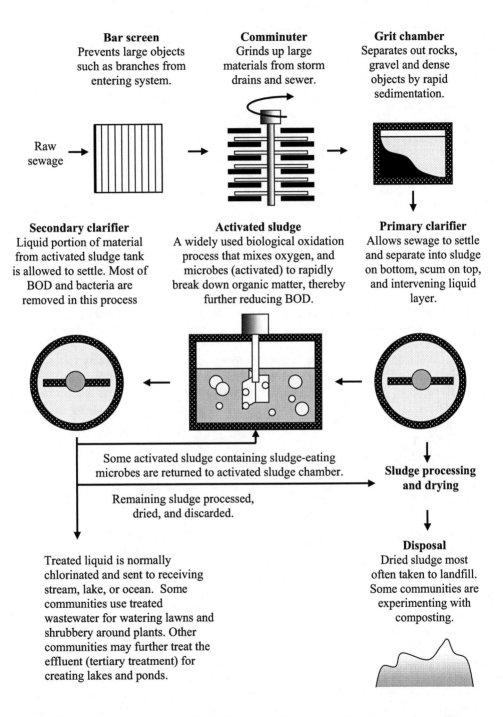

Bar screen
Prevents large objects such as branches from entering system.

Comminuter
Grinds up large materials from storm drains and sewer.

Grit chamber
Separates out rocks, gravel and dense objects by rapid sedimentation.

Raw sewage

Secondary clarifier
Liquid portion of material from activated sludge tank is allowed to settle. Most of BOD and bacteria are removed in this process

Activated sludge
A widely used biological oxidation process that mixes oxygen, and microbes (activated) to rapidly break down organic matter, thereby further reducing BOD.

Primary clarifier
Allows sewage to settle and separate into sludge on bottom, scum on top, and intervening liquid layer.

Some activated sludge containing sludge-eating microbes are returned to activated sludge chamber.

Remaining sludge processed, dried, and discarded.

Sludge processing and drying

Treated liquid is normally chlorinated and sent to receiving stream, lake, or ocean. Some communities use treated wastewater for watering lawns and shrubbery around plants. Other communities may further treat the effluent (tertiary treatment) for creating lakes and ponds.

Disposal
Dried sludge most often taken to landfill. Some communities are experimenting with composting.

Figure 7.8. Schematic of a Typical Municipal Wastewater Treatment Plant. (Source: Moore, 1999).

Changes to natural features have a large impact on the amount of rainfall that becomes storm water runoff. One of the major impacts is the development of land, which adds impervious surfaces. An impervious surface is basically a hardened surface – rooftops, parking areas, roadways, etc. Impervious surfaces do not allow rainfall to infiltrate into the soil surface as occurs on natural terrain, so more of the rainfall becomes storm water runoff.

Storm water runoff can have a number of impacts. As development and imperviousness increase in an area, the natural capacity of the soil and vegetation to take up rainfall decreases and more rainfall becomes storm water runoff. This can produce negative impacts by causing erosion of land areas and stream banks, by causing or increasing flooding, and also by carrying pollutants to surface waters.

As development activities occur and human activities increase in an area, various pollutants are deposited on surfaces where they can be picked up and carried by storm water runoff this is especially true on impervious surfaces where pollutants can easily be washed off.

Storm water runoff may be carried through natural or man-made drainage ways or conveyance systems. In some cases storm water runoff leaves a site spread out over a large dispersed area as "sheet flow." It may also be conveyed through natural ditches, swales, and natural drainage features. In most developing and urbanizing areas storm water is conveyed through a system of catch basins and pipes commonly referred to as a storm sewer system.

Unfortunately everyone is not currently aware. As an example, many times people assume that storm water runoff that enters a storm sewer system is being routed to some type of treatment process before it makes its way to our surface waters. In a lot of cases this is not occurring and the storm sewer system is designed simply to capture the storm water and convey it to the nearest surface water.

B. TYPES OF POLLUTANTS

The Table 7.2 summarizes common storm water pollutants and also provides information on potential sources of these pollutants and types of impacts they may cause.

C. TYPES OF CONTROL MEASURES

Mechanisms for controlling storm water runoff impacts can be grouped into two categories of activities.

The first category is preventative measures. These measures work to reduce the impacts of storm water runoff through changes in design, operation, or management to minimize or prevent the generation of runoff and the contamination of runoff from pollutants. Preventative measures include land use management practices, which look at methods to do better planning of the way land uses are located within a jurisdictional area or on a specific project site to avoid impacts, and source reduction practices, which focus on locating the sources of pollutants and implementing design and operational changes that minimize or completely remove these sources. Preventative measures can be very efficient and effective because they are implemented in a manner that will keep pollutants from ever getting into storm water.

Table 7.2. Common Storm water Pollutants, Sources, and Potential Impacts. (Source: North Carolina Division of Water Quality, 2001).

COMPONENT AND IMPACT
Sediment
Sediment is often viewed as the largest pollutant load associated with storm water runoff in an urban setting. Loadings are exceptionally high in the case of construction activity.
Sediment is associated with numerous impacts in surface waters, including increased turbidity, effects on aquatic and benthic habitat, and reduction in capacity of impoundments.
A number of other pollutants often attach to, and are carried by, sediment particles.
Nutrients
The nutrients most often identified in storm-water runoff are phosphorus and nitrogen.
In surface waters, these nutrient loads can lead to heavy algae growth, eutrophication (especially in impoundments), and low dissolved oxygen levels.
Nutrients are input into the urban system in a variety of ways, including landscaping practices (commercial and home) and leaks from sanitary sewers and septic systems.
Organic matter
Various forms of organic matter may be carried by storm-water in urban areas.
Decomposition of this material by organisms in surface waters results in depleted oxygen levels. Low levels of dissolved oxygen severely impact water quality and life within surface waters.
Sources of organic matter include leaking septic systems, garbage, yard waste, etc.
Bacteria
High bacterial levels may be found in storm water runoff as a result of leaking sanitary systems, garbage, pet waste, etc.
The impacts of bacteria on surface waters may affect recreational uses and aquatic life as well as presenting possible health risks.
Oil and grease
Numerous activities in urban areas produce oil, grease, and lubricating agents that are readily transported by storm water.
The intensity of activities, including vehicle traffic, maintenance and fueling activities, leaks and spills, and manufacturing processes within an urban setting contribute heavily to the level of these pollutants present in adjacent surface waters.
Toxic substances
Many toxic substances may potentially be associated with urban storm-water, including metals, pesticides, herbicides, and hydrocarbons.
They may affect biological systems, and accumulate in bottom sediments of surface waters.
Heavy metals
Heavy metals such as copper, lead, zinc, arsenic, chromium, and cadmium may be typically found in urban storm-water runoff.
Metals in storm-water maybe toxic to some aquatic life and may accumulate in aquatic animals.
Urban sources of metals in storm-water may include automobiles, paints, preservatives, motor oil, and various urban activities.
Temperature
Storm-water runoff increases in temperature as it flows over an impervious surface. In addition, water stored in shallow, unshaded ponds and impoundments can increase in temperature.
Removal of natural vegetation (such as tree canopy) opens up water bodies to direct solar radiation.
Elevated water temperatures can have an impact or the ability of a water body to support certain fish and aquatic organisms.

The second category is control measures. These are devices that are put in place to capture storm water flows and provide management of the storm water through filtering, infiltration, detention, or some related process that works to remove pollutants from the storm water. These measures may be limited in their ability to remove some pollutants efficiently and may be fairly costly. Control measures also require commitment to long-term operation and maintenance to assure that the measures continue to function properly.

D. TYPES OF CONTROL ACTIVITIES

Many of our daily activities have the potential to cause storm-water pollution. Any situation in which activities can add to the types of pollutants that may be picked up and carried by storm-water runoff is an area that should be considered in your attempts to minimize impacts. The list of items below is certainly not all-inclusive, but it gives an idea of things citizens can do to help control storm-water pollution:

1. Maintain buffer areas around stream segments to protect stream banks and to provide a mechanism for pollutant removal.
2. Minimize impervious areas to reduce runoff.
3. Design all new construction to prevent or minimize runoff and storm water pollution - a major component here is planning up front in the design process to consider and manage potential storm-water problems.
4. Practice "good housekeeping" by keeping areas clean of potentially harmful pollutants. This also may involve changing activities or practices if they have potential impacts.
5. Use lawn care practices that protect water quality - minimize the use of fertilizers and pesticides, and when used, do so in a safe manner.
6. Properly use and store household materials and be aware of and make use of local recycling and collection centers to handle household wastes.
7. Remember that materials poured or placed on the ground, streets, driveways, etc. can be picked up and carried by storm-water runoff to our surface waters.
8. Report any pollution, illegal dumping, or soil erosion that you see to the appropriate authorities.
9. Get involved with local efforts for public education, water quality monitoring, stream cleanup, recycling, etc.

IX. WATER QUALITY CRITERIA: STANDARDS AND REGULATIONS

In Figure 7.9, the relationship of water quality criteria, water quality standards and effluent standards is depicted. Water quality criteria are scientific determinations to quantify water quality in terms of its physical, chemical, and biological characteristics for such specific uses as: (1) public water supplies, (2) recreation and aesthetics, (3) freshwater and marine aquatic life and wildlife, (4) agricultural, and (5) industrial.

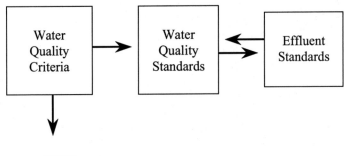

USES
1. Public water supplies
2. Recreation and Aesthetics
3. Freshwater and Marine Aquatic and Wildlife
4. Agricultural
5. Industrial

Figure 7.9. Relationship of Water Quality Criteria, Water Quality Standards and Effluent Standards. (Source: Masters, 1974).

Water quality standards are legal plans established by a governmental authority as a program for water pollution prevention. Water quality standards should be primarily based on water quality criteria, although economics and politics do enter into the standard setting procedure. Finally, the water quality standards will directly impact on what the effluent standards will be from point sources of pollution, and the effluent standards will impact directly on the water quality standards for a particular use.

An example of a water quality standard for a particular use is the National Interim Primary Drinking Water Regulations as set by the U.S. Environmental Protection Agency (Table 7.3, 7.4, and 7.5). Except for the microbiological standards, raw water source would have to have nearly the same maximum contaminant levels as the finished water because the conventional water treatment techniques of coagulation, sedimentation, filtration and disinfection do little to remove the non-organic and organic chemicals and radioactivity. The bacteria decompose the organic matter under aerobic conditions. After about six hours of aeration and bacterial digestion of the organic matter, the effluent passes on to a secondary settling tank where the bacterial masses are removed by sedimentation.

After sedimentation, some of the bacteria (sludge) are recycled back to the aeration tank to keep the digestion process going, and the remainder of the sludge from the secondary settling tank and the sludge from the primary settling tank is removed for processing and disposal. The combination of primary and secondary treatment will remove about 90% of the BOD and 90% of the suspended solids.

Another secondary treatment process is the trickling filter. After primary settling, the effluent will be sprinkled over a circular bed of rocks, which are covered, with a layer of slime teaming with bacteria. The bacteria digest the organic matter in the same fashion as the activated-sludge process. However, the trickling filter process is not quite as efficient in removing BOD and solids when compared to activated-sludge.

After secondary treatment, the effluent is generally passed through a chlorine contact chamber before it goes into the receiving water. The purpose for chlorinating the effluent is to kill off the pathogens before they get out into the environment. However, some scientists feel chlorinated effluents pose a greater environmental/health impact through the formation of chlorinated hydrocarbons.

Table 7.3. Interim National Secondary Drinking. Water Regulations. Secondary Maximum Contaminant Levels (SMCL). (Source: Conway, 1998).

Contaminant	SMCL
Chloride	250 mg/L
Color	15 color units
Copper	I mg/L
Gorrosivity	Noncorrosive
Foaming agents	0.5 mg/L
Hydrogen sulfide	0.5 mg/L
Iron	0.3 mgIL
Manganese	0.05 mg/L
Odor	3 threshold odor number
pH	6.5—8.5
Sulfate	250 mg/L
TDS	500 mg/L
Zinc	5 mg/L

Table 7.4. Volatile Organic Chemical Additions To Primary Drinking Water Regulations in Table Above. (Source: Conway, 1998).

Contaminants	MCL (mg/L)	MCLG (mg/L)
Benzene	0.005	0
Carbon Tetrachloride	0.005	0
p-Dichlorobenzene	0.075	0.075
1,2-Dichloroethane	0.005	0
1,1-Dichloroethylene	0.007	0.007
1,1,1-Trichloroethane	0.2	0.2
Trichloroethane	0.005	0
Vinyl Chloride	0.002	0

Table 7.5. National Primary Drinking Water Standards. (Source: Nadakavukaren, 2000).

Contaminant	MCL (mg/L)	Contaminant	MCL (mg/L)
Acrylamide	*	Glyphosate	0.7
Alachlor (Lasso)	0.002	Gross Alpha Particle Activity	15 pCi/L
Aldicarb (3)	0.003	Heptochlor (H-34, Heptox)	0.0004
Aldicarb Sulfone (3)	0.002	Heptochlor Epoxide	0.0002
Aldicarb Sulfoxide (3)	0.004	Heterotrophic Plate Count	**
Antimony	0.006	Hexachlarobenzene	0.001
Asbestos	7 MFL ᵀ	Hexachlorocyclopentadiene	0.05
Atrazine (Atranex, Crisazina)	0.003	Lead	ττ
Arsenic	0.05	Legionelba	**
Barium	2	Lindane	0.0002
Benzene	0,005	Methoxychlor (DMDT, Marlate)	0.04
Benzo [a] Pyrene (PAH)	0.0002	Monochlorobenzene	0.1
Beryllium	0.004	Mercury	0.002
Beta Particle & Photon Emitters	4 mrem/yr	Nickel	--
Cadmium	5	Nitrate (as nitrogen)	10
Carbofuran (Furadon 4F)	0.04	Nitrite (as nitrogen)	1
Carbon Tetrochloride	0.005	Total Nitrate/Nitrite	10
Chlordane	0.002	Oxamyl (Vydote)	0.2
ChromiumS ram urn	0.1	Pentachlorophenol	0.00 1
Copper	ττ	Picloram	0.5
Cyanide	0.2	Polychlorinated Biphenyls (PCBs)	0.0005
2, 4-D (Formula 40, Weeder 64)	0.07	Radium 226 & Radium 228	5 pCi/L
Dalapon	0.2	Selenium	0.05
Di (2-ethylhexyl) adipate	0.4	Simazine	0.004
Di (2-ethylhexyl) phthalate	0.006	Styrene	0.1
Dibromochloropropane (DBCP)	0.0002	Sulfate	500 mg/L
o-Dichlorobenzene	0.6		(proposed)
p-Dichlorabenzene	0.075	2, 3, 7, 8-TCDD (Dioxin)	0.00000003
1, 2-Dichloroethane	0.005	Tetrachloroethylene	0.005
1, 1 –Dichloroethylene	0.007	Thallium	0.002
cis-1, 2-Dichloroethylene	0.07	Toluene	1
Trans-1, 2-Dichloroethylene	0.1	Total Coliforms	None
Dichloromethane	0.005	Total Trihalomethanes	0.1
1, 2-Dichloropropane	0.005	Toxaphene	0.003
Dinoseb	0.007	2, 4, 5-TP (Silvex)	0.05
Diquat	0.02	1, 2, 4-Trichlorobenzene	0.07
Endothall	0.1	1, 1, 1 -Trichloroethane	0.2
Endrin	0.002	1, 1, 2-Trichloroethane	0.005
Epichlorohydrin	*	Trichloroethylene	0.005
Ethylbenzene	0.7	Turbidity	**
Ethylene dibromide	0.00005	Vinyl Chloride	0.002
Flouride	4	Viruses	**
Giardia Lamblia	**	Xylenes	10

(*) Each Public Water System must certify annually in writing to the state that when acrylamide and epichlorohydrin are used in drinking water systems, the combination of dose and rnonomer level does not exceed the levels specified.

(ᵀ) MFL is million fibers per liter.

(ττ) Lead and copper rule: treatment technique which requires water systems to take top water samples from homes with lead pipes or copper pipes with lead solder and/or with lead service lines. If more than 10 percent of these samples exceed an action level of 1.3 mg/U for copper or 0.015 mg/L for lead, the system is triggered into additional treatment.

(**) These contaminants are regulated under the Surface Water Treatment Rule.

X. <u>ENGINEERED PROCESSES OF TREATMENT OF WATER</u>

The treatment of waters to make them suitable for subsequent use requires physical, chemical, and biological processes. These processes may take place in nature. When natural processes cannot be ensured of a desired quality, these processes need to be engineered in water treatment plans (Figure 7.10).

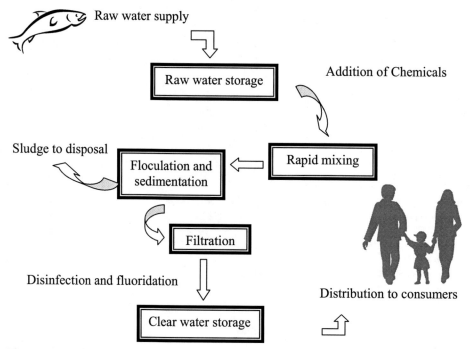

<u>Figure 7.10.</u> Principle Steps in the Water Purification Process.   (Source: Gomez & Phillips, 1997).

Engineering processes are increasingly necessary, in part because the contamination that impairs the quality of water is increasingly human-made and resistant to nature's purification process and in part because of growth of population and its activity in the face of fixed natural resources. The processing steps used for purifying water for drinking are described below, while those used for treating wastewater are described under Bacterial Examination of Drinking Waters.

A. <u>DISTILLATION</u>

Evaporation and condensation maintain the hydrologic cycle. Engineered distillation is used for desalination and for other applications where special water quality may be needed. Distillation produces the purest water of any of the processes listed, with only volatile organics persisting.

B. GAS EXCHANGE

Oxygen is added to waters, and dissolved gases such as carbon dioxide and hydrogen sulfide are removed. This helps in reducing taste and odors and may also assist in the oxidation of iron and manganese, making them more easily removable. Aeration is an important natural process, helping to restore water quality in polluted rivers and other bodies of water. It is also used in water purification and wastewater treatment.

C. COAGULATION

Colloidal and suspended particles are brought together to form large *flocs* that settle more easily. This occurs in nature in lakes and other bodies of water, but it is an important process in water purification and is aided by the addition of coagulants such as alum (aluminum sulfate) or synthetic polymers. The floc is then removed by sedimentation, filtration, or both.

D. FLOCCULATION

In nature, mixing is induced by the velocity of flow in rivers or by wind-, thermal-, or density-induced currents in lakes. This mixing causes interparticle contact. In treatment plants, flocculation is engineered and aids, with the process of coagulation, in the formation of large-floc particles that are more easily removed.

E. SEDIMENTATION

Under the action of gravity, particulates, including bacteria, settle to the bottom. Because the settling velocities of these small particles are low, turbulence or swift currents interfere with sedimentation so that the process is effective only in slow-moving bodies of water such as lakes. In engineered works, special tanks that minimize extraneous currents are used, encouraging the settling of the smallest and most dense particles. Coagulation assists in sedimentation.

F. FILTRATION

Water passes through granular media, and fine particulates are removed by the adhesion to the grains and by sedimentation in the pore spaces. Removal of particles by filtration is not accomplished by straining, as the particles removed are generally much smaller than the spaces between the grains of the medium. In some instances biological growth on the filter helps with the removal of particles and assists with biochemical degradation of the adsorbed organic matter. Natural filtration occurs as water percolates through the soil.

G. ADSORPTION

While some adsorption takes place in filtration, often special media designed to adsorb contaminants may be used. Activated carbon, both in granular form as filters and in powdered form as an additive to water, is used to adsorb taste and odors and a wide variety of organic chemicals.

H. Ion Exchange

Resins, both natural and synthetic, are used to remove specific ions. The most common are zeolites used for removing calcium and magnesium, two hardness-producing ions, and replacing them with sodium.

I. Disinfection

A wide variety of disinfection procedures is available for the destruction of microorganisms that may cause disease. Sterilization is not intended or necessary. The most common disinfection procedure is chlorination.

Other processes are available for specific purposes, such as treatment to help prevent corrosion and processes for the handling of the solids (sludge) that accumulate in treatment. The handling and disposal of sludge is a difficult problem, particularly at wastewater treatment plants where the sludge is often noxious and can constitute a health hazard. Other processes may be required for the removal of specific substances such as ammonia, phosphorus, radioactivity, or specific contaminants. In general, one or more of the unit processes mentioned will be used.

Where the aim is potable water, the selection of the treatment process is dependent on the quality of the water source. For example, ground waters may require only aeration and disinfection, while heavily polluted surface waters may require all the processes. Community wastewaters, except for the presence of industrial wastewater discharges, tend to be much the same, and the treatment processes are selected to provide an effluent that protects the receiving water and the subsequent uses to which the water may be put. If the effluent is to be discharged into an ocean, fewer processes are likely to be required than if the effluent is intended for discharge into a small, fragile stream or for reuse for non potable purposes.

XI. WASTEWATER COLLECTION AND DISPOSAL

In common with other living organisms, humans discharge to the environment waste substances that, in turn, re-energize the endless cycle of nature. With urbanization and industrialization, waste products have increased in volume and in kind, and their impact on the environment has intensified.

Human wastes are discussed under two headings: so-called night soil and wastewaters. Each exerts its influence on specific environmental resources; night soil, principally on the soil; water-carried wastes, principally on water; but both, in some degree on the atmosphere and in some places or in some ways on soil and water together. Some of the effects on the environment have, in turn, reacted on our health and general well being.

The expression **night soil** is used to describe human body wastes, excreta, or excrement, or the combination of feces and urine voided by humans. The terms itself derives from the practice of carting away accumulations of human ordure at night. Night soil is one of several components of urban refuse in parts of the developing world. In industrialized countries, except in parts of Japan, night soil no longer exists as such, because excreta are flushed away by water into sewerage systems.

The disposal of night soil is a problem of economy, convenience, general cleanliness, and personal hygiene. The danger of exposure to infectious diseases is proportional to the concentration of the causative agents, which tends to be high in countries that do not yet have sewerage systems. The unsightliness of excrement does not injure the public health and neither do the odors disseminated by decomposing urine and feces. Yet they are offensive to the senses and interfere with the enjoyment of an otherwise attractive environment. From this standpoint alone, their elimination is important.

Night soil is the source of a wide variety of GI infections. Its safe disposal has important public health implications, and it is understandable why this has become a concern of official health agencies even though needed operations are commonly left to other departments of local government.

The following five water pollution regulations have had the greatest impact in reducing pollutant discharges to navigable waters in the United States and/on preventing adverse health effects:

1. Federal Water Pollution Control Act of 1972 (P.L. 92-500) established a national goal to eliminate pollutant discharges. The goal was to be attained by having industries and municipalities use:

    a. Best practicable technology (BPT); and
    b. Best available technology (BAT) that is economically achievable.

   Enforcement of point sources of pollution was to be accomplished through a permit system called the National Pollutant Discharge Elimination System (NPDES).
2. The Safe Drinking Water Act of 1974 (P.L. 93-523) requires EPA to set standards for substances found in the nation's drinking water which may have any adverse effect on the health of persons.
3. The Toxic Substances Control Act of 1976 (P.L. 94-469) allows EPA to regulate existing chemical hazards not covered by other environmental laws. New chemicals with the exception of food additives, drugs, pesticides, alcohol and tobacco require a pre-market evaluation as mandated by this Act.
4. The Resource Conservation and Recovery Act 1976 (PA, 94-580) allows EPA to protect against groundwater contamination from the improper disposal of hazardous and non-hazardous wastes.
5. The Clean Water Act of 1977 (P.L. 95-271) has the following major provisions:
   BPT for Municipal Treatment Facilities and for Industries.
   Industrial pollutants were classified into the following three categories:

    a. **Conventional pollutants** defined as biological oxygen demand (BOD) suspended solids, fecal coliforms, pH and others must be controlled using best conventional technology.

b. **Toxic pollutants** as identified by the 1977 Act, must be controlled by applying BAT. EPA may add or substract from the list of identified toxic pollutants.

c. **Nonconventional pollutants** are those not classified by EPA as either conventional or toxic. Dischargers must use BAT.

XII. BIBLIOGRAPHY

Conway, J.B. (1998). Water Quality Management. In R.B. Wallace (Ed.), <u>Public Health and Preventive Medicine 14th Edition</u> (pp.737-763). Stamford, CT: Appleton & Lange.

Gomez, H.F., Phillips, S.D. (1997). Water Pollution. In M.I. Greenberg, R.J. Hamilton, & S.D. Phillips (Eds.), <u>Occupational, industrial, and Environmental Toxicology</u> (pp. 437-449). St. Louis: MO: Mosby.

Hill, D.J. (2001). Sewage and Animal Waste. In L. Williams, & R. Langley (Eds.), <u>Environmental Health Secrets</u> (pp. 38-42). Philadelphia, PA: Hanley & Belfus, Inc.

Masters, G.M. (1974). <u>Introduction to Environmental Science and Technology</u>, John Wiley and Sons, New York.

Moeller, D.W. (1997). <u>Environmental Health Revised Edition</u> (126-148). Cambridge, MA: Harvard University Press.

Moeller, D.W. (1997). <u>Environmental Health Revised Edition</u> (149-169). Cambridge, MA: Harvard University Press.

Moore, G.S. (1999). <u>Living with the Earth: Concepts in Environmental Health Science</u> (9.1 – 9.39). Boca Raton, FL: Lewis Publishers.

Nadakavukaren, A. (2000). <u>Our Global Environment: A Health Perspective 5th Edition</u> (pp. 529-559).Prospect Heights, IL: Waveland Press, Inc.

Nadakavukaren, A. (2000). <u>Our Global Environment: A Health Perspective 5th Edition</u> (pp. 561-621). Prospect Heights, IL: Waveland Press, Inc.

North Carolina Division of Water Quality. (2001). Storm water Runoff. In L. Williams, & R. Langley (Eds.), <u>Environmental Health Secrets</u> (pp. 54-57). Philadelphia, PA: Hanley & Belfus, Inc.

US Environmental Protection Agency. (1976). <u>National Interim Primary Drinking Water Regulations</u> (EPA-570/9-76-003), Washington, D.C.

Williams, L.K. (2001). Chemical and Microbiological Groundwater Contaminants. In L. Williams, & R. Langley (Eds.), <u>Environmental Health Secrets</u> (pp. 43-47). Philadelphia, PA: Hanley & Belfus, Inc.

Yassi, A., Kjellstrom, T., de Kok, T., Guidotti, T. (2001). <u>Basic Environmental Health</u> (209-241). New York, NY: Oxford University Press.

CHAPTER

8

SOLID / HAZARDOUS WASTE AND RODENTS, INSECTS, AND PESTS

I. INTRODUCTION

Prior to 1976, there was no federal legislation to effectively control the disposal of wastes upon the land. Many wastes were discarded on the land to prevent violating emerging air and water laws.

EPA determined that in 1976 only 35% of 16,000 landfills surveyed were in compliance with state and local laws. Many sites were uncontrolled landfills or dumps. Problems related to dumps were the following:

1. Rats and flies that transmit disease (rats-plague, Trichinosis, rabies, rat fever; flies - typhoid, cholera, dysentery, tuberculosis, intestinal worms),
2. Burning,
3. Contamination of ground and surface waters,
4. Odors, and
5. Toxic chemicals or hazardous chemicals [This was a multimedia contamination with health effects such as poisoning (direct and through drinking water)].

Prior to 1976, large quantities of hazardous wastes (< 90%) generated by industry were disposed of by environmentally unsound methods such as: 1) dump or unsecured landfills (unlined, etc.), 2) unlined surface impoundments, 3) deep well injection, and 4) uncontrolled incineration.

Only 10% of industrial waste was disposed of with proper methods such as: 1) secured landfills, 2) neutralization/solidification, 3) recovery for reuse, and 4) controlled incineration.

EPA documented over 400 cases of environmental and human health damage from mismanagement of hazardous waste such as: 1) groundwater pollution, including drinking water, human poisonings, 2) surface water pollution, including impact on biota (fish kills, bioaccumulation, etc.), 3) direct human poisonings (dermal contact), 4) air emissions of volatile chemicals, and 5) explosions (some major), and fires.

So, in 1976 the Resource Conservation and Recovery Act (RCRA) was passed to insure the proper handling of wastes from wastes disposed of from homes to industrial wastes (nuclear wastes regulated by the Nuclear Regulatory Commission).

Wastes have been generated since the human race was born. These wastes included food scraps, sewage, broken tools, animal parts, and pottery. However, the amount of waste generated was very little because of the scarcity of materials and goods.

But as societies evolved and our ability to extract raw materials and produce goods grew, products correspondingly grew more sophisticated and complex, as did the composition and volume of our wastes. Mining by-products, acids, and heavy metal wastes, in addition to traditional human wastes, were produced at an ever-increasing rate to fulfill increasing demands. Although the Industrial Revolution of the late 1800s brought unsurpassed wealth, it also brought a new generation of wastes, whose management received scant attention. Finally, the unprecedented explosion of synthetic organic chemicals during this century increased both the volume and toxicity of wastes.

Although we can produce products and goods that were unthinkable a few decades ago, our increased waste production is not as impressive - from increased amounts of food packaging to highly radioactive waste that remains hazardous for millions of years. Additionally, our ability and desire to manage the unwanted by-products of this production waste has lagged far behind our technological achievements. Our knowledge of the health and environmental effects of the mismanagement of waste also has been deficient.

Waste management has caused problems for society throughout its history. Improperly disposed trash attracted vermin and disease-carrying insects (such as malaria and typhus) in addition to pathogens (bacteria and viruses) that were a serious health threat. The focus of the initial settlement of America on locating lands adjacent to navigable waterways for trade and protection encouraged dumping waste in the water and letting the current transport it downstream. Although such dumping reduced the health hazard of those dumping, it impacted both the receiving river as well as those people downstream, although the health and environmental impact from garbage was relatively limited (human sewage presented the most serious threat).

But the dramatic rise in synthetic organic chemical production following World Wars I and II soon presented additional, far more serious threats to health and the environment. Large quantities of chemicals, with their unknown effects, were being discharged into the air, water, and land. During the early 1960s, the public began to question the safety of managing waste by discharging it into the air or dumping it into rivers. As a result, Congress passed the Federal Water Pollution Control Act and the Clean Air Act to control these discharges. Although discharges into water and air were reduced, wastes still had to go somewhere. Thus, reliance on land disposal increased, often on land thought to be substandard (such as wetlands, floodplains, and former rock quarries). During the mid-1970s, contaminated groundwater from land-disposed hazardous waste and the discovery of Love Canal, Kentucky's Valley of the Drums, and other abandoned waste sites demonstrated that the lack of a national waste management program was the remaining loophole allowing **uncontrolled** releases of pollutants to the environment. As a result, the federal government began to establish a comprehensive waste management program that has reduced the amount of waste generated, increased recycling, and established safer disposal techniques.

Until World War II most solid or municipal waste took the form of garbage, yard waste (leaves, grass clippings, tree limbs), newspapers, cans and bottles, coal and wood ashes, street sweepings, and discarded building materials. Most such waste was not considered hazardous, and it was simply transported to the local land disposal facility or "dump," where it was periodically set on fire to reduce its volume and to discourage the breeding of insects and rodents. Because this practice often led to windblown debris and unsightly disposal facilities, and because people recognized the need for a technically sounder method of disposal, it was gradually replaced by the sanitary landfill, where municipal waste was buried in the ground. As long as windblown debris and fires were contained, material was covered over and sealed daily (so that breeding and habitation by insects and rodents were controlled), and contamination of nearby groundwater supplies was avoided, the sanitary landfill was considered an acceptable method of disposal.

With the development of a throwaway society and an unprecedented demand for new products, the volume of solid waste has increased enormously. Within the United States, the quantity of municipal solid waste rose from 2.7 pounds per person per day in 1960 to 4.3 pounds in 1990. Today the average person in this country annually produces 1,000-

1,500 pounds of municipal solid waste, including almost 100 pounds of plastics - more municipal solid waste per capita than in any other industrialized nation. Vastly larger quantities of similar non-hazardous wastes are produced by industry. At the same time, the composition of the waste has changed. Solid waste today contains many materials (such as plastics) that are not readily degradable and toxic materials - primarily various types of chemical waste produced by industry - that can contaminate soil and groundwater indefinitely if not properly disposed of.

In a similar manner, the amount of **hazardous waste** generated has been undergoing dramatic change, increasing from about 0.5 million metric tons per year at the time of World War II to some 300 million metric tons in 1993 - more than one ton of hazardous waste per person per year. In addition, industry annually discharges some 18 billion pounds (9 million tons) of toxic chemicals directly into the air, water, or land or into deep underground injection wells. The chemical and petroleum industries currently generate more than 70 percent of the hazardous waste in the United States; the rest comes from a wide range of other industries. In total, about 6 billion tons of waste are produced in the United States each year.

About two-thirds of the municipal solid waste produced is sent to sanitary landfills for disposal. However, many existing disposal sites are being filled and phased out. In 1980, there were about 16,000 active sanitary landfills in the United States; by 1995, the number had decreased to about 3,000. In fact, much of the heavily populated East Coast ran out of acceptable landfill space. Although this trend is partially due to the growing difficulty of establishing new facilities, it is also a response to the increasing stringency of federal regulations and a recognition of the benefits of establishing larger, better designed and operated disposal facilities on a regional basis.

The disposal of waste is increasingly becoming a worldwide problem. The best example is China. China is entering an era of economic development complete with fast food, single use disposable items, and a throwaway culture. Throwing trash out the window into the river or onto the streets is so commonplace, that no one is surprised. Garbage and rubbish floats down China's rivers, chokes its canals, flies out of passenger train windows, and creates mountains of trash. China is not alone in this disregard for proper disposal. The constant influx of rural people to the city of Nairobi has doubled its population in the last 10 years and overwhelmed its ability to provide basic services such as rubbish collection. Littering the streets with solid waste is commonplace, and heaps of uncollected stinking, fly and rodent-infested garbage appear everywhere. Once renowned as "The Green City in the Sun," Nairobi is now riddled with heaps of uncollected garbage and is called by many "The Stinking City in the Sun." The failure to properly manage the solid wastes in Nairobi is thought to be contributing to the increased incidence of shigellosis, paratyphoid, and cholera. Such diseases are easily spread as accumulating garbage has clogged drainage systems, flooding the cities, polluting water sources, and converting the Nairobi River into an open sewer devoid of higher life forms.

There are a number of reasons given for the indiscriminate dumping, including poor management of finances and resources, a lax attitude of city employees, and little concern among residents for the cleanliness of their city. The value systems of people moving to Nigeria, or Wuhan, China, or many other areas of the world, change in the face of economic development and industrialization. China was once a culture of thrift, where rags and cloth diapers were re-used and where national cleanliness was monitored and enforced. Now it is giving way to a hurried, money-driven, throwaway society. This is not unusual for cities. Cities have historically been centers for filth and disease. Cities in Western Europe such as England were disease-ridden centers of filth up until the 19th century. It was the norm to cast garbage, rubbish, and bodily wastes out the windows onto the streets below, or leave them on the floor about the living space. The consequence of increasing refuse, filth, insects and rodents resulted in disease outbreaks of enormous consequences such as the bubonic plague or "black death" that ravaged Europe in the 13th and 14th centuries. The relationship between disease outbreaks and accumulated filth gradually clarified in the eyes of municipal leaders so that by the early 1900s efforts were undertaken in Europe and North America to improve sanitation.

One of the major efforts was directed at promptly collecting urban wastes and dispersing them at some distance from the population so as to reduce the probability of disease. This normally meant dumping the collected refuse on the outskirts of town. Unfortunately, much of the world continues to follow this pattern of refuse disposal which: 1) invites the proliferation of rodents and insects; 2) becomes a source of contamination to groundwater; 3) pollutes ambient air when combusted; 4) facilitates the spread of debris around the dumping site; 5) lowers property values around the site; and 6) encourages the spread of disease from microorganisms and toxic chemicals. It has only been within recent years that the United States has adopted waste management policies that recognize the need for safer and more effective methods of collecting, storing, transporting, and disposing of the unusable or unwanted materials generated by society.

A large percentage of municipal solid waste (MSW) was thrown into open dumps up through the early 1970s, with very little recycling occurring. Larger communities with diminishing open land for dumping opted to construct incinerators. There were more than 300 municipal incinerators operating in the U.S. during the 1960s. The introduction of strict air quality regulations in the 1970s caused many of the incinerators to close as they represented major sources of air pollution. These same regulations imposed restrictions on the burning of open dumps. During the mid-1970s, incineration capacity declined, open dumps disappeared, and the generation of MSW increased dramatically. During the same period, the recovery of materials, such as from recycling, grew very slowly. The federal government passed regulations in 1976, which forbade open dumping while introducing the concept and use of the sanitary landfill. This law is known as the **Resource Conservation and Recovery Act (RCRA)** (pronounced "rickra") of 1976 (P. L. 94-580). There are three distinct programs under RCRA. **Subtitle D** encouraged states to develop comprehensive plans for the management of solid wastes with emphasis on those of a non-hazardous nature, such as household wastes. **Subtitle C** was designed to control the improper disposal of hazardous waste through a manifest process known as the "**cradle-to-grave**" approach. **Subtitle I** was designed to minimize the contamination of groundwater from underground storage tanks through leak detection requirements, mitigation and prevention of leaks, and new performance standards for underground storage tanks. Subtitle D was soon found to be inadequate despite regulations, which dictated the conditions for the proper siting, construction, and management of sanitary landfills. Nearly 94 percent of 17,000 land disposal sites surveyed in the mid-1970s failed to meet minimum requirements. The consequences included substantial odors and debris, contamination of groundwater, proliferation of pests, and other environmental pollution problems.

Seeing the need for additional control over the disposal of solid wastes, Congress passed the **Hazardous and Solid Waste Amendments Act of 1984 (P.L. 98-616).** This provided strict requirements for the proper siting of landfills to minimize surface and groundwater pollution. However, in an effort to achieve an improved and sustainable waste management program, the USEPA promulgated new **RCRA Subtitle D** landfill requirements that went into effect in October of 1993. The landfills were to be constructed with double liners, systems for collecting the liquids percolating through the wastes **(leachate),** groundwater monitoring wells, and methane venting and detection systems. The costs for sitting and operating landfills escalated dramatically as the number of landfills diminished in the face of rapidly growing amounts of MSW. Not only has the population of the United States increased markedly since the 1960s, but a person in the United States today generates more than 4.3 pounds of refuse per day compared to 2.7 pounds in 1960. This exceeds 1500 pounds per person per year, more than any other country. The problem of diminishing refuse disposal capacity has been further exaggerated by community opposition to landfill siting which has become known as the "not in my backyard" (NIMBY) syndrome. The cost for a truck to unload its waste at a landfill **(tipping fee)** has approached $65-$100 per ton in the Northeast United States making other disposal alternatives more attractive. Although sanitary land filling continues to be among the most widely used methods of disposal, the USEPA's Agenda for Action endorsed the concept of integrated waste management by which MSW is reduced or managed through several different practices that include:

1. Source reduction (including reuse of products and backyard composting of yard trimmings);
2. Recycling of materials (including composting); and
3. Waste combustion (preferably with energy recovery) and land filling.

Federal regulations classify wastes into three different categories, based on hazard criteria: 1) **nonhazardous**, 2) **hazardous**, and 3) **special**. **Nonhazardous wastes** are those that pose no immediate threat to human health and/or the environment, for example, municipal wastes such as household garbage and many high-volume industrial wastes. **Hazardous wastes** are of two types: (a) those that have characteristic hazardous properties, i.e., **ignitability**, **corrosivity**, or **reactivity**, and (b) those that contain leachable toxic constituents. Other hazardous wastes include liquid wastes, which are identified with a particular industry or industrial activity. The third category from industry is classified generically as **special wastes** by origin, and are regulated with waste-specific guidelines. Examples include **mine spoils**, **oil-field wastes**, **spent oils**, and **radioactive wastes**. In the United States, all hazardous wastes are regulated under **Subtitle C of RCRA**.

There are many types of wastes, with various physical characteristics and origins. (Figure 8.1). They includes:

1. **Hazardous waste** - Primarily industrial waste that meets the legal definition of hazardous and thus must be managed in accordance with special federal regulations.

2. **Industrial waste** - This category of waste comprises industrial waste that is **not** legally defined as hazardous; it includes manufacturing waste, mining waste, coal combustion waste, and oil and gas production waste.
3. **Municipal solid waste** - Garbage and trash that is generated by households, schools, offices, and similar facilities.
4. **Medical waste** - Waste generated by hospitals, laboratories, universities, morgues, and dental clinics.
5. **Radioactive waste** - All wastes that exhibit radioactivity, including spent nuclear fuel, high-level and transuranic radioactive waste from weapons production, low-level radioactive waste, and uranium mill tailings from the processing of uranium ore.

Based on the best available data, the estimated total amount of waste generated is presented in Table 8.1 and Figure 8.2. Also included are examples of each waste category and the applicable federal laws.

The EPA estimates that approximately 197.5 million tons of waste legally defined as hazardous are produced annually by approximately 195,000 generators. (Seventy-nine percent of hazardous waste is generated by the chemical industry.) However, this data is from the 1989 reporting year that was released in 1993. In 1990, the EPA expanded the definition of hazardous waste. The EPA has estimated that the current generation rate is between 300 and 700 million tons of hazardous waste. However, this will not be confirmed until 1995, when the 1991 data is released (hazardous waste generators report every other year).

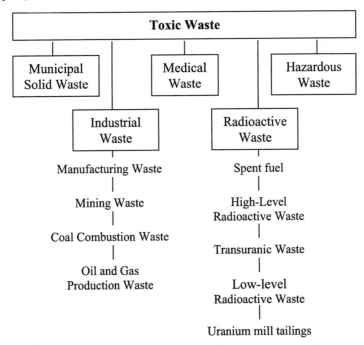

Figure 8.1. The Universe of Wastes. (Source: Wagner, 1994).

Table 8.1. Waste Categories, Laws, and Amounts*. (Source: Wagner, 1994).

Waste category	Amount generated (per year)	Examples	Applicable federal laws	Per capita generation rate
Hazardous waste**	196,500,866 tons	Industrial wastes exhibiting certain hazardous and toxic characteristics	Resource Conservation and Recovery Act	4.3 lbs./day
Industrial waste Manufacturing waste Mining waste Coal combustion waste Oil and gas production waste	6,500,000,000 tons 1,810,000,000 tons 1,000,000,000 tons 3,700,000,000 tons	Wastewater, non-hazardous waste, scraps, waste rock and tailings, chemicals	Resource Conservation and Recovery Act	142.5 lbs./day 39.7 lbs./day 21.9 lbs./day 81.0 lbs./day
Municipal solid waste	164,000,000 tons	Garbage, paper, packaging, food scraps	Resource Conservation and Recovery Act	4.3 lbs./day
Medical waste	500,000 tons	Syringes, body parts, laboratory animals	Medical Waste Tracking Act	1 oz./day
Radioactive wastes Spent fuel High-level radioactive waste Transuranic waste Low-level radioactive waste Uranium mill tailings	2,106 tons 2,474 yd^3 NCG 150,157 yd^3 471,000 yd^3	Nuclear power generation wastes, nuclear weapons wastes, industrial wastes, and mining and ore processing wastes	Atomic Energy Act, Nuclear Waste Policy Act, and the Low-Level Radioactive Waste Policy Act	

*   The amounts provided are estimates based on the sources listed below. However, it is important to note that although they are expressed as annual amounts, the amounts may differ. For example, the only data available for oil and gas wastes is 1985, whereas 1991 data exist for municipal solid waste. NCG = Not currently generated.

**   The only national data on hazardous waste generated in the United States is from 1989, which was released in 1993. However, the definition of hazardous waste was expanded in 1990. Thus, the quantity is currently estimated to be between 300 and 700 million tons.

More than 90 percent (by weight) of waste designated as hazardous is wastewater (water used in industrial processes that becomes contaminated). Often, this wastewater is fairly dilute, but contains enough regulated constituents to render it hazardous. The remaining 10 percent includes inorganic solids (heavy metals, contaminated soil), organic liquids (solvents), and sludges (treatment residues) from air- and water-pollution-control devices.

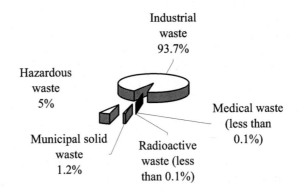

Figure 8.2. The Universe of Wastes by Percentages. (Source: Wagner, 1994).

II. MUNICIPAL SOLID WASTE

A. INTRODUCTION

The USEPA's Office of Solid Waste uses a materials flows methodology to estimate the amounts of municipal solid waste (MSW) generated. This methodology is based on production data (by weight) for both materials and products in the waste stream and is adjusted for imports and exports. Materials in MSW include paper and paperboard, yard trimmings, food wastes, plastics, glass, metal, and wood wastes.

Municipal solid wastes (MSW) may also be categorized by the products generated, which include: durable goods (e.g., appliances), non-durable goods (e.g., newspapers), containers and packaging, food wastes and yard trimmings, and miscellaneous organic wastes. Such wastes generally come from residential, commercial, institutional, and industrial sources.

Wastes may be classified by their physical, chemical, and biological characteristics. An important classification criterion is their consistency. Solid wastes are waste materials having less than approximately 70 percent water. This class includes municipal solid wastes such as household garbage, industrial wastes, mining wastes, and oil field wastes. **Liquid wastes** are usually wastewaters, including municipal and industrial wastewaters that contain less than 1 percent suspended solids. Such wastes may contain high concentrations (greater than 1 percent) of dissolved species, such as salts and metals. **Solid waste**, as defined under the Resource, Conservation, and Recovery Act (RCRA) is any solid, semisolid, liquid, or contained gaseous materials discarded from industrial, commercial, mining, or agricultural operations and from community activities. **Solid waste** includes garbage, construction debris, commercial refuse, sludge from water supply or waste treatment plants, material from air pollution control facilities, and other discarded materials. Solid waste does not include solid or dissolved materials in irrigation return flows or industrial discharges. **Sludge** is a class of wastes intermediate to solid and liquid wastes. Sludges usually contain between 3 and 25 percent solids, while the rest of the material is water-dissolved species. These materials, which have a slurrylike consistency, include municipal sludges, which are produced during secondary treatment of wastewaters, and sediments found in storage tanks and lagoons

During the 1970s, heavy rains raised the groundwater level and turned Love Canal region in Niagara Falls, New York into a muddy swamp which mixed with some of the 19,000 tons of toxic wastes buried in the abandoned canal by Hooker Chemical Company. The chemically-laced ooze seeped into basements, onto playgrounds, and over lawns creating a storm of protests, accusations of severe health effect, and costs of over $37 million to relocate families from the area, and another $30 million to aid families. More than $150 million and 12 years have been spent on clean-up efforts. Love Canal became a major turning point in directing public attention to other chemical wastelands scattered across the country in abandoned warehouses, manufacturing facilities, landfills, and processing plants. In 1982, scientists recommended a government buyout of Times Beach, Missouri after waste oil dealer Russell Bliss sprayed the dirt roads in 1971 with dioxin-laced oil to keep the dust down. The events at Love Canal and Times Beach are not unique.

The Escambia treating company near a Pensacola, Florida neighborhood closed its doors years ago, but now a toxic mess piled in a 60 foot mound by the USEPA sits in the neighborhood since 1991, covered only with a polyethylene bag. This is a black, working-class neighborhood and the citizens felt that their backyards were being contaminated by dioxin and chemical preservatives such as creosote and pentachlorophenol. The USEPA announced in 1996 it was planning to spend $18 million to relocate people from 158 houses and 200 apartments making it the largest move since Love Canal and Times Beach which took place more than a decade earlier. Agency officials acknowledged that they had to consider **environmental justice** in the decision.

The idea of environmental justice developed from studies that indicated minorities were being subjected to environmental pollutants disproportionately. This prompted President Clinton to issue an executive order in 1994 that decreed agencies must address the notion of environmental justice when considering the disposal of hazardous wastes. Additionally, the order required minorities be given a voice in environmental regulation and that the cleanup of the worst toxic waste sites in minority areas be given priority.

In the early and mid-seventies, cases of acute lymphocytic leukemia began to surface in the town of Woburn, Massachusetts. Although no conclusive link was established between discarded organochlorine chemicals appearing in the drinking water and elevated leukemia levels, the involved companies agreed to pay nearly $70 million in cleanup costs. The story, as written by Jonathan Harr, became a best seller titled **A Civil Action**, and a film starring John Travolta released in early 1999. These events point to increased public awareness and concern about hazardous wastes as one of the major environmental challenges. The USEPA estimates that in excess of 270 million tons of hazardous waste are generated every year in the United States, with most of it produced by the petrochemical industry. Discarded or released hazardous substances have contaminated surface and groundwater, soil, and air. Drinking water has been contaminated, food sources polluted, and wildlife habitats destroyed or compromised.

The piles of refuse and unsightly, unsanitary conditions that quickly accumulate during the garbage workers' strikes that occasionally plague some cities provide a dramatic illustration of the importance to public health of regular, frequent urban refuse collection. Any breakdown in this essential service, particularly during the warmer months of the year, can result in odor and litter problems or in the rapid growth of fly and rat populations. To prevent such problems, the Public Health Service recommends that refuse be collected twice weekly in residential areas and daily from restaurants, hotels, and large apartment complexes. This is particularly important during the peak of the summer fly-breeding season when eggs may hatch in less than a day and larval stages can be completed in three to four days. Historically, because the public has been far more concerned that refuse be regularly removed than with what happens to it once the garbage truck rounds the nearest corner (the "out of sight, out of mind" philosophy), municipal solid waste budgets have traditionally allocated a significantly greater proportion of their resources to refuse collection than to disposal.

B. CURRENT WASTE DISPOSAL OPTIONS

1. Sanitary Landfilling

In recent decades, most municipalities seeking an economically feasible yet environmentally acceptable alternative to open dumping have opted for sanitary landfills. A sanitary landfill differs from an open dump in that collected refuse is spread in thin layers and compacted by bulldozers. When the compacted layers are 8 - 10 feet deep, they are covered with about 6 inches of dirt, which is again compacted. At the end of each working day another thin layer of soil is placed over the fill to prevent litter from blowing about, to keep away insect and rodent pests, and to minimize odor problems. When the landfill has reached its ultimate capacity, a final earth cover two feet deep is placed over the entire area and the land can then be used for a park, golf course, or other kinds of recreational facilities.

When properly sited, well designed, and efficiently operated, a sanitary landfill can be perfectly adequate means of urban refuse disposal, free from offensive odors, vermin, or pollution problems. Unfortunately, in the past most so-called "sanitary" landfills were not well sited, properly designed, or well run. As a result, many landfills caused environmental contamination problems little different from those of open dumps and made sanitary landfills unwelcome neighbors wherever they were located. In the mid-1970s it was reported that of 17,000 land disposal sites surveyed, 94% failed to meet the minimum requirements of a sanitary landfill - requirements that in the 1970s were far less stringent than those prevailing today.

The new public focus on MSW concerns sparked intensive efforts by local and state officials to develop new, more sustainable waste management strategies for the decades ahead - and to insist that new and existing landfills be better designed and operated than the earlier facilities responsible for so many environmental horror stories. A major step toward the latter objective was EPA's promulgation of its new RCRA SubtitleD landfill requirements, now in effect nationwide. Mandating that all landfills install groundwater monitoring wells and methane detection systems, Subtitle D has sharply increased the cost of landfill operations but has also ensured that leachates or potentially explosive gases migrating from the fill don't go unnoticed and neglected. Requirements that new cells within a landfill be constructed with double liners and a leachate collection system to remove standing water means that new MSW landfills will be virtually indistinguishable in design from land disposal facilities licensed to accept hazardous wastes. Compliance with such requirements, of course, is expensive and owners of many smaller landfills opted to go out of business rather than invest the sums necessary to continue operations under the new regulations.

2. Source Reduction

The best and cheapest way of managing wastes is not to produce them in the first place. Accordingly, policies of reducing wastes at their source are top-ranked in every priority listing of waste management options. First raised as a possible approach for dealing with U.S. solid waste problems at a 1975 EPA-sponsored Conference on Waste Reduction, the goal of conserving materials and energy through waste prevention or by reducing the volume or toxicity of wastes generated was given little more than lip service until recently. The present sense of urgency to relieve pressures on existing disposal facilities has prompted a more serious look at the potential for source reduction strategies, which most advocates estimate could cut present urban waste streams by about 5%. Approaches to source reduction variously target consumers, manufacturers, or government and can include either voluntary or mandatory components.

Appealing to consumers to use their considerable purchasing power in a more environmentally aware manner has been a key component of source reduction efforts for years. By shopping selectively - buying only the amount of a product that will be used, choosing items without excessive amounts of packaging, buying products that have fewer toxic ingredients than comparable items used for the same purpose, avoiding single-serve disposable packages, or participating in waste exchanges (yard- or garage-sales might be regarded as an effective source reduction strategy!) are all ways of reducing the garbage we throw away. Another approach involves substituting reusable consumer items for single-use throwaway products - cloth napkins and terry towels instead of paper ones; china or plastic dishes instead of paper plates; handkerchiefs instead of Kleenex; cloth diapers in lieu of Pampers (the 3 million tons of dirty disposable diapers thrown away in the U.S. each year make up 1.4% by volume of the entire MSW stream). Backyard composting of kitchen scraps and garden debris, as well as "grasscycling" - allowing grass clippings to fall and decompose on the lawn or using them for mulch - are other examples of waste reduction that can easily be practiced by individuals.

3. Recycling

More broadly referred to as resource recovery - any productive use of what would otherwise be a waste material requiring disposal - recycling and composting are ranked in second place, after source reduction and reuse, on the EPA's list of most environmentally desirable strategies for municipal solid waste management. Perceived by many environmentally aware citizens as "the right thing to do" and by local officials as a way of extending the remaining lifespan of existing land disposal facilities (thereby postponing politically prickly decisions regarding the siting of new landfills or incinerators), recycling of MSW has made impressive gains since the late 1980s. In its

1999 report on "The State of Garbage in America," **RioCycle** magazine reported that recycling rates, including composting, reached their highest levels ever - 31.5% of all MSW generated in the U.S., nearly four times the level attained in 1990.

Recycling, of course, is not a new phenomenon. An earlier generation of Americans diligently recycled during World War II, when saving valuable resources to aid in the war effort was widely regarded as a patriotic duty. However, interest in resource conservation waned during the prosperous 1950s and 1960s and only revived with the emergence of the ecology movement and the energy "crisis" of the 1970s. At that time increased emphasis on recycling was promoted primarily for its very real ecological benefits:

Resource conservation - recycling reduces pressure on forest resources and extends the nation's supply of nonrenewable mineral ores.

Energy conservation - recycling consumes 50 - 90% less energy than manufacturing the same item from virgin materials.

Pollution abatement - manufacturing products from secondary rather than virgin materials significantly reduces levels of pollutant emissions. For example, recycling scrap metal, as opposed to processing iron ore in a coke oven, reduces particulate emissions by 11 kg/metric ton and eliminates the mining wastes generated in extracting iron ore and coal. Recycling aluminum has an even greater environmental impact - both air pollution and energy use are thereby cut by 95%.

If disposal costs increase, the rate of recycling can be expected to increase. With current low disposal costs in many areas, there is little incentive for recycling. In addition, increased demand for the products of recycling are necessary to make any progress. This is partially driven by economics and will take federal government action to eliminate tax subsidies for the timber, mining, and extraction industries that prevent recovered materials from competing for market share.   In addition, purchasing preferences that set minimum recycled content requirements for certain products can drive markets in favor of more recovery.

There must be a way to build into our process a strategy that promotes cost-effective solid waste management. Local government officials must have facts presented to them that are easy to understand and are politically palatable. We must realize that solid waste management is competing with all other locally funded programs, and, again, be realistic with our expectations.

4. Composting

Since the late 1980s, proliferation of state mandates prohibiting the land filling of yard wastes has led to an explosive increase in municipal composting facilities in the United States. By 1999, 21 states had enacted such bans and over 3,800 yard waste composting facilities were operating in every U.S. state except Alaska (bans on the land filling of yard wastes have also contributed to booming sales of mulching mowers; results from a four-year demonstration project conducted by the Rodale Institute concluded that use of mulching mowers produces healthier lawns with fewer weeds and no thatch buildup). While a number of European countries have long recognized that composting of organic household waste can reduce the amount of refuse requiring disposal, consideration of composting as a viable waste management alternative in the United States is a much more recent phenomenon. Even though readily decomposable food and yard wastes make up nearly 25% of the U.S. urban waste stream (considerably more during the warmer months of the year, less during the winter), perceived lack of demand for the finished product, plus the ease and low cost of land filling, led city officials to dismiss composting as an impractical venture.

That attitude has now been transformed by the realization that it makes little sense to devote valuable landfill space to grass clippings and autumn leaves when such materials could be converted into a useful and environmentally beneficial product. Nor are yard wastes the only potentially compostable materials in MSW. By 1999, nineteen cities hosted mixed waste composting plants that process the entire organic portion of residential and commercial wastes - food scraps, soiled paper, etc. - removing only noncompostable (but still recyclable) glass, metal, and plastics, as well as any hazardous materials. Though questions have been raised about the quality of mixed waste compost and thus its acceptability to mid-users; efforts to educate citizens on the importance of source separation have helped to prevent contamination of the final product and to avoid the loss of potentially compostable materials.

A form of resource recovery, composting utilizes natural biochemical decay processes to convert organic wastes into a humus-like material, suitable for use as a soil conditioner. Although its nutrient content is too low to consider it a fertilizer, compost greatly improves soil structure and porosity, aids in water infiltration and retention, increases soil aeration, and slows erosion. Co-composting of yard wastes with municipal sewage sludge (another increasingly difficult-to-dispose-of waste product), now being practiced in a number of communities, enhances the nitrogen content of the finished product and makes it more valuable for agricultural uses.

A variety of methods for converting wastes to compost are currently in use, ranging from the low-tech, relatively inexpensive windrow technique, where long rows of wastes are piled outdoors and mechanically turned periodically to aerate the mass, to highly sophisticated, expensive in-vessel operations or processes in which pumps mechanically aerate windrows ("**aerated static pile**"), hastening decay and eliminating the need for frequent turning.

Choice of the most appropriate composting method depends on the needs and resources of the community in question: if land is abundant and funding scarce, the windrow method may be the best option - though it often requires two or three years for complete breakdown of wastes to occur if the piles are turned only once or twice annually. If available space is at a premium and rapid turnover of wastes desirable, a community might be wise to choose a more high-tech method, provided it can afford the considerably higher price tag associated with such facilities. Whatever the technology, the composting process consists of four basic steps:

Preparation - incoming wastes are shredded to a relatively uniform size; in most composting operations, nonbiodegradable materials such as glass, metal, plastics, tires, and so on are separated from the compostable wastes. In some composting operations, sewage sludge or animal manures are added to the refuse at this point.

Digestion - microbes naturally present in the waste materials or special bacterial inoculants sprayed on the refuse are utilized to break down organic waste materials. While digestion may be either aerobic or anaerobic, aerobic systems are generally preferred due to shorter time periods required and fewer odor problems. In aerobic decomposition, heat given off by microbial respiration raises the temperature in the windows well above the 1400° F necessary to kill fly eggs, weed seeds, or pathogenic organisms.

Curing - after digestion of simpler carbonaceous material's is complete, additional curing time is allowed to permit microbes to break down cellulose and lignin in the waste.

Finishing - to produce an acceptable finished product, compost may be put through screens and grinders to remove non-digested materials and create a uniform appearance. Some composting facilities bag or package the finished product to facilitate marketing or distribution.

While the public rightly regards composting as an environmentally desirable method of organic waste management, composting facilities do not always make good neighbors. Some have been forced to close due to problems with objectionable odors-problems that are gradually being solved as operators compare notes and learn techniques for managing trouble-free facilities. Another public health issue related to composting operations is their potential to emit bioaerosols, tiny airborne particles of microorganisms whose inhalation has been blamed for ailments ranging from a runny nose and watery eyes to flu-like symptoms. Bioaerosols, such as spores of the ubiquitous fungus **Aspergillus fumigatus**, were first cited as a potential environmental health concern in 1992 when a New Jersey epidemiologist testified before Congress about potential health risks to persons living within a two-mile radius of composting sites. Since that time bioaerosols have attracted intensive scrutiny and have prompted organized community opposition to siting of compost facilities in several localities. Representatives of the composting industry argue that any fears are vastly exaggerated, stating that public exposure to **Aspergillus** emissions from composting are negligible when the process is performed correctly.

A report jointly sponsored by the EPA, USDA, NIOSH, and the Composting Council tends to support industry's contention. Conceding that exposure to bioaerosols could be life-threatening if inhaled by individuals with suppressed immune systems, the report nevertheless points out that the level of such particles is no higher in the vicinity of composting operations than in the general environment. A person is just as likely to inhale **A. fumigatus** spores while mowing the lawn, raking leaves, or cleaning the attic as by living near a composting facility. Experts report that **Aspergillus** at composting sites originates primarily from the storage of bulking agents such as wood chips, with airborne spores being released at the time of initial mixing (the steam rising off the top of windrows does not appear to be a major source). Operational considerations such as moisture and dust control and minimization of handling can significantly mitigate bioaerosol emissions. While authorities agree that more research is needed, the general consensus at present is that bioaerosols do not present concerns serious enough to warrant a reconsideration of municipal composting operations.

In the past, the difficulty of finding outlets for municipal compost was a major stumbling block in convincing local officials to consider composting as a waste management strategy. In recent years, however, cities' marketing efforts and increased public awareness of compost's desirability as a soil conditioner have created sufficient demand among landscaping firms, nurseries, parks departments, and home gardeners to provide a ready outlet. This growing willingness to use compost, coupled with improvements in composting technology and a national need to curtail the flood of urban refuse destined for landfill space, suggests that municipal composting will constitute an increasingly significant waste management alternative in the years ahead.

5. Waste Combustion

Prior to passage of the 1970 Clean Air Act, burning of urban refuse at large municipal incinerators was the waste disposal method of choice in a number of communities where the high cost of land, unavailability of suitable sites, or neighborhood opposition to siting made landfilling unfeasible. By the 1960s, almost 300 municipal incinerators were operating in the United States. As the decade of the 1970s ushered in an era of strict air quality control regulations, however, most of these incinerators closed down, unable to comply with the new emission standards. Studies indicated that in some large cities, close to 20% of all particulate pollutants were coming from municipal incinerators.

By the end of the 1990s, incineration was the management option for only 7.5% of U.S. municipal solid wastes, a figure considerably lower than predicted just a few years earlier. During the 1980s, as the nation's mounting garbage woes assumed center stage in the environmental policy debate, interest in burning as an attractive waste management option was revived by the advent of a new generation of incinerators: **waste-to-energy (WTE)** plants. These facilities not only burn refuse, thereby reducing its volume by 80 - 90%, but also capture the heat of combustion in the form of salable electricity or process steam.

From an environmental standpoint, the euphoria that in the 1980s web corned WTE incinerators as the ideal solution to our disposal dilemmas is now giving way to a more cautious appraisal, as concerns are raised about possible toxic air emissions, especially dioxins, furans, and heavy metals (e.g. lead, cadmium, and mercury). Proponents of the technology insist such problems can be minimized through good emission controls and proper plant operation; in 1991 tighter emissions limitations required by Clean Air Act Amendments for municipal incinerators were approved by EPA, requiring that facilities install state-of-the-art equipment to control acid gases, metal particulates, and organic products of incomplete combustion, such as dioxin. Smokestacks are now being fitted with acid gas scrubbers, baghouse filters for trapping metal particulates, and activated carbon injection systems for capturing mercury vapors. By utilizing advanced combustion controls, plant operators can maintain furnace temperatures high enough to prevent dioxin formation and to ensure a more complete burn.

Disposal of the considerable volumes of incinerator ash generated by large WTE facilities has been another contentious issue. Incineration is not a complete waste management method; in general, for every three tons of refuse burned, a ton of ash remains, requiring disposal.

Nevertheless, opponents remain wary, fearing that cities opting for incineration are going to find they've simply traded one set of environmental problems for another. Perhaps the major question regarding the future of WTE incineration, however, is financing their construction and operation.

The future role of WTE incineration in a comprehensive waste management strategy thus depends on a number of economic and political considerations, including trends in landfill tipping fees (increases make incineration more cost-competitive and vice-versa). WTE combustion remains the most important MSW management method in

Japan and a number of European countries. However, given the current abundance of landfill capacity in the U.S. and the large discrepancy between per unit disposal charges at landfills versus incinerators, it is unlikely that the percentage of MSW managed by combustion will increase significantly in the years immediately ahead.

III. HAZARDOUS WASTE

A. INTRODUCTION

Hazardous waste has been defined as a myriad of substances that causes toxicity to living organisms. For all practical purposes, toxic waste and hazardous waste are interchangeable. Traditionally, when discussing radioactive or medical waste, the term "mixed waste" is used. Toxic substances occur naturally in soil, water, and air; however, thousands of toxic substances are anthropogenic. The anthropogenic substances are of particular concern because of the quantities that are produced, their dissemination and persistence, and because, historically, their release into the environment has not been well controlled. Furthermore, most anthropogenic compounds are organic and are readily absorbed by living organisms.

In the 1976 Resource Conservation and Recovery Act (RCRA), Congress legally defined **hazardous waste** as "any discarded material that may pose a substantial threat or potential danger to human health or the environment when improperly handled" (Figure 8.3). EPA has established a two-tier system for determining whether a specific waste is subject to regulation under current hazardous waste management laws: If the substance in question is among the more than 500 wastes or waste streams itemized in Parts 261.31 - 33 of the Code of Federal Regulations, it will automatically be subject to regulation as a hazardous waste. Wastes may be placed on the list because of their ability to induce cancer, mutations, or birth defects; because of their toxicity to plants; or because even low doses are fatal to humans. However, the Administrator of EPA can exercise a wide measure of discretion in deciding whether to list a particular waste, so a number of potential carcinogens, mutagens, and teratogens are not yet listed as officially "hazardous."

B. IDENTIFICATION OF HAZARDOUS WASTES

According to RCRA regulations, to be considered a hazardous waste, a material first must be classified as a solid waste. A solid waste is defined as garbage, refuse, sludge, or other discarded material (including solids, semisolids, liquids, and contained gaseous materials). If a waste meets the solid waste definition, it must then be determined if the waste is hazardous. There are thousands of wastes that can be hazardous for many different reasons. Determining which wastes are hazardous is an ongoing process influenced by new research, new and improved testing, and health concerns. RCRA regulations identify hazardous wastes based on one or more of its dangerous properties or characteristics.

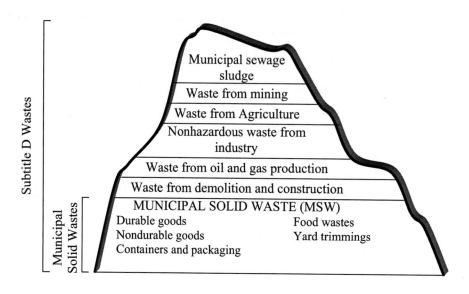

Figure 8.3. Municipal Solid Wastes as a Component of RCRA Subtitle D wastes. (Source: Moore, 1999).

The Environmental Protection Agency, the federal agency that is responsible for establishing and enforcing RCRA regulations has also determined that some specific wastes are hazardous and have incorporated them into published lists. These "listed" wastes are known to be harmful to human health and the environment when not managed properly; regardless of the concentrations of hazardous constituents they contain, these wastes must be handled according to the hazardous waste regulations.

The Environmental Protection Agency (EPA) has published a list of approximately 450 wastes that have been predetermined to be hazardous; these wastes are subject to the federal requirements for managing hazardous waste. The listing of a hazardous waste is based on its potential to affect human health or the environment, toxicity to laboratory animals, persistence in the environment, and damage case history.

In addition to the wastes listed in the federal code, any waste which exhibits one or more of the following characteristics is defined as hazardous and subject to regulation:

Toxic - wastes such as arsenic, heavy metals such as lead and mercury, or certain synthetic pesticides are capable of causing either acute or chronic health problems. Toxic wastes are harmful or fatal when ingested or absorbed. When toxic wastes are disposed of on land, they can leach through the ground and pollute the groundwater. Toxicity is identified through a laboratory rest known as the Toxicity Characteristic Leaching Procedure (TCLP), which was designed to mimic the leaching process and other conditions that occur when wastes are buried in a typical municipal landfill. The regulations require a facility to apply the TCLP to its hazardous waste samples and determine whether the leachate contains any of 40 different toxic chemicals in amounts above the specified regulatory levels. The regulation describing the toxicity characteristic is codified at 40 CER 261.24.

Ignitable - organic solvents, oils (including gasoline), plasticizers, industrial alcohols, furniture polish and paint wastes are examples of wastes that are hazardous because they have a flashpoint less than 60 °C (140 °F) or because they tend to undergo spontaneous combustion. These are liquids capable of burning or causing fire. The resultant fires are dangerous not only because of heat and smoke, but also because they can disseminate toxic particles over a wide area. Ignitable substances can irritate the skin, eyes, and lungs and may give off harmful vapors.

   Corrosive - substances with a pH of 2 or less or 12.5 and above can eat away at standard container materials or living tissues through chemical action (such as burning human tissue on contact) and are termed corrosive. Such wastes, which include acids, alkaline cleaning agents, some chlorides, fluorides, acids, and battery manufacturing residues, present a special threat to waste haulers who come into bodily contact with leaking containers.

   Reactive - obsolete munitions, peroxides, isocyanates, cyanides, and chlorine wastes from the manufacturing of dynamite or firecrackers, and certain chemical wastes such as picric acid are hazardous because of their tendency to react vigorously with air or water or to explode and generate toxic flames. Many people have been injured in their homes by mixing chlorine bleach and ammonia when cleaning. Chlorine bleach and ammonia are reactive and create a poisonous gas (chloramine and chlorine gas) when they come into contact with each other.

The lists of hazardous waste are organized into three categories:

   Source-specific wastes: This list includes waste from specific industries such as petroleum refining, wood preserving, and chemical manufacturing. These wastes typically include sludges, spent catalysts, and residues and wastewater from treatment and production processes in specific industries.

   Nonspecific source wastes: This list identifies generic wastes commonly produced by manufacturing and industrial processes. Examples include halogenated solvents used in cleaning and degreasing and wastewater treatment sludges from electroplating processes.

   Commercial chemical products: This List includes specific discarded commercial chemical products, off-specification products, container residues, and spill residues of any of these. Examples include chloroform, creosote, acids, and pesticides.

C. REQUIREMENTS FOR HANDLING HAZARDOUS WASTE

Generation - Many industries, both large and small, generate hazardous wastes during the manufacture of their products. For example, industries that manufacture plastics, chemicals, paint, petroleum products, wood products, metal products, and many other products all produce hazardous wastes. Companies and local businesses that use many of these products, such as print shops, gas stations, dry cleaners, hospitals, laboratories, and auto repair shops, may also create hazardous wastes. There are hundreds of types of businesses in all parts of the country, in rural areas and in urban ones, in industrial parts of towns and in neighborhoods, that produce hazardous and toxic wastes, as well as treat, store, and dispose of these wastes. Hazardous wastes are also generated in the home as a result of the use of products such as paint, mineral spirits, paint thinner, batteries, oil, and cleaning solvents.

The regulations vary based on the volume of hazardous waste generated or managed. In general, the hazardous waste generator must comply with storage standards for tanks and drums, labeling and marking requirements, safety and spill-response measures, recordkeeping requirements, and must periodically report to the EPA (or the state) the type and amount of hazardous waste generated and shipped offsite.

Generators must ensure that the waste is handled properly and must keep track of the waste when it is moved from where it is produced to treatment, recycling, storage, or disposal facilities.

The tracking system requires the generator to package and label the waste properly for transportation and to prepare a manifest (list of cargo) that must travel with the waste when it is transported. The generator is ultimately responsible (cradle-to-grave liability) for the proper management of its hazardous waste regardless of who treats, stores, or disposes of it in the future. The generator, the transporter, and the treatment, storage, and disposal facility all must sign and keep a copy of the manifest as they handle the waste.

Transportation - Those who transport hazardous wastes must register with the EPA and obtain an identification number, as must generators and other hazardous waste management facilities. Transporters must make sure that the waste is properly contained and labeled, in accordance with the federal Department of Transportation shipping requirements, that a manifest accompanies the waste, and that precautions and plans are in place in case of a spill.

Treatment, Storage, Disposal - Facilities that treat, store, or dispose of hazardous wastes must meet a number of stringent requirements and safety standards and must obtain a permit to operate. EPA regulations lay out detailed operating requirements for specific types of treatment, storage, and disposal facilities, such as landfills and incinerators, to minimize the threat of harm from their activities. For example, hazardous waste landfills are required to have liner systems to prevent leaks from entering the underlying soil and groundwater. Treatment facilities use different processes to recover material from the waste for reuse, to change the waste to make it less hazardous or nonhazardous, or to reduce the volume of the waste. They are required to have site safety plans or contingency plans should a release occur.

Household Hazardous Waste - Although hazardous wastes produced from households such as old pesticides, paints, acids, cleaners, and used oils are not regulated, they should be disposed of properly. Many communities provide collection centers or pickup services. Contact your local waste collection facility to see if they provide a collection center for household hazardous wastes and watch your local newspaper for "Household Hazardous Waste Disposal Days." Public service announcements on television and radio also help promote such events. In addition, local gas stations may recycle used motor oils and old automobile batteries.

Special Training for Handling Hazardous Waste - All personnel who have duties involving hazardous wastes, or have the potential to handle hazardous waste, must be formally trained to perform their duties. They must also be trained in emergency procedures and they must be able to respond effectively to an emergency. Training records must be kept by the facility and a review of the training must be conducted annually. Generators and treatment, storage, and disposal facilities are required to be prepared in case of a fire, explosion, or release of hazardous waste and to maintain and operate their businesses to minimize these risks. A copy of the contingency plan, which describes staff response in case of a fire, explosion, or release, must be distributed to local police, fire departments, hospitals, and emergency response teams so that they can be prepared to respond as well.

Because hazardous waste is subject to special federal controls, its ultimate disposition is strictly regulated. A person generating hazardous waste may elect to manage hazardous waste with the following methods:

1. Reclamation
2. Treatment
3. Incineration
4. Storage
5. Disposal

D. Methods of Hazardous Waste Disposal

Historically, the largest percentage of hazardous wastes have been disposed of on land, primarily because land disposal, particularly prior to government regulation of hazardous waste management, was by far the cheapest disposal option. During the mid-1970s, for example, almost half of all hazardous wastes, the majority of which were in the form of liquids or sludges, were simply dumped into unlined surface impoundments, technically referred to as "pits, ponds, or lagoons," located on the generators' property (even today, approximately 96% of all hazardous wastes generated in this country are treated or disposed of at the site where they are generated; only 4% of all hazardous wastes are sent off-site for management). These wastes eventually evaporated or percolated into the soil, often resulting in groundwater contamination. Other wastes, about 80% of the total, were buried in sanitary landfills, easily subject to leaching, and another 10% were burned in an uncontrolled manner. None of these methods would be in compliance with current regulations.

Although many citizens are convinced that no methods exist for the safe disposal of hazardous wastes, a number of new technologies have been developed which avoid most of the shortcomings inherent in past hazardous waste management practices. All such methods, not surprisingly, are considerably more expensive than simply dumping wastes in a pit or a municipal landfill, and thus were not widely utilized until strict regulatory action was taken by Congress. A listing of legal hazardous waste disposal options would include the following.

Secure Chemical Landfill - Generally, the cheapest method of hazardous waste disposal is the so-called "**secure**" chemical landfill, a specially designed earthen excavation constructed in such a way as to contain dangerous chemicals and to prevent them from escaping into the environment through leaching or vaporization. In the past, secure landfills frequently differed from sanitary landfills only in that they were topped with a layer of clay to keep water out of the trenches in which chemical drums had been placed. This of course did not prevent chemical seepage from contaminating water supplies. Under current RCRA standards, a secure chemical landfill must be located above the 100-year floodplain and away from fault zones; it must contain double liners of clay or synthetic materials to keep leaching to a minimum; a network of pipes must be laid to collect and control polluted rainwater and leachate accumulating in the landfill; and monitoring wells must be installed to check the quality of any groundwater deposits in the area (surface water supplies must also be monitored by the landfill operator). In spite of these precautions, most experts agree that there is no way to guarantee that sometime in the future contaminants will not migrate from the landfill site. Liners eventually crack; soil can shift or settle. Since many chemical wastes remain hazardous more or less indefinitely, serious pollution problems can occur many years after a secure chemical landfill has been closed and forgotten. Many authorities feel that although chemical landfills are legal, they are the least acceptable method of managing hazardous wastes.

Deep Well Injection - The use of deep wells for waste disposal dates back to the late 19th century when the petroleum industry employed this method to get rid of salt brine, but its use for liquid hazardous waste disposal began only during the 1940s. A number of industries, most notably petroleum refineries and petrochemical plants, now utilize this disposal method. Commercial deep well injection currently is practiced only in the Midwest and in Texas and neighboring states, although many other injection wells operated by private firms solely for the disposal of their own wastes are widely scattered across the United States. The process involves pumping liquid wastes through lined wells into porous rock formations deep underground, well below any drinking water aquifers (Figure 8.4). Some critics point out that cracks in the well casing or undetected faults in the earth, which intersect the disposal zone could result in outward migration of wastes. EPA contends that deep wells are safe, provided that they are constructed, operated and maintained in accordance with agency regulations.

Various Chemical, Physical, or Biological Treatment Processes - Processes that render wastes non-hazardous or significantly reduce their volume or toxicity have assumed major importance in recent years, particularly as more and more "land bans" have been implemented, prohibiting the land filling of untreated wastes. With economic motivation spurring invention, a number of promising new technologies are now in the pilot project phase or fully operational, promising safer, more effective ways of cleaning up past mistakes and ensuring that wastes currently being generated are properly managed.

Physical methods include **evaporation** to concentrate corrosive brines, **sedimentation** to separate solids from liquid wastes, **carbon adsorption** to remove certain soluble organic wastes, and **air-stripping** to remove volatile organic compounds from groundwater.

Chemical techniques involve processes such as **neutralization** to render wastes harmless, sulfide **precipitation** to extract certain toxic metals, **oxidation-reduction** processes to convert some metals from a hazardous to a non-hazardous state, and **stabilization/solidification**, in which the waste material is detoxified and then combined with a cement-like material, encapsulated in plastic, blended with organic polymers, or combined with silica to form a solid, inert substance which can be disposed of safely in a landfill or incorporated into road beds.

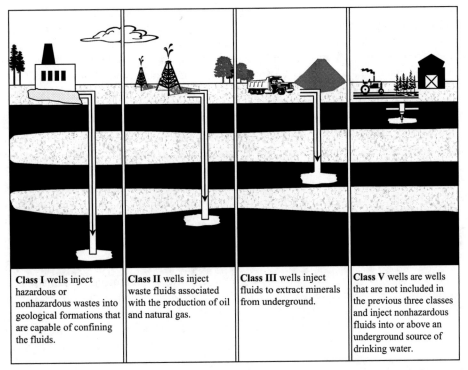

| Class I wells inject hazardous or nonhazardous wastes into geological formations that are capable of confining the fluids. | Class II wells inject waste fluids associated with the production of oil and natural gas. | Class III wells inject fluids to extract minerals from underground. | Class V wells are wells that are not included in the previous three classes and inject nonhazardous fluids into or above an underground source of drinking water. |

Figure 8.4. Injection Wells and Underground Sources of Drinking Water. (Source: EPA, 1998).

Another innovative technology is **in-situ vitrification** (ISV), a process that relies on large amounts of electricity (about 750 kilowatt-hours per ton of soil) delivered by giant electrodes fixed at several locations in the soil surrounding the area undergoing cleanup. Suitable for detoxifying soils contaminated with toxic organics (e.g. chlorinated pesticides), heavy metals, or radioactive wastes, ISV actually melts the soil as the electricity flows through it, fusing the toxics into a solid block of glassified material, similar to natural obsidian. The solidified material can simply be left in place, no longer posing any environmental threat.

Bioremediation - Based on the ability of microbes, fungi, or plants to break down or absorb organic pollutants or toxic metals, bioremediation is increasingly used for cleanup of oil spills and remediation of contaminated soil and groundwater. The largest number of projects utilizes various species of naturally occurring bacteria.

Controlled Incineration - Because burning at very high temperatures actually destroys hazardous wastes (as opposed to storing them out of sight underground as is essentially the case with various land disposal methods), most hazardous waste management experts regard controlled incineration as the best and, in some cases, the only environmentally acceptable means of disposal. In spite of its relatively high cost compared to other hazardous waste management options, controlled incineration is assuming increased importance, as land disposal regulations grow more restrictive. Waste generators, fearful of legal liability if their wastes migrate from a land disposal site, are increasingly likely to choose a management method that ensures total waste destruction. A controlled incinerator burns at temperatures ranging from 750-3000°F with wastes, air, and fuel being thoroughly mixed to ensure complete combustion. Afterburners, which are part of the incineration system, destroy any gaseous hydrocarbons, which may have survived the initial incineration process, while scrubbers and electrostatic precipitators remove pollutant emissions from the stack gases. In 1999, EPA further tightened nationwide standards for air emissions from hazardous waste combustors. The 20 commercial incinerators, 18 cement kilns, and 134 other facilities throughout the country which burn hazardous wastes were required to achieve a 70% reduction in dioxins and furans as well as reductions in mercury and lead emissions up to 86% by 2002. The technologies employed to lower concentrations of these pollutants will also reduce emissions of particulates, carbon monoxide, hydrocarbons, hydrochloric acid, and other toxic metals. The stringent requirements were justified as necessary to protect the health and environment of the 37 million U.S. residents living in the vicinity of hazardous waste combustors.

Waste Exchanges - The ideal way to manage hazardous materials would be to recycle them, thus preventing their entry into the waste stream and eliminating the disposal problem. This is the idea, which prompted the establishment of waste exchanges, which act as helpful third parties in establishing contact between waste generators and potential waste users. For example, a paint manufacturer, faced with the problem of how to dispose of hazardous sludges from a mixing operation, contacts a waste exchange and is referred to another company which willingly purchases the sludge to use as a filler coat on cement blocks. Thus, the paint manufacturer avoids the high cost of disposal in a secure chemical landfill or controlled incinerator and also makes a modest profit on the sale of the waste. The buyer, too, is pleased with the arrangement because a needed raw material is obtained for a lower price than unused filler would have cost; and society is well served because a potentially hazardous substance has been prevented from entering the environment. The waste exchange concept originated in Europe where the first such program began in the Netherlands in 1972.

Bioremediation - Bioremediation is a method for using the activities of microorganisms and/or plants to transform organic or inorganic compounds that may be harmful to humans, animals, plants, or the environment to compounds that are less harmful. In many instances toxic compounds may becompletely degraded to their simple inorganic components, such as carbon dioxide, nitrate, and chloride ions. This is termed **mineralization**.

Many bacteria and fungi that normally occur in soil, groundwater or surface water have the ability to transform organic or inorganic compounds. Some of the microbes are aerobic, i.e., they oxidize compounds using oxygen as the electron acceptor, similar to the way we use oxygen for our sustained activities. Some specialized microbes can use sulfate or nitrate as the electron acceptor. Other microorganisms carry out their transformations by an anaerobic process, i.e., they use one organic compound as the electron acceptor in order to oxidize another compound.

For millions of years common soil and water microbes have carried out the degradation of dead plants and animals, releasing the common inorganic substances that make up the organic compounds. When the inorganic substances are released back into the soil and water, they can be reused for plant growth. Without this activity we would be choked in a mass of dead material. Plants, shrubs, and trees contain a great variety of complex organic chemicals that are very similar to some of the toxic compounds that have been manufactured for industrial use. Microbes normally encounter these compounds only at low concentrations; the compounds are often bound to complex lignins and tannins from plant material or to humic compounds in soils. This ability of microbes to transform a great variety of compounds has been very useful for the treatment of hazardous chemicals.

For thousands of years, farmers have used bioremediation for the degradation of plants and wastes by plowing the wastes into the soil or setting up compost piles. More recently, waste water lagoons, anaerobic digesters, and activated sludge treatment systems have been used to treat sewage. Degradation of the organic matter prevents oxygen depletion in the receiving streams. A process has been developed using microbial activity to oxidize ammonia to nitrate; denitrifying bacteria then change the nitrate to nitrogen gas. This removal of the excess nitrogen has helped to prevent massive algal blooms in some streams, ponds, and lakes.

Degradation of petroleum wastes, especially gasoline and diesel fuel, by land treatment, slurry reactors, and **in situ** treatment has been the most widely used bioremediation process around the world. Only in the past two decades have we learned that many more exotic compounds may be degraded by bioremediation.

Land farming (also termed **soil tillage**) is the treatment of soils containing hazardous organic compounds by rototilling or mixing using a farm tractor and then tilling the contaminated soil so that air is available for microbial biodegradation of organic compounds. The soil water content is adjusted to be optimum for microbial activity (generally 25-45% of the soil moisture holding capacity).

Nutrients such as nitrogen and phosphorous fertilizer may be added to enhance the growth and activities of the microbes. This is especially beneficial when neither the soil nor the contaminants contain any easily available nitrogen or phosphorus necessary for the growth of the microbes that will carry out the bioremediation. The advantage of this type of treatment is that when there is sufficient space, large amounts of soil may be treated at one time. Earth-moving equipment and tractors and tillage equipment may be very large and many acres of excavated soil may be treated at once. The depth of soil is usually 6 - 10 inches for each lift to be treated to ensure good aeration. Mixing is often done once per week to ensure that all the contaminated soil is well mixed with the bacteria, nutrients, and air.

In situ bioremediation is the treatment of contaminated groundwater or soil by microbial activity without excavation of the contaminated soil or removal of the contaminated groundwater. This may be useful in many instances because the contaminants remain below the surface and cannot volatilize or cause harmful effects to surrounding lands or animals. In situ bioremediation may be aerobic, anaerobic, or anaerobic followed by an aerobic stage.

There are several distinct methods of carrying out this activity. **Bioventing** is a method whereby air is slowly drawn through the soil. Vacuum pumps are placed in wells located in the contaminated zone and operated at only a slight vacuum. This encourages air to move through the soil to these wells. Nutrients may be added to the contaminated soil. This process is not very expensive. It does require that the soil not be waterlogged (that would prevent the movement of the air). Also, in general the contaminants must be those that can be degraded by the microorganisms present in the soil. This process has been used extensively by the U.S. Air Force to cleanup soils contaminated by jet fuel spills and gasoline spills where trucks were refueled.

Biosparging - Biosparging is the method of getting air into contaminated groundwater by using compressor pumps to force air out through outlets placed below the groundwater table in wells located upgradient to the contamination. This air then becomes absorbed into the groundwater and will flow down-gradient though the contaminated zone. Nutrients can also be added to the water that will flow through the contaminated zone. Water has only a limited capacity to hold oxygen and much of the air pumped into the water comes right out at the injection well and does not get to the contaminated area. Therefore, many bioremediation firms are adding hydrogen peroxide directly to the water in order to increase the amount of oxygen present in the water as it enters the contaminated plume area. The level of hydrogen peroxide added must be kept to less than 50 or 100 mg of hydrogen peroxide per liter of water in order to prevent the hydrogen peroxide from killing the microbes necessary for the biodegradation. Hydrogen peroxide is relatively expensive, so treatment tests are often performed in the laboratory to determine whether this added expense is beneficial. Hydrogen peroxide may cause rapid precipitation of iron in soils containing large amounts of ferrous iron. Such precipitates have even clogged soils and have blocked movement of the water through the soil. Thus care is required where such precipitation can occur.

Phytoremediation - Phytoremediation is a process using plants for the treatment of contaminated soil and groundwater. The plants may actually transform some compounds; they may instead accumulate some compounds, preventing the subsequent down-gradient travel of those compounds, or the plants may provide an environment for improved biodegradation as compared to soil without plants. This increased microbial activity in the rhiozosphere of plants and trees is well known to soil microbiologists.

Plants provide oxygen to the soil through their roots, and often root exudates contain sugars and other compounds that stimulate microbial growth. Growth of plant roots also helps create conditions beneficial to the movement of water and air through the soil. Extensive research is presently being undertaken in the U.S. EPA Superfund Innovative Technology Evaluation Program (SITE) to evaluate where phytoremediation is beneficial. Where the effects of phytoremediation are mainly the uptake by plants without plant destruction (such as the uptake and accumulation of metals in plants or trees). Then the plants or trees must be harvested after the appropriate period of growth and then disposed at a site where the hazardous wastes contained will not cause any problems. Otherwise, degradation of the plant material at the growth site will release the hazardous compounds back into the soil or groundwater.

Biomineralization of Heavy Metals - Biomineralization is a process involving formation of complex metal aggregates with silicates, oxides, and carbonates; the process appears to be initiated and influenced by microbial activity. It is believed that this activity may have been important in the formation of some natural ore deposits. The process was first encountered in studies of cyanide in waters and spoil heaps found in the mining industry.

Work is presently underway to test the process in soil columns with soils contaminated in one case with lead and in another case with arsenic. Formation of complex stable mineral compounds reduces the danger of the leaching of metals from the spoil heaps or soil and subsequent contamination of groundwater or drinking water.

E. MANAGING WASTE AND ITS IMPACTS

Government should provide education and guidance to citizens and to businesses on solid waste management issues and related topics of importance, to include planning, waste reduction, and resource recovery, so that these parties can effectively plan for and participate in future solid waste issues affecting them and their communities.

Further, government should promote enhancement of infrastructure, information, and economic support relating to resource recovery, especially in the area of markets for recovered materials.

It appears that a lot of the local governments are contracting with solid waste contractors and consultants in just about every aspect of solid waste - from disposal to reduction and recycling and from planning to engineering and operations.

We should give serious consideration to the "bioreactor" or "perpetual landfill" technology in the very near future. This technology involves operating a landfill to optimize the degradation of waste, capturing the methane generated for fuel, and removing stabilized, decomposed material for application as soil additive, while availing the disposal "cell" for another round of waste placement and treatment. Similarly, we may soon consider the practicality of bioremediation and reclamation of some of the existing older landfills. This may involve new thinking, new regulatory controls, new environmental concerns, and government subsidies to prove these technologies.

As with any pollution control technology, there are inherent risks in managing wastes. Unlike air pollution and surface water pollution, the impacts from wastes are usually localized, because wastes are typically concentrated in discrete areas, such as a landfill or surface impoundment, and because it is more cost effective to consolidate waste than to spread it out over vast areas. Thus, a collection of drums or a landfill may have a large volume of wastes, but the potential for the waste to spread out over a large area is often limited by the physical barriers of the waste management unit (liners) and the underlying soil. Conversely, the localized hazard presented by this material tends to be much higher than other sources of pollution. Thus, waste is more of a "hot spot" - that is, a localized source of contamination.

Before 1980 (the effective date of federal waste management regulations), wastes were generally managed improperly in poorly constructed waste management units or dumped into open pits, such as old rock quarries. Thus, there were serious localized occurrences of groundwater, surface water, soil, and air pollution, as shown in Figure 8.5. Since 1980, a number of strict regulations have been enacted to control the releases of most wastes. Such controls include the requirement for liners in landfills, banning of liquids and untreated hazardous waste in landfills, mandated liability for improper waste management, forced reliance on treatment instead of disposal, and increased controls on incineration. Not all wastes are subject to these controls.

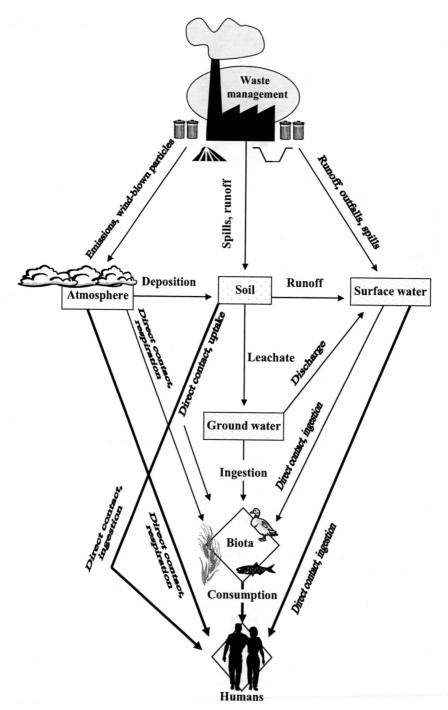

<u>Figure 8.5.</u> Impacts of Improper Waste Management on the Environment. (Source: Wagner, 1994).

Although proper management and control of hazardous wastes can reduce the dangers, a lot can still go wrong. The most technologically advanced landfills we build will probably leak someday. Tanks used for storing chemical and petroleum products can leak and catch fire. Transportation accidents such as train crashes and overturned trucks can occur during transport of hazardous waste and hazardous substances. Accidental releases can occur during industrial processes. Because treating and disposing of hazardous waste are expensive and involve serious legal responsibilities, there are many cases of intentional and illegal dumping along roadsides, in sewer systems, and in abandoned warehouses. Hazardous wastes can end up in our rivers and streams, our air, and our drinking water. They can contaminate our food and poison plants, animals, and humans. We can breathe vapors from hazardous liquids or from contaminated water while taking a shower. We can eat fish, fruits, vegetables, or meats that have been contaminated through exposure to hazardous wastes.

Small children often eat soil or household materials that may be contaminated, such as paint chips containing lead. If a hazardous waste comes into direct contact with our skin it may be absorbed. The most common type of exposure is from drinking contaminated water. Exposure to hazardous wastes can result in serious illnesses, an increased risk of cancer, birth defects, and death.

In Florida, two children were killed when they were playing in a neighborhood dumpster where hazardous waste had been thrown in with ordinary garbage. Advances in technology have improved our ability to treat and dispose of hazardous waste, and many environmental laws are in place to help ensure hazardous waste is managed properly, but the best way to prevent harm to people or the environment is to simply not produce hazardous waste.

The EPA has established a national policy that places the highest priority on reducing the volume and/or toxicity of hazardous waste through source reduction and recycling. Hazardous waste generators are required to have a waste minimization program in place to reduce the volume or quantity and toxicity of generated waste to the extent economically practicable. Better manufacturing processes are producing less waste, and fewer hazardous ingredients are being included in manufacturing processes. Some wastes are being recycled and others are immobilized so they cannot be released into the environment.

Having laws and regulations does not ensure that people are abiding by them. Facility inspections by federal and state officials are the primary tool for ensuring compliance with the hazardous waste laws. All hazardous waste generators and treatment, storage, and disposal facilities are subject to compliance inspections, which may be announced or unannounced. Inspections must be conducted annually at all federally or state-operated facilities and at least once every 2 years at each treatment, storage, and disposal facility. Individuals and companies that do not comply with hazardous waste regulations can face legal penalties. The EPA or a state can impose these penalties. For a minor violation, the EPA or a state may simply tell a facility that it is not complying with the rules and that legal action will be taken if the owner does not comply within a certain period of time. For severe violations or in cases in which the same violation has been repeated, a facility may face fines of up to $25,000 for every day past the deadline that it fails to comply. The facility's operations can also be suspended or the operators can face criminal charges in court and go to jail. Facilities are also financially responsible for cleaning up when they have contaminated the environment. To achieve greater compliance, the EPA and the states have issued several policies to provide incentives for businesses voluntarily to evaluate their own compliance and disclose violations, and to provide assistance to businesses in complying with the regulations. By helping businesses understand the regulations, and by providing certain incentives for compliance, the number of businesses in violation of the laws is reduced and public health and the environment are better protected.

RCRA, as well as other environmental statutes, provides ongoing opportunities for public involvement in all facets of the program. Citizens can take legal action against a person or company not complying with the regulations, or against the EPA or a state for not properly enforcing the rules. Citizens are also given the opportunity to voice their concerns about new rules and new facilities seeking a permit to operate in their community.

When citizens recognize potential hazardous waste problems and illegal dumping, they should contact the National Response Center at 1-800-424-8802 or their state or local government environmental protection or health agency if they detect the following signs of hazardous waste releases or illegal dumping:

1. Drums in the woods, on roadsides, on abandoned property, in empty buildings, or in city or county landfills.
2. Odors that smell like turpentine, paint, fingernail polish, glue, rotten eggs, or any tar chemical odor.
3. Discolored soil with dead vegetation along roadsides, in abandoned lots or fields, around vacant buildings, or beside streams and rivers. Abandoned warehouses or factories with leaking drums or wastelike material.
4. Sludgelike material or ooze on the ground.

For questions concerning hazardous waste or location of a hazardous waste sites near one's home, they should contact their state environmental protection agency, their local EPA regional office, or the RCRA hazardous waste hotline (1-800-424-9346). The hotline is open Monday through Friday, 9:00 a.m. to 6:00 p.m. eastern standard time. Information is also available on the internet at http://www.epa.gov.

F. LAWS AND REGULATIONS GOVERNING HAZARDOUS WASTE

1. RCRA

The Resource Conservation and Recovery Act (RCRA) of 1976 is the federal statute that defines hazardous waste and regulates its generation, storage, treatment, and disposal. RCRA gave the U.S. Environmental Protection Agency (EPA) the responsibility of establishing regulations, as well as the authority to enforce these regulations, to ensure the safe treatment, storage, and disposal of hazardous waste. EPA regulations require that all waste generators (those who produce waste) evaluate their waste to determine if it exhibits any of four specific hazardous characteristics or if it is specifically named on one of the hazardous waste lists. Once a waste has been determined to be hazardous, RCRA's "cradle-in-grave" system for managing hazardous waste requires that it be managed safely and tracked from the moment it is generated until the moment it is properly disposed. Those who generate, transport, treat, store, or dispose of hazardous waste are subject to RCRA regulations. The hazardous waste regulations are found in Title 40, Code of Federal Regulations, Chapter I, Subchapter I, Parts 260-281. In addition to active hazardous waste sites regulated under RCRA, some sites have abandoned hazardous waste, and ownership is unclear or unknown.

In these situations, control and cleanup are handled under the Comprehensive Environmental Response, Compensation, and Liability Act of 1980 (CERCLA), commonly known as "Superfund."

2. Superfund

Spurred by public demands that something be done to alleviate problems caused by old, leaking dumpsites, Congress in December of 1980 enacted the **Comprehensive Environmental Response, Compensation, and Liability Act (CERCLA**, dubbed the "**Superfund**") authorizing the expenditure of $1.6 billion over a five-year period for emergency cleanup activities and for the more long-term containment of hazardous waste dump sites (the legislation, however, did not include funds to compensate victims for health damage incurred by exposure to such sites - an issue which was the focus of considerable debate). EPA, in cooperation with the states, was charged with compiling a **National Priority List (NPL)** of sites considered to be sufficiently threatening to public health or environmental quality to make them eligible for Superfund cleanup dollars. These funds can be used either to remove hazardous substances from the site (a process which may also include temporary relocation of people in the area and provision of alternative water supplies) or for remedial measures such as storage and confinement of wastes, incineration, dredging, or permanent relocation of residents (Table 8.2).

Table 8.2. "Top 20" Most Prominent Toxic Substances Found at NPL Sites. (Source: Nadakavukaren, 2000).

Lead	Cadmium	Trichloroethylene	DDE
Arsenic	PCBs	DDT	Arochlor 1242
Mercury	Benzo(a)pyrene	Arochlor 1254	Dibenzo(a,h)anthracene
(metallic)	Chloroform	Hexochlorobutodiene	Hexavalent chromium
Benzene	Benzo(b)fluoranthene	Arochlor 1260	Dieldrin
Vinyl			
chloride			

Ranking based on: 1. Frequency at NPL sites, 2. Toxicity, and 3. Exposure hazard to humans.

The original Superfund bill expired in September 1985, and in spite of public demands for speedy reauthorization so that cleanup work could proceed without interruption, the law was not renewed until late the following year. Extreme congressional dissatisfaction with the excruciatingly slow rate of progress during Superfund's first years led to several significant changes in the 1986 **Superfund Amendments and Reauthorization Act (SARA)**.

EPA was given mandatory deadlines for initiating site-specific cleanup plans and remediation activities. Concerned that previous cleanup actions represented little more than moving contaminated wastes from one site to another site, which would itself then become eligible for Superfund status, Congress specified a preference for cleanup actions which "permanently and significantly" reduce the volume, toxicity, or mobility of hazardous substances. This mandate has given a major impetus to development of treatment or disposal technologies (e.g. mobile incinerators which can be moved from one Superfund site to another) which permit hazardous wastes to be destroyed or detoxified on site, thereby avoiding the risks of transporting such wastes to another facility where they might cause future problems.

While Americans (60 million of whom live within four miles of a Superfund site) generally support the concept of cleaning up our hazardous waste mistakes of the past, there has been considerable criticism regarding the pace of site cleanups. By mid-1999, the number of officially listed or proposed NPL sites had grown from an original 400 to 1,225. However, after more than a decade and a half of on-site work and the expenditure of many billions of dollars by government and industry, construction had been completed (i.e. all cleanup equipment was in place) at 432 sites and just 176 others had been completely remediated and taken off the NPL, indicating they no longer present a threat to human health or the environment.

Passionate disputes also rage over the extent of remediation necessary - "How clean is clean enough?" Critics complain that it makes no sense to spend millions of dollars to remove every last trace of contamination on a site destined to be paved over for a parking lot; it is quite likely that future amendments to the law will permit cleanup decisions to be based, at least in part, on the probable future use of the site. As EPA Administrator Carol Browner once remarked, "there will be different levels of clean." Undoubtedly, the most controversial feature of the Superfund program has been its liability provisions, based on the philosophically sound "**the polluter pays**" principle, but which has resulted in fully one-quarter of all Superfund dollars spent thus far going to pay legal fees. While business interests are demanding fundamental changes in what they regard as inherently unfair provisions, environmental advocates strongly support the status quo, insisting that concerns about "**Superfund liability**" alone have caused generators to be much more conscientious about managing their wastes in a responsible manner and have given major impetus to serious efforts toward pollution prevention. As evidence, such advocates point to the fact that between 1987 and 1991, the chemical industry alone reduced its output of toxic wastes by 35%, largely in response to future liability considerations.

Finally, there is the question of cost. Close to one-quarter of EPA's entire budget has been allocated to Superfund. The Agency estimates it will cost at least $28 billion to clean up the sites currently on the NPL - and sees an additional 4,800 sites as likely candidates for listing in the years ahead. Although Superfund legislation mandates that 10% of site cleanup costs be paid by the state in which the site is located and requires that an attempt be made to find the "**potentially responsible party**" (PRP) who caused or contributed to the problem in order to recover cleanup expenses through litigation, the federal government will continue to bear much of the financial burden for site remediation efforts. The ultimate future of the Superfund program obviously will depend on the continued willingness of taxpayers to support the detoxification of America's hazardous waste dumpsites.

Before the 1980s, it was common practice for industries and municipalities to haul the wastes to a depression in the ground, dump them, and cover them. In years previous to that, many local landfills weren't even covered with soil. In many cases, drums of toxic wastes were simply stored in piles on-site. Many of these sites were abandoned, forgotten, and even built on, as neighborhoods expanded with the pressures of a rapidly increasing population. Then the buried toxic sludge began to appear, as rusted 55 gallon drums seeped their contents into the soil to contaminate groundwater, or work their way to the surface where the true drama of poisonous mud and rusted containers could be seen.

The term "Superfund" is attributed to the fact that the bill created a trust fund financed primarily by excise taxes on chemicals and oil, and an environmental tax on corporations. The liability rules applied include: **retroactive liability**, **joint and several liability**, and **strict liability** (Figure 8.6). This may force individuals, companies, organizations (entities) to pay for cleanups that have had little or no part in causing the damage. In practice, state or federal agency personnel will attempt to identify entities with the largest pockets (most financial resources) as PRPs.

Such rules have been held responsible for 36 to 60 cents of every dollar spent in Superfund going to legal and other transactional costs.

There are presently nearly 33,000 hazardous waste sites that have come under Superfund authority. The NPL was established because sites vary in size, hazardous substance content, containment, and degree of threat to the surrounding populations and environment. The USEPA established a **hazard-ranking system (HRS)** based on the estimated hazard potential of the hazardous waste site. The factors used to make this estimate include the waste characteristics (toxicity, quantity, solubility, reactivity); the distance to the local population; and the proximity to surface and groundwater, and drinking water supplies. Other factors include the level of containment such as the condition of the containers (i.e., are the drums rusted?), and whether there are leachate collection systems or liners. The NPL is updated annually.

Environmental groups buttressed by a large contingent of concerned citizens charged that RCRA was not being vigorously enforced. These actions caused Congress to respond by passing the Superfund Amendments and Reauthorization Act of 1986 (SARA), which increased the program's funding to $85 billion, and provided new and stricter standards. A series of delays, lawsuits, and accusations followed, demanding that the Superfund program be repaired. Superfund had spent $13.8 billion of taxpayer money and $12 billion of private sector money since 1980 to clean only 291 sites by 1996. This cost was expected to escalate to $42 billion in the next 70 years to clean up an estimated total of 2,300 NFL sites. At the end of 1995, the tax authorization for Superfund expired. The balance of some $6 billion in the Hazardous Substance Superfund Trust Fund is being supported by:

1. Taxes on domestically produced and imported oil;
2. A tax on feedstock chemicals;
3. A corporate environmental income tax; and
4. General revenues, reimbursements, penalties, and interest on the trust fund.

Strict Liability: The government needs to prove only involvement at a waste site. Negligence or strict causation is not necessary to establish liability.

Joint and Several Liability: Any involved party can be legally responsible for cleaning up a site no matter what the degree of involvement. In practice, liability is often apportioned .

Retroactive Liability: The PRPs can be held liable for releases resulting from actions before Congress enacted CERCLA in 1980.

Figure 8.6. Definitions of liability under Superfund. (Source: Moore, 1999).

The reauthorizing of the Superfund law has been very contentious as evidenced by a flurry of reform bills introduced in both houses. The major arguments center around the issue of liability. The pending bills exempt small businesses from liability for actions that occurred prior to the Superfund law and provide liability relief for panics that contribute only small amounts of waste. The bills stress more cost-effective clean-up strategies by the USEPA and give greater control to states. Additionally, the amount of damages that can be recovered from harming natural resources is limited. Proponents of the bills argue that liability issues discourage the development of brownfields, which are abandoned and underused commercial and industrial properties. Opponents feel the bills will permit businesses to pollute with reduced liability, and will shift economic liability to the taxpayers. Less stringent cleanup requirements would result in great exposures and risks to the public, and permit natural resources to remain polluted. Regardless of the outcome of pending legislation, current efforts of Superfund are widely supported, and there has been significant progress in recent years cleaning up sites.

In fiscal year 1997, the USEPA listed 1,405 sites which were distributed over 6 different stages involved in the cleanup process. Nearly 500 of the 1,405 sites listed were in the stage of construction completion with nearly 55 sites where remedial assessment had not yet started Figure 8.7. According to Carol Browner, Director of USEPA, as of September 1998, 1100 sites are undergoing or have completed cleanup construction, with 400 of the worst sites completed. Two-thirds of the completed cleanups were accomplished within the previous four years, and there is a commitment by the USEFA to clean up an additional 500 sites by the year 2,000. The most recent listing (February 10, 1998) shows there are 1,191 sites on the NFL, reflecting the removal of cleanup completions. If you would like to know of Superfund sites near you, you can search for local Superfund sites with the "Site information" page at <http://www.epa.gov./superfund/sites/index.htm>. To locate Superfund sites across the country try <http://www.epa.gov/superfund/sites/npl.htm>.

Numbers of NPL sites in 1997

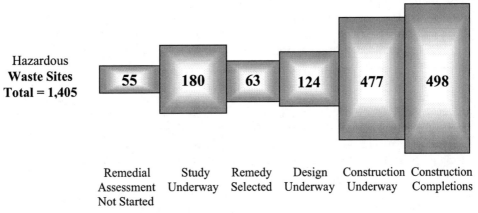

Hazardous
Waste Sites
Total = 1,405

| 55 | 180 | 63 | 124 | 477 | 498 |

| Remedial Assessment Not Started | Study Underway | Remedy Selected | Design Underway | Construction Underway | Construction Completions |

Figure 8.7. Site Remediation Progress at NPL sites. (Source: Moore, 1999).

3. Other Laws Protecting People From Hazardous Waste Besides RCRA

To ensure adequate protection of human health and the environment from exposures to hazardous waste and contaminants, Congress enacted several major environmental statutes to address hazardous waste problems. These include media-specific statutes that limit the amount of waste released into a particular environmental medium, such as air or water, and other statutes that directly control the production of certain products and protect workers managing hazardous waste. The following statutes have been enacted:

1. Clean Air Act
2. Clean Water Act
3. Safe Drinking Water Act
4. Emergency Planning and Community Right-to-Know Act
5. Federal Insecticide, Fungicide, and Rodenticide Act
6. Marine Protection, Research, and Sanctuaries Act
7. Occupational Safety and Health Act
8. Comprehensive Environmental Response, Compensation, and Liability Act
9. Toxic Substance Control Act

G. ILLEGAL DUMPING

Illegal dumping continues to be a problem. As long as there is an economic advantage to dump waste in the woods and avoid a disposal fee, there will be illegal dumping.

Strong enforcement at the local level is a necessary piece of the puzzle. A requirement that any construction or demolition job obtain a permit, and that the permit will specify that the contractor must provide receipts for proper disposal prior to allowing occupancy, would aid in solving the problem. A permit fee or fee on problematic materials could generate funds for cleanup of illegal dumps.

Landfill disposal of waste results in the potential for environmental degradation, potential restrictions on future use of the land, and waste of valuable natural and manufactured resources.

Health effects of landfill air emissions, neighborhood nuisance issues (such as noise, traffic, dust, etc.), landfill fires and toxic releases from unscreened hazardous materials, and facility releases to air and water of contaminants now and in the future are the most frequently raised concerns. The issue of **"environmental justice"** is raised with increasing frequency as minority communities look around and realize that they are facing these health, safety, and nuisance situations at an apparent inordinate level relative to their more affluent neighbors.

It is getting more difficult to gain local approval for any type of landfill site. Everyone has a reason why a landfill should not go "**in my back yard**," and local officials are pressured not to issue special use or zoning permits that allow landfills. Even established sites may be revisited by local government in respect to items such as environmental discrimination, or encroachment of residential development. This could cause problems with economically available landfill capacities for the future in many urban areas. The fear of groundwater contamination and restrictions on future uses of the sites (such as development) could cause additional siting difficulty in the future.

The landfills of today have more environmental safeguards compared to those of a decade ago. The state-of-the-art for landfills includes bottom liners for liquid (leachate) containment, leachate leak detection systems, leachate collection and treatment systems, and landfill gas emission control systems. Municipal waste landfills now require financial commitments to long-term monitoring, maintenance, and corrective action programs.

Due to pressures imposed by federal and state regulations, landfill siting woes, and economies of scale, private waste management firms are gaining an increasing level of control over landfill operations. The trend toward privatization of solid waste services, regionalization of landfills, and closing of numerous public facilities has resulted in increased use of transfer stations to bring waste from ever-increasing distances into private landfills.

H. WASTE MANAGEMENT CONCERNS FOLLOWING A NATURAL DISASTER

Natural disasters can result in failed facilities and infrastructure with resultant disposal capacity shortfalls or environmental releases. Considerable debris can result from demolished forest, vegetation, and buildings. Contamination can result from demolished structures and their potentially hazardous contents. Potential for fires can result from growing piles of debris awaiting processing and proper disposal. Spoiled foods from supermarkets, distributors, and farms as well as decomposing livestock and wildlife carcasses can result in increased proliferation of disease vectors. Planning for such disasters is a critical public health need in many areas of the country.

I. CONTAMINANTS IN WILDLIFE

The terms "**environmental toxicology**" and "**ecotoxicology**" are both commonly used to describe the study of contaminant effects on widlife and the environment. However, the term "**ecotoxicology**" more accurately describes this scientific discipline because it is broadly defined to include both the effects on humans and the effects on the environment and its living components.

Because of the direct and indirect linkages between environmental health and human health, wildlife species serve as valuable sentinels or indicators of environmental pollutants that may ultimately affect human health. Previous studies have shown that the effects of toxic contaminants on wildlife may provide early warning signals of hazards to humans. In addition, many species of wildlife, such as various freshwater and marine fish, are consumed by humans as food and therefore represent a direct link for the dietary transfer of accumulated contaminants.

Wildlife and other biological organisms accumulate contaminants from their surroundings by several routes of exposure, including oral intake through the diet, direct contact with their outer protective coverings (skin, feathers, fur, or membranes), and respiratory activities through air or water. This process of net accumulation of contaminants into or onto wildlife and other organisms from all sources, including air, water, and solids, is called **bioaccumulation**.

When accumulated contaminants are passed from one trophic level to another by the dietary route (e.g., from prey to predator), and result in an increased concentration in the next higher trophic level, this process is referred to as **biomagnification.**

The persistent environmental contaminants that readily bioaccumulate in wildlife and biomagnify through food webs are of paramount concern for producing adverse effects on both wildlife and human populations. This group of contaminants includes persistent organic pollutants (POPs) such as the organochlorine pesticides aldrin, dieldrin, endrin, chlorophenyl (DDT) and trichloroethanes metabolites DDE and DDD, chlordane, heptachlor, mirex, and toxaphene.

Industrial chemicals such as polychlorinated biphenyls (PCBs) and hexachlorobenzene (which formerly was also used as a pesticide); and industrial by-products such as the dioxins and furans. Also included in this group of contaminants of concern are inorganic pollutants such as mercury, cadmium, lead, and selenium.

Contaminants that resist environmental degradation, persist in the environment for decades, travel long distances in the atmosphere, and associate with lipids (fatty tissue) are generally more capable of bioaccumulation and biomagnitication.

These contaminants largely include the lipophilic (fat-loving) persistent organic pollutants.

The globally transported pollutant mercury is also a major concern for bioaccumulation and biomagnification because when the inorganic form of the metal enters the aquatic environment, it is transformed by resident bacteria, under certain environmental conditions, to the highly toxic organic form, methylmercury.

Methylmercury is lipid soluble, but not lipophilic. This means that it can readily cross biological membranes and cause toxicity, but that it does not accumulate in fats.

Methylmercury accumulates in axial or skeletal muscle through its association with sulfhydryl groups on proteins and readily accumulates in organisms such as fish, which leads to biomagnification through the food web.

The classic example of known adverse effects of a contaminant on wildlife populations occurred in the 1960s and 1970s through the combined effects of the organochlorine pesticide DDT and its metabolites DDE and DDD on raptorial and fish-eating birds.

Birds that feed at higher trophic levels (bald eagles and peregrine falcons) are especially sensitive to these contaminants because DDT and DDE, with their ability to accumulate in lipids and to resist environmental degradation, biomagnify through the food web. When birds were exposed to these chemicals at relatively high dietary concencrations, the calcium-dependent ATPases in the shell gland were inhibited, resulting in eggshell thinning and increased risk of egg breakage. These effects led to widespread reproductive failure, population decline, and the eventual listing of bald eagles and peregrine falcons as endangered species in the United States.

Standards have been established for individual contaminants. These are legal limits permitted by each state for a specific contaminant level and natural resource use. For example, the water-quality standard to protect aquatic life from cadmium exposure in nontrout waters of North Carolina is 2.0 parts per billion (ppb).

Success has clearly been demonstrated by the recovery of raptorial and fish - eating birds that had been adversely affected in the 1960s by the organochlorine pesticide DDT, which was banned from use in the United States in 1972.

Birds such as the bald eagle and peregrine falcon, which were most severely impacted and subsequently placed on the endangered species list, have recovered to the point where they have recently been removed from the endangered species list.

There remains however, certain situations and areas in which wildlife species continue to be adversely affected by chemical contaminants, and their populations are in decline.

For example, the hypoxic zone in the Gulf of Mexico is largely devoid of fish and wildlife because of nutrients and other contaminants emanating from the Mississippi River and its upstream tributaries.

The oral (dietary) route of exposure is of greatest concern and consists largely of the health risks associated with consuming contaminated fish and shellfish.

The mercury contamination of fish and shellfish in Minamata Bay, Japan in the 1950s resulted in over 700 cases of human mercury poisoning and numerous deaths.

The poisoning was traced to a vinyl chloride factory where inorganic mercury salts were used as catalysts in the commercial production of vinyl chloride and acetaldehyde from acetylene.

After the mercury was discharged from the plant, bacteria in the aquatic sediments and waters of Minamata Bay converted inorganic mercury to the highly toxic form, methylmercury. Methylmercury was then accumulated by fish and shellfish, which were later consumed by humans.

In the United States, the individual states, the four U.S. Territories, and the Native American Tribes have the responsibility for protecting their residents from the adverse health risks associated with consuming contaminated, noncommercially caught fish and wildlife. They accomplish this by issuing consumption advisories that address the risks for the general population and also for sensitive subpopulations such as children, pregnant women, and women of childbearing age. These advisories inform the public that high concentrations of a specific contaminant have been found in fish and wildlife from a given area and make recommendations for limiting or avoiding consumption of this species.

Contact your state health department or other appropriate environmental regulatory agency. In many states, a list of fish and wildlife consumption advisories (or information on how to obtain one) is often contained in the state fishing and hunting regulations that are distributed when fishing and hunting licenses are purchased.

Although consumption advisories were issued for a total of 46 different chemical contaminants in 1998, the majority (99%) involved the five bioaccumulative contaminants of mercury, PCBs, chlordane, dioxins, and DDT (and metabolites DDE and DDD).

Of these advisories, nearly 68% were issued for mercury contamination of fish and shellfish.

There is not a method of cleaning or cooking fish that will reduce the amount of mercury consumed in a meal. Almost all (95-99%) of the mercury in fish is in the form of methylmercury, which is tightly bound to proteins in the fish muscle (the portion that is consumed).

Neurotoxicity is the greatest concern from overexposure to methylmercury. Symptoms in both children and adults include impairment of peripheral vision; disturbances in sensation such as "pins and needles" feelings and numbness, which usually occur in the hands, feet, and around the mouth.

Incoordination of movements; impairment of speech, hearing, and walking; and mental disturbances. Because methylmercury readily penetrates the blood-brain and placental barriers, the developing fetus is especially sensitive to the neurotoxic effects of methylmercury.

Skinning and trimming fish to remove fatty areas along the back, sides, and belly can reduce the levels of some lipophilic contaminants, such as PCBs and dioxins, by 20-50%. Cooking techniques (broiling, baking, or grilling) that allow the fat to drip off can reduce the PCB and dioxins levels even further. Poaching and deep-fat frying remove some contaminants, but pan frying removes few contaminants.

The adverse health effects from eating fish contaminated with PCBs are difficult to evaluate because the potential links between long-term, low-level exposure and demonstrated human health problems are unclear. However, studies have shown that certain susceptible populations, such as specific ethnic groups, sport-fish anglers, the elderly, pregnant women, children, fetuses, and nursing infants, continue to be exposed to high levels of PCBs through fish and wildlife consumption and have a greater risk for health problems.

These studies also indicate that overexposure to PCBs may result in reproductive dysfunction, neurobehavioral and developmental deficits in newborns and school-aged children who were exposed **in utero**, systemic effects such as liver disease and diabetes, effects on the thyroid and immune systems, and increased risk of cancer (e.g., non-Hodgkin's lymphoma).

Wildlife consumption advisories have been issued by several States for turtles, frogs, various waterfowl species (including mergansers, wood ducks, and the American coot), and moose organ meat (liver and kidney).

IV. PESTS, ANIMAL BITES, RODENTS, AND INSECTS

A. INTRODUCTION

There are about 170 different species (kinds) of mosquitoes, about 80 species of ticks, about a dozen species of spiders, and assorted bugs, chiggers, caterpillars, mites, wasps, bees, and hornets that will either sting or bite people in the United States. Some also transmit diseases to people and animals.

There are several viral diseases (called arboviruses) transmitted to people by mosquitoes in the United States. Western equine encephalitis is a disease spread from wild birds to horses and humans by mosquitoes west of the Mississippi River; Eastern equine encephalitis is similar but usually occurs east of the Mississippi River.

LaCrosse encephalitis (a member of the California group of arboviruses) occurs in the north central to east central U. S. and is spread from wild rodents to humans; St. Louis encephalitis occurs in the south and midwest. West Nile virus appeared in the northeastern U.S. in 1999. People occasionally acquire other unusual arboviruses, such as Cache Valley virus, which is a disease of wild and domestic ruminants. Yellow fever was once a common mosquito-transmitted arbovirus in the U. S., particularly in seaports. A very serious arboviral disease, dengue (breakbone fever), has begun to reappear in the southwestern U. S. after an absence of many decades. Malaria has also begun to show up in isolated outbreaks in a number of states. The continuing influx of people from tropical countries, where many arboviral diseases are common, means that we can probably expect to see more cases of mosquito-transmitted diseases hitherto unknown or uncommon in the U. S. This emphasizes the need for better disease surveillance and reporting and for better mosquito control efforts.

Repellents work fairly well for most biting arthropods (mosquitoes, ticks, chiggers, black-flies, etc.) if they are used according to label directions. The length of protection can vary a lot, depending on the strength of the active ingredient [usually N, N-diethyl-m-toluamide (DEET)], the amount applied, the amount of repellent you wash off by sweating or getting wet, and the kind of pest you are trying to repel. Tick repellents containing permethrin should never be applied to the skin, just to the clothing. You must be very careful when applying repellents to children! Read and follow directions on the container very carefully!

The stinging hymenopterans are usually mobile, fast, aggressive, and inflict painful, even life-threatening, stings. They are best left alone, if possible, and managed with care if you must manage them at all. Be aware that some people can suffer fatal anaphylactic reactions to the stings. It is estimated that 0.3-3% of the population may experience an anaphylactic reaction to an insect sting. Anaphylaxis may be fatal if not immediately treated. Individuals with a known history of severe insect reaction should carry an anaphylactic prevention kit with them at all times.

On average, approximately 150-160 people die as a result of an animal-related injury yearly. Hymenoptera (bees, wasp, fire ants, yellow jackets) are responsible for 50-60 deaths per year. Snake bites cause fewer than 10 deaths per year and spider bites cause about 4-5 deaths per year. However, worldwide, snakebites cause thousands of deaths yearly. Of the approximately 120 species of snakes, about 20 are venomous. It is estimated that about 45,000 snakebites occur yearly, of which 8000 are inflected by venomous snakes. Approximately 20% of all bites by venomous snakes show no evidence of envenomation.

Dog bites are very common. It is estimated that annually in the U. S. there are 4.7 million dog bites. Dog bite injuries result in an estimated 330,000 emergency department visits, nearly 6000 hospitalizations, and 17 deaths yearly. The total costs of injury is estimated to be at least $235-250 million.

A zoonotic disease is an infectious disease transmissible between vertebrate animals and humans. Approximately 200 zoonotic diseases are known to exist and the number is growing.

Examples include rabies, tularemia, pasteurellosis, erysipeloid, staphylococcosis, streptococcosis, rat bite fever, herpes B virus, and seal finger, to name a few. Many of these are potentially fatal if medical evaluation is delayed. All animal bites should be immediately evaluated by a physician.

Scientists estimate that there are 10 million insect species in the world. Of these, nearly 1 million have been identified, including more than 100,000 species of butterflies and moths, over 100,000 species of ants, bees, and wasps, and almost 300,000 species of beetles. About 4,000 new varieties are discovered each year. Some, such as the honeybee and silkworm, bring financial benefits; in fact, honeybees are responsible for the pollination of $10 billion worth of agricultural products (for example, oranges, apples, alfalfa, and almonds) in the United States each year. Other insects (such as the butterfly and lightning bug) are aesthetically pleasing. Still others, however (flies, mosquitoes, boll weevils, corn borers, termites, and locusts) are destructive and even dangerous to humans. The mosquito, in particular, is the vector (transmitter) for a wide range of disease agents. The common housefly and the cockroach are also thought to be implicated in a number of human diseases.

Rodents too are known transmitters of disease agents and represent a major challenge to environmental health. It is estimated that in the United States there are 125 million rats, or one for every two people. Table 8.3 lists rodents, as well as various insect and noninsect vectors, and the diseases they can transmit. These vectors and vector hosts have major public health, social, and economic impacts throughout the world.

As with rodents, the control of insects requires knowledge of their characteristics, including their life cycles and breeding habits, as well as their role as vectors of disease.

Each year insects infect multitudes of people with diverse agents of disease; some of the more prominent are summarized in Table 8.4. Mosquitoes alone cause millions of new cases of malaria worldwide each year. Many of these cases are in Africa, where the disease causes an estimated 2 million deaths annually; in Central and South America, the number of deaths averages about 25,000 each year. Half of these are children, often under the age of 5 years. In addition, an estimated 90 million people throughout the world have lymphatic filariasis, an infection caused by a parasitic worm transmitted by mosquitoes. In fact, filariasis is one of the most rapidly spreading diseases.

Table 8.3. Some Serious Pest-Borne Diseases of Humans. (Source: Moeller, 1997).

Disease	Causative Agent	Vector	Method of Infection
African sleeping sickness	Tryponosome	tsetse fly	bite
Cholera	bacterium, Vibrio cholerae	housefly	contamination of foods
Dengue fever	Virus	Aedes mosquito	bite
Dysentery, amoebic	Protozoon	housefly	contamination of foods
Dysentery, bacillary	bacterium, Shigella sp.	housefly	contamination of foods
Encephalitis	Virus	Culex mosquito	bite
Lyme Disease	spirochete bacterium Borrelia burgdorferi	deer tick	bite
Malaria	protozoon, Plasmodium vivax	Anopheles mosquito	bite
Onchocerciasis (River blindness)	Parasitic worm, Onchocerca volvulus	black flies	bite
Plague	bacterium, Posteurella pestis	Oriental rat flea and other fleas	bite or contact with infected rodents
Rocky Mountain spotted fever	Rickettsia Rickettsia rickettsi	American dog tick	bite
Typhoid fever	bacterium, Salmonella typhi	housefly	contamination of food and water
Typhus	rickettsia, Rickettsia prowazeki	human body louse	contamination of bite and abrasions
Yellow fever	Virus	Aedes mosquito	bite

Table 8.4 Global Impacts of Tropical Disease Infections. (Source: Moeller, 1997).

Disease	Insect vector	Number of countries affected	Number of people infected (millions)	Total population at risk (millions)
Malaria	Mosquitoes	103	270	2.100
Lymphatic filariasis	Mosquitoes	76	90	900
River blindness	Black flies	34	17	90
Chagas'disease	Triatomine (kissing bugs)	21	16-18	90
Leishmaniasis	Sandflies	80	12	350

B. Sources of Discomfort

Itching, buzzing, creeping, and crawling may not seem like serious concerns, but the creatures responsible have been driving people to distraction for millennia and have been the targets of a great deal of pesticide use in recent decades. Some of the major villains involved in producing acute human discomfort, if not illness, include the following.

Lice - Head lice, body lice, and crab lice are all human parasites that can cause severe itching, secondary infections, and scarred or hardened skin. Lice are typically associated with people living in crowded conditions where opportunities for bathing and laundering clothes are limited. With the introduction of DDT following World War II, the incidence of lice infestations dropped to low levels. As the use of this insecticide became restricted, however, cases of head lice among schoolchildren have been increasing.

Fleas - Aside from the flea species, which transmit the deadly plague bacterium (see next section), fleas commonly found on domestic animals can cause severe irritation, loss of blood, and discomfort. Although most fleas prefer to feed on their animal host, they frequently bite humans if the normal host is absent. Such bites can be extremely painful and may cause swelling and a reddening of the skin.

Mites - These tiny insect relatives are responsible for the serious skin condition known as scabies, as well as a number of other forms of dermatitis such as "grocers' itch," acquired by handling mite-infested grain products, cheese, dried fruits, and so on. Mites that normally live as ectoparasites on birds may become very serious pests of humans when they migrate in large numbers into homes after starlings or sparrows leave their nests. For this reason, householders should discourage birds from nesting on eaves or windowsills or other locations in close proximity to homes. **Chiggers,** a type of mite inhabiting many parts of the southern or Midwestern United States, can cause extreme skin irritation lasting for a week or more when they attach themselves to a human host, usually around the waist or armpits.

Bedbugs - Hiding during the day in mattresses, bedsprings, cracks in the wall, and so on, bedbugs cause many a sleepless night and produce large, intensely itchy welts on sensitive victims. Fortunately they are not known to transmit any disease.

Spiders - Though many people harbor an irrational antipathy toward spiders, the vast majority of these eight-legged creatures are quite harmless to humans. Even the fearsome - looking tarantula - the loathsome villain in many a B-grade Hollywood thriller - is actually rather docile. Now widely sold as pets, tarantulas can be handled with ease and rarely bite; even when they do, their venom is of little harm to most people. Only three U.S. species present any real danger: the **black widow** (female only), the **brown recluse** (both sexes), and the **aggressive house spider** (males more venomous and , more likely to bite than females).

In addition to the above, the buzzing of flies, mosquitoes, gnats, cicadas, June bugs, or wasps - even when these insects are not carrying disease organisms - can provoke extreme annoyance. Certain plant species also, particularly poison ivy and its relatives, have been prime targets of chemical herbicides because of the intensely irritating rash which contact with these plants can produce.

C. VECTORS OF DISEASE

Public health practitioners, along with farmers, were among the first to greet the introduction of synthetic chemical pesticides with great enthusiasm. Compounds such as DDT were viewed as perhaps the ultimate weapon in freeing humanity from the threat of a number of insect- or rodent-borne diseases responsible for millions of deaths and illnesses each year. Quite appropriately, the first use to which DDT was put involved the wartime dusting of refugees in Italy to curb an outbreak of typhus fever. The success of this effort led to extensive spraying campaigns in many parts of the world against the vectors of such dreaded killers as malaria, yellow fever, river blindness, bubonic plague, and encephalitis. Although the medical community's high hopes for complete eradication of the carriers of these diseases have proven overly optimistic, pesticide use has played a significant role in lowering death rates and improving public health in many parts of the world. Some pests of particular public health importance include mosquitoes, flies, body lice, rat fleas, and ticks.

Mosquitoes - Mosquitoes have probably been responsible for more human deaths than any other insect, though their role as disease-carriers was not recognized until late in the 19th century. Worldwide, even today millions of people become ill each year due to such mosquito-borne ailments as malaria, yellow fever, dengue, filariasis, and encephalitis.

Flies - Many species of flies, particularly the common housefly, are important carriers of serious gastrointestinal diseases such as typhoid fever, cholera, dysentery, and parasitic worm infections due to their habit of feeding on human and animal wastes. If such wastes contain pathogenic organisms, the fly can pick these up either on the sticky pads of its feet or on its body hairs or mouthparts and mechanically transmit them to humans when it alights on food materials. Fly vomitus and feces also frequently contain pathogenic bacteria that can inoculate human food, multiply rapidly in the food medium, and subsequently result in outbreaks of intestinal diseases when people consume the food.

Cockroaches - Contrary to common belief, cockroaches have not been implicated as important vectors of infectious disease, even though laboratory, studies have repeatedly shown these insects harbor a wide range of pathogenic microbes on their feet and can mechanically transmit these organisms to food.

Body Lice - Body lice can be a source of intense discomfort, but they are of special public health concern because they are vectors of several serious epidemic diseases. Typhus fever, characterized by elevated temperature, severe headache, and a rash, has been a major killer in past centuries, particularly during wartime when perhaps as many soldiers died from typhus as from swords or bullets. The rickettsial pathogen responsible for the disease is passed from louse to human by the feces of the insect, not its bite. When a person infested with lice scratches the affected area, minor abrasions on the skin permit entry to the rickettsia.

Other lice – Other lice, after feeding on a person infected with typhus, ingest the pathogen and spread it as they move from person to person. This method of transmission explains why typhus outbreaks are most prevalent when people are living together in crowded, unsanitary conditions. Insecticidal dusting of louse-infested persons has proven to be an effective method for controlling the spread of typhus fever. Two other louse-borne diseases, also most common during wartime but with much lower fatality rates than typhus, are trench fever and causing fever.

Rat Fleas - Aside from the enormous economic damage caused by rats, these pests are of great public health concern because they are vectors of a number of diseases, the most deadly of which is plague (the "Black Death" of medieval times). In September 1994 the first major plague outbreak in half a century terrorized residents of the Indian city of Surat, killing more than 50 people. Even before the Surat incident, plague rates had been steadily rising worldwide since the early 1980s. The vast majority of recent plague victims (90% of total cases reported) have been in Africa, predominantly in the nations of Madagascar and Tanzania, while Brazil, Peru, Myanmar, and Vietnam account for most of the remainder.

Ticks - Among our most common parasites, ticks are a source of profound annoyance to campers, hunters, dog owners, and livestock raisers who frequently discover themselves or their pets providing a blood meal to these tiny pests. Ticks are far more than a nuisance, however. They are vectors of several serious human diseases such as Rocky Mountain spotted fever, a condition that frequently results in death within two weeks and which, contrary to its name, is not restricted to mountainous areas but is found throughout the continental United States, with the largest number of cases being report from North and South Carolina.

V. BIBLIOGRAPHY

Cope, G.W. (2001). Contaminants in Wildlife. In L. Williams, & R. Langley (Eds.), Environmental Health Secrets (pp. 130-133). Philadelphia, PA: Hanley & Belfus, Inc.

Environmental Protection Agency (EPA). (1998, April). National Water Quality Inventory: 1996 Report to Congress.

Lewis, R.F. (2001). Bioremediation. In L. Williams, & R. Langley (Eds.), Environmental Health Secrets (pp. 79-84). Philadelphia, PA: Hanley & Belfus, Inc.

Moeller, D. W. (1997). Rodents and Insects. Environmental Health (pp.196-216). Cambridge, MA, and London, UK: Harvard University Press.

Moeller, D. W. (1997). Solid Waste. Environmental Health (pp.170-195). Cambridge, MA, and London, UK: Harvard University Press.

Moore, G.S. (1999). Solid and Hazardous Waste. Living with the Earth: Concepts in Environmental Health Science (pp. 11.1 – 11.40). Boca Raton, FL: Lewis Publishers.

Moore, G.S. (1999). The Trouble with Pests. Living with the Earth: Concepts in Environmental Health Science (pp. 6.1 - 6.41). Boca Raton, FL: Lewis Publishers.

Moore, S.H. (2001). Hazardous Waste. In L. Williams, & R. Langley (Eds.), Environmental Health Secrets (pp. 67-71). Philadelphia, PA: Hanley & Belfus, Inc.

Nadakavukaren, A. (2000). Pests and Pesticides. Our Global Environment: A Health Perspective 5th Edition (pp. 269-316). Prospective Heights, IL: Waveland Press, Inc.

Nadakavukaren, A. (2000). Solid and Hazardous Wastes. Our Global Environment: A Health Perspective 5th Edition (pp. 623-682). Prospective Heights, IL: Waveland Press, Inc.

Newton, N.H. (2001). Pests and Animal Bites. In L. Williams, & R. Langley (Eds.), Environmental Health Secrets (pp. 189-192). Philadelphia, PA: Hanley & Belfus, Inc.

Parker, C.M. (2001). Indoor and Outdoor Shooting Ranges. In L. Williams, & R. Langley (Eds.), Environmental Health Secrets (pp. 145-147). Philadelphia, PA: Hanley & Belfus, Inc.

Prete, J.P. (2001). Solid Waste Management. In L. Williams, & R. Langley (Eds.), Environmental Health Secrets (pp. 63-66). Philadelphia, PA: Hanley & Belfus, Inc.

Shear, T.H. (2001). Desertification. In L. Williams, & R. Langley (Eds.), Environmental Health Secrets (pp. 58-62). Philadelphia, PA: Hanley & Belfus, Inc.

Wagner, T. (1994). Managing our wastes. In T. Wagner (Ed.), In our Backyard: A Guide to Understanding Pollution and Its Effects (pp 126-183). New York, NY: Van Nostrand Reinhold.

CHAPTER

9

FOOD QUALITY

I. INTRODUCTION

Food is a fundamental human need, a basic right, and a prerequisite to good health. The human body depends on the energy, protein, vitamins, and minerals that are found in a variety of foods to survive and remain strong. Studies in Europe in the 1920s showed that in general the poor were short, thin, and suffered from ill health. Their health improved and children grew taller if they were given a diet rich in protein, energy, and vitamins. This diet became the standard for good health and the "balanced diet" became common terminology. A balanced diet could be guaranteed if people ate a plentiful and varied supply of different foods - for example, protein foods derived from animal products or soybeans, energy foods rich in carbohydrate or fat, and protective foods, such as vegetables and fruits, that are rich in vitamins and some minerals (Figure 9.1).

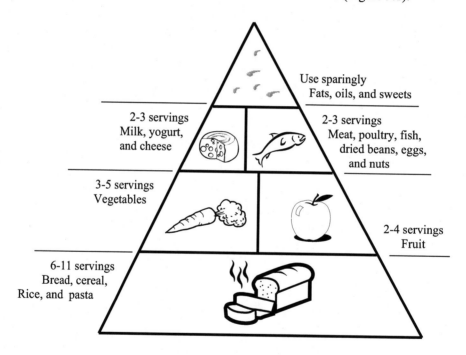

Figure 9.1. Food Pyramid – Guides for a Healthy Diet. (Source: Moeller, 1997).

A variety of nutrients are required by humans to maintain healthy metabolic function. The primary component of our diet is **energy**, expressed as calories or joules. **Energy requirement** is the amount of energy needed to maintain health, growth, and an appropriate level of physical activity. Although the number of calories required varies greatly among individuals, depending on their size, age (all of which influence basal metabolic rate), and level of physical activity maintained, it is commonly based on balancing intake with output. If energy intake and expenditure are not in balance, this imbalance will result in changes in body mass. The conditions of being underweight or overweight both have adverse effects on human health. The health effects of malnutrition and specific deficiency disorders are described below. **Obesity**, defined as a state characterized by excess body fat, is a common cause of severe morbidity and diminished longevity. An association has been found between obesity and hypertension, diabetes, the formation of gallstones, breast cancer, and endometrium cancer.

Centuries before microorganisms were first observed under a microscope, their effects on foods were evident to primitive people. Humans learned by experience that fresh foods changed in taste, odor, and appearance with the passage of time. They acquired a liking for certain changes, particularly the alcoholic and lactic acid fermentations, and developed empirical methods of inducing them to add variety to their diet and to preserve seasonal foods for later use. They recognized other changes as spoilage and avoided the spoiled foods as unpalatable or associated with sickness. The ill effects often were attributed to evil spirits, to gods such as Bacchus, or to the influence of the moon and stars.

During the last century scientists recognized the ubiquity and variety of microorganisms and their immense power to decompose food, cause disease, and create new products. On the basis of the pioneering work by Louis Pasteur, Robert Koch, Joseph Lister, Nicholas Appert, and their colleagues, evidence was accumulated to show that microorganisms occur in nature almost everywhere in greater abundance and variety than any other form of life. Not only did scientists show that specific bacteria, yeast, and molds cause particular kinds of fermentation, proteolysis, and fat decomposition, but they also identified the resulting acids, gases, toxins, and other end-products and determined the conditions that would prevent or promote various types of microbial action. These scientists helped to establish the basic principles of food preservation and sanitation on which the U.S. food processing and service industries depend for the preparation of safe, wholesome products. Bacteria, yeast, and molds play leading roles in the food industry, both in the production of foods such as bread, sauerkraut, cheese, and wine, and in the destruction of foods as a result of rotting and spoilage.

As foods appear in nature, they are essentially free of microorganisms. Microorganisms and other contaminants may be found on the food's surface, but only under unnatural conditions are microorganisms found below the skin or protective outer layer. Some experts think that without the outer skin, microorganisms would invade human bodies so rapidly that within weeks no one would be left on earth. Meats, fruits, and vegetables are similar to humans in that their skin is a protector. If the skin or peeling is cut or removed, microorganisms invade and cause them to rot or deteriorate.

Adding to the above complexities, food no longer is grown where it is consumed, nor is it consumed the day it is harvested. Little of the food served in New York City is grown in New York City or even in that state. The food is shipped many miles from where it is grown to where it is served. Shipping requires time. The food may lie in supermarkets for days before it is sold. Then it may remain in people's dwellings for several days. The longer the food is stored, the greater is the risk of contamination with pathogens and, obviously, the greater the risk of spoilage.

Usually from the time a product leaves a farm until a consumer purchases it, the agricultural industry is responsible for keeping the product as fresh as possible. If it spoils during this time, the industry takes a loss. Therefore, the food industry is interested in the ways and, techniques of keeping the product from spoiling or losing its appeal to buyers. This is why the food industry conducts most of the food research done today. It seeks additional ways to keep food from losing its nutritive value, to make it more appealing to potential purchasers, to enable a longer shelf life and to enhance its flavor, texture, and color.

Given the central importance of food in our personal environment, one would expect it to be an aspect of our lives that we control. Yet this is far from the case. In recent years both the number of individuals affected and the number of food poisoning outbreaks have been increasing. **Salmonella enteritidis**, for instance, showed a fourfold increase in outbreaks from 1973 to 1987. Some of the increase may be a result of better reporting; nevertheless, food poisoning in the United States is grossly underreported despite the best surveillance efforts. The reported data could well be the tip of the iceberg; most foodborne diseases occur as isolated or sporadic events rather than as part of large dramatic outbreaks that attract the attention and investigative resources of public health authorities. Exacerbating the situation is the fact that many victims do not seek medical care. Current estimates are that the consumption of contaminated food causes some 6.5 million cases of preventable disease and some 9,000 deaths annually in the United States.

As is well known, food is essential to life and many foods are known to have ingredients that are beneficial to health. In fact, dietary factors are implicated in the cause and prevention of a variety of ailments, including cancer, coronary heart disease, birth defects, and cataracts. Strong evidence indicates that the consumption of vegetables and fruits protects against these diseases; however, the active constituents have not been completely identified. Whether fat per se is a major cause of disease is a question being debated. However, many nutritionists believe that the consumption of saturated fats probably increases the risk of coronary heart disease. One conclusion from existing epidemiologic evidence is that many individuals in the United States have suboptimal diets and that the potential for disease prevention via improved nutrition is substantial.

In recognition of the important role that diet can play in the health of the public, the Department of Agriculture has developed a "food pyramid", which provides advice on what people should eat. Foods at the bottom of the pyramid - grains, vegetables, and fruit - should be consumed in larger quantities than those at the top-meat and dairy products, fats, oils, and sweets. The highest listed numbers of daily servings are for tall, active men; the lowest are for short, inactive women.

The focus in this chapter will be on contaminants that are commonly found in food, their effects on health, and the steps that must be taken in the preservation and handling of food to assure its safety. Aside from objectionable materials, such as rust, dirt, hair, machine parts, nails, and bolts, the contaminants found in food fall into two broad categories:

1. Biological agents, such as bacteria, viruses, molds, antibiotics, parasites, and their toxins, which can cause a wide range of illnesses; and
2. Chemicals, such as lead, cadmium, mercury, sodium, phosphates, nitrites, nitrates, and organic compounds, which can have both acute and chronic health effects. Such contaminants can gain access to the food chain at any of a multitude of stages during growing, processing, preparation, or storage.

Although the expression "food poisoning" is generally applied to any disease caused by food, a more appropriate rubric is "foodborne disease." This designation includes not only true "poisonings," such as from the metabolic products (toxins) produced by certain microorganisrns while they multiply in food (e.g., **Staphylococcus aureus)**, but also foodborne"infections" such as salmonellosis.

The potential for large-scale foodborne outbreaks has never been greater. A major reason is our increasing reliance on massive, centralized food production and processing, combined with extensive distribution. Any contamination in that chain, even low-level or infrequent contamination, could result in the exposure of thousands, whereas contamination of foods processed in the home, where foods were primarily processed generations ago, exposed relatively few individuals. The technological advances in industry that freed homemakers from food production and processing have not always been coupled with advances that assured food safety.

In addition, the epidemiology of foodborne diseases has changed in recent years there is:

1. Increasing globalization of our food supplies,
2. Increasing consumption of raw or minimally processed foods, particularly of fruits, vegetables, and grains (and less consumption of meat and other high fat foods), and
3. Increasing consumption of food outside the home, in fast-food and other restaurants.

As the production/processing/distribution/preparation of foods has grown in complexity, so too have the opportunities for contamination. When contamination occurs today, sporadic illnesses tend to be widely dispersed, whereas the proverbial church supper outbreak of the past (but still occurring today, of course) caused high attack lines in localized settings.

The consuming public has also changed:

1. The population of elderly persons has increased markedly in absolute numbers (and in older age there is decreased resistance to infection through waning - immunity and less stomach acid), and
2. There is an ever-expanding population of other individuals who are immunocompromised (by AIDS, cancer, chemotherapy for a number of conditions, diabetes mellitus, and others). Such individuals are susceptible to a greater range of microorganisms and become ill with smaller doses. It is for these reasons that humans have become the "ultimate bioassay" for low-level contamination of pathogens in our food supply.

II. <u>TYPES OF FOODBORNE ILLNESS</u>

Contrary to popular consumer perception about the risk of chemicals in foods, major hazards associated with foodborne illness are clearly of biological origin. The Centers for Disease Control and Prevention (CDC) has published recent summaries of foodborne diseases by etiology for the years 1983 through 1992. CDC groups foodborne disease agents in four categories: bacterial, parasitic, viral, and chemical (Table 9.1).

Table 9.1 Major Foodborne Illnesses. (Source: Moeller, 1997).

Illness	Causative Agent	Food Usually Involved	Incubation Period
Foodborne Parasites			
Trichinellosis	Trichinella spiralis	Pork	8-15 days
Giardiasis	Giardia lamblia	Raw salads and vegetables	7-10 days
Amebiasis(amebic dysentery)	Entamoeba histolytica	Food contaminated with fecal matter	2-4 weeks
Bacterial Infections			
Salmonellosis	Salmonella typhimurium and enteritidis	Eggs, chicken, pork, beef	12-36 hours
Shigellosis(bacillic dysentery)	Shigella dysenteriae	Moist food, milk, dairy products	1-3 weeks
Streptococcal sore throat and scarlet fever	Beta-hemolytic streptococcus	Milk products, egg salad	1-3 days
Viral Infections			
Viral hepatitis	Hepatitis A	Sandwiches, salads	28-30 days
Foodborne Toxins			
Paralytic shellfish poisoning	Dinoflagellates(neurotoxins)	Shellfish	Up to 24 hours
Cancer	Aspergillus flavus (mycotoxins)	Peanuts, corn, cereal grains	Years
Staphylococcal food poisoning	Staphylococcus aureus	Meat, poultry, custards, salad dressings, sandwiches	2-4 hours
Botulism	Clostridium botulinum	Home-canned vegetables, fruit	12-36 hours
Gastroenteritis	Clostridium perfringens	Meat, poultry, vegetables, spices	10-12 hours
Diarrhea	Escherichia coli	Meat, poultry, shellfish, watercress	24-72 hours

Greater than 95 percent of all reported outbreaks of foodborne illnesses are caused by microorganisms or their toxins. Fully 97 percent of reported cases are likewise linked to a microbial source. Only around 3 percent of the outbreaks and less than 1 percent of cases can be truly linked to chemical (heavy metals, monosodium glutamate, and other chemicals) contamination of foods. Furthermore, 97 percent of reported deaths are due to microbial sources.

Investigations of a reported foodborne outbreak begin with the determination of the mean incubation time and symptoms. Often, the pathogen or chemical is not detected. In such cases, the incubation time can be used to narrow the range of possibilities and rule out certain causes. The unconfirmed outbreaks are classified as follows:

Incubation Time	Probable Agent
< 1 hour	Chemical
1- 7 hours	S. aureus
8 -14 hours	C. perfringens
>14 hours	other

A. BACTERIAL INFECTIONS

Bacterial agents are by far the leading cause of illness, with total numbers estimated as high as 6.5 to 33 million cases per year and deaths as high as 9,000 annually in the United States. Costs are estimated to be $3 to 8 billion annually in medical expenses and lost productivity. The high incidence of bacterial foodborne disease is paralleled in other developed countries.

Predominant bacterial infections transmitted via foods are salmonellosis, campylobacteriosis, yersiniosis, vibriosis, and shigellosis. Most are Gram-negative rod-shaped organisms that are inhabitants of the intestinal tract of animals. That foods of animal origin are primary causes of foodborne gastroenteritis is thus not surprising. Indeed, federal and most state regulatory agencies consider foods of animal origin (meat, poultry, eggs, fish, shellfish, milk, and dairy products) potentially hazardous foods. One look at epidemiological data confirms this suspicion.

Foodborne bacterial hazards are classified based on their ability to cause infections or intoxications. Foodborne infections are usually the predominant type of foodborne illness reported. Foodborne outbreaks most often occur with foods prepared at food service establishments and at home. Improper holding temperatures and poor personal hygiene were the leading factors contributing to reported outbreaks.

Bacterial hazards are further classified based upon the severity of risk. Severe hazards are those capable of causing widespread epidemics. Moderate hazards can be those that have potential for extensive spread, with possible severe illness, complication, or sequelae in susceptible populations. Mild hazards can also cause outbreaks but have limited ability to spread. Those involved with food production, processing, and service should pay careful attention to controlling these biological hazards by:

1. Destroying or minimizing the hazard,
2. Preventing contamination of food with the hazard, or
3. Inhibiting growth or preventing toxin production by the hazard.

Control steps are described in later sections of this chapter. When investigating foodborne disease outbreaks, the most important factor is time. Prompt reporting of an outbreak is essential to identifying implicated foods and stopping potentially widespread epidemics. Initial work in the investigation should be inspection of the premises where the outbreak occurred. Look for obvious sources, including sanitation and worker hygiene. Food preparation, storage, and serving should be carefully monitored. Interview those involved in the outbreak. Obtain case histories of victims and healthy individuals. Discuss health history and work habits of food handlers. Collect appropriate specimens for laboratory analysis, including stool samples, vomitus, and swabs of rectum, nose, and skin. Attempt to collect suspect foods, including leftovers or garbage if necessary. Specific tests for pathogens or toxins will depend on potential etiological agents and food type. Analysis of data should include case histories, illness specifics (incubation time, symptoms, and duration), laboratory results, and attack rates. All foodborne disease outbreaks should be reported to local and state health officers and to the CDC.

1. Salmonellosis

Salmonellae are among the most prevalent of zoonotic infectious agents. Raw meat and raw meat products frequently harbor salmonellae (poultry more commonly than pork; pork more commonly than beef). Foodborne **Salmonella** infection, however, can be prevented by adequate heating to destroy these pathogens and avoidance of cross-contamination after heating. On the other hand, raw produce such as sprouts has caused **Salmonella** outbreaks; and, sprouts are not commonly washed in homes or restaurants. The ultimate sources of such contaminations have not been identified but may relate to contact of sprout seeds or plants with animals or their wastes. Occasionally, infected food handlers are implicated in outbreaks as sources of contamination, but more often they represent additional cases, having eaten the same foods as their customers. Any "responsibility," however, lies in their not having eradicated (through proper heating, etc.) the salmonellae introduced into their establishments in the raw meat and meat products that were implicated. While low-level contamination of foods with **S. aureus** is unavoidable and, in itself, poses no threat, there can be no tolerance of any level of **Salmonella** contamination in foods ready for serving.

The infective dose for **Salmonella** infection is most commonly given as 10^5 organisms but can be as high as 10^9 or 10^{10}, depending on the serotype and the host. However, past volunteer studies to determine the infectious dose were limited by several factors: they were often done on healthy young males with laboratory strains that could have lost their virulence; they failed to assess minimal infective doses; and they used few volunteers at the lower dose levels. Much lower infective doses, of $=10^3$ total organisms ingested, have been estimated from observations in the "more natural" setting of recent food-borne outbreaks. Specifically, 60 to 2300 organisms per 100 g of food were estimated in raw hamburger that caused **S. newport** infection, less than 100 organisms per 100 g of chocolate candy that caused **S. eastbourne** infection, less than 10 organisms per 100 g in Schwan's ice cream in the 1994 **S. enteritidis** outbreak estimated to have affected more than 200,000 persons nationwide, and less than 1 organism per 100 g of cheddar cheese that caused **S. heidelberg** infection. A comprehensive review of the infective dose of **Salmonella** in both volunteers and outbreak settings has been published.

It is recognized that gastric acid protects against ingested enteric pathogens such as salmonellae. This can explain why infants (and the aged) can be infected by relatively low doses: they may normally lack stomach acid. The reason why the foods listed above may have caused disease in presumably healthy, young adults despite low-level **Salmonella** contamination probably relates to their high fat content, which protects the salmonellae from gastric acid and allows salmonellae to reach the less hostile, alkaline duodenum. Milk (and ice cream) has high fat content and, if contaminated, pose an additional risk. Since these are fluids, they quickly pass into the duodenum (unless consumed with solid food) and escape acid contact. The large Riverside, California, waterborne outbreak of 1965 was due to low-level contamination (MPN of 17 salmonellae per liter) of water that, as a fluid, could similarly reach the duodenum after short gastric contact time.

2. Vibriosis

Other important foodborne diseases deserve comment. **Vibrio parahaemolyticus** is one of the leading causes of foodborne disease in Japan, but it was not identified in the United States until 1969. Most outbreaks have been traced to crustaceans taken from warm coastal marine waters that were either inadequately cooked or subsequently recontaminated by raw shellfish or surfaces and implements that had contact with raw fish or shellfish. The incubation period is about 12 hours; onset is generally acute; and symptoms resemble those of salmonellosis. Recovery is usually complete in 2 to 5 days. Special media (thiosulfate citrate bile salts sucrose agar (TCBS)) should be used when this disease is suspected. Other **Vibrio** species (which contaminate 5 to 10 percent of shellfish in the U.S. market) cause disease too. The most virulent is **V. vulnificus**, which is fatal in more than 50 percent of those who develop bacteremia. At greatest risk of serious **V. vulnificus** infection are those with liver disease (such as from alcoholism), reduced stomach acid (naturally occurring or therapeutically induced), acquired immunodeficiency syndrome (AIDS), and other conditions with compromised immunity. These individuals, especially, should avoid eating raw or undercooked shellfish. Cholera, due to **V. cholerae** serogroup 1, has occurred in the United States from a variety of imported foods that were transported by international travelers; but cases have also been traced to Gulf Coast shellfish.

3. Escherichia coli

Escherichia coli can be grouped into five categories by differences in virulence properties, epidemiology, and clinical syndromes. These are enteropathogenic E. coli (EPEC), enteroinvasive E. coli (EIEC), enterotoxigenic E. coli (ETEC), enteroadherent E. coli (EAEC), and enterohemorrhagic E. coli (EHEC). The latter is most commonly represented by E. coli 0157:H7. Symptomatic and asymptomatic human carriers are believed to be a principal reservoir and source of EPEC, EIEC, ETEC, and EAEC strains involved in human illness, whereas the primary reservoir for coli 0157:H7 appears to be dairy cattle. Ground beef (hamburger) and, less commonly rare roast beef, and raw cow's milk, and, recently, even raw apple juice have been implicated in outbreaks due to E. coli 0157:H7. E. coli 0157:H7 cannot be identified by routine stool cultures but requires plating on sorbitol-MacConkey agar (SMAC) where this strain cannot ferment sorbitol within 24 hours as most E. coli can. Infection with E. coli 0157:H7 is followed by hemolytic uremic syndrome (HUS) 5 to 10 percent of the time, particularly in children with bloody diarrhea. On the other hand, about 90 percent of cases of HUS probably result from E. coli 0157:H7 infection. Antibiotic treatment of that infection may be a predisposing factor for developing HUS.20 Studies of retail meat and poultry in the United States and Canada have revealed E. coli 0157:H7 in 4 to 30 percent of ground beef and in about 2 percent of pork, poultry, and lamb samples. Accordingly, concern about E. coli 0157:H7 disease should provide one additional reason to avoid consumption of raw milk and undercooked meats, especially hamburgers. Recent outbreaks from raw, unpasteurized apple juice and from dry, fermented salami indicate the unusual tolerance of coli 0157:H7 to acidic pH values =4.6. A huge outbreak in widespread areas of Japan in 1996 that involved more than 10,000, particularly schoolchildren, defied efforts to identify a cause although one or more items in school lunches were suspected and probably responsible. The interstate outbreak from salami in 1994 indicated the infectious dose of E. coli 0157:H7 can be less than 50 organisms. At such low doses, secondary person-to-person transmission can easily occur, as they have in day care centers and custodial institutions.

4. Yersiniosis

Yersinia enterocolitica infection has been recognized for years in other areas of the world, especially Scandinavia and Japan. While outbreaks have suggested the possibility of foodborne transmission, specific food items have not been incriminated until recently. These include not only unprocessed "natural" products such as tofu, raw milk, and raw pork but also pasteurized milk and pasteurized products probably contaminated by the addition of ingredients after pasteurization (chocolate milk). Generally, **Y. enterocolitica** is destroyed by standard pasteurization; but, if it is present in great numbers, some **Yersinia** may survive pasteurization and multiply during refrigeration. In one large multistate outbreak due to pasteurized milk, symptoms in children included abdominal pain (suggestive of acute appendicitis, which prompted appendectomies), fever, and diarrhea; many adults, however, presented with pharyngitis and had throat cultures positive for **F. enterocolitica**. Since this pathogen grows best at 75 to 77°F (24 to 25°C), it maybe missed when stools, foods, and pharyngeal swabs are cultured at the usual 99°F (37°C).

5. Campylobacteriosis

Campylobacter jejuni, formerly known to veterinarians as **Vibrio fetus**, has become recognized as an important cause of enteritis in humans and also of Guillain-Barre syndrome. In developed countries it has been isolated from the stools of 3 to 14 percent of patients evaluated for diarrhea, but it is rarely isolated from healthy individuals. Transmission occurs through contaminated food and water, as well as from person to person. The apparent incubation period is 2 to 10 days. The organism has been found in pets, domestic livestock, and fowl (live and dressed). Investigations in the United States have implicated raw milk, raw clams, raw hamburger, raw and undercooked chicken, untreated water, and even municipal water supplies. The epidemiology of this pathogen is similar to that of **Salmonella** (for which chicken is also a common vehicle), and where reporting is compulsory, the incidence of **C. jejuni** infection commonly surpasses that of salmonellosis. Selective media, vacuum jar, and an incubator set at 109°F (43°C) have made this zoonotic infection an important addition to the growing list of enteric pathogens.

6. Listeria monocytogenes

Listeria monocytogenes is commonly found in the environment and in raw food. Studies in the United States and Europe have shown it to be present in 15 to 20 percent of ground beef, in 15 to 80 percent of poultry and in a small percentage of ready-to-eat processed foods including such dairy products as soft cheeses. Moreover, unlike other foodborne pathogens, this organism continues to grow at refrigerated temperatures (4°C, 39°F), and so the degree of contamination increases with storage. The infectious dose is unknown, but it is presumably less for immunosuppressed persons, pregnant women, and the elderly. Although most cases are sporadic (1 to 10 per million people per year), common-source outbreaks have occurred and have implicated several commercial foods: cole slaw, pasteurized milk, and soft cheeses. Case-control studies have implicated uncooked hot dogs and undercooked chicken. A World Health Organization (WHO) informal working group on food-borne listeriosis has concluded that total elimination of **Listeria** from all food is impractical, if not impossible, but that control procedures should be carried out at all possible points during processing. The group recommended withdrawal of foods from market in two situations:

1. When the contents of sealed packages are contaminated despite treatment to eliminate Listeria and
2. When foods have been implicated in human cases of listeriosis.

7. Shigellosis

Four species are associated with food-borne transmission of dysentery, **Shigella dysenteriae, Shigella flexneri, Shigella boydii,** and **Shigella sonnei**. The disease is characterized with an incubation period of 1 to 7 days (usually less than 4 days). Symptoms include mild diarrhea to very severe with blood, mucus, and pus. Fever, chills, and vomiting also occur. Duration is long, typically 4 days to 2 weeks. *Shigella* **spp**. have a very low infectious dose of around 10 cells. Foods most often associated with shigellosis are any that are contaminated with fecal material, with salads frequently implicated. Control is best focused on worker hygiene and avoidance of human waste.

8. Other Bacterial Foodborne Infections

Many other bacteria have been linked to foodborne diseases including **Plesiomonas shigelloides** (raw seafood), **Aeromonas hydrophila** (raw seafood), **Arizona hinshawii** (poultry), **Streptococcus pyogenes** (milk, eggs), and perhaps **Enterococcus faecalis**. Their contribution to foodborne illness appears to be minimal but they may contribute to opportunistic infections.

B. VIRAL INFECTIONS

Foodborne viral infections are uncommonly reported. Poliomyelitis appears to have been the first human viral disease for which a food vehicle was reported (in 1914, in association with raw milk), but there have been no polio foodborne outbreaks reported since 1949. Though hepatitis A is an uncommon cause of foodborne disease, a 1988 outbreak associated with raw shellfish from the Shanghai area of China that affected nearly 300,000 gives hepatitis A the distinction of causing the "largest" foodborne outbreak recorded?' Other foodborne illnesses of proven viral etiology include tickborne encephalitis virus, ECHO 4, and, most importantly of late, Norwalk agent and other small round structured viruses (SRSVs) in the calicivirus family. The Norwalk group probably caused many past outbreaks previously designated as "gastroenteritis of undetermined etiology" or "acute infectious nonbacterial gastroenteritis (AING)" but was not identified until modern diagnostic methods, particularly immune electron microscopy, became available. But inasmuch as the necessary viral diagnostic capability to detect SRSVs exists at only a few centers and since stools collected only during the first 2 days of illness contain a sufficient number of viral particles to be detected, these important causes of foodborne outbreaks will continue to escape detection, and cases will continue to be passed off as "stomach flu" or "intestinal flu." The incubation period for Norwalk-like viruses is 24 to 48 hours; onset is abrupt; symptoms can include nausea, vomiting, abdominal cramps, diarrhea, headache, and sometimes low-grade fever; the duration is generally 1 to 2 days. The secondary attack rate among contacts of cases is notably higher than in other foodborne infections. While viruses belonging to about seven groups (**rotaviruses, parvoviruses, adenoviruses, caliciviruses, enteroviruses, astroviruses,** and **coronaviruses**) commonly cause human gastroenteritis, are shed in stools, and have the potential to contaminate food, it has primarily been the SRSVs of the calicivirus group that have been repeatedly identified in common-source outbreaks of gastroenteritis.

The two basic mechanisms for the contamination of food by viruses that infect the intestinal tract are (a) "indirect" contamination by growing of filter-feeding shellfish in fecally contaminated waters or by irrigating or washing produce by polluted water and (b) "direct" contamination of food, primarily by feces but sometimes by vomitus, by a food handler with poor personal hygiene. Once contamination has occurred, the question is whether the virus will retain infectivity. Unlike bacterial pathogens, viruses do not multiply (or produce toxins) in food.

1. Infectious Hepatitis

Hepatitis A virus is a fairly common infectious agent having an incubation period of 10 to 50 days, mean 25 days. Symptoms include loss of appetite, fever, malaise, nausea, anorexia, and abdominal distress. Approximately 50 percent of cases develop jaundice that may lead to serious liver damage. The duration is several weeks to months. The infectious dose is quite low, less than 100 particles. The long incubation period and duration of the disease means that affected individuals will shed virus for a prolonged period. Foods handled by an infected worker or those that come in contact with human feces are likely vehicles (raw shellfish, salads, sandwiches, and fruits). Filter-feeding mollusks concentrate virus particles from polluted waters. Control is achieved by cooking food, stressing personal hygiene, and by avoiding shellfish harvested from polluted waters.

2. Enteroviruses

Coxsackie, ECHO, and Norwalk viruses, and rotavirus, astrovirus, **Calicivirus**, **Parvovirus**, and adenovirus are being implicated with increasing frequency as agents of foodborne disease. Other viruses most certainly are involved but our ability to isolate them from infected consumers and foods is limited. The incubation period is typical for infectious organisms, 27 to 60 hours. Symptoms are usually mild and self-limiting and include fever, headache, abdominal pain, vomiting, and diarrhea. Duration is from 1 to 3 days. The infectious dose for these agents is thought to be very low, 1 to 10 particles. Foods associated with transmission of viral agents are raw shellfish, vegetables, fruits, and salads. Control is primarily achieved by cooking and personal hygiene.

C. PARASITES

1. Helminths

a. Nematodes (Roundworms)

Trichinosis is caused by the migration of the larva of the worm, **Trichenella spiralis**, through the body and by their encystment in muscle tissue. The source is primarily infected pork, although beef, bear, and walrus have also been implicated. Incubation is usually about 9 days after ingestion. The migration can cause severe eye problems, high fever, and muscle pain. The severity of the disease is extremely variable. Prevalence has been estimated to be from 2 - 10% of the U.S. population based upon autopsy.

b. Cestoda (Tapeworms)

Tapeworm - beef, pork, and fish tapeworms may be acquired from flesh infected with larvae. The larvae develop into the adult tapeworm in the human intestine. A serious complication of the pork tapeworm infection, cysticercosis, may develop due to auto-infection with the eggs passed in human feces. The ingested eggs hatch and penetrate the human intestine and the larva or cysticerci develop in subcutaneous tissue, striated muscle, or other organs. Consequences may be serious when larvae localize in the ear, eye, CNS, or heart.

2. Protozoa

Amoebic dysentery (**Entamoeba histolytica**) is transmitted via water and food contaminated with human sewage, or by rats, flies, and cockroaches. Foods eaten raw and insufficiently washed are often implicated. The incubation period is 5 days or longer and is most often 3 to 4 weeks.

Giardiasis (**Giardia lamblia**) is transmitted in much the same manner, except that vector transmission has not been found. The average incubation time is 9 days. Giardiasis is an extremely debilitating disease due to prolonged diarrhea and severe weight loss.

D. FOODBORNE INTOXICATIONS

Food-borne microbial intoxications are caused by a toxin in the food or production of a toxin in the intestinal tract. Normally the organism grows in the food prior to consumption. There are several differences between foodborne infections and intoxications. Intoxicating organisms normally grow in the food prior to consumption, which is not always true for infectious organisms. Organisms causing intoxications may be dead or nonviable in the food when consumed; only the toxin need be present. Organisms causing infections must be alive and viable when food is consumed. Infection-causing organisms invade host tissues and symptoms usually include headache and fever. Toxins usually do not cause fever and toxins act by widely different mechanisms.

1. Staphylococcal Food Poisoning

a. History

The work of in 1930 established staphylococci as a cause of food poisoning. They isolated **Staphylococcus aureus** in pure culture from a cake implicated in an outbreak; when cell-free filtrates prepared from broth cultures of the isolate were fed to volunteers, symptoms like those in the outbreak resulted. Eight enterotoxins have been identified, and a ninth may exist. These toxins easily resist boiling for 30 minutes or more. It is the heat-stable, preformed toxin, not **S. aureus** organisms per se, that causes staphylococcal food poisoning. The target organ is the gut.

b. Symptoms

Symptoms usually appear 2 to 4 hours after ingestion; the range is 1 to 6 hours. Onset is generally abrupt and maybe violent. Salivation, nausea vomiting, abdominal cramps, prostration, diarrhea (diarrhea less often than vomiting), and occasionally hypertension occur. There is generally no fever or chills but patients may experience a subjective feeling of fever from the flushing and perspiration that accompany vomiting, and a subsequent chilly sensation as perspiration evaporates. Acute gastrointestinal symptoms commonly last several hours but generally less than a day; weakness may persist for another 1 or 2 days. Death in otherwise healthy individuals is rare. The intensity of symptoms has prompted surgical exploration (for suspected appendicitis) in sporadic, severe cases.

c. Sources of Contamination

Staphylococci are widely distributed in nature, and humans are a natural reservoir **S. aureus** can colonize normal, healthy skin as well as the normal oronasopharynx, but the organism can be especially abundant in purulent discharges of an infected finger, hangnail, cut, bum, eye, or chronic infections of the nasal sinuses. Individuals with acne, boils, carbuncles, and common colds may be heavy shedders as well. Cows with infected udders also pose a health hazard if their milk is not promptly refrigerated. Foods implicated in staphylococcal food poisoning generally require much handling and are characteristically rich in protein (e.g., custards and cream fillings, sliced and chopped meats). Occasionally, surprising foods are implicated such as the extensive, widespread 1989 outbreak due to canned mushrooms imported from the People's Republic of China.

d. Prevention

The three principal requirements for the production of sufficient enterotoxin to cause disease are:

1. The food must be contaminated with enterotoxin-producing staphylococci;
2. The food must be a good growth medium and
3. The food must be held at an improper temperature (such as ambient room) for several hours.

Prevention depends on eliminating sources of contamination and practicing safe food handling: workers with purulent discharges, common colds, etc., should be excluded from food preparation. The actual food handling time should be reduced to an absolute minimum. Foods should be at room temperature no longer than necessary, preferably under 1 hour, and then should be kept hot ($\geq 140°F$, $60°C$) or cold ($=40°F$, $4°C$), and covered to exclude dust.

2. Clostridium Perfringens Food Poisoning

a. History

While it was suggested earlier in this century that **C. perfringens** (**C. welchii**) caused food-borne disease, it was not until the classic paper by Hobbs et al. in 1953's that **C. perfringens** received attention. Since then it has become recognized as one of the most common foodborne diseases in developed countries. The organism is a common, anaerobic, spore-forming rod that exists widely in nature and can frequently be recovered from raw meats and meat products. Five toxicological types (A to E) are recognized; types A and C cause human gastroenteritis. Type A also causes gas gangrene, and type C, necrotic enteritis ("pigbel"). Of the several toxins and enzymes produced by **C. perfringens** type A, the important one appears to be alpha toxin, which includes the enzyme lecithinase, **C. perfringens** produces both heat-resistant spores and heat-sensitive spores; the latter predominate in nature, but it is the heat-resistant strains that are most often associated with outbreaks of food-borne poisonings.

b. Typical Setting of C. Perfringens Poisoning

With rare exceptions the implicated food is a meat dish prepared in advance, and in bulk, for a large group such as a banquet or institutional population, in such a way that anaerobic and thermal conditions existed to permit germination of spores that survived initial cooking. These spores are heat shocked (activated) to germinate as soon as the cooling mass reaches a suitable temperature. Young vegetative cells continue to multiply, depending on temperature, storage time, and the nature of the food (liquid masses of meat such as stews can provide especially good anaerobic conditions). With generation times as short as 9 minutes under optimal conditions, a critical dose of disease-producing **C. perfringens** (several million organisms or a concentration of organisms $=10^5$/g of food) can readily result. If the mass is too large to cool quickly during subsequent refrigeration, multiplication can continue in the refrigerator and can also resume on subsequent rewarming if not carried out at temperatures inhibitory to growth ($=140°F$, $60°C$). In summary, the cooking of meats and poultry in huge quantities, prolonged storage at room temperature, slow cooling, and insufficient reheating are typical features in **C. perfringens** outbreaks.

c. The Disease

After an incubation period of approximately 12 hours (range: 6 to 24), abdominal cramps and diarrhea develop. Occasionally, nausea is reported, but vomiting and fever are typically absent. The disease is so mild that medical consultation is rarely sought; for most, the illness lasts only a day or less. In elderly debilitated patients, however, the disease can be severe, and deaths have been reported.

d. Prevention

Outbreaks of **C. perfringens** foodborne disease would not occur if cooked foods were eaten after initial cooking, while still hot. If it is absolutely necessary to prepare large amounts of food several hours or days before its intended use, the cooked food should not be held at room temperature to cool. Instead, it should be chilled rapidly to a temperature of 40°F (4°C), preferably in a walk-in refrigerator with forced air circulation. To speed the cooling process, the meat, gravy, or stew should be placed in a freezer compartment or divided into shallow containers to induce more rapid heat transfer in the refrigerator. The meat may be served cold, but if it is to be served hot, it should be rewarmed to 165°F (74°C) as quickly as possible. Cold meat slices may be covered with boiling-hot gravy immediately before serving, but the habit of pouring warm gravy on sliced meat and putting both in a warming oven with temperature below 140°F (60°C) is to be condemned. The expression "Keep hot foods hot and cold foods cold" is worth emphasizing for **C. perfringens**, as well as for other organisms responsible for foodborne diseases.

3. Botulism

a. History

Botulism was first recognized as a disease entity early in the nineteenth century and was named for sausage (from the Latin **botulus)**, which was often implicated in the earliest outbreaks. Since then a host of other improperly preserved foods (fish, vegetables, fruit) have caused disease, but the name has been retained. Van Ermengem first identified the causative organism in 1895. Its neurotoxins (simple proteins) are among the most deadly of all known poisons.

Three forms of botulism are now recognized according to the site of toxin production by **Clostridium botulinum** (although a fourth category, "undetermined," exists for those cases not easily categorized):

1. Classic foodborne botulism, the form with which most health workers are familiar, results from the ingestion of preformed botulinal toxin in improperly preserved food. Interest in foodborne botulism far exceeds its importance as a cause of extensive illness (less than 2000 cases reported in the United States since 1900 and only about 10 cases per year in recent decades).
2. Wound botulism results from local tissue infection and in situ toxin production by **C. botulinum**; it was first reported in 1951. This form of botulism is rarely documented; approximately 100 cases have been reported worldwide through 1995. California, alone, has reported 80 of those cases, and most of those related to injecting drug use (particularly of Mexican "black tar" heroin) in the 1990s.
3. Infant botulism results from colonization of the gut lumen by **C. botulinum** with subsequent in vivo production of toxin. This third form of botulism was first recognized in 1976 and, by 1995, more than 1400 cases had been identified worldwide. Some "undetermined" cases of botulism in adults have been considered adult forms of infant botulism, occurring particularly in those who have had altered intestinal anatomy and physiology.

b. Clostridium botulinum

Clostridium botulinum is a Gram-positive, strictly anaerobic, spore-forming bacillus whose natural habitat is the soil. Eight toxigenic types have been identified but, in humans, the disease is almost always caused by A, B, or E toxins and rarely by F or G. These toxins prevent the release of acetylcholine at cholinergic synapses. The most notable effect is flaccid paralysis because of the interruption of nerve impulses at the myoneural junction. The spores of **C. botulinum** are ubiquitous, and except for those infants who develop infant botulism for reasons still unknown, the spores are not otherwise dangerous when ingested. Indeed, since spores are so widely distributed in soil and dust, they could be ingested every time fresh produce is eaten. Toxin is elaborated, however, when spores that survive improper food preservation germinate in anaerobic conditions. Boiling readily destroys botulinal toxin, once formed, but most botulinum spores are not promptly destroyed by boiling; they require temperatures of 240°F (116°C) for destruction.

c. The Disease

In foodborne botulism, signs and symptoms of intoxication appear 6 hours to 8 days (most typically 12 to 48 hours) after ingestion of contaminated food. Those with the shortest interval to onset (less than 24 hours) generally are most severely affected. The initial symptoms are frequently ptosis, blurred or double vision, and dry, sore throat. Progressive descending paralysis, usually but not always symmetrical, may then develop. After impairment of cranial nerve function (which causes diplopia and poor accommodation, dysphagia, dysphonia, and inability of neck muscles to support the head), paralysis of the respiratory muscles and of the extremities may ensue. Conspicuously absent are objective sensory abnormalities, altered mental status, and fever. Gastrointestinal symptoms are frequently but not necessarily present and may precede or accompany neurological symptoms; constipation is common after paralysis develops. The case fatality ratio for classic foodborne botulism was formerly about 60 percent, but in recent years it has been less than 30 percent. Respiratory paralysis is generally the immediate cause of death. If vital functions can be maintained, full neurological recovery can be expected, although convalescence may be slow and weakness may last for months.

The clinical picture in wound botulism is like that in foodborne botulism, but there is more likely to be fever (secondary to wound infection) and less likely to be early gastrointestinal complaints. With some exceptions, cases to date have primarily involved wounds of an extremity, and the median interval between injury and symptoms of botulism has been 6 days. An increasing proportion of recent cases has been reported in injecting drug users, particularly by "skin popping" or by intramuscular injections. The resulting abscess formation and associated devitalized/scar tissue provide a favorable milieu for the establishment and multiplication of injected anaerobes such as **C. botulinum**.

In the typical case of **infant** botulism requiring hospitalization, the child is 3 months old, and the first symptom is usually constipation, followed by lethargy, poor sucking and swallowing, and then generalized weakness and hypotonia. The infant appears "floppy." The case fatality rate in children hospitalized for infant botulism in the United States is less than 3 percent; however, it has been shown that some cases of sudden infant death syndrome (SIDS) can be attributed to infant botulism.

d. Foods Involved

Most cases of foodborne botulism are caused by home-preserved foods that received some preliminary heat treatment as by canning or smoking. More recently, however, major restaurant-associated outbreaks have involved foods that were not preserved in the usual sense, for example, previously baked potatoes used for potato salad, chopped garlic in oil, and sauteed fresh onions. Store-bought refrigerated foods that were not kept refrigerated after purchase have also caused botulism outbreaks. Inadequately rewarmed foods have also been implicated, such as commercial potpies and home-prepared meat loaf that were kept in gas ovens, with only the pilot light on, for many hours after initial cooking. Despite the publicity given to commercial foods, about 90 percent of all outbreaks in recent years have been due to improper home canning rather than commercial canning. Home canning at temperatures insufficient to destroy spores is the usual problem. For vegetables, a pressure cooker that can reach temperatures of 240°F (116°C) is necessary. Resistance of spores to heat sterilization is reduced at a low pH, and this is why highly acid fruits are rarely implicated in outbreaks and why acidification of home-canned vegetables (with vinegar or lemon juice) is recommended before pressure cooking as an extra measure of protection.

In the United States, most botulinal poisonings are due to home-canned vegetables or fruits, rarely meats; but in Europe, most cases are due to sausages, smoked or preserved meats, and fish. Foods spoiled by some types of **C. botulinum** are frequently foul smelling and vile tasting, especially when proteolytic strains of the organism are involved. Jar lids or can tops may be swollen from gas produced by **C. botulinum**, but this is not invariably the case.

For those infants who develop botulism, it is likely that there are multiple sources of gastrointestinal colonization since botulinal spores are ubiquitous in the environment. To date, toxin has not been found in any food fed to infants with botulism. **C. botulinum** spores, however, have been found in up to 10 percent of honey samples surveyed and in honey that had been fed to patients.

e. Distribution

Spores of **C. botulinum** exist in soil throughout the world. In nations where home canning is discouraged (e.g., England) or where fresh fruits and vegetables are available year round and there is little home canning (as in tropical Third World countries), botulism outbreaks are rare. Additionally, some cases may go undiagnosed in some developed and in most developing countries because laboratory tests to diagnose the disease are not generally available.

In the United States, more than 50 percent of outbreaks have been reported from five western states. California alone has reported 33 percent of the national total. There is a distinct geographical distribution of botulinal toxin types: type A outbreaks predominate west of the Mississippi River, type B occurs primarily in eastern states, and type E is reported primarily from Alaska and the Great Lakes area. This correlates with the types of spores found in these respective regions. Most outbreaks in Europe are due to type B, and in Japan most are due to type E.

Wound botulism has been reported primarily from the United States which has reported more than 90 percent of the world's cases. The diagnosis should be considered when characteristic features of botulism develop in a person with a wound, particularly of an extremity (not necessarily suppurative), where food cannot be incriminated.

Infant botulism, as of December 1996, has been recognized on all inhabited continents except Africa. More than 1300 of the world's 1400+ laboratory-confirmed cases have been identified in the United States, where it was first recognized. As medical awareness of this disease entity increases throughout the world, the incidence and importance of infant botulism worldwide will probably exceed that of classic foodborne botulism, as it has in the United States.

f. Prevention

For foods canned at home, attention must be given to the necessary time, pressure, and temperature to ensure destruction of **C. botulinum** spores. Vegetables should generally be acidified before they are pressure cooked and should be reboiled for at least 3 minutes, with stirring, before serving. Although the toxin is readily destroyed by boiling, foods with off-odors should not be consumed or "taste tested" and cans or bottles with bulging lids, whether home canned or commercial, should not be opened. Foodborne botulism is a public health emergency; local public health authorities should be notified immediately of any presumed case so that efforts can be initiated to confirm the diagnosis, locate other cases and impending cases, determine the food source, and confiscate all existing food containers. Notification of even suspected cases is a legal requirement in most states. Until the epidemiology of infant botulism is better delineated, no recommendations can be given except that honey should not be fed to infants, especially since this is not an essential food. The only practical way to prevent wound botulism from the injection of illicit drugs is to stop such injections.

4. Bacillus cereus

Bacillus cereus poisoning has been recognized for decades in Europe, but the first fully documented episode in the United States occurred in 1969. At least two clinical syndromes exist. The first is like staphylococcal food poisoning in that it has a median latency period of only 2 hours and produces primarily upper gastrointestinal symptoms. The vehicle for this form has most commonly been fried rice served in Chinese restaurants, where the rice had previously been steamed or boiled and then left unrefrigerated for hours or days before it was mixed with egg or pork and quickly stir-fried before serving, The second syndrome resembles **C. perfringens** poisoning in that it has a median latency period of 10 hours and produces primarily lower gastrointestinal symptoms. A variety of foods have been implicated in this type of illness. In both syndromes, disease is generally mild and lasts only a few hours. Diagnosis can be confirmed by the isolation of 10^5 if **B. cereus** organisms per gram of food from epidemiologically implicated food and also by fecal culture. The prevalence of *B. cereus* in control subjects will be much less than in patients. The organism produces at least two enterotoxins - one is heat stable and causes vomiting, and the other is heat labile and causes diarrhea. **B. cereus** is widely distributed in soil and in raw, dried, and processed foods. In one survey, 52 percent of 1500 food ingredients were positive for **B. cereus**. Foods with low colony counts (e.g., $=10^3 g$) probably pose no problem if they are handled properly and refrigerated promptly after cooking.

E. POISONOUS PLANTS AND ANIMALS

Mushrooms and grains contaminated with the fungus, Ergot, are the most common plants, which may cause foodborne intoxications. Scombrotoxin and ciguatoxin found concentrated in warm water ocean fish have been found to cause outbreaks each year since the CDC began surveillance. Scombroid poisonings are primarily due to dolphin (machi-machi) and are mostly found to be restaurant-associated. Ciguatera poisonings are more likely acquired at home due to ingestion of amberjack, grouper, or snapper.

F. TOXIC CHEMICALS

Chemical food poisoning may result from eating foods that have been contaminated accidentally or deliberately with toxic chemicals. The contaminant may be inorganic or organic, naturally occurring or human made. The soluble salts or oxides of such heavy metals as antimony, cadmium, copper, tin, and zinc can cause abrupt and severe gastrointestinal symptoms, typically in a setting where foods or beverages of high acid content have reacted chemically with the metal containers in which they were prepared or stored. The latency period is characteristically short (about 15 minutes). The explosive vomiting that occurs generally eliminates enough of the chemical from the gastrointestinal tract so that systemic toxicity is rarely a problem. Treatment is symptomatic and supportive, antiemetics should be avoided to prevent gastrointestinal retention of toxic ions and potential systemic absorption. A greater threat to life is posed by foods poisoned with insecticides and rodenticides. These chemicals are all too often kept in kitchens where they are mistaken for flour, salt, sugar, baking powder, and other food ingredients. Such chemicals include arsenic, barium carbonate, sodium fluoride, and silver polishes containing cyanide and mercury. Preventive measures are obvious; such chemicals should be labeled poisonous and kept out of food handling areas and away from children.

Contamination with heavy metal salts occurs occasionally in commercial food items with catastrophic consequences. In 1955 more than 12,000 Japanese children were poisoned by arsenic tainted Morinaga dry milk, and more than 130 died. A study of survivors 15 years later showed them to be shorter and to have lower IQs, more central nervous system disorders (epilepsy, brain damage, reduced hearing), and other mental and physical defects than control subjects had. Another catastrophic incident due to a commercial product occurred in Morocco in 1960 when 10,000 people became ill (6000 suffered paralysis) after they had consumed cooking oil adulterated with turbo-jet lubricating oil containing 3 percent triorthocresyl phosphate. Table 9.2 lists some of the many chemicals, which are found in foods. These chemicals largely originate from human processes.

1. Packaging Materials

Chemical poisoning from packaging materials can cause illness and death within 30 minutes. Substances such as plasticizers, stabilizers, and inks can migrate from the packaging to the food causing illness. Exposure to these substances is usually exceptionally low, and the chemicals tend to be non-toxic. In the United States commercial packaging materials are tested for chemical migration and can be considered safe. There are a few chemical contaminants of this nature that are worth mentioning.

a. Antimony

Antimony leaches into foods stored in chipped enamel containers. Acidic foods such as lemon juice will cause antimony to leach out into the product. The ingestion of antimony can cause complications of the gastrointestinal, cardiovascular, and hepatic systems.

b. Cadmium

Cadmium, which is used as a plating material for trays and containers, is also leached into food from containers by acidic conditions. Chronic exposure to cadmium can lead to kidney damage. Cadmium accumulates in both the liver and the kidneys.

Table 9.2 Some Of The Many Chemicals Originating from Human Processes That May Be Found in Food. (Source: Moore, 1999).

Unintended Chemicals in Food
Insecticides
DDT, parathion, pyrethrum, arsenicals, others.
Fungicides
Dithiocarbamates, mercurials, others.
Herbicides
Carbamates, chlorphenoxy cpds (2, 4-D),
Bipyridyls
Fertilizers
Nitrogen, others.
Treatments and Supplements
Food additives and veterinary drugs.
Accidental and inadvertent
Mercury, PCBs, lead, dioxin. Aluminum
and cadmium from kitchenware.
Migration from packaging
Plasticizers, stabilizers such as
alkylphenols, printing inks, tin, and lead.
Chemicals resulting from processing or preparation
Polycyclic aromatic hydrocarbons
(PAHs), nitrosamines, mutagens.

2. Chemical Poisoning

Sources of Infection: Gastroenteritis may be caused by ingesting toxic chemicals present in food or drinks. Chemicals may be ingested in several ways:

1. Ingestion of fruits and vegetables with residual insecticide on their surfaces.
2. Use of utensils for cooking or storing food or drink from which toxic chemicals may leach out.
3. Mistaken use of a toxic chemical in the preparation, seasoning, or sweetening of food.
4. Deliberate and malicious contamination of food by a person for some irrational reason.
5. Ingestion by children believing them to be drinks.
6. Pollution of water while treating farmland or spraying fruit trees.

a. Symptoms

In most instances the triads of gastroenteritis - vomiting, abdominal cramps, and diarrhea - are the predominant symptoms. Vomiting rids the stomach of the food or fluid containing the irritating chemical.

b. Chemicals Most Frequently Encountered

(1) **Sodium fluoride**: An insecticide used for eliminating cockroaches. It has been mistaken for flour, sugar, baking soda, and salt in the preparation of food.

(2) **Sodium Nitrite and Sodium Nitrate**: Used in curing and preserving meat; can be mistaken for salt. Causes cyanosis, a bluish discoloration of the skin resulting from deficient oxygenation of the blood.

(3) **Metallic Poisoning**: Caused by cooking acid foods such as apples, and storing sour drinks (lemonade, orange juice) in certain types of pots, trays, or pitchers. If gray cooking enamelware is used, antimony present in the enamel may leach out and cause lead poisoning. Acid foods cooked in copper pots may leach copper. Drinking water running through lead pipes and acid foods kept in lead vessels will leach out quantities of the metal and cause lead poisoning. Infants may poison themselves by gnawing lead paint from window sills, particularly in old houses.

(4) **Pesticides**: Chemical insecticides are lethal to insects and also are harmful to humans if ingested. Some of them, when fed to laboratory animals, have been found to be carcinogenic and others teratogenic (capable of causing abnormalities in the fetus). Leafy vegetables should be washed before ingestion.

(5) **Silver Polish**: A number of silver polishes contain cyanide. If not washed sufficiently to remove residues of the polish, eating with these utensils may result in gastroenteritis.

G. RADIONUCLIDES

Radiation is introduced into the food chain naturally from mineral deposits beneath the Earth's surface or from the atmosphere in the form of ultraviolet and cosmic rays. Radiation from these sources is emitted at low levels tolerable by plant and animal life. Radionuclides, which are deposited in the environment accidentally or intentionally as a direct result of human activity, are of much greater concern. The levels that result from these activities are tens to hundreds of times higher than those normally encountered by plant and animal life. Exposure to radiation at high levels has the potential to cause in-eversible damage to whole organ systems, genetic mutations or deformities in offspring. If the central nervous system is damaged, symptoms of disorientation, convulsions, and lack of muscle coordination are experienced.

The fallout from the Chernobyl accident of 1986 deposited Cesium 137 (137Cs) and Iodine 131 (131I) throughout the northern hemisphere. The isotopes 137Cs and 131I are absorbed by plants through the roots and foliage, which are in turn used as feed for farm animals. Humans ingest these radionuclides directly from the consumption of fruits and vegetables or indirectly by consuming meat and dairy products. There is recent concern that the concrete vault meant to contain the Chernobyl radioactivity is crumbling and the danger of additional radioactive leakage is eminent. While we are aware of the dangers that arise from fallout, nuclear weapon testing continues to be a concern. Recently, India and Pakistan conducted a series of nuclear weapons tests in an attempt to achieve the upper hand in an arms race. Although the nuclear testing are underground and usually in remote areas where there is little or no agricultural activity, radioactive plumes may travel across national boundaries where fallout could still pose a significant threat to human populations.

H. PHYSICAL HAZARDS

Consumers frequently report physical defects with foods, of which presence of foreign objects predominate. Glass is the leading object that consumers report and is evidence of manufacturing or distribution error. Most physical hazards are not particularly dangerous to the consumer, but their obvious presence in a food is disconcerting. Most injuries are cuts, choking, and broken teeth. Control of physical hazards in foods is often difficult, especially when these hazards are a normal constituent of the food, such as bones and shells. Good manufacturing practices and employee awareness are the best measures to prevent physical hazards. Metal detectors and x-ray machines may be installed where appropriate.

III. FOOD ADDITIVES

More controversial than the accidental, often unavoidable, food contaminants are the approximately 2,800 food additives, substances intentionally added to food to modify its taste, color, texture, nutritive value, appearance, resistance to deterioration, and so forth. The years since the end of World War II witnessed explosive growth of the food chemical industry, as food processors responded to public demand (or occasionally created public demand) by promoting a host of new products - convenience foods, frozen foods, dehydrated foods, ethnic foods, and low-calorie foods. Many of these products could not exist in a world free of additives. Nevertheless, a great many people are automatically suspicious of additives with long, unfamiliar, often unpronounceable names; reading the list of ingredients on virtually any supermarket package, can, or bottle seems a bit like a quick tour of a chemical factory. However, there's nothing inherently evil about using additives, provided that the chemical in question has no adverse effect on human health and performs a useful function.

Many substances that can technically be termed "additives" have been in use for thousands of years - sugar, salt, and spices constitute just a few examples. Some additives come from natural sources; lecithin, derived from soybeans or corn, is used as an emulsifier to achieve the desired consistency in products such as cake mixes, non-dairy creamers, salad dressings, ice cream, and chocolate milk. Other food additives are factory made but are chemically the same as their natural analogs. The synthetic vitamins and minerals added to foods to improve nutritive value are examples of these; identical in chemical composition to natural vitamins and minerals found in food, they are preferentially used because they are less expensive and more readily available. Such synthetic additives frequently are more concentrated, more pure, and of a more consistent quality than some of their counterparts in the natural world.

The use of synthetic vitamins and minerals in food over the past half century has had a profound impact on public health in the United States, virtually eliminating certain deficiency diseases that in former years afflicted large numbers of Americans. The addition of vitamin D to milk, iodine to table salt, and niacin to bread has relegated rickets, goiter, and pellagra, respectively, to nearly nonexistent status in this country. Other additives perform such useful functions as retarding spoilage, preventing fats from turning rancid, retaining moisture in some foods and keeping it out of others.

Most people don't quarrel about additives used for these purposes. What does concern many scientists and laypersons alike is that a not-insignificant number of chemicals are used as food additives for purely cosmetic purposes— and many of these have been shown to be toxic, carcinogenic, or both.

Until 1958, food processors wishing to use a new additive were free to do so unless the FDA could prove that the additive in question was harmful to human health. With the passage of the Food Additives Amendment to the Food, Drug, and Cosmetic Act in that year, the situation was reversed: the manufacturer of any proposed food additive or new food-contact chemical (e.g. packaging materials, equipment liners) now has to satisfy the FDA that the product is safe before it can be approved for use. Proof of safety must include such considerations as: 1) the amount of' the additive that is likely to be con-sinned along with the food product; 2) the cumulative effect of ingesting small amounts of the additive over a long period of time; and 3) the potential for the additive to act as a toxin or a carcinogen when consumed by humans or animals. The FDA can rescind approval at any time if new information indicates that the additive in question is unsafe.

While protection of public health is the main intent of the Food Additives Amendment, the law is also designed to prevent consumer fraud by prohibiting the use of preservatives that make foods look fresher than they really are. A case in point is the regulation forbidding the use of sulfites on meats, since these restore the red color, deceptively lending a just slaughtered appearance to a variety of meat products. On the other hand, sodium nitrite, another additive recognized for its ability to "fix" the red color of fresh meats, can legally be added to meat, fish, and poultry because its primary purpose is to act as a preservative, deterring both spoilage and botulism, a deadly disease caused by the presence of a bacteria] toxin. Because it is now known that nitrites can react with other compounds in food to produce nitrosamines, substances known to be carcinogenic, food processors wishing to use the additive must take precautionary measures to severely limit nitrosamine formation.

Undoubtedly the section of the Food Additives Amendment that has generated the most heated controversy in recent years is the Delaney Clause, which flatly prohibits the use in food of any ingredient shown to cause cancer in animals or humans (people who question why the FDA bans certain moderately carcinogenic food dyes yet takes no action against cigarettes have to be reminded that the Delaney Clause pertains solely to carcinogenic food additives, not to carcinogens in general; if a food processor should propose to add cigarette smoke as a flavoring to, say, cured meats, this would undoubtedly be prohibited under the Delaney Clause). While many environmental groups feel that the Delaney Clause constitutes the public's sole line of defense against the deliberate addition of carcinogens to the nation's food supply, critics charge that the "zero tolerance" standard implicit in this mandate is unrealistic and an example of regulatory overkill which fails to recognize enormous advances in analytical techniques since the Delaney Clause was enacted in 1958. Whereas the best efforts at chemical analysis during the 1950s yielded results in the parts per million range, today's monitoring devices routinely detect the presence of chemical residues in the parts per trillion. New evidence for the existence of threshold levels of exposure for at least some carcinogens has added fuel to the debate as well (when the Delaney Clause was enacted it was presumed that any amount of exposure to a carcinogen, no matter how small, could result in cancer). The Food Quality Protection Act attempted to address these concerns to a limited extent when it amended the Delaney Clause in 1996 by excluding pesticide residues in processed food from regulation as food additives. The revised mandate now permits EPA to approve a tolerance level for residues of a carcinogenic pesticide so long as the agency determines that doing so presents a "negligible risk" (defined as no more than one cancer death per one million population) to consumers. For all other food additives, the "**zero tolerance**" standard explicit in the Delaney Clause remains intact and continues to generate heated debate.

Since many hundreds of food additives were already in widespread use at the time the 1958 amendment was passed, a portion of this legislation exempted such substances from the rigorous safety testing demanded for new additives. Instead, additives already in common usage were designated "**generally regarded as safe (GRAS)**" and placed on what is referred to as the GRAS list. In order to remove a food additive from the GRAS list, the FDA must demonstrate that the substance in question is harmful. Original screening of existing food additives to determine whether they should be placed on the GRAS list was done rather haphazardly, and by the 1970s it was recognized that longtime usage is no firm guarantee of safety. More thorough studies of certain substances included on the GRAS list have resulted in withdrawal of approval for the use of such once-common food additives as cyclamates (artificial sweeteners suspected of being carcinogenic); safrole (mutagenic and carcinogenic extract of sassafras root, formerly used to give root beer its characteristic flavor); and a number of coal-tar dyes (long used as food colorings but delisted because they were shown to be carcinogenic or to cause organ damage).

Numerous other additives still on the GRAS list are considered of dubious safety by many researchers, yet remain in use due to lack of conclusive evidence or because of industry pressure on FDA regulators. Critics of current policy insist that food additives require a higher standard of care than other environmental chemicals and shouldn't be used if they present a health risk. They base this judgment on the fact that everyone is exposed to chemicals in food, not only those who voluntarily assume the risk. Varying levels of susceptibility among individuals and the effects of simultaneous exposure to other chemicals, including synergistic effects, have to be taken into consideration. Both MSG (monosodium glutamate), a flavor enhancer that can cause the headache, dizziness, nausea, and facial flushing sometimes referred to as "**Chinese Restaurant Syndrome**," and a group of sulfur-containing compounds known collectively as "sulfites" or "sulfiting agents," added to certain foods, drugs, and wine to prevent discoloration and spoilage, are examples of food additives that serve a useful purpose and pose no danger to the majority of consumers but which can provoke severe allergic reactions among a sizeable minority of sensitive individuals. Because of the vast processed food market, any miscalculation of risk can have far-reaching implications on a public, which assumes and expects that special care is being taken with the nation's food supply. Nevertheless, although some health authorities recommend avoiding foods containing nonessential additives (such as artificial colors and flavorings) wherever possible, little evidence exists at present to indicate that the health of Americans is suffering due to the chemical food additives currently in use.

Ironically, while questions dealing with the safety of chemical additives generate most of the public's concern regarding food quality these days, most cases of illness or death due to food involve a number of old-fashioned food-borne diseases commonly referred to as "food poisoning." Food poisoning can result from a variety of causes, including Natural Toxins in Food.

The Food and Agricultural Organization and World Health Organization (WHO) define a food additive as a nonnutritive substance added intentionally to food, generally in small quantities, to improve its appearance, flavor, texture, or storage properties. Some of the additives used in foods are identified below.

1. **Vinegar** is used to lower the pH, thereby inhibiting the growth of microorganisms.
2. **Sugar** is used to enhance taste and nutritive value and to kilt bacteria by plasmolysis (shrinking of the bacterium cytoplasm as a result of loss of water).
3. **Salt** is used to enhance taste and nutritive value. It also induces plasmolysis. Salt has **potassium iodide** added to prevent simple goiter.
4. **Nitrates** give a rich color to meats. They are allowable in concentrations less than 200 parts per million (ppm), but in larger doses they reduce the ability of hemoglobin to carry oxygen and produce methemoglobinemia. Nitrates also may react to produce neurosamines, which cause concern about cancer.
5. **Formaldehyde**, formerly used as a preservative for milk and occasionally other foods now is prohibited by the laws of practically all nations.
6. **Salicylic acid**, formerly used extensively in jams, juices, and other sweets as a preservative now is prohibited in the United States.
7. **Potassium permanganate** is used on the surface of meat to hide evidence of decomposition.
8. **Benzoic acid and benzoate of soda** are weak germicides used in tomato catsup. They are allowable in concentrations up to 0.1 percent in certain foods.
9. **Borax and boric acid**, formerly used to preserve meats, milk, butter, oysters, clams, fish, sausage and other foods, are no longer allowed.
10. **Sulfites**, which act as an antiseptic and color preserver in red meats, are prohibited but frequently are found on ground meat or dusted lightly on wrapping paper and meat blocks.
11. **Cinnamon cloves** and **mustard** have antiseptic powers and are used as preservatives, as well as seasoning and flavoring.
12. **Additives used for seasoning** and **flavoring** include ginger, pepper, nutmeg, and garlic, among many others.
13. **Propionates** retard mold growth in bread.
14. **Nutrient supplements** are vitamins and minerals added to foods to improve their nutritive value. For example, thiamine (Vitamin B_1), riboflavin (Vitamin B_2), niacin, and iron must be added to bread if it is to be called enriched."
15. **Bleaching and maturing agents.** Freshly milled flour has a yellowish color caused by small quantities of pigments. Bleaching agents change the yellow pigment to white.

16. **Sulfur dioxide** is allowable for bleaching if it is labeled properly. It is not a preservative.

17. **Benzoyl peroxides** are used for bleaching agents.

18. **Coloring agents**. Today's consumer expects food to have a characteristic and appetizing color. To obtain this, substances may be added to correct the color change undergone during processing.

19. **Carotene**, an extract from carrots, often is added to products such as margarine to give the desired colon.

20. **Synthetic colors** are used frequently in soft drinks, cordials, frozen desserts, puddings, meat casings and many prepared mixes. A number of synthetic colors and dyes have been banned from use by the FDA.

21. **Leavening agents** are substances used to make foods light in weight.

22. **Yeasts** produce carbon dioxide by fermentation; thus, holes occur in breads and other yeast products.

23. **Baking soda**, when heated, releases carbon dioxide, which forms holes in bread and other baked products.

24. **Baking powder** contains baking soda, an acid salt, and starch. When water is added, the acid reacts with sodium bicarbonate in the soda to produce carbon dioxide. The starch then absorbs the water.

25. **Antioxidants** prevent an undesirable change in food when exposed to the air. An example is fresh sliced apples, which will turn brown upon being exposed to oxygen. Lemon, orange, and pineapple juices contain sorbic acid (Vitamin C) and are good antioxidants. Therefore, one can dip sliced apples in these juices to keep the apples from turning brown as readily. The darkening of some fruits and vegetables results from a type of oxidation known as "enzymatic browning." If these foods are bruised or cut and subsequently exposed to air, the tissue turns dark. Therefore, many times antioxidants are added to retain the natural color. Fats and oils become rancid as a result of oxidation. Butylated hydroxyanisole, sugar dioxide, propyl gallate, and thiodipropions acid are a few examples of antioxidants. They may not exceed *0.005* percent of total food content.

26. **Emulsifiers** often are added to attain consistency. For example, water and oil will not mix, but if an emulsifier is added, they will mix and stay mixed. Some examples are diglycerides from the glycerolysis of edible fats or oils, monosodium phosphates, and propylene glycol.

27. **Stabilizers** in small amounts account for the smooth, uniform tenure and flavor of many foods. Stabilizers are added to chocolate milk to prevent the chocolate particles from settling to the bottom, and to peanut butter to prevent separation. They also are used in ice cream to increase the viscosity of the ingredients and help prevent the formation of crystals. Some examples of stabilizers are agar-agar, carob bean gum, and guar gum.

28. **Thickeners** form a gel. Some fruits contain enough natural thickeners to form a gel - for example, berries and apples from which we make jams and jellies. Pectin and gelatin are good examples of thickeners.

29. **Sequestrants.** The word "sequester" means to set apart or to separate. Many fats and oils contain traces of iron- or copper. The sequestants keep these elements inactivate or allow their removal. Sequestrants also play a role in the soft drink industry, tying

up calcium, magnesium, and the like, preventing them from precipitating out in the beverages.

30. **Humectants** are used to keep moisture in foods. Before humectants were known to exist, people - had to buy a coconut, for example, and use it immediately. Now we can buy soft, fluffy, shredded coconut.

31. **Nonnutritive sweeteners** are of great benefit to persons who must limit their intake of ordinary sweets. They add only sweetness, not calories or other food value. Saccharine is a good example.

An egg is a good example of a multi-purpose additive. It serves as a thickener in custards, as a leavening agent to incorporate air in baked goods, as a catalyst in candies, and as an emulsifier in solids. Eggs add color, richness, and flavor to many foods, yet eggs are made of only natural elements. Liquid pasteurized eggs are recommended because raw eggs contain **Salmonella enteritidis** in the yolk when they are laid.

Population growth and our modern way of life have made food additives necessary. If regulated and controlled, food additives are not harmful. Thanks to the official enforcing agencies, we now can eat our food knowing that the additives have been tested and proven nontoxic to humans in the concentrations in which they are added.

IV. <u>FOOD POISONING</u>

A. <u>INTRODUCTION</u>

The widely prevalent notion that all "natural" foods are safe and nutritious is a dangerous misconception. The faddish trend toward "living off the land" by collecting and eating various types of wild plants has led to a surge in food poisoning cases, according to some local public health officials. The fact is that there are many common plants, both wild and cultivated, that are poisonous, capable of causing ailments ranging from mild stomach disorders to a quick and painful death if consumed by the unwary. In addition, certain marine fish and shellfish species may contain toxins that induce severe illness or death.

Favism is a disease caused by eating fava beans. The fava bean (vicia fava) is a main diet item in Mediterranean countries, grown and consumed by people of Italian descent. The danger stems from a nucleoside (vicine) that causes hemolysis. Blood in urine is a symptom. After insufficient cooking, lima beans, sweet peas, kidney beans, Jack beans, navy beans, and soybeans have been found to contain hemagglutinin, capable of agglutinating red blood cells. During the warm months, when the plankton Convaulax grows copiously, it turns the water red. Mussels that feed on the diatoms become poisonous. During "red tide", the plankton contain a strong alkaloid so poisonous that a few milligrams may prove fatal to humans within 5 to 30 minutes. Certain fish are poisonous as they contain a naturally occurring neurotoxin – not to mention mercury, and other poisons, from polluted water. Several types of fish are capable of causing poisoning in humans. Some examples of plants or animals capable of causing a toxic reaction if eaten include the following.

B. POISONING

1. Scombroid fish poisoning

Scombroid fish poisoning results from the ingestion of spoiled fish, primarily of the suborder **Scombroidei** (e.g., tuna, mackerel). Inadequate or delayed refrigeration at sea of fish taken from temperate and tropical waters results in overgrowth of bacteria *(***Proteus morganii***,* among others) that normally comprise the microflora of fish. These bacteria metabolize histidine and degrade the protein of fish flesh to produce scombrotoxin, which consists of histamine and other amines. Since orally administered histamine has no effect in humans, perhaps co-contaminants like cadaverine, putrescine, and other products of fish decomposition enhance the toxic action of histamine by inhibiting histaminases in the human intestine. (Similarly, drugs such as isoniazid, which inhibit histamine-detoxifying enzymes, have evoked reactions to low levels of histamine normally found in such foods as cheese). Scombroid fish poisoning is sometimes misdiagnosed as "fish allergy." Symptoms develop about 30 minutes after eating and include a peppery sensation of the tongue, rash, flushing (sometimes urticaria), pruritus, headaches, dizziness, periorbital edema, thirst, nausea, vomiting, diarrhea, and abdominal cramps. Some of these symptoms resemble histamine reaction and respond to antihistamine therapy. Laboratory studies of implicated fish frequently show "honey-combing" (a sign of decomposition), bad odor, and histamine levels =50 mg/100 g. Scombrotoxin is heat stable and can withstand the temperatures used in canning; commercially canned fish has been implicated in several international outbreaks.

2. Ciguatera poisoning

Ciguatera poisoning can be caused by more than 400 species of fish that are primarily bottom-dwelling shore fish caught near reefs between 35°N and 35°S latitude. In the United States, 90 percent of outbreaks are reported from Hawaii and Florida and are due mostly to grouper, red snapper, and barracuda. Ciguatoxin is actually produced by certain dinoflagellates attached to algae on coral reefs. Small fish feed on the algae and are, in turn, eaten by larger bottom-dwelling shore fish and so on up the food chain. The larger fish are more toxic than smaller ones; organs such as liver, intestines, and gonads are the most toxic parts. The median latency period is 5 hours, and the median duration of symptoms is 8 days. Besides gastrointestinal symptoms of abdominal cramps, nausea, vomiting, and diarrhea, there may be numbness and paresthesia of lips and tongue, paresthesias of the extremities, metallic taste, arthralgia, myalgia, blurred vision, temporary blindness, and paradoxical temperature sensation. In those with life-threatening disease there may be hypotension, bradycardia, cranial nerve palsies, and respiratory paralysis. Therapy is primarily supportive, although intravenous mannitol has been reported to produce dramatic improvement. Tocainide, an orally effective lidocaine analog, has also been reported of value (presumably by blocking the toxic effect of ciguatoxin). Prevention is difficult; ciguatoxic fish do not appear or taste spoiled, and ordinary cooking does not destroy the heat-stable toxin. Unusually large reef fish should be avoided, especially their liver and roe.

3. Paralytic shellfish poisoning

Paralytic shellfish poisoning   is caused by the ingestion of filter-feeding bivalve mollusks (e.g., mussels and clams) that had previously ingested (without adverse effect) toxic dinoflagellates of **Alexandrium** sp. (formerly **Gonyaulax sp**.) and concentrated the neurotoxin saxitoxin in their tissues. Symptoms in humans usually begin about 30 minutes after eating, with paresthesias of the mouth, lips, face, and fingertips; then, in more severe cases, dysphagia, dysphonia, ataxia, weakness, paralysis, and occasionally respiratory arrest occur. Treatment is supportive and should include efforts to remove unabsorbed toxin from the gut. Fortunately, even in severe cases, symptoms disappear completely in 1 to 2 days. A standardized mouse bioassay is used for demonstrating and quantifying toxin in shellfish. Toxic dinoflagellates bloom in waters above 30°N and below 30°S latitude and sometimes impart a reddish color to the water - the so-called red tide. Regulatory agencies monitor shellfish and impose quarantines on harvesting them, when deemed necessary to protect the public health.

4. Cyclospora cayetanensis

Cyclospora cayetanensis (previously known as blue-green algae, cyanobacteria, and "big **Cryptosporidium***")* is a recently characterized coccidian parasite. Before 1996, only three outbreaks (all in the 1990s) had been reported in the United States. In the spring of 1996, however, a great number of outbreaks involving more than 1000 laboratory-confirmed cases occurred in states east of the Rocky Mountains. Investigations implicated fresh raspberries probably imported from Guatemala, but it was not possible to trace back to the farm(s) of origin or identify the mechanism(s) of contamination. Whether animals can serve as sources of infection is also unknown. The usual incubation period is about 1 week and the symptoms and protracted course are reminiscent of giardiasis. Diagnosis is by demonstration of **Cyclospora** oocysts in stool by modified acid-fast stain (the cysts are twice the size of **Cryptosporidia***).* Treatment is possible with trimethoprim-sulfamethoxazole. Produce eaten raw should be thoroughly washed but this may not entirely eliminate risk, and some fruits, such as raspberries, don't tolerate washing without becoming macerated.

5. Mushroom poisoning

Mushrooms constitute a gourmet's delight, provided, of course, that the item in question is a nonpoisonous variety. **Mushroom poisoning** can be produced by 50 species among the 2000 that are known. The problem is that there is no simple rule of thumb for distinguishing between those wild forms that are safe and those that are not. Although only a relatively few of the thousands of species found in North America are poisonous, they may look very much like nonpoisonous species and frequently even grow together. Even trained mycologists confuse toxic varieties with edible ones because of the extensive variations and intergradations between species; contrary to popular belief, there are no simple field tests to aid in differentiation. Mushroom poisons are conveniently divided into two categories based on their latency period: the delayed onset group and the rapid onset group. The most deadly types tend to have delayed onsets of at least 6 hours.

These include **Amanita phalloides, Amanita verna,** and certain **Galerina** species, which cause 90 percent of all deaths from mushrooms and produce heat-stable cyclic polypeptides toxic to kidneys and liver. One species of the amanitas is called the "**Death Angel**" and grows commonly in "fairy rings" in woods and on lawns. Just one or two bites of these alkaloid-containing amanitas can be fatal to an adult. Typically a biphasic illness is seen. There may be sudden onset of severe nausea, vomiting, bloody diarrhea, abdominal pain, and cardiovascular collapse 6 to 20 hours after ingestion. After a short phase of improvement, painful, tender hepatomegaly with jaundice and oliguria may develop. Confusion, coma, and convulsions are common. Death ensues in 30 to 50 percent of cases. There is no specific antidote for **Amanita** intoxication; treatment is mostly supportive but should include purgation and high enemas to remove unabsorbed toxin. Experimental or invasive treatment including hemodialysis or hemoperfusion, repeated doses of activated charcoal given orally, cytochrome c, penicillin, corticosteroids, or thioctic acid (which is available from the FDA) have not been subjected to controlled studies to confirm effectiveness. An algorithm for treating mushroom poisoning has been proposed.

The rapid onset group (2 hours or less) includes mushrooms that contain hallucinogens that produce psychotropic, LSD-like effects that begin minutes after eating as well as mushrooms with muscarinic effects of salivation, perspiration, lacrimation, increased bronchial secretions, abdominal pain, miosis, nausea, vomiting, diarrhea, and bradycardia beginning about 1 hour after ingestion. Atropine is a specific antidote for this intoxication. Other mushroom poisons primarily cause gastric irritation, produce disulfiram-like effects, or produce states resembling alcoholic intoxication.

6. Chinese Restaurant Syndrome

Chinese Restaurant Syndrome sometimes follows ingestion by those susceptible to monosodium glutamate (MSG), a flavor enhancer especially popular in Chinese restaurants. Illness typically begins 20 to 30 minutes after exposure and can include a flushed or burning sensation of the neck and face, perspiration, a heavy feeling in the precordial area, palpitations, headache, and lacrimation. Since absorption of MSG is rapid when the stomach is empty, the first course of a meal - typically soup - is a common vehicle. Susceptible individuals, who can be sensitive to just 2 g of MSG, should avoid eating foods containing MSG, especially on an empty stomach.

In 1981 an epidemic of a new illness tentatively designated "**toxic oil syndrome**" (**TOS**) occurred in Spain and resulted in 20,000 cases and 300 deaths. It was traced to the ingestion of unlabeled, illegally marketed rapeseed oil that had been denatured with aniline and further treated to remove the aniline before it was fraudulently sold to the public as pure olive oil. As yet unidentified toxic agents were probably produced during the illegal refining process but the resulting disease, which affected multiple organ systems in progression, suggested either a continued body burden of toxin(s) or, more probably, the triggering of a chronic autoimmune process. Unique was the common progression of disease through an initial phase of febrile pneumonia-like symptoms sometimes with rash, followed late in the first month by gastrointestinal problems and striking eosinophilia, and about 100 days after onset in severely affected cases by profound neuromuscular manifestations (myalgia, atrophy of major muscle groups, and contractures). In late 1989 a new disease, designated **eosinophilia-myalgia syndrome** (**EMS**), was identified. It shares many clinical features of the intermediate and chronic phases of TOS. In EMS a striking association has been found with oral preparations of L-tryptophan-containing products.

7. Methylmercury Poisoning

The hazard of **methylmercury poisoning** was dramatized in Japan. Those who consumed fish taken from Minamata Bay, which had received direct factory discharges of methylmercury, subsequently developed Minamata disease which was frequently fatal. Methylmercury poisoning may take weeks, months, and possibly even years before symptoms are manifest, and unlike poisoning from inorganic mercury, it primarily affects the central nervous system, especially the cerebellum and cerebrum, where damage is usually irreversible. Symptoms can include paresthesia, ataxia, emotional lability, blindness, deafness, and in those most severely affected, stupor, coma, and death. It is not generally appreciated that discharges of even relatively inoffensive metallic mercury can be converted via biological methylation to methylmercury by bottom-dwelling bacteria. These bacteria are then consumed by plankton, which are consumed by small fish, and these by larger fish, and so on up the food chain until humans fall victim. Human exposure can sometimes be more direct. Alkyl mercury compounds have been used for years as a fungicidal seed dressing. Although such seeds are meant for planting purposes only, they have occasionally been consumed by people who were unaware of the danger or were driven by starvation. In 1971, 80,000 tons of methylmercury-treated wheat and barley were imported by Iraq for planting. Some of the grain was used, however, in the preparation of homemade bread and resulted in 6000 hospital admissions and 400 deaths. Similar outbreaks were reported from Pakistan and Guatemala.

V. <u>SURVEILLANCE AND INVESTIGATION OF FOODBORNE DISEASES</u>

The surveillance of foodborne diseases has traditionally aimed at disease control through:

1. Identification and removal of contaminated products from the commercial market,
2. Identification and correction of improper food handling practices both in commercial establishments and in the home,
3. Identification and treatment of cases and carriers of foodborne disease, and
4. Knowledge of disease causation, trends, new etiologic agents, and their food vehicles.

In the data published by the Centers for Disease Control and Prevention (CDC) summarizing foodborne diseases in the United States in recent years, about 500 outbreaks have been reported annually. In only about 40 percent of these was a cause identified; of these, it has been bacterial about 75 percent of the time, chemical 20 percent, parasitic 3 percent, and viral 2 percent of the time. Most outbreaks of unknown etiology have had incubation periods of more than 15 hours and many had secondary cases, suggesting an infectious cause; many of these were probably viral but laboratory capability to diagnose

Norwalk-like agents is still not widely available. Most cases of bacterial origin involve **Salmonella, Staphylococcus,** and **Clostridium perfringens**. Accordingly, an appreciation of the different clinical features and incubation periods of these three diseases is important in the investigation of foodborne outbreaks. If a judgment as to probable cause can be made early in an epidemic investigation, then one can better decide on the most appropriate specimens and methods to select for study, and how far back in time to inquire about food exposures.

Procedures for the investigation of foodborne disease outbreaks are detailed in a monograph published by the International Association of Milk, Food, and Environmental Sanitarians, Inc. Some general points merit emphasis. Interviews with food handlers, patients, and control subjects should be conducted as soon as possible: memories fade, people scatter, and the suspect foods may be discarded and unavailable for study or, worse, consumed by others. The investigator should appreciate the urgent necessity to collect the facts and materials that may not be practical or sometimes even possible to obtain at a later time.

In a relatively small outbreak, an effort should be made to question all who were exposed, whether ill or not, for symptoms and food consumption history. To identify the responsible food(s), a retrospective cohort study design is commonly used. Rates of illness in those who ate specific food items (the "attribute" or "characteristic') are calculated and compared with the rates of illness in those who did not eat those items. The implicated foods generally have the highest attack rates. More important, however, is that when rates for eaters and noneaters are compared, the implicated foods show the greatest differences in attack rates. The difference is called the "attributable risk," or the rate of disease that can be attributed to the food under consideration. Alternatively, "relative risks" may be calculated by comparing, as a ratio, the rate of illness in those exposed to specific foods to the rate of illness in those not exposed. If the relative risk is significantly greater than 1.0, there may be an association between food exposure and illness. CDC has developed a popular software program called Epi Info for analyzing data collected in foodborne and other outbreak investigations. The necessity of interviewing well people in order to incriminate a particular food is illustrated by the item root beer, which might have been suspected as the cause of the outbreak. More ill people had root beer than any other item; in fact, all ill people had drunk some. However, it is evident that root beer was also consumed by nearly all those who remained well. The reason it was so popular is that it was the only drink available.

One might think that the association of illness with a particular implicated food should be "perfect" (i.e., all those who ate it must have become sick, and all those who got sick must have eaten it), but there are several reasons why this is rarely so:

1. The implicated food may not be contaminated throughout,
2. Host susceptibility varies,
3. Dosage (the quantity consumed) vanes,
4. Food histories may contain reporting errors through faulty recall, uncertainty, or lying; there may also be errors in recording,
5. Those who report illness but no exposure to the incriminated food may have coincidental, unrelated illness or secondary infection when the outbreak is due to

infection (e.g., **Salmonella**); alternatively, illness may be due to trace contamination of other foods or utensils by the implicated food.

If an outbreak is large and it is not possible to interview all participants, a random sample should be selected and questioned for symptoms and food exposure history. The data can be arranged in prospective fashion and similarly analyzed.

On the other hand, outbreaks can also be studied in a case-control fashion; and, in fact, there may be no alternative to case-control studies when the overall attack rate is low. In such situations the frequencies with which specific food items were selected by patients are compared with the frequencies in controls; that is, the so- called "food preference" rates are compared and odds ratios calculated. Food preference rates can also be effectively used when recall for specific food items is compromised as can occur in patients ill with diseases that have especially long incubation periods, such as hepatitis A.

The remainder of this chapter briefly describes the prevention of foodborne illness including food quality assurance, food safety, sanitation, and regulation.

VI. PREVENTION OF FOODBORNE ILLNESS

A. INTRODUCTION

The causes of foodborne illness can be the food itself, the personnel who handle the food, equipment used to pick, process and/or serve food, and the environment and/or facilities used in the processing, transport, storage, and preparation of food.

Certain foods are poisonous in and of themselves, while any food can serve as a simple vehicle on or in which the organisms and chemicals discussed above are carried due to contamination from people, sewage, or vectors. Certain foods, however, are more conducive for the support and multiplication of pathogens and thus are potentially more hazardous. These are perishable foods of animal origin, such as milk, milk products, eggs, meat, poultry, fish, and shellfish. No plant or animal product will ever be sterile, however, the introduction of human pathogens must be prevented.

Processing as used here includes any activity involved in getting raw food from the field or slaughterhouse to the table. Processes, which prevent foodborne illness, are those that take the growth characteristics of the organisms into account. Bacteria grow exponentially. They are also stressed by environmental conditions such as a rapid temperature change from cold to warm. Fortunately, this stress results in what is known as a "lag phase" of growth from 2 to 4 hours during which the organisms are multiplying very slowly or not at all. One of the main goals of food processing, therefore, is to prevent foods, especially hazardous foods, from remaining at temperatures conducive to growth for longer than 4 hours. Two hours is recommended for a margin of safety.

Proper time - temperature control is also important during canning, pasteurization, and cooking of food. High temperatures are used to destroy bacterial cells and spores, viruses, and to inactivate enzymes and other chemicals, which may cause spoilage or illness. Processing must be designed so that sufficiently high temperatures are reached in all parts of the food for sufficient time to achieve the desired destruction. Pasteurization is accomplished for milk by heating to 161°F for 15 continuous seconds or 145°F for 30 continuous minutes. Temperatures and times for both canning and freezing are specific both to the food and the process since they are based on the characteristics of the food (e.g., pH) and of the pathogen or toxin, most likely to be found in a particular food.

Food which has been properly heated or cooked may still be contaminated during processing directly by food - handling personnel. Contamination from personnel is consistently identified as the second leading factor involved in outbreaks.

There are federal bacterial standards only for milk and milk products, frozen cream pies, and gelatin. There are also standards for "filth," such as insect parts and rodent hairs. These objects do not constitute a direct health hazard, but rather serve as an indicator of the hygiene practices within a food-processing establishment. Due to the difficulty in determining a meaningful standard and actually enforcing that standard for all of the food consumed, food protection is regulated by equipment, temperature, and personnel practices specifications.

B. FOOD QUALITY ASSURANCE

To ensure high quality of the food supply, a number of parties must play specific roles. The main actors include the government, consumers, and the food industry. The government is responsible for the establishment of standards or codes of practice as well as the enforcement of laws and regulations. Furthermore, it should encourage the food industry to undertake voluntary measures to improve food safety, such as providing advice and guidance. Consumers in turn should be well aware of the quality of the food they buy, prepare, and consume and should adopt appropriate practices of food handling at home. At the industry level, all segments, including agriculture, should establish some system for safety assurance of their products and employ appropriate procedures and technologies.

The flow of raw food materials to actual consumption is schematically presented in Figure 9.2, including the accompanying hazards and risks. In principle, the same flow scheme applies to both the food industry and to locally produced foods for private consumption, although in the latter case the food processing, storage, and transport stages will be relatively short. In such a situation, adequate monitoring of food quality is usually more difficult to achieve. All steps in this process and possible preventive measures for ensuring food quality at various stages are briefly presented here.

C. FOOD SAFETY

The objective of food processing and preparation is to provide safe, wholesome, and nutritious food to the consumer. The responsibilities for accomplishing this objective lie with every step in the food chain, beginning with food production and continuing through processing, storage, distribution, retail sale, and consumption. Producing safe food is a continuum, where each party has certain obligations to meet and certain reasonable expectations of the other parties involved in the process. No single group is solely responsible for producing safe food, and no single group is without obligations in ensuring the safety of food.

Production of Raw Materials ⇓	Hazards: -Nutrients -Natural toxins -Microbial toxins -Environmental contaminants
Food Processing ⇓	Hazards: -Reaction products -Contaminants -Additives
Storage and Transport ⇓	Hazards: -Chemical contamination -Microbial contamination
Food Preparation ⇓	Hazards: -Chemical contamination -Microbial contamination
Food Consumption ⇓	Risks: -Intoxication by chemical contaminants -Foodborne infections -Food poisonong

Figure 9.2. Flow Scheme of Food Production to Food Consumption. (Source: Yassi, 2001).

Food producers have a reasonable expectation that the food he or she produces will be processed in such a manner that further contamination is minimized. Food producers are an integral part of the food production system, but are not solely responsible for food safety. It is not practical to deliver fresh unprocessed food that is completely free of microorganisms, whether the food in question is apples or livestock. The environment in which the food is produced precludes the possibility that uncontaminated food can be grown or produced. However, appropriate methods can be used to reduce, to the extent possible, this level of background contamination. Alternately, producers have an obligation to use these same reasonable practices to prevent hazards from entering the food chain. As an example, when dairy cattle are treated with antibiotics for mastitis, producers have an obligation to withhold milk from those animals from the normal production lot. Milk from these animals must be withheld for the specified withdrawal time, so that antibiotic residues will not occur in milk delivered to dairies. In contrast, production of salmonellae-free poultry in the United States has been an elusive goal for poultry producers. While it is not a reasonable expectation for producers to deliver salmonellae-free birds to poultry processors, it is reasonable to expect producers to use good management practices to minimize the incidence of **Salmonella** within a flock.

Food processors have reasonable expectations that raw materials delivered to the processing facility are of reasonable quality and not contaminated with violative levels of any drugs or pesticides. In addition, processors have a reasonable expectation that processed food will be properly handled through the distribution and retail chain, and that it will be properly prepared by the consumer. The latter is particularly important, as processors have responsibility for products because they are labeled with the processor's name, even though the food is no longer under processor control once it leaves the processing facility. Processor obligations are to process raw foods in a manner that minimizes growth of existing microorganisms as well as minimizes additional contamination during processing. These obligations extend from general facility maintenance to the use of the best available methods and technologies to process a given food.

Clearly, consumers have an important role in the microbiological safety of foods. However, it is not reasonable to expect every consumer to have a college degree in microbiology. Consumers have a reasonable expectation that foods they purchase have been produced and processed under hygienic conditions. They also have a reasonable expectation that foods have not been held under unsanitary conditions, or that foods have not been adulterated by the addition of any biological, chemical, or physical hazards. In addition, consumers have an expectation that foods will be appropriately labeled, so that the consumer has information available on both composition and nutritional aspects of products. These expectations are enforced by regulations that govern production, processing, distribution, and retailing of foods in the United States. The vast majority of foods meets or exceeds these expectations, and the average consumer has relatively little to be concerned with regarding the food they consume.

Some consumers have advocated additional expectations, which may or may not be reasonable. For example, some would argue that raw foods should be free of infectious microorganisms. Initially, this would appear to be reasonable; however, in many cases, technologies or processes do not exist in a legal or cost-effective form to ensure that raw foods are not contaminated with infectious agents. Two recent examples are the outbreaks of **Cyclospora** epidemiologically linked to imported raspberries and **Escherichia coli** O157:H7 in raw ground beef. With the exception of irradiation, technologies do not exist to ensure that either of these foods would be absolutely free of infectious agents while stilt retaining desirable characteristics associated with raw food. Therefore, in some cases, the expectation that raw foods should be free of infectious agents may not be reasonable.

Consumers have several obligations regarding food safety. As part of the food production to consumption chain, consumers have similar obligations to food processors. Namely, not holding foods under unsanitary conditions prior to consumption and not adulterating foods with the addition of biological, chemical, or physical agents. Improper food handling can increase food-borne illness risks by allowing infectious bacteria to increase in numbers or by allowing for cross- contamination between raw and cooked foods. In addition, consumers have an obligation to use reasonable care preparing foods for consumption, as do personnel in food service operations. As an example, consumers should cook poultry until it is "done" (internal temperature at or above 155°F) to eliminate any concerns with salmonellae.

Consumer education on the basics of food safety in the home should be a priority. Every consumer should understand that food is not sterile, and that the way food is handled in the kitchen may affect the health of individuals consuming it. Although our long-term goal is to reduce or eliminate food-home disease hazards, in the near term we need to remind consumers of what some of the potential risks are and how consumers can avoid them. In the end, it is the consumers who decide what they will or will not eat.

D. SANITATION

Sanitation is the fundamental program for all food processing operations, irrespective of whether they are converting raw products into processed food or preparing food for final consumption. Sanitation affects all attributes of processed foods, from organoleptic properties of the food to the safety and quality of the food itself. From a food processor's perspective, an effective sanitation program is essential to producing quality foods with reasonable shelf lives. Without an effective program, even the best operational management and technology will ultimately fail to deliver the quality product that consumers demand.

Sanitation programs are all-encompassing, focusing not only on the details of soil types and chemicals, but on the broader environmental issues of equipment and processing plant design. Many foodborne microorganisms, both spoilage organisms and bacteria of public health significance, can be transferred from the plant environment to the food itself. Perhaps one of the most serious of these microorganisms came to national and international attention in the mid 1980s, when **Listeria monocytogenes** was found in processed dairy products. **Listeria** was considered to be a relatively minor veterinary pathogen until that time, and not even considered a potential foodborne agent. However, subsequent research demonstrated that **L. monocytogenes** was a serious human health concern and, more importantly, was found to be widely distributed in nature. In many food processing plants, **Listeria** was found to be in the general plant environment, and subsequently efforts have been made to improve plant sanitation, through facility and equipment design as well as focusing more attention on basic cleaning and sanitation.

1. Sanitary Plant Design

Some of the basic considerations of food plant design include the physical separation of raw and processed products, adequate storage areas for nonfood items (such as packaging materials), and a plant layout that minimizes employee traffic between raw and processed areas. While these considerations are easily addressed in newly constructed facilities, they may present challenges in older facilities that have been renovated or expanded. Exposed surfaces, such as floors, walls, and ceilings, in the processing area should be constructed of material that allows for thorough cleaning. Although these surfaces are not direct food contact surfaces, they contribute to overall environmental contamination in the processing area. These surfaces are particularly important in areas where food is open to the environment, and the potential for contamination is greater when temperature differences in the environment result in condensation. As an example, a large open cooking kettle will generate some steam that may condense on surfaces above the kettle. This condensate may, without proper design and sanitation, drip back down into the product, carrying any dirt and dust from overhead surfaces back into the food. Other obvious considerations are basic facility maintenance as well as insect and rodent control programs, as all of these factors may contribute to contamination of food.

2. Sanitary Equipment Design

Many of the same considerations for sanitary plant design also apply to the design of food processing equipment. Irrespective of its function, processing equipment must protect food from external contamination and from conditions that will allow existing bacteria to grow. The issue of condensate as a form of external contamination has already been raised. Opportunities for existing bacteria to reproduce may be found in the so-called dead spaces within some equipment. These areas can allow food to accumulate over time under conditions that allow bacteria to grow. These areas then become a constant inoculation source for additional product as it moves through the equipment, increasing the bacteriological population within the food. Other considerations of food equipment design include avoiding construction techniques that may allow the product to become trapped within small areas of the equipment, creating the same situation that occurs in the larger dead spaces within the equipment. As an example, lap seams that are tack welded provide ample space for the product to become trapped. Not only does this create a location for bacteria to grow and contaminate the food product, it also creates a point on the equipment that is difficult, if not impossible, to clean.

3. Personnel

A final element in food plant sanitation programs is the personnel who perform the sanitation operations as well as the employees who work in the processing area. Sanitation personnel should be adequately trained to understand the importance of their function in the overall processing operation in addition to the training necessary to properly use the chemicals and equipment necessary for them to perform their duties. Personnel who are actually involved in processing operations should also understand the necessity for proper cleaning and sanitation and not simply rely on the sanitation crew to take care of all issues. In addition, all employees must be aware of basic issues of personal hygiene, especially when they are in direct contact with food or food processing equipment. Some key elements, such as hand washing and wearing clean clothing and gloves, should be reemphasized on a periodic basis. This information has been outlined by the U.S. Food and Drug Administration in the Good Manufacturing Practices section of the Code of Federal Regulations.

4. Cleaning and Sanitizing

Cleaning and sanitizing processes can be generically divided into five separate steps that apply to any sanitation task. The first step is removal of residual food, waste materials, and debris. This is frequently referred to as a "dry" cleanup. The dry cleanup is followed by a rinse with warm (48 to 55°C) water, to remove material that is only loosely attached to surfaces and to hydrate material that is more firmly attached to surfaces. Actual cleaning follows the warm water rinse, which usually involves the application of cleaning chemicals and some form of scrubbing force, either with mechanical brushes or with high-pressure hoses. The nature of the residual food material will determine the type of cleaning compound applied. After this, surfaces are rinsed and inspected for visual cleanliness. At this point, the cleaning process is repeated on any areas that require further attention. Carbohydrates and lipids can generally be removed with warm to hot water and sufficient mechanical scrubbing. Proteins require the use of alkaline cleaners, while mineral deposits can be removed with acid cleaners. Commercially available cleaning compounds generally contain materials to clean the specific type of food residue of concern, as well as surfactants and, as necessary, sequestrants that allow cleaners to function more effectively in hard water.

When surfaces are visually clean, a sanitizer is applied to reduce or eliminate remaining bacteriological contamination. Inadequately cleaned equipment cannot be sanitized, as the residual food material will protect bacteria from the sanitizer. One of the most common sanitizing agents, widely used in small- and medium-sized processing facilities, is hot water. Most regulatory agencies require that, when hot water is used as the sole method of sanitization, the temperature must be at or above 85°C. While heat sanitization in effective, it is not as economical as chemical sanitizers because of the energy costs required to maintain the appropriate temperature. Chlorine-containing sanitizers are economical and effective against a wide range of bacterial species and are widely used in the food industry. Typically, the concentrations of chlorine applied to equipment and surfaces are in the 150- to 200-ppm range. Chlorine sanitizers are corrosive and can, if improperly handled, release chlorine gas into the environment.

Iodine-containing sanitizers are less corrosive than chlorine sanitizers, but are also somewhat less effective. These sanitizers must be used at slightly acidic pH values to allow for the release of free iodine. The amber color of iodine sanitizers can give an approximate indication of concentration, but can also leave residual stains on treated surfaces. Quaternary ammonium compounds (QACs) are non- corrosive and demonstrate effective bactericidal action against a wide range of microorganisms. These sanitizers are generally more costly and not as effective as chlorine compounds, but they are stable and provide residual antimicrobial activity on sanitized surfaces. Food processing plants will frequently alternate between chlorine and QAC sanitizers to prevent development of resistant bacterial populations or will use chlorine sanitizers on regular production days and then apply QACs during periods when the facility is not operating (for example, over a weekend).

E. REGULATION

1. National Executive Agencies

Responsibility for regulating food is diffused among several national executive agencies (FDA, USDA, EPA, FTC, ICC, DOD, DOC, DOI, State Department), Congress federal courts, and state and local agencies:

a. FDA regulates most food substances, monitors pesticides, and enforces pesticide tolerances set by EPA,
b. USDA regulates meat and poultry,
c. EPA registers pesticides and sets tolerances for pesticides,
d. FTC monitors advertising claims,
e. ICC sets safety standards for food transportation,
f. DOD is an independent food safety authority,

g. DOC/DOI regulates marine and fishery production,
h. State Department regulates exports and imports,
i. Congress legislates and interprets food laws, e.g., suspension of FDA's saccharin ban,
j. Courts interpret food laws, e.g., FDA's ban on DES was overturned.

A food substance will be regulated differently depending on its assignment to one of 8 major categories of substances as currently defined by the Food, Drug, and Cosmetic Act. These categories are not mutually exclusive and regulatory efforts frequently become complicated and confusing.

2. Historical development of food laws

1906- Pure Food and Drugs Act- first federal food law. It prohibited the marketing of any food containing an "added" poisonous or deleterious substance that "may render such article injurious to health". It did not authorize the USDA to regulate naturally occurring harmful substances or to require premarket proof of safety.

1938- Food, Drug, and Cosmetic Act divided substances into those "added" and those "not added." To ban either of these two types of substances from food, the FDA had to prove it was toxic and unnecessary in food. The Act did not require premarket proof of safety. FDA could permit the use of unavoidable poisonous substances that were required to produce food which would otherwise be banned.

1947- Insecticide, Fungicide, and Rodenticide Act required all pesticide products to be registered before they were marketed.

1954- Pesticide Chemical Amendments to FDC Act authorized FDA to set tolerances for pesticide residues on raw agricultural commodities.

1958- Food Additives Amendment to FDC Act prohibited use of new food additives until manufacturer established safety and FDA issued regulations specifying conditions of use. The FDA cannot consider benefits in deciding how to regulate these substances. "Food additive" refers to substances (including radiation) used in production, manufacture, processing, holding, packaging, preparation, and transport. For example, direct food additives include flavors, antioxidants, and emulsifiers (3lb/person/year, 1975 estimate). Indirect food additives include impurities in direct additives (OTS, CHA), migrants from packaging materials (vinylchloride, acrylonitrile), and processing solvents (trichloroethylene). The amendment contains the anticancer clause: "no additive shall be deemed to be safe if it is found to induce cancer when ingested by man or animal, or if it is found, after tests which are appropriate for the evaluation of the safety of food additives, to induce cancer in man or animal." Frequency, severity, and dose considerations are not required. No threshold of effect is assumed. The amendment defined several classes of food substances as not being food additives: GRAS substances, prior sanction substances, pesticides, color additives, and animal drugs.

GRAS (generally recognized as safe) status was based primarily on long use before 1958, e.g. flavors, sucrose, salt, corn syrup, dextrose, MSG, formerly saccharin and cyclamate. GRAS substances can be used in any amount in any food. Few GRAS substances were subjected to complete toxicity testing. After the cyclamate ban in 1970, the entire list was reviewed and 4% of the hundreds of GRAS substances were re-classified as regulated food additives.

Prior sanctioned substances are those given FDA or USDA permission for use prior to 1/1/58, e.g. nitrite/nitrate (1925), antioxidants, stabilizers, and chemicals; used in food packaging. Toxicological evaluation was generally not required.

1960- Color Additive Amendment to FDC Act authorized FDA to set safe limits on the amounts of colors which may be used in foods, drugs, and cosmetics and to require manufacturers to retest previously listed colors. Contains the Delaney anticancer clause.

1968- New Animal Drug Amendment to the FDC Act authorized the use of carcinogenic animal drugs if no residue is found in any edible portion of animals or products derived from them.

1972- Environmental Pesticide Control Act gave EPA authority to set about 6000 tolerances for pesticides. The manufacturer must demonstrate that the product will not pose unreasonable adverse effects on the environment after economic, social, and environmental costs and benefits are accounted.

All of the preceding legislation has resulted in eight categories of food substances which have unique safety criteria:

a. **An added poisonous substance** which is required in the production of food or which cannot be avoided by good manufacturing practice, e.g. mercury & PCB's in fish, PBB's in animal products. FDA sets **"action levels"** for these,

b. **A food additive**, e.g., saccharin, vinyl chloride, beta-naphthylamine, and trichloroethylene. FDA establishes conditions of use for these substances,

c. **A GRAS substance**, e.g. salt, sugar, vinegar,

d. **A prior sanction substance**, e.g. nitrites in meat and poultry, caffeine in soft drinks,

e. **A pesticide chemical,** e.g. heptachlor, DDT,

f. **A color additive**, e.g. Red 2, 40,

g. **An animal drug residue**, e.g. nitrofuran and DES residues in beef,

h. **A naturally occurring poisonous substance**, e.g. solanine in potatoes, oxalic acid in rhubarb, aflatoxin in peanuts. In some cases FDA sets "action levels."

Several regulatory groups, from local and state agencies to international agencies, are involved in the regulation of food safety and quality standards. Since there is tremendous variation within and between local and state agencies, this discussion is confined to the national and international agencies that regulate food. At the national level, two federal agencies regulate the vast majority of food produced and consumed in the United States, namely, the U.S. Department of Agriculture (USDA) and the Food and Drug Administration (FDA).

F. U.S. DEPARTMENT OF AGRICULTURE

The USDA has responsibility for certification, grading, and inspection of all agricultural products. All federally inspected meat and meat products, including animals, facilities, and procedures, are covered under a series of meat inspection laws that began in 1906 and have been modified on several different occasions, culminating in the latest revisions in 1996. These laws cover only meat that is in interstate commerce, leaving the legal jurisdiction of intrastate meats to individual states. Key elements in meat inspection are examination of live animals for obvious signs of clinical illness and examination of gross pathology of carcasses and viscera for evidence of transmissible diseases. The newest regulations also require the implementation of a hazard analysis critical control point (HACCP) system and microbiological testing of carcasses after chilling. Eggs and egg products are also covered by USDA inspection under the Egg Products Inspection Act of 1970. This act mandates inspection of egg products at all phases of production and processing. All USDA inspection is continuous; that is, products cannot be processed without an inspector or inspectors present to verify the operation.

G. FOOD AND DRUG ADMINISTRATION

The FDA has responsibility for ensuring that foods are wholesome, safe, and have been stored under sanitary conditions, as outlined by the Food, Drug and Cosmetic Act of 1938. This act has been amended to include food additives, packaging, and labeling. The last two issues relate not only to product safety and wholesomeness, but also to nutritional labeling and economic fraud. The FDA is also empowered to act if pesticide residues exceed tolerances set by the Environmental Protection Agency. Unlike USDA inspection, FDA inspection is discontinuous, with food processing plants being required to maintain their own quality control records while inspectors themselves make random visits to facilities.

H. MILK SANITATION

Perhaps one of the greatest public health success stories of the twentieth century has been the pasteurization of milk. The U.S. Public Health Service drafted a model milk ordinance in 1924, which has been adopted by most local and state regulatory authorities and has become known as the PMO (Pasteurized Grade A Milk Ordinance). This ordinance covers all phases of milk production, including but not limited to animal health, design and construction of milk processing facilities, equipment, and most importantly, the pasteurization process itself. The PMO sets quality standards for both raw and processed milk, in the form of cooling requirements and bacteriological populations. The PMO also standardizes the pasteurization requirements for fluid milk, which ensures that bacteria of public health significance will not survive in the finished product. From a historical perspective, it is interesting to note that neither the public nor the industry initially embraced pasteurization, but that constant pressure from public health officials finally succeeded in making this important advance in public health almost universal.

I. INTERNATIONAL ADMINISTRATION

The Codex Alimentarius Commission, created by the Food and Agriculture Organization and the World Health Organization, has the daunting task of implementing food standards on an international scale. These standards apply to both general and specific food categories and also set limits for pesticide residues in foods. Acceptance of these standards is voluntary and at the discretion of individual governments, but acceptance of the standards requires that the country apply them equally to both domestically produced and imported products. The importance of international standards is growing daily as international trade in food expands. Many countries find that they are both importing and exporting foods, and a common set of standards is critical in establishing trade without the presence of nontariff trade barriers.

J. HAZARD ANALYSIS CRITICAL CONTROL POINT SYSTEM (HACCP)

In confronting the challenge of how best to ensure the safety of food supplies from biological, chemical, or physical hazards, government regulators and food industry quality assurance personnel alike have traditionally relied on an approach that involved periodic inspections of food processing facilities (e.g. mills, slaughterhouses, canneries, bakeries, supermarkets, restaurants, etc.) and random end-product analyses. The mandated inspection system for meat and poultry still relies on visual examination, the inspector touching and sniffing carcasses to detect signs of disease or spoilage. Most food safety experts decry this approach as outdated and completely useless for identifying the presence of the foodborne pathogens that constitute today's most urgent food quality concerns. The ineffectiveness of trying to protect public health in this manner through sole reliance on efforts to detect problems after-the-fact is attested by the continued prevalence of foodborne disease.

In recent years a paradigm shift has been occurring in the way regulatory agencies approach foodborne disease prevention. Moving away from a nearly century-old reactive food safety strategy, regulators are turning instead to a science-based concept called the Hazard Analysis and Critical Control Point system, or **HACCP** (pronounced "**hassip**").

The basic concept of HACCP was developed in the early 1960s as a joint effort to produce food for the space program. The U.S. Air Force Space Laboratory Project Group, the U.S. Army Natick Laboratories and the National Aeronautics and Space Administration contributed to the development of the process, as did the Pillsbury Company, which had a major role in developing and producing the actual food products.

The concept like so many other innovations of the late 20th-century American life, originated with the space program. In the late 1930s, NASA asked the Pillsbury Company to produce a food that could be eaten by astronauts in orbit. Such an undertaking presented a number of challenges, none more daunting than the imperative of ensuring that any food developed be 100% free of microbial, chemical, or physical contamination. The potentially disastrous consequences of a food poisoning outbreak inside a space capsule had to be avoided at any cost.

Pillsbury scientists realized that only a proactive preventive system could provide the high degree of safety assurance required. Pillsbury spent the following decade developing and refining its concept and in 1971 adopted the HACCP approach in its own facilities. That same year the FDA awarded Pillsbury a contract to conduct classes for its employees on the HACCP system, and in 1973 the company published the first comprehensive document on HACCP principles as a training manual far FDA personnel. By the early 1980s a number of U.S. food companies, following Pillsbury's example, had established their awn HACCP programs, but HACCP's wider application in the public sector remained extremely limited. In 1980, several federal agencies requested that the National Academy of Sciences examine the potential applications for microbiological criteria in food. The result was a 1985 NAS publication that strongly recommended the application of HACCP in regulatory programs, stating that HACCP "provides a more specific and critical approach to the control of microbiological hazards in foods than that provided by traditional inspection and quality control approaches."

Since that time, the HACCP system has evolved and been refined, but still focuses on the original goal of producing food that is safe for consumption.

Since development, HACCP principles have been used in many different ways. However, recent interest in the system has been driven by changes in the regulatory agencies, specifically the USDA Food Safety and Inspection Service (FSIS) and the U.S. Food and Drug Administration. The USDA-FSIS recently revised the regulations that govern meat inspection to move all federally inspected meat plants to a HACCP-based system of production and inspection. The FDA has also changed the regulations for fish and seafood, again moving this to a HACCP-based system for production. It is likely, given current trends by federal agencies, that most commercially produced foods will be produced under HACCP systems within the next 10 years.

The goal of a HACCP system is to produce foods that are free of biological, chemical, and physical hazards. HACCP is a preventative system, designed to prevent problems before they occur, rather than trying to fix problems after they occur. Biological hazards fall into two distinct categories, those that can potentially cause infection and those that can potentially cause intoxications. Infectious agents require the presence of viable organisms in the food and may not, depending on the organisms and the circumstances, require that the organism actually reproduce in the food. As an example, **E. coli** O157:H7 has an extremely low infectious dose for humans (possibly less than 100 viable cells), and as such, the mere presence of the bacterium in foods is a cause for concern. In contrast, organisms involved in intoxications usually require higher numbers of the organism in the food to produce sufficient amounts of toxin to cause clinical illness in humans. However, some of the toxins involved in foodborne diseases are heat stable, so that absence of viable organisms in the food is not necessarily an indication of the relative safety of the food. **S. aureus** is a good example, where it typically requires greater than 1,000,000 to 10,000,000 cells per gram of food to produce sufficient toxin to cause illness in humans. However, because the toxin itself is extremely heat stable, cooking the food will eliminate the bacterium but not the toxin, and the food can still potentially cause an outbreak of foodborne illness.

Chemical hazards include chemicals that are specifically prohibited in foods, such as cleaning agents, as well as food additives that are allowed in foods but only at regulated concentrations. Foods containing prohibited chemicals or food additives in levels higher than allowed are considered adulterated. Adulterated foods are not allowed for human consumption and are subject to regulatory action by the appropriate agency (USDA or FDA). Chemical hazards can be minimized by ensuring that raw materials (foods and packaging materials) are acquired from reliable sources that provide written assurances that the products do not contain illegal chemical contaminants or additives. During processing, adequate process controls should be in place to minimize the possibility that an approved additive will be used at levels not exceeding maximum legal limits for both the additive and the food product. Other process controls and Good Manufacturing Practices (GMPs) should also ensure that industrial chemicals, such as cleaners or lubricants, will not contaminate food during production or storage.

Physical hazards are extraneous material or foreign objects that are not normally found in foods. For example, wood, glass, or metal fragments are extraneous materials that are not normally found in foods. Physical hazards typically affect only a single individual or a very small group of individuals, but because they are easily recognized by the consumer, are a source of many complaints. Physical hazards can originate from food processing equipment, packaging materials, the environment, and employees. Physical contaminants can be minimized by complying with good manufacturing practices and by employee training. While some physical hazards can be detected during food processing (e.g., metal by the use of metal detectors), many nonferrous materials are virtually impossible to detect by any means, and so control often resides with employees.

Development of a HACCP plan begins with the formation of a HACCP team. Individuals on this team should represent diverse sections within a given operation, from purchasing to sanitation. The team is then responsible for development of the plan. Initial tasks that the team must accomplish are to identify the food, method of distribution, the consumer, and intended use of the food. Having done this, the HACCP team should construct a flow diagram of the process and verify that this diagram is accurate.

The development of a HACCP plan (Figure 9.3) is based on seven principles or steps in logical order. With the flow diagram as a reference point, the **first principle or step** is to conduct a hazard analysis of the process. The HACCP team identifies all biological, chemical, and physical hazards that may occur at each step during the process.

Once the list is completed, it is reviewed to determine the relative risk of each potential hazard, which helps identify significant hazards. Risk is the interaction of likelihood of occurrence with severity of occurrence. As an extreme example, a sudden structural failure in the building could potentially contaminate any exposed food with foreign material. However, likelihood of the occurrence of such an event is small. In contrast, if exposed food is held directly below surfaces that are frequently covered with condensate, then the likelihood of condensate dripping on exposed food is considerably higher. An important point in the determination of significant hazards is a written explanation by the HACCP team regarding how the determination of "significant" was made. This documentation can provide a valuable reference in the future, when processing methods change or when new equipment is added to the production line.

The **second step** in the development of a HACCP plan is the identification of critical control points (CCPs) within the system. A CCP is a point, step, or procedure where control can be applied and a food safety hazard can be prevented, eliminated, or reduced to acceptable levels. An example of a CCP is the terminal heat process applied to canned foods after cans have been filled and sealed. This process, when properly conducted according to FDA guidelines, effectively eliminates a potential food safety hazard, **Clostridium botulinum**.

Once CCPs have been identified, the **third step** in the development of a HACCP plan is to establish critical limits for each CCP. These limits are not necessarily the ideal processing parameters, but the minimum acceptable levels required to maintain the safety of the product. Again, in the example of a canned food, the critical limit is the minimum time and temperature relationship to ensure that each can has met the appropriate standards required by FDA.

The **fourth step**, following in logical order, is to establish appropriate monitoring requirements for each critical control point. The intent of monitoring is to ensure that critical limits are being met at each critical control point. Monitoring may be on a continuous or discontinuous basis.

HAZARD CRITICAL CONTROL POINT (HACCP) SYSTEM
Assess the Hazards • Identify potentially hazardous foods. • Follow the flow of food to assess hazards at receiving, storing, preparing, cooking, holding, serving, cooling, and reheating. • Estimate risks.
Identify Critical Control Points (CCPs) • Develop procedure and flowcharts showing the flow of food and all of the CCPs.
Set up Procedures and Standards for CCPs • Standards must be met at each CCP and should be: measurable, based on fact, correct for the recipe, clear directions with specific actions.
Monitor CCPs • Check to see if standards are met. Employees should be involved in process. Standards must be met.
Take Corrective Actions • If standard not met, correct it. • Have specific steps for correction.
Set Up Record-Keeping System • Blank forms near equipment where they are to be used. • Notebooks to write down actions. • Flowcharts and recipes near work areas.
Verify That the System Works • Identify and assess all hazards. • CCPs selected. • Standards set with monitoring and schedules. • Corrective actions in place. • Monitoring being done. • Flaws or omissions corrected. • Monitoring equipment calibrated.

Figure 9.3. The Seven Key Principles of HACCP. (Source: Moore, 1999).

Presence of a physical hazard, such as metal, can be monitored continuously by passing all of the food produced through a metal detector. Alternately, presence of foreign material can be monitored on a continuous basis by visual inspection. Discontinuous inspection may involve taking analytical measurements, such as temperature or pH, at designated intervals during the production day. Some analytical measurements can be made on a continuous basis by the use of data recording equipment, but it is essential that continuous measures be checked periodically by production personnel.

The **fifth step** in the development of a HACCP plan is to establish appropriate corrective actions for occasions when critical limits are not met. Corrective actions must address the necessary steps to correct the process that is out of control (such as increasing the temperature on an oven) as well as addressing disposition of the product that was made while the process was out of control. A literal interpretation of the HACCP system and a CCP is that when a CCP fails to meet the critical limits, then the food product is potentially unsafe for human consumption. As a result, food produced while the CCP was not under control cannot be put into the normal distribution chain without corrective actions being taken to that product. Typically this means that the product must be either reworked or destroyed, depending on the nature of the process and the volume of product that was produced while the CCP was out of control. This argues for frequent monitoring, so that the actual volume of product produced during each monitoring interval is relatively small.

The **sixth step** in the development of a HACCP plan is the establishment of effective record-keeping procedures. In many respects, a HACCP plan is an elaborate record-keeping program. Records should document what was monitored, when it was monitored and by whom, and what was done in the event of a deviation. Reliable records are essential from both a business and regulatory perspective. From the business perspective, HACCP records allow a processor to develop an accurate longitudinal record of production practices and deviations. Reviewing HACCP records may provide insight on a variety of issues, from an individual raw material supplier whose product frequently results in production deviations, to an indication of an equipment or environmental problem within a processing plant. From a regulatory perspective, records allow inspectors to determine if a food processor has been fulfilling commitments made in the HACCP plan. If a processor has designated a particular step in the process as a CCP, then the processor should have records to indicate that the CCP has been monitored on a frequent basis and should also indicate corrective actions taken in the event of a deviation.

The **final step** in the development of a HACCP plan is verification. Verification can take many forms. Microbiological tests of finished products can be performed to evaluate the effectiveness of a HACCP plan. Alternately, external auditors can be used to evaluate all parts of the HACCP plan to ensure that the stated goals and objectives are being met. A HACCP plan must also be periodically reviewed and updated to reflect changes in production methods and use.

K. FOOD PRESERVATION

1. Principles of Food Preservation

Principles of food preservation rely on preventing or delaying microbial decomposition. This can be accomplished by using asepsis or removal. Preventing growth or activity of microbes with low temperatures, drying, anaerobic conditions, or preservatives can also be done. Killing or injuring microbes with heat, irradiation, or some preservatives is certainly effective. A second principle is to prevent or delay self-decomposition, which is done by destruction or inactivation of enzymes (blanching) or by preventing or delaying auto- oxidation (antioxidants). The last principle is to prevent physical damage caused by insects, animals, and mechanical forces, which prevents entry of microorganisms into food. Physical barriers (packaging) are the primary means of protection. To control microorganisms in foods, many methods of food preservation depend not on the destruction or removal of microbes but rather on delaying the initiation of growth or hindering growth once it has begun.

For food preservation to succeed, one must be able to manipulate the microbial growth curve. Many steps can be done to lengthen the lag phase or positive acceleration phase of a population. These steps include: (a) prevent introduction of microbes by reducing contamination (fewer numbers gives a longer lag phase); (b) avoid addition of actively growing organisms that may be found on unclean containers, equipment, and utensils; and (c) create unfavorable environmental conditions for growth. The last step is the most important in food preservation and can be done by low water activity, extremes of temperature, irradiation, low pH, adverse redox potential, and by adding inhibitors and preservatives. Some of these steps may only damage or injure microorganisms; hence, the need for multiple barriers becomes essential. For each of these steps to be effective, other factors should be considered. For example, the number of organisms present determines kill rate. Smaller numbers give faster kill rates. Vegetative cells are most resistant to lethal treatments when in late lag or stationary phase and least resistant when in log phase of growth.

Normal microflora of foods are characterized by food type and growing and handling practices. Foods of plant origin have flora on outer surfaces. Animals too have flora on surfaces, but also have intestinal flora and secretion flora. Outside sources, such as soil, dust, water, humans, and equipment, can be significant sources of disease-causing microbes. Use of diseased animals for foods is dangerous because they often carry human pathogens. It should be noted that the inner tissues of plants and animals are generally sterile; however, cabbage inner leaves have lactobacilli and animal intestinal tracts have numerous microbes. Pathogens found on fruits and vegetables are from soil origin (**Clostridium Bacillus**) or from contaminated water, fertilizer, or food handlers. Some grain and nut products are naturally contaminated in the field with mycotoxin-producing molds. Soil is also a source of contamination of foods from animal origin. Animal feces can harbor coliforms, **C. perfringens**, enterococci, and enteric pathogens. Milk from infected udders (mastitis) can carry disease causing **Streptococcus pyogenes** and S. **aureus**. Nonmastitic udders can shed **Brucella**, **Rickettsia**, and viruses.

Outside sources of contamination that are not normally associated with food can be important in terms of food safety. Soil and dust contain very large numbers and a large variety of microbes. Many microorganisms responsible for food spoilage come from these sources. Contamination is by direct contact with soil, water, or by airborne dust particles. Air can carry microorganisms from other sources such as sneezing, coughing, dust, and aerosols. Pathogens, mold spores, yeast, and spoilage bacteria can be then disseminated. Organic debris from plants or animals is an excellent source. Microorganisms can grow on walls, floors, and other surfaces and act as a source of contamination during food processing and preparation. Airborne particles can be removed by filtration or by electrostatic precipitation.

Treated sewage may be used for fertilizer, although due to large amounts of toxic compounds such as heavy metals it is not used often for this purpose." Sewage can be an excellent source of pathogens including all enteric Gram-negative bacteria, enterococci, **Clostridium**, viruses, and parasites. Sewage that contaminates lakes, streams, and estuaries has been linked to many seafood outbreaks. In addition, water used for food must be safe for drinking and must be treated and free of pathogens. Furthermore, water must not contain toxic wastes. Water in food processing is typically used for washing, cooling, chilling, heating, ice, or as an ingredient. Stored water (reservoirs) and underground water (wells) are usually self-purifying.

Numbers and types of microorganisms found in foods depends on: (a) the general environment from which the food was obtained, (b) quality of raw food, (c) sanitary conditions under which the food was processed or handled, and (d) adequacy of packaging, handling, and storage of foods. The Hurdle Concept uses multiple methods (multibarrier approach) to food preservation and is the most common. Examples include pasteurized milk (heat, refrigeration, and packaging) or canned beans (heat, anaerobiosis, and packaging).

2. Asepsis/Removal

Keeping microorganisms out of food is often difficult during food production. Processing and postprocessing are much easier places to apply asepsis. Protective covering of foods such as skin, shells, and hides are often removed during processing, thereby exposing previously sterile foods to contaminating microbes. Raw agricultural commodities normally carry a natural bioburden upon entering the processing plant. Packaging is the most widely used form of asepsis and includes wraps, packages, cans, etc.

Removal of microorganisms from foods is not very effective. Washing of fruits and vegetables can remove some surface microorganisms. However, if wash water becomes dirty, it can add microbes to the food. Trimming is an effective way to remove spoiled or damaged pans. Filtration is good for clear liquids (juices, beer, soft drinks, wine, and water) but is of little value for solid foods. Centrifugation, such as used in sedimentation/clarification steps, is not useful for removal of bacteria or viruses.

3. Modified Atmosphere Conditions

Altering the atmosphere surrounding a food can be a useful way to control microbes. Examples include packaging with vacuum, CO_2, N_2, or combinations of inert gases with or without oxygen. Some CO_2 accumulation is possible during fermentations or vegetable respiration. It is important to note that vacuum packaging can lead to favorable environments for proliferation of anaerobic pathogens such as **Clostridium botulinum**.

4. <u>High-Temperature Preservation</u>

Use of high-temperature processing is based on destroying microbes, but it may also injure certain thermoduric microbes. Not all microorganisms are killed, i.e., spore formers usually survive. Other barriers are combined with a thermal process to achieve adequate safety and product shelf life. Commercial sterilization used in the canning process usually destroys all viable microbes that can spoil the product. Thermophilic spores may survive but will not grow under normal storage conditions.

Several factors affect heat resistance of microorganisms in foods. Species variability and the ability to form spores, plus the condition of the microbial population can affect heat resistance. Environmental factors, such as food variability and presence of other preservative measures employed also dictate thermal resistance. For example, heat resistance increases with decreasing water activity. Hence, moist air heating is better than dry heating. High-fat foods tend to increase resistance of cells. The larger the initial number of microorganisms present means a higher heat resistance. Older (stationary phase) cells are more resistant to heat than are younger cells. Resistance increases as growth temperature increases. A microbe with a high optimum temperature for growth will generally have a high heat resistance. Addition of other inhibitors, such as nitrite, will decrease resistance. Likewise high-acid foods (pH less than 4.6) will not generally support growth of pathogens. There is a time-temperature relationship that is a very important factor governing heat resistance of a microbial population. As temperature increases, the time needed for a given kill decreases. The relationship is dependent on type and size of food container. Larger containers require longer process times. Metal conducts heat better than glass, which can lower process times.

Microorganisms are killed by heat at a rate nearly proportional to the numbers present. This is a log order of death, which means that under a constant temperature the same percentage of a population will die at a given time interval regardless of the population size. For example, 90 percent die in 30 seconds, 90 percent of remaining in the next 30 seconds, and so on. Thus, as the initial number of organisms increases, then the time required for the reduction of all organisms at a given temperature also increases. Food microbiologists express this time-temperature relationship by calculating a number of constants. D value is the time required to reduce a population by one log cycle at a given temperature. Thermal death time (TDT) is the time needed to kill a given number of organisms at a given temperature. Thermal death point (TDP) is the temperature needed to kill a given number of organisms at a set time (usually 10 minutes; D_{10}).

In food canning, the time-temperature profile must be calculated for each size of container, for each food type, and for each retort used. When done correctly, these time-temperature conditions provide a large margin of safety since one rarely knows the numbers and types of microbes in a given container, but one must assume that **C. botulinum** is present. To ensure safety, inoculated pack studies are done using **Clostridium sporegenes** PA 3679, which is six times more heat resistant than **C. botulinum**. A known number of PA 3679 are added to cans fitted with thermocouples. Cans are then processed to 120°C (250°F) and held for various time periods. Survivors are enumerated to construct a thermal death curve for that particular food and a D value calculated. For canned foods a 12D margin of safety is used. Thus, heat at a given temperature is applied for a time equal to D times 12 log cycle reductions of PA 3679. Therefore, if a can had 10^9 spores only 1 in 1000 cans would have a viable spore. Thus, the probability of survival for **C. botulinum** would be 1 in 10^{12} if a can is heated at 250°F for 3 minutes. A minimum botulinum cook is one where every particle of food in a container reaches 250°F and remains at that temperature for at least 3 minutes.

Several factors affect heat transfer and penetration into food packages. Food type (liquids, solids, size, and shape) determine mixing effects during heating. Conduction occurs with solid foods (pumpkin) and results in slow heat transfer because there is no mixing of contents. Convection gives liquids (juice) faster heat transfer due to mixing by currents or mechanical agitation, Combination of conduction and convection is observed with particles in liquid (peas), though heating is primarily by convection and depends on viscosity of liquid component. Container size, shape, and composition are important. Tall thin cans transfer heat faster than short round cans. Large cans take longer than small cans. Metal (tin, steel, and aluminum) containers transfer heat faster than glass, resulting in shorter process times. Plastics can have rapid heat transfer due to thinness. Retort pouches, which are laminates of foil and plastic, have rapid heat transfer; however, pinhole problems can occur. Preheating foods prior to filling containers and preheating retort will shorten process time. Rotation or agitation of cans during processing increases convection, giving faster heating.

Canning is the preservation of foods in hermetically sealed containers, usually by heat treatments. The typical sequence in canning is as follows. Freshly harvested good-quality foods are washed to remove soils. Next, a blanch or mild heat treatment is applied to set color of fruits and vegetables, inactivate enzymes, purge dissolved gases, and kill some microorganisms. Clean containers are then filled to leave some head space. Hot packing is filling with preheated food to give faster processing, although cold packing can be done. Containers are sealed under vacuum then placed into a retort. The retort is sealed and heated with pressurized steam. After heating, cans should be rapidly cooled to avoid overcooking and to prevent growth of thermophiles. Cooling is done by submerging cans in a sanitized water bath, which can cause problems if pinhole leaks are present, allowing water to enter containers.

Less severe heat processing is pasteurization, which usually involves heating at less than 100°C. Pasteurization has two purposes, to destroy all pathogens normally present in a product and to reduce numbers of spoilage microorganisms. This thermal process kills some but not all microorganisms present in the food. Pasteurization is used when more rigorous heat treatments might alter food quality. For example, overheated milk will coagulate, brown, and burn. Pasteurization should kill all pathogens normally associated with the product. This is useful when spoilage microorganisms are not heat resistant and when surviving microbes can be controlled by other methods. Another reason for pasteurization is to kill competing microorganisms to allow for a desirable fermentation with starter cultures. Pasteurization is used to manufacture cheeses, wines, and beers. Milk pasteurization may use three equivalent treatments. Low-temperature long time (LTLT) treatment uses 145°F (63°C) for 30 minutes. High temperature short time (HTST) uses 161°F (72°C) for 15 seconds. Ultra high temperature or ultrapasteurized (UHT) uses 138°C for only 2 seconds. UHT processes are used for shelf-stable products.

Heating at or below 100°C involves most cooking temperatures. Baking, roasting, simmering, boiling, frying (oil is hotter but internal temperature of food rarely reaches 100°C) are examples of cooking methods. All pathogens are usually killed except spore formers. Microwaving does not exceed 100°C and can result in uneven heating. Microwave cooking should allow an equilibration time after removal from the oven for more even heating.

5. Low-Temperature Preservation

Low temperatures retard chemical reactions, and refrigeration slows microbial growth rates. Freezing prevents growth of most microorganisms by lowering water activity. Several psychrotrophic pathogens (**Listeria monocytogenes, Yersinia enterocolitica,** and nonproteolytic **Clostridium botulinum**) are able to multiply at refrigeration temperatures. Among factors influencing chill storage, temperature of the compartment is critical. Temperature of food products should be held as low as possible. Relative humidity should be high enough to prevent dehydration but not too high to favor growth of microorganisms. Air velocity in coolers helps to remove odors, control humidity, and maintain uniform temperatures. Atmosphere surrounding food during chill storage can affect microbial growth. Modified atmosphere packaging can help ensure safe chill-stored foods. Some plant foods respire, resulting in removal of O_2 and release of CO_2. Ultraviolet irradiation can be used to kill microorganisms on surfaces and in the air during chill storage of foods.

For chill storage to be effective in controlling microorganisms, the rate of cooling should be done rapidly. Temperature should be maintained as low as possible for refrigerated foods (less than 40°F). Thawing of frozen foods presents special problems because drip loss provides ample nutrients for microorganisms. In addition, thawing should be done as rapidly as possible and the food used as quickly as possible to avoid opportunity for microbial growth. Often, thawing is done at room temperature over many hours, which can lead to exposure of surfaces to ambient temperatures for extended periods. Another problem is incomplete thawing of large food items (turkeys). By cooking a large item that is not completely thawed, the internal temperature may not reach lethal levels to kill even the most heat- sensitive enteric pathogen. In fact, a spike in the number of salmonellosis and camplyobacteriosis outbreaks occurs every Thanksgiving and Christmas holidays because of consumption of undercooked turkey and stuffing.

6. Drying

Foods can be preserved by removing or binding water. Any treatment that lowers water activity can reduce or eliminate growth of microorganisms. Some examples include sun drying, heating, freeze drying, and addition of humectants. Humectants act not by removing water but rather by binding water to make it unavailable to act as a solvent. Humectants in common use are salt, sugars, and sugar alcohols (sorbitol). Intermediate moisture foods are those that have 20 to 40 percent moisture and a water activity (a_w) of 0.75 to 0.85. Examples include soft candies, jams, jellies, honey, pepperoni, and country ham. These foods often require antifungal agents for complete stability.

7. **Preservatives**

Food preservatives can be extrinsic (intentionally added), intrinsic (normal constituent of food), or developed (produced during fermentation). Factors affecting preservative effectiveness include:

(a) Concentration of inhibitor; (b) kind, number, and age of microorganisms (older cells more resistant); (c) temperature; (d) time of exposure (if long enough some microbes can adapt and overcome inhibition); and (e) chemical and physical characteristics of food (water activity, pH, solutes, etc.). Preservatives that are cidal are able to kill microorganisms when large concentrations of the substances are used. Static activity results when sublethal concentrations inhibit microbial growth.

Some examples of inorganic preservatives are NaCl, nitrate and nitrite, and sulfites and SO_2. NaCl lowers water activity and causes plasmolysis by withdrawing water from cells. Nitrites and nitrates are curing agents for meats (hams, bacons, sausages, etc.) to inhibit **C. botulinum** under vacuum packaging conditions. Sulfur dioxide (SO_2), sulfltes (SO_3), bisulfite (HSO_3), and metabisulfites (S_2O_5) form sulfurous acid in aqueous solutions, which is the antimicrobial agent. Sulfites are widely used in the wine industry to sanitize equipment and reduce competing microorganisms. Wine yeasts are resistant to sulfites. Sulfites are also used in dried fruits and some fruit juices. Sulfites have been used to prevent enzymatic and nonezymatic browning in some fruits and vegetables (cut potatoes),

Nitrites can react with secondary and tertiary amines to form potentially carcinogenic nitrosamines during cooking; however, current formulations greatly reduce this risk. Nitrates in high concentrations can result in red blood cell functional impairment; however, at approved usage levels they are safe. Sulfiting agents likewise can cause adverse respiratory effects to susceptible consumers, particularly asthmatics. Therefore, use of these two classes of agents is strictly regulated.

A number of organic acids and their salts are used as preservatives. These include lactic acid and lactates, propionic acid and propionates, citric acid, acetic acid, sorbic acid and sorbates, benzoic acid and benzoates, and methyl and propyl parabens (benzoic acid derivatives). Benzoates are most effective when undissociated; therefore, they require low pH values for activity (2.5 to 4.0). The sodium salt of benzoate is used to permit ease of solubility in foods. When esterifled (parabens), benzoates are active at higher pH values. Benzoates are primarily used in high-acid foods (jams, jellies, juices, soft drinks, ketchup, salad dressings, and margarine). They are active against yeast and molds, but minimally so against bacteria. They can be used at levels up to 0.1 percent.

Sorbic acid and sorbate salts (potassium is most effective) are effective at pH values less than 6.5 but at a higher pH than benzoates. Sorbates are used in cheeses, baked or nonyeast goods, beverages, jellies, jams, salad dressings, dried fruits, pickles, and margarine. They inhibit yeasts and molds, but few bacteria except **C. botulinum**. They prevent yeast growth during vegetable fermentations and can be used at levels up to 0.3 percent.

Propionic acid and propionate salts (calcium is most common) are active against molds at pH values less than 6. They have limited activity against yeasts and bacteria. They are widely used in baked products and cheeses. Propionic acid is found naturally in

Swiss cheese at levels up to 1 percent. Propionates can be added to foods at levels up to 0.3 percent.

Acetic acid is found in vinegar at levels up to 4 to 5 percent. It is used in mayonnaise, pickles, and ketchup, primarily as a flavoring agent. Acetic acid is most active against bacteria, but has some yeast and mold activity, though less active than sorbates or propionates. Lactic acid, citric acid, and their salts can be added as preservatives, to lower pH, and as flavorants. They are also developed during fermentation. These organic acids are most effective against bacteria.

Some antibiotics may be found in foods. Although medical compounds are not allowed in human food, trace amounts used for animal therapy may occasionally be found. Bacteriocins, which are antimicrobial peptides produced by microorganisms, can be found in foods. An example of an approved bacteriocin is nisin, which is allowed in process cheese food as an additive. Some naturally occurring enzymes (lysozyme and lactoferrin) can be used as preservatives in limited applications where denaturation is not an issue. Some spices, herbs, and essential oils have antimicrobial activity, but such high levels are needed that the food becomes unpalatable. Ethanol has excellent preservative ability but is underutilized because of social stigma. Wood smoke, whether natural or added in liquid form, contains several phenolic antimicrobial compounds in addition to formaldehyde. Wood smoke is most active against vegetative bacteria and some fungi. Bacterial endospores are resistant. Activity is correlated with phenolic content. Carbon dioxide gas can dissolve in food tissues to lower pH and inhibit microbes. Developed preservatives produced during fermentation include organic acids (primarily lactic, acetic, and propionic), ethanol, and bacteriocins. All added preservatives must meet government standards for direct addition to foods. All preservatives added to foods are GRAS, generally recognized as safe.

8. Irradiation

Foods can be processed or preserved with a number of types of radiation. Nonionizing radiations used include ultraviolet, microwave, and infrared. These function by exciting molecules. Ionizing radiations include γ-rays, x-rays, β-rays, protons, neutrons, and α-particles. Neutrons make food radioactive, while β-rays (low-energy electrons), protons, and α-particles have little penetrating ability and are of little practical use in foods. Ionizing γ-rays, x-rays, and high-energy electrons produce ions by breaking molecules and can be lethal to microorganisms.

Ultraviolet (260 nm) lamps are used to disinfect water, meat surfaces, utensils, air, walls, ceilings, and floors. UV can control film yeasts in brines during vegetable fermentations. UV effectiveness is dose dependent. Longer exposure time increases effectiveness. UV intensity depends on lamp power, distance to object, and amount of interfering material in its path. For example, humidity greater than 60 percent reduces intensity. UV will not penetrate opaque materials and is good only for surface decontamination. Infrared heats products, but has little penetrating power. Microwaves cause rapid oscillation of dipole molecules (water) and result in the production of heat. Microwaves have excellent penetrating power. However, there are problems with the time-temperature relationship because microwaves cause foods to reach hot temperatures too quickly. Also, microwave-treated foods rarely exceed 100°C. Thus, instances of microbial survival in these foods has been reported.

X-rays have excellent penetrating ability but are quite expensive. They are not widely used in the food industry. γ-Rays from radioactive sources (Cs^{135} and Co^{150}) have good penetration and are widely used to pasteurize and sterilize foods. Electron beam generators also are gaining appeal as ionizing sources of radiation to process foods. Food irradiation is much more widespread in countries other than the United States. There is much untapped potential to use ionizing radiations to reduce or eliminate microbial pathogens in foods. This technology remains underexploited due to consumer wariness about the safety of the technology.

9. Fermentation

A number of foods use beneficial microorganisms in the course of their processing. Bread, cheeses, pickles, sauerkraut, some sausages, and alcoholic beverages are made by the conversion of sugar to organic acids, ethanol, or carbon dioxide. These three byproducts not only serve as desirable flavors but also provide a significant antimicrobial barrier to pathogens. There have been instances where poorly fermented foods have been linked to foodborne illness.

Furthermore, cheese made from unpasteurized milk has a distinctly higher risk of carrying pathogens than cheese made from pasteurized milk. Proper acid development and avoidance of cross-contamination are essential control steps in manufacturing fermented foods. Alcoholic beverages have not been linked to food-borne disease other than excess consumption leading to ethanol toxicity.

VII. BIBLIOGRAPHY

Metcalf, S.W. (2001). Environmental Biomarkers and Biomonitoring. In L. Williams, & R. Langley (Eds.), Environmental Health Secrets (pp. 214-218). Philadelphia, PA: Hanley & Belfus, Inc.

Metcalf, S.W. (2001). Food Sanitation. In L. Williams, & R. Langley (Eds.), Environmental Health Secrets (pp. 204-208). Philadelphia, PA: Hanley & Belfus, Inc.

Metcalf, S.W. (2001). Foodborne Illnesses. In L. Williams, & R. Langley (Eds.), Environmental Health Secrets (pp. 209-213). Philadelphia, PA: Hanley & Belfus, Inc.

Moeller, D. W. (1997). Food. Environmental Health (pp. 103-125). Cambridge, MA, and London, UK: Harvard University Press.

Moore, G.S. (1999). Environmental Degradation and Food Security. Living with the Earth: Concepts in Environmental Health Science (pp. 3.1 – 3.53). Boca Raton, FL: Lewis Publishers.

Moore, G.S. (1999). Foodborne Illness. Living with the Earth: Concepts in Environmental Health Science (pp. 8.1 – 8.47). Boca Raton, FL: Lewis Publishers.

Nadakavukaren, A. (2000). Food Quality. Our Global Environment: A Health Perspective 5th Edition (pp. 317-353). Prospective Heights, IL: Waveland Press, Inc.

Yassi, A., Kjellström, T., de Kok, T., & Guidotti, T. L. (2001). Food and Agriculture. In A. Yassi, [et al](Eds.), <u>Basic Environmental Health</u> (pp. 242-280). New York, NY: Oxford University Press, Inc.

CHAPTER

10

ENERGY, RADIATION, AND NOISE

I. ENERGY

A. INTRODUCTION

Energy can have direct and indirect, beneficial and detrimental, effects on health. It is essential for socioeconomic development. Without it, communities would not be able to cook their food, and would be more susceptible to infections and food poisoning. Nor could they maintain systems for heating, transportation, communication, and the production of materials. Energy is required for basic human needs (heating, lighting, cooking), agriculture (irrigation, mechanization), urbanization (basic services), transportation and industrial production.

The patterns of energy use and production are key characteristics of all societies. The challenge is to produce the amount of energy needed while imposing the least possible health risk and environmental detonation. The availability of energy often determines the nature of a region's socioeconomic development. For development to be sustainable, energy sources must also be dependable, safe, and environmentally sound.

It is widely accepted that an assessment of the total risk of an energy source must include an evaluation of all the risks across the **energy cycle:**

1. Material acquisition and construction,
2. Emissions from material acquisition and energy production,
3. Operation and maintenance,
4. Energy back-up systems,
5. Energy storage systems,
6. Transportation, and
7. Waste management.

Various forms of development require many forms of development, resulting in a number of trends in global energy consumption. Overall, energy consumption increased by about 2.2 % per year before 1950; between about 1950 and 1970, energy consumption increased by 5.2% per year; but since the energy crisis in the 1970s, the demand for energy has slowed back to an increase of 2.3% per year. The total energy consumption over the period of 20 years (1973-1993) was 49% greater than in the previous 20 years.

Energy is critical for society to survive and prosper. We need it to power our transportation systems, grow our food, heat our homes and workplaces, operate our factories, and ensure our high living standard. However, this high standard of living and productivity have increased our energy dependence.

This dependence in part can be attributed to a seemingly abundant supply of inexpensive energy. The United States is the world's largest energy producer and consumer, and our energy use pattern is heavily influenced by economic growth, land area, low population density, climate, and transportation habits. For example, the United States currently spends 11.2 percent of its gross national product on energy, compared to Japan's 5 percent expenditure.

Though energy has many benefits, it also has many costs, such as its impacts on human health and the environment. Society generally has focused only on the most visible impact - air pollution from the actual burning of fuel - and not on land, surface water, and groundwater pollution resulting from mining, exploring, producing, processing, transporting, and storing energy sources as well as from disposing post-combustion wastes.

All the energy we currently use produces some negative environmental or human health impacts. Even renewable resources have environmental impacts and require energy input, though these impacts and inputs may be much less than those of fossil fuels. For example, to produce fuel from corn (ethanol or ethyl alcohol), fertilizers and pesticides are necessary to grow the corn. In addition, harvesting, transporting, storing, and processing corn into fuel all require energy inputs, which themselves produce pollution. As this example shows, to fully understand the impacts of energy, we must consider not just the impacts from burning the fuel, but rather analyze the full environmental costs of each energy option across the life of the option (that is, account for the effects of extracting it, processing it, using it, and disposing of it). This is called **life-cycle analysis** because it considers the additional impacts from obtaining the energy source and disposing of the post-combustion wastes.

In 1992, the United States consumed 81.51 quadrillion British thermal units ("**quads**") of energy, an 81% increase since 1960, by the sources in Table 10.1 (the percentages in parentheses represent the amount of energy supplied by that source). One Quad is equal to 10^{15} Btu.

Table 10.1 Sources of Energy. (Source: Wagner, 1994).

Sources of Energy	quads	Percentages
Petroleum	32.72	36.7
Natural gas	20.16	22.6
Coal	18.81	21.1
Nuclear	6.54	7.3
Hydroelectric	3.08	3.4
Other sources (Solar, geothermal, wind, and biomass)	2.8	3.1

The British thermal unit (Btu) is the accepted standard for comparing the heating values of fuels. One Btu equals the quantity of heat required to raise the temperature of one pound of water one degree Fahrenheit. As shown in the previous list, the majority of our energy is supplied by nonrenewable fossil fuels (that is, once used, they are gone forever), with a much smaller percentage supplied by so-named "**renewable sources**." As shown in Figure 10.1, the primary uses of energy in the United States are:

1. Electricity (secondary energy) production-37 percent
2. Transportation-27 percent
3. Industry-24 percent
4. Residential-12 percent

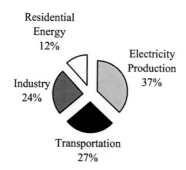

Figure 10.1. Energy Uses in the United States. (Source: Wagner, 1994).

B. ENERGY RESOURCES

The fuels that are available to meet the world's energy needs fall into two broad categories:

1. **Renewable** Resources - (like solar, wind, waterpower and geothermal energy)
2. **Non-renewable** Resources - (like fossil fuels and nuclear fuels)

The sources of energy are the following: fossil fuels, nuclear fuels, geothermal energy, and solar energy.

1. Fossil Fuels

They are the best examples of non-renewable sources. The remaining worldwide and domestic supplies of these three fuels are estimated to be about as followed:

a. **Natural Gas** – perhaps five or more decades, however new supplies are being discovered, and the total recoverable reserves are probably not known at this time.
b. **Coal** – perhaps two to four centuries, US has abundant reserves.
c. **Oil (petroleum)** – perhaps three to five decades, more than half of these resources are located in the Middle East.

2. Nuclear Fuels

They are another example of non-renewable sources. The energy available from existing US sources of uranium, if consumed exclusively in the current generation of boiling-water and pressurized-water nuclear power plants, is estimated to be equal to that available through the combustion of the existing sources of natural gas or petroleum.

3. Geothermal Energy

Although geothermal energy is available in enormous quantities, it is difficult to tap and is limited to certain geographic areas, most of which are remote from population and industry.

4. Solar Energy

Offers tremendous potential for meeting the world's energy needs. Sources are hydropower, tidal power, windpower, heat pumps, photovoltaic pumps, trees and agricultural crops. Potential applications of solar energy extend far beyond the above examples. In developing countries the sun is used for heating and distilling water, for drying crops, and for heat engines such as the sofretes pump, manufactured in France. In urban areas the trees planted around a house can promote not only comfort but also energy conservation. Deciduous trees, for example, shade a house in the summer and permit sunlight to warm it in the winter. And trees directly absorb greenhouse gases, such as carbon dioxide.

The types of solar energy resources:

a. **Hydropower** – one of the most common sources of solar energy, a prominent example being the enormously successful series of hydroelectric power plants that were constructed by the Tennessee Valley Authority on major waterways in the south central US during the mid-twentieth century
b. **Tidal Power** – another source of solar energy, tidal power is manifested in the rise and fall of the ocean tides.
c. **Wind-Power** – although windmills have been used for centuries on an individual basis to pump water, few multiunit wind-powered stations were developed in the US until recently.
d. **Heat Pumps** – instead of burning natural gas or oil to provide heat, the heat pump uses electricity to collect and concentrate the latent in the ambient air or ground that has been warmed by solar radiation.
e. **Photovoltaic Systems** – use of solar collectors to provide power for small appliances.
f. **Trees and Agricultural Crops** – in many parts of the world, the primary source of fuel for cooking and heating is firewood, the growing use of wood as a source of energy, however, has led to the wholesale destruction of hardwood forests in many areas.

C. HEALTH AND ENVIRONMENTAL IMPLICATIONS

Each increase in energy production and use, or transfer from one energy mode to another, will produce changes in public health and the ambient environment (Table 10.2). Occupational morbidity and mortality are associated with fuel mining or drilling, transport to the point of combustion, and power generation or other fuel use. Emissions of particulate matter, SO_2 and nitrogen oxides (NO_2) from power plants and CO and NO_x from automobiles and trucks are potential health hazards in the ambient environment.

Table 10.2. Environmental Effects of Energy Use and Production. (Source: Wagner, 1994).

Energy Source	Uses	Impacts to Land	Impacts to Water	Impacts to Air	Impacts to Human Health	Impacts to Environment	Future Use
Coal	Electricity	Disturbed land and erosion from mining, solid waste generation	Acid drainage from mines, siltation, thermal pollution	High amounts of sulfur dioxide, nitrogen oxides, particulates, carbon monoxide	Respiratory effects from air pollutants, black lung (miners) disease	Aquatic organisms adversely affected by acid deposition and acid mine	↑
Petroleum	Transportation, heating, electricity	Disturbed land for drilling and support activities, brine wastes from production, oil	Oil spills, brine spills, leaks into ground-water	Nitrogen oxides, sulfur dioxides, carbon dioxide, acid deposition carbon monoxide	Respiratory effects from air pollutants; contaminated water is moderately	Aquatic organisms and vegetation adversely affected by acid deposition	↓
Natural gas	Heating, residential electricity	Land distur-bance from pipeline construction and drilling operations	Minimal	Carbon dioxide, carbon monoxide and hydrogen sulfide	Few known effects	Few known effects	↑
Nuclear	Electricity	Disturbed land from mining, erosion, tailings from mines, releases from fuel	Releases of hot water, releases of radioactive cooling water, contamina-tion of ground-water	Radio-active gases, but minimal	Respiratory and internal effects from mining, none detectable in normal	All living organisms are potentially adversely affected by radiation	Stable
Hydro-electric	Electricity	Loss of wildlife habitats and fertile farmland from flooding	Flooding, increased water temperature, siltation	Negligible	Negligible	Decreased spawning opportunities for migratory fish and impacts	Stable

Natural gas is relatively clean burning, and if transported by pipeline, relatively safe. However, the recent trend toward transport of liquefied natural gas by tanker poses an increased potential fire and explosion threat.

Nuclear power does not produce the types of pollutants associated with fossil fuel combustion. However, the thermal operating characteristics of nuclear plants stress construction materials and equipment much more than in conventional plants. In addition, the wastes are highly radioactive and will require safe storage for time intervals of thousands of years. Also of continuing concern are the occupational hazards of uranium mining (a much higher incidence of lung cancer in smoking miners than in control groups) and, although generally well-monitored, the longterm exposure of construction workers and plant operators to radiation.

Other environmental problems associated with fossil fuel combustion include atmospheric CO_2 buildup and the production of sulfates and nitrates leading to acid rain. When fossil fuels are burned one of the major end products is CO_2.

Acid rain is apparently the result of the conversion of SO_2 and NO_x gases from combustion processes into particulate sulfates and nitrates, and the subsequent absorption of these materials into rain water. Lakes in Scandinavia, Eastern Canada and the Northeastern U.S. have been identified as having acid levels too high to permit fish life.

D. MINERAL RESOURCES

The U.S. demand rate is much greater than would be expected based on population alone. Sixty one percent of nickel, 75% of tin and 100% of the U.S. manganese demand were imported in 1976. On the other hand, much of the world's known mineral resources are located in developing countries. The public health implications of mineral mining are similar to those for various fuels. However, since the resources are often located elsewhere, it is that population which must endure much of the health cost of production.

E. ENERGY AND MINERAL CONSUMPTION

Whenever fuels are burned or products containing minerals discarded (e.g., old car bodies), there is an energy cost corresponding to the decrease in the organization of matter. This energy cost is sometimes referred to as an increase in entropy; its existence is referred to as the Second Law of Thermodynamics. Essentially it is a way of describing the inefficiencies, which occur during any energy transfer.

Some processes are more inefficient than others. For instance the internal combustion engine in an automobile has an efficiency of about 25% while that of a diesel bus is approximately 38%. Energy which is used to meet inefficiencies can never be recovered and so must be regarded as a net loss to our future use. So, in general, our interest is in fostering efficient systems of energy and mineral use.

Many of our resources are wasted because after one use they are discarded. Very little recycling is actually carried out in the U.S. compared to the resources we use. For instance only about 21% of paper, 7% of aluminum, 3% of glass and none of plastics or wood are recovered from consumer residential and commercial solid waste.

Developing economies are faced with the problem of having inadequate resources or inadequate means of extracting and processing, or both. And, for those who do possess resources, much is siphoned off to more developed countries. In addition, as development proceeds, it is only with great difficulty that an emerging country can avoid the pollution problems experienced in the past by industrial nations.

A variety of scenarios have been proposed for the world's energy future. The most optimistic of these require significant changes in American lifestyle and an understanding of how our energy demands affect the rest of the world. Conservation, recycling, and the prudent use of renewable resources are important consequences of this realization. The alternative is an abrupt decline in non-recoverable resources with all the social inequity and friction that this entails.

F. ENERGY PRODUCTION CONSUMPTION

Conventional sources of energy for the industrially developed countries of the world include fossil fuels, such as coal, oil gas and wood, nuclear fuels, and geothermal and hydropower. Meeting energy needs and protecting the environment are inseparable goals. The mining of coal, for example, can lead to chronic diseases and injuries among miners and to degradation of the environment (as is often the case in strip mining); the drilling, acquisition, and transportation of oil can lead to spills that contaminate vast areas of land, water, or both; and the use of gasoline in cars leads to air pollution and smog. Internationally, the production and use of oil can lead to conflicts among nations and even to wars. The generation of electricity through either hydropower or the consumption of fossil or nuclear fuels leads to air pollution, problems of waste disposal, and other effects on the environment. Additional concerns in terms of the burning of fossil fuels include the long-range impacts, such as acidic deposition and global warming.

Conservation can play a substantial role in meeting energy needs. One of the most obvious places to practice conservation is the home, where one-sixth of the energy consumed in the United States is currently used. Newer generations of technology are leading to far more efficient ways to light, cool, and heat dwellings, and to more efficient home appliances. Conservation measures have been incorporated into the construction techniques for new buildings. Yet even actions such as these are not always without negative impacts; as an example, tighter, energy-efficient buildings have led to increased indoor radon concentrations and the "**sick building syndrome**". Even the use of solar energy involves occupational health problems in the manufacture of photovoltaic cells, and injuries or deaths to home owners who fall while cleaning solar panels on the roofs of their houses.

After years of consuming energy resources as if they were unlimited, policymakers today recognize that continued health and safety would be possible only if these resources, particularly the supplies of nonrenewable fossil fuels, are carefully managed, conserved, and protected. The urgency of coping with this situation in the United States is illustrated by the fact that this country is only about 6 percent of the world's population, consumes 30 percent of the world's energy. In fact, domestic sources of oil have been depleted to the extent that this nation now imports more than half of the oil it consumes. The seven largest countries of the Organization for Economic Cooperation and Development (OECD) consume over 40 percent of the world's production of fossil fuels.

G. ENERGY USES IN THE UNITED STATES

Making long-range plans for meeting energy needs requires detailed knowledge of current energy sources and how they are being utilized.

The uses of energy in the three major sectors are summarized below:

1. The **industrial sector** accounts for 38 percent of end-use energy consumption, relying on a mix of fuels. Of the energy it consumes, industry uses 70 percent to

provide heat and power for manufacturing. In all, it uses 25 percent of the nation's petroleum, half of that as feedstocks.

2. This country devotes 36 percent of its end-use energy consumption to the **transportation** of people and goods. Virtually all of this energy consists of petroleum products that power automobiles, trucks, ships, airplanes, and trains. In fact, almost 200 million automobiles are in use, approximately three for every four members of the U.S. population. Over the past 44 years, the transportation sector's consumption of petroleum has more than tripled, but because of energy conservation and other measures, growth was slower in the 1980s and 1990s than in previous decades.

3. The **residential** and **commercial sector** accounts for 26 percent of U.S. end-use energy consumption. Of the total, almost 40 percent is used in the form of electricity. A typical house contains five basic energy-consuming items: central heating system, hot-water heater, cooking stove, refrigerator, and lighting system. Most of the energy consumption in commercial buildings is for space heating and cooling, lighting, and office equipment. Although many uses of energy are beyond the control of the average person, individuals can contribute in many ways to conserving energy in the home, when commuting to work, and in the office.

Individuals can contribute to energy conservation in many ways:

Home:
Weather-stripping doors and caulking windows.
Closing damper when fireplace not in use.
Setting the thermostat at lowest comfortable setting during winter and at highest comfortable setting in summer.
Appliances turned off when not in use.

Workplace:
Electronic equipment (PCs, printers, copiers, fax machines) accounts for about 8% of direct electricity use. Through Energy Star Computers Program, EPA is encouraging manufacturers to develop desktops, PCs and monitors that go into a standby mode automatically after a period of inactivity.

Resistance to conserve energy has occurred in spite of campaigns and rebate programs to encourage the purchase and use of energy-efficient products, because:

1. **Skepticism** - consumers do not trust manufacturers claims relative to energy savings that new technology will provide.
2. **First Cost** - many energy-efficient products have high purchase price.
3. **Savings difficult to measure** - it is difficult for customers to identify how and to what degree a new energy-saving appliance will reduce their electric bill.
4. **Poor aesthetics** - new appliances often are not pleasing to the eye.
5. **Requirements for change in behavior** - new products that require consumers to change their behavioral patterns are often rejected in marketplace.

6. **Market-related issues** - consumers sometimes find that retailers do not stock adequate supplies of the newer energy-efficient models.

H. ENVIRONMENTAL IMPACTS

The environmental impact of electricity-generating plants, like coal and oil plants, where smoke is clearly visible, and nuclear power plants, are both highly controversial.
The demand for electricity continues to grow. In 1973 - 1988, the use of electricity in US increased over 50%.

Methods of generating electricity with environmental impact: 1. Hydroelectric Power, 2. Geothermal Energy, and 3. Nuclear or Fossil fuels.

1. Hydroelectric Power

Harnessing waterpower on a major scale involves the construction of a dam on a river or stream, thereby a lake is formed, and the potential energy in the water is used to turn turbines and generate electricity. Large scale projects can alter the environment and people's lives drastically, bringing many risks and benefits. Dams can also have serious effects on ocean fish, such as salmon, sturgeon, steelhead, and striped brass that spawn in freshwater streams. More than 400 people where killed in the failure of the Malpassest Dam (France) during a flood in 1959.

2. Geothermal Energy

The use of geothermal energy has a variety of environmental impacts. Pressure in pressurized hot-water reservoirs is often a result of the weight of the overlying land; withdrawal of the water can lead to subsidence.

3. Nuclear and Fossil Fuels

Facilities that generate electric power with nuclear fuels use similar processes as those that employ fossil fuels. To avoid thermal pollution of water sources, many electric utilities have equipped their power plants with cooling towers, which release the excess heat into the atmosphere instead of into a lake or river.

Fossil-fueled and nuclear-fueled power plants have environmental impact at five stages: a. fuel acquisition, b. fuel transportation, c. power plant releases, d. processing and disposal of spent fuel or ashes, and e. power transmission.

a. Fuel acquisition

The acquisition of fossil fuels has considerable environmental impact, like in the case of coal and oil it is largely related to the volumes required. **Example:** A standard 1,000-megawatt electric (MWe) power plant requires more than 2 million tons of coal or more than 500 million gallons of oil per year. Strip mining of coal pollutes the air dust and defaces the earth's surface if the land is not restored to its original state after the mining is completed.

b. Fuel transportation - Example:

A standard 1,000-MWe coal-fired electric power plant requires about 8,000 tons of fuel per day, enough to fill at least 100 railroad cars. Much of the oil consumed in the US is obtained overseas. Tanker accidents are common, like Exxon Valdez in Alaska in the spring of 1989 that released more than 10 million gallons of oil into Prince William Sound and onto nearby beaches. Ocean shipment of natural gas poses similar problems.

c. Power Plant Releases

Fossil-fueled plants release sulfur oxides, nitrogen oxides, carbon monoxide, and some naturally occurring radioactive material originally present in the fuel. A plant fueled by natural gas has less impact on the environment than a plant fueled by either coal or oil. In a **BWR (boiling water reactors)**, the water is heated by the fuel and converted into steam, and this steam turns the turbine. In a **PWR (pressurized-water reactors)**, the water heated by the reactors is kept under sufficient pressure that it is not converted into steam.

Examples of particulate emissions by:

Coal-Fired Plant - Releases requiring the largest dilution are the particulates for which the EPA standard is 50 $\mu g/m^3$
Oil-Fired Plant - the controlling pollutant is sulfur dioxide (SO_2), for which the EPA standard is 80 $\mu g/m^3$
Gas-Fired Plant - the controlling pollutant is nitrogen dioxide (NO_2), for which EPA limit is 100 $\mu g/m^3$.

Natural processes remove pollutants such as SO_2, NO_2 and particulates from the atmosphere.
Factors should be taken into account in an overall evaluation of the environment and public health impact of electric power plant: Fossil fuel facilities, contribute to acidic deposition, through the release of sulfur and nitrogen compounds, and the global warming as a result of the release of carbon dioxide.
When all factors are taken into account (including the atmospheric pollution associated with the processing of spent fuel), it appears that a nuclear-powered plant has far less environmental impact than a plant fueled by oil or natural gas.

d. Processing and Disposal of Spent Fuel or Ashes

Nuclear-powered plants are superior in terms of airborne releases, but produces 30-50 tons of spent fuel per year. The spent fuel is intensely radioactive and poses significant problems of radiation protection and waste disposal.

e. Power Transmission

The type of power plant has no effect on the efficiency with which electricity is distributed to consumers. An estimated 12-20% of the electricity generated in US is lost during transmission.

Electricity-generating facilities are undesirable, but essential to the quality of modern life. Electricity is necessary to:

1. Clean the air,
2. Operate the water purification and sewage treatment plants,
3. Dispose of old automobiles,
4. Recycle other types of solid waste,
5. Power appliances, and
6. Reduces accidents on highways and crimes in cities by better lighting.

Conservation can reduce the overall demand for energy. The challenge is to educate people to use energy efficiently and conservatively, and to encourage the commercial sector to design, construct, and operate generating stations that function at maximum efficiency with minimal impact on the environment

II. RADIATION

A. IONIZING RADIATION

1. Definition

Simply put, radiation is energy in transit. If the radiation energy is of sufficient strength to eject orbital electrons when it interacts with a target material, then it is classified as "ionizing" (Figure 10.2).

The term comes from the definition of ionization, which is the process of ejecting an orbital electron from an electrically balanced atom. The threshold for ionization is important for a number of reasons, but predominantly because the event can cause the breakage of chemical bonds.

For example, when water molecules are exposed to ionizing radiation, they can break into their constituent elements and possibly reform into hydrogen peroxide, which can cause cellular damage. The ionization event can also result in breakage of DNA chains in the cell nucleus, possibly resulting in cell death or mutation.

2. Main Types of Ionizing Radiation

Ionizing radiation may either be particulate or waveform. Particulate radiations can be either charged or uncharged. The most commonly encountered charged particle radiations are alpha particles and beta particles. Alphas resemble the nucleus of a helium atom, consisting of four neutrons: two positively charged protons and two neutrally charged neutrons.

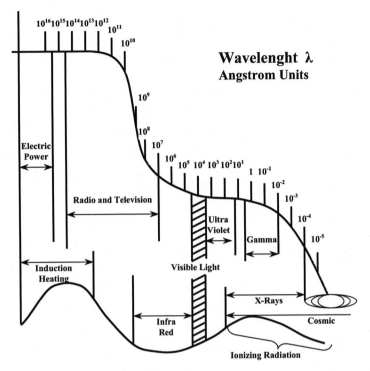

Figure 10.2. Electromagnetic Waveform Radiations.

An alpha, a relatively massive particle with a +2 charge has the potential to cause significant biological damage but cannot travel very far. Thus, from a safety standpoint, alpha radiation is of greatest concern when sources are incorporated into the body.

Beta radiation is also a charged particle, but smaller in size, resembling something more like an electron. Thus this particle can travel greater distances, and if energetic enough can be a safety concern even if outside the body.

A third particulate radiation, neutron radiation, is an uncharged particle. Depending on the energy possessed, these particles can have great penetrating abilities and thus can cause biological damage.

Two electromagnetic waveform radiations are x-rays and gamma rays. X-rays are formed outside of the nucleus of an atom and can travel great distances. Gamma rays arise from transformations from within a nucleus, but are essentially identical to x-rays once formed and emitted. Because of their waveform, these radiations can represent a biological concern when either inside or outside the body.

3. Sources of Ionizing Radiation

Ionizing radiation is used in a wide variety of settings. Applications include medicine, for the purposes of both diagnostic and therapeutic treatments; industry, for level gauges and thickness measurements; and research, for molecular tracers and imaging tools. Common consumer products that include sources of radiation include household smoke detectors, some lantern mantels for camping lanterns, and self-luminous watches and exit signs.

4. Definition of Radioactivity and an Isotope

Whereas radiation is merely energy in transit, radioactivity is the characteristic of certain materials to emit radiation spontaneously. Unlike an x-ray machine that requires an external power source for the emission of radiation, a material that is radioactive emits radiation without any outside source of energy.

An isotope is a version of an element that has the same number of protons as the natural element, but different number of neutrons. In some cases, this variability can result in the isotope atom being unstable, and thus radioactive. For example, ^{12}C is the stable form of carbon, with 6 protons and 6 neutrons. ^{14}C is a radioactive isotope of carbon, with 6 protons and 8 neutrons.

5. The Concept of Half-Life

Half-life is the amount of time it takes for half of the radioactive atoms of a particular isotope to undergo energy emission or decay. Half-lives can range from microseconds to millions of years.

6. Typical Doses of Radiation Received

The earth is radioactive and people are exposed to radiation from a number of sources everyday. Therefore, it is appropriate to answer the question "What are the typical doses of radiation received by an average American?" by starting with the amount of radiation dose the average American receives every day just being alive. This number is approximately 300 millirem/year, of which 200 is due to radon and its subsequent decay products, and the remainder due to man-made sources such as medical applications and consumer products.

Individuals occupationally exposed to radiation as a part of their jobs are permitted to receive up to 5000 millirem/year to the whole body. There are also specific occupational limits for the lens of the eye (15,000 millirem/year), extremities and skin (50,000 millirem/year), the general public (100 millirem/year), and a fetus in the workplace (500 millirem/9-month gestation period). Most occupationally exposed individuals do not receive these levels because the rules governing radiation safety also require that doses be maintained "as low as reasonably achievable," or **ALARA**. This standard of excellence has helped maintain doses to workers and the general public to very low levels. Individuals charged with overseeing the safe use of radiation sources are called "health physicists," and can serve as an excellent source of additional information regarding sources of radiation.

7. Occupations at Highest Risk of Radiation-Related Accidents

Although a number of occupations involve working with radiation sources, industrial radiography is the occupation that historically has been the work environment with the most reported radiation-related incidents. In this job, workers use high-activity radioactive sources of penetrating radiations to analyze the integrity of metal, concrete, and other materials. High activities of gamma-emitting sources such as ^{137}Cs, ^{60}Co, or ^{192}Ir are necessary to penetrate these dense materials.

Incidents can usually be traced to worker error, when safety procedures are overlooked and monitoring is not performed. For instance, if the radiation source is not safely retracted into its shielded holder, significant doses can be inadvertently delivered.

8. Pathways of Radiation Exposure

The different radiation exposure pathways can be described by using a source of radioactive material as an example. Suppose an ^{192}Ir source is used for medical treatment or industrial radiography. With the source encapsulated in its original container, gamma radiations emitted from the source can penetrate the human body. Then suppose the container or the source were somehow damaged such that radioactive material became dispersible. If contaminants in the form of dust or particles are incorporated into the body by ingestion or inhalation, the dose is delivered internally as well. Consideration of these two pathways of exposure is important in order to ensure the implementation of appropriate safety assessments and measures.

9. Principal Health Effects

For high doses of radiation, acute concerns include effects on the blood and digestive systems. High doses to the lens of the eye may result in cataract formation. For low chronic doses, the principal health effects are an increased risk of cancer.

10. Prevention of Radiation Exposure

In addition to education and awareness, three primary actions can be taken to minimize radiation exposure:

a. **First**, the amount of time near any source of radiation should be reduced to the minimum necessary;
b. **Second**, the distance from the source should be maximized, because the exposure is reduced exponentially as one moves away from a source;
c. **Third**, shielding materials can be used to further reduce the dose.

The type of shield used varies with the type of radiation encountered. The most penetrating radiations are usually shielded with lead and concrete.

11. Handling of Radioactive Waste

Wastes containing radioactive materials with relatively short half-lives can be stored for a period of decay and then disposed of as nonradioactive. This includes nearly all waste generated in nuclear medical departments.

Waste containing longer half-life isotopes or higher levels of radioactivity are typically shipped for permanent burial, sometimes after an interim treatment step of compaction, solidification, or incineration. In certain cases, very small amounts of radioactive materials can be released to the environment, but only under very controlled conditions. For example, patients undergoing nuclear medicine diagnosis or treatment may release small amounts of radioactivity via normal bodily functions and discharges. Such releases are allowed because the amounts of activity are low and the half-lives of the isotopes used in these techniques are usually quite short.

B. NONIONIZING RADIATION

1. Definition

Again, radiation is energy in transit. To knock out orbital electrons when it interacts with material, then it is classified as "non- ionizing" electromagnetic radiation.

Electromagnetic radiation is a form of energy that arises when electric charges are accelerated. Moving electric charges can generate electric and magnetic fields (EMFs) in space. The electric charges move back and forth as an alternating current in a length of wire, such as electromagnetic radiation generated by a television tower. This radiation leaves the source as electromagnetic waves and travels at the speed of light. These waves have the physical characteristics of frequency and wavelength, and can be reflected, refracted, and absorbed when they interact with matter. Electromagnetic radiation is either ionizing (x-rays or gamma rays) or nonionizing.

2. Types of Nonionizing Radiation

Nonionizing radiation makes up the major portion of the electromagnetic spectrum, and includes **ultraviolet (UV)**, **visible (vis)**, **infrared (IR)**, **laser (UV, Vis, and IR** with coherent wave energy), **radiofrequency**, **microwave**, and **extremely low frequency (ELF) /very low frequency (VLF)** radiation.

3. Typical Sources and Examples of Nonionizing Radiation

a. **Ultraviolet** (welding, mercury vapor lamps, tanning beds, sterilization)
b. **Visible light** (high-intensity lamps, projectors, spotlights, floodlights)
c. **Infrared** (heating sources, glassblowing, molten metal)
d. **Lasers** (light pointers, bar code readers, surveying and microsurgery tools, telecommunications)
e. **Radiofrequency** (broadcasting and telecommunications, cell phones, radar, product heating, sterilization, medicine)
f. **Microwave** (radar installations, broadcast stations, microwave ovens, diathermy)
g. **ELF/VLF** (power lines, electrical appliances, motors, video display terminals)

4. People Exposed to Nonionizing Radiation

Every individual on earth, even in the remotest locations, is exposed to varying low levels of nonionizing radiation. The radiation not only comes from natural sources such as the sun and Earth, but also from the rapidly and ever increasing man-made sources such as telecommunications, navigational equipment, medical equipment, and power transmission lines.

5. Difference of Biological Effects of Ionizing Radiation Versus Nonionizing

Ionizing radiation such as gamma rays has very different biological effects compared to nonionizing radiation such as microwaves. When the molecules of a cell are ionized, very reactive compounds called free radicals are formed and can damage the essential parts of a cell. Most of the damage to the cell can be repaired, but with higher doses, some damage is not repaired and stays with the cell. Nonionizing radiation, with its longer wavelengths, lacks the energy to ionize the contents of cells.

It also appears not to be able to damage DNA like ionizing radiation can and generally has not been shown to cause irreversible changes that accumulate over time. Although overall healing or "thermal effects" are the best-documented biological changes resulting from nonionizing radiation, there are definite acute and chronic effects on the skin and eyes as well as possible effects on the immune system and other "nonthermal effects."

Some specialized heating effects that occur only at specific or resonance frequencies have been reported. Body resonance occurs when the wavelength of the radiation is about as long as the body.

The EMF energy can be concentrated in some areas and cause local hot spots and it is even possible to experience localized burns and electric shocks. These specific heating effects are important because some organs, particularly the testes and eyes, are especially sensitive to heating.

6. Controversies Surrounding Nonionizing Radiation

Ionizing radiation has long been very controversial. In contrast, recent studies show that nonionizing radiation issues are more of a cause for concern by the general public.

Some of the more controversial sources include high-tech equipment:

Nonionizing Radiation and Video Display Terminals - Many studies show that the extremely low-frequency exposure associated with workplace video display terminals is not an identifiable health risk for workers or even for pregnant workers. Most of the health problems, concerns or complaints about VDTs usually turn out to be ergonomic issues.

Microwaves and Cardiac Pacemakers - Microwaves and other forms of nonionizing radiation can cause heating in the human body. During the early stages of pacemaker use, genuine concerns about the effects of microwaves on their operation were prevalent.

These concerns have been shown to be false because of the inherent shielding designs of the pacemakers and years of safe operation. There has never been a documented case of pacemaker failure due to microwave radiation.

The "thermal response" to microwaves depends on the total amount of energy absorbed by the tissue; the intensity, duration, pattern, and frequency of the radiation; and the size, shape, and the composition of the body in terms of bone, fat, and muscle. The human body is designed to withstand normal heating with slight changes in body temperature, depending on factors such as age, physical condition, outside temperature and humidity, physical activity, and clothing.

EMF heating only lasts as long as the body is exposed to the nonionizing radiation, with body temperatures returning to normal resting levels shortly after cessation of any exposure. Even at higher levels where heating is greater than the body can tolerate and injury results, generally this effect cannot be felt because much of the radiation penetrates and heats tissues well below the skin and sensory perception. Because of this any warm feeling of heat cannot be used as a reliable warning of an overexposure.

Tanning Booths Versus Natural Sunlight - Many commercial tanning bed operators believe their systems are much safer than natural sunlight. However, the experts warn that artificial tanning light is still ultraviolet radiation and has nearly all of the risks of natural sunlight and maybe even more.

Tanning beds and sunlight darken the skin by delivering ultraviolet radiation to its surface, causing the cells to make extra darkening pigment. The operators maintain that tanning lamps emit only "safe" ultraviolet A (**UVA**) rays, as opposed to the sun's broad spectrum of UV (**A, B,** and **C**). UVB radiation is believed to be the most carcinogenic component of sunlight. However, studies have raised concerns about UVA radiation too. The longer wavelengths in UVA radiation penetrate the skin more deeply than UVB radiation, and because UVA is less effective at tanning the skin than UVB, higher doses are required for a "good" tan.

More than a half million cases of skin cancer develop annually in the United States, in normally healthy people. These figures indicate that the malignancies are indeed related to UV exposure. It should be strongly recommended that a sunscreen be used during exposure to natural sunlight and that the use of artificial tanning devices be curtailed or avoided altogether.

Problem with Laser Points - The problem with laser pointers is essentially one of misuse, primarily by minors. They are being used in many instances as toys rather than hazardous instruments. The pointers were designed to "point out" important information on a screen during lectures and training sessions.

Unfortunately, they have been misused in public gatherings and are a very real eye hazard because they have enough power (Class 2) to cause damage under certain conditions. There is also concern by law enforcement officers about their misuse because the beam produced is similar to that in weapon sighting devices.

III. NOISE

A. DEFINITIONS

1. Noise

Noise is any unwanted sound. The noise may be unwanted because it interferes with speech and hearing, because it is intense enough to damage hearing, or because it is otherwise annoying. Noise is described in terms of sound; thus we need to describe sound.

2. Sound

Sound can be described as a propagating disturbance through a physical medium. From a noise pollution perspective, sound is induced by a vibrating source and travels through air in the form of sound waves. These waveforms may be described in terms of frequency, amplitude, and pattern.

3. Frequency

The frequency of a waveform is the number of times per second the waveform oscillates. These oscillations per second are measured in Hertz (Hz). The human ear has a wide range of response, from 20 to 20,000Hz. Most sound contains a broad spectrum of frequencies.

However, some sounds contain only one frequency. These sounds are referred to as pure tones. Some sounds also have a dominant waveform or one that has significantly higher amplitude compared to the other waveforms.

4. Amplitude and Measurement of Sound Pressure

The amplitude is the sound pressure or the difference between background atmospheric pressure and the pressure with the sound present. Sound pressure is measured in decibels (dB). The decibel scale is logarithmic and as such is not linear. For example, every 3dB increase results in a doubling in the sound pressure. Sound pressure level (**SPL**) is measured using a sound level meter (**SLM**). A Type 2 SLM or better is typically used.

5. Use of Weighting Scales in Measuring Sound

Sound levels may be measured using different weighting scales. Weighting scales were developed to better evaluate human exposure to sound. The most commonly used scales are "A" and "C."

The A scale is most commonly used to measure human sound exposure. It has been weighted to be reflective of the human ear's response by reducing the effects of low and high frequencies.

The C-weighting network weighs the frequencies between 70 and 4000 Hz uniformly. Due to the weighting characteristics of the A and C scales, a comparison of decibel levels measured for the same noise source can help determine if the source has a significant low-frequency component. It is also possible to measure sound pressure levels within octave bands.

6. Octave Band

An octave is a spectrum of frequencies in which the center frequency is the square root of twice the lower cutoff frequency, and an upper cutoff frequency that is twice the lower cutoff frequency. When the center frequency is 1000Hz, the lower cutoff frequency is 1000Hz divided by the square root of 2, or 1000/1.414, which equals 707 Hz. The upper frequency would be 1000 times 1.414 or 1414Hz.

B. ANALYSIS OF AN OCTAVE BAND

Measuring of decibels within octave bands has traditionally been performed using an Octave Band or Third Octave Band Analyzer. Octave band analysis is of particular interest when searching for control techniques.

The use of noise data loggers (dosimeters) has allowed the accumulation of data over a wide spectrum of criteria. The data loggers can interface with a computer, so data can be reviewed in a time reflective manner. These dosimeters allow for analysis of data based on high and low sound levels and the times when they occur, average sound pressure levels, and a graphic time-sensitive analysis of sound pressure levels over the sampling time.

C. EFFECTS OF NOISE

1. Factors That Impact a Community's Response to Noise Pollution

A variety of factors can influence a community's response to a noise source in their neighborhood. The response may be more dramatic when a noise source moves into a previously quiet neighborhood.

According to the Environmental Protection Agency (EPA), the following factors may impact a community's response to noise pollution and should be considered when performing a community risk assessment:

a. History of prior exposure to the noise source,
b. Time of day and time of year of exposure,
c. Attitude toward the source,
d. Whether the residents believe they are being treated fairly,
e. Duration, frequency, presence of pure tones, and intensity,
f. Outdoor noise levels prior to intrusion of source and when source is not operating,
g. Interference with outdoor activities, and
h. Socioeconomic status and education level.

2. Adverse Health Impacts of Environmental Noise Exposure

As with many adverse health impacts, the dose determines the health impact. The adverse health impacts for environmental exposures are less well documented and defined compared to occupational noise exposure.

Environmental noise exposures are typically less than occupational noise exposures. Recreational activities such as shooting, mowing grass, using a chain saw, and other similar activities can produce sound levels equivalent to occupational exposures and cause hearing loss. Persons participating in such activities should wear hearing protection.

Noise can impact humans in several ways. Health ramifications such as hearing loss, permanent and temporary threshold shifts (hearing loss attributable to noise alone), ear pain, and tinnitus (ringing in the ears) are typically associated with occupational and not environmental/community noise. In contrast, interference with speech, perception of noise, performance effects, effects on residential behavior, annoyance, sleep disturbance, psychophysiological effects, and mental health effects may be associated with environmental/community noise.

3. Sleep Disturbance Impacts Associated With Environmental Noise Exposure

The primary noise-induced sleep disturbances are manifested as difficulty in falling asleep, changes in sleep pattern or depth, and awakenings. Noise during sleep can induce physiological effects such as increased blood pressure, increased heart rate, increased finger pulse amplitude, vasoconstriction, changes in respiration, and cardiac arrhythmia.

Secondary effects of nighttime noise exposure can be measured on the morning or day after the exposure. These secondary effects may include fatigue, mood changes, perceived poor sleep quality, and changes in performance.

4. Psychophysiological Effects of Noise

Noise has been postulated to act as a general stressor and may lead to changes in blood pressure, heart rate, and vasoconstriction. Community studies focusing on noise as a risk factor for cardiovascular disease have shown a tendency for increased blood pressure for persons living near airports or on streets with higher levels of noise as compared with controls. Other studies have tended to show much weaker associations when major risk factors for hypertension are considered.

5. Regulations Governing Community Noise Pollution

There is no regulation governing community noise on a national basis. The EPA Noise Control Act of 1972 established a means to coordinate federal research in noise control, authorized the establishment of noise emissions standards for products distributed in commerce, and provided a means of providing information to the public with respect to noise emission and reduction for such products.

A few states do have noise regulations, but for the most part community noise regulations are promulgated by counties, cites, or other local governing bodies.

The EPA did present a Model Community Noise Control Ordinance in 1975. In reality, noise control ordinances vary in exposure levels, times of day, and measurement methods. The EPA does provide a recommendation for sound exposures. This recommendation will require some definition of terms:

The equilavent sound level (L_{eq}) is the A-weighted sound level that is equivalent to an actual time-varying sound level; L_{eq} may also be described as the equivalent continuous sound level (in decibels) for the sound energy averaged over *a* specific time. Day-night sound level (L_{dn}) is the A-weighted equivalent sound level for a 24-hour period, with 10 dB added to nighttime levels (10PM to 7AM).

6. Noise Control Measures

It is generally easier to implement noise controls at the design level. This would be true whether one is speaking about the design of a piece of machinery or of a manufacturing plant. The control measures required are dependent on the sound level and the frequency.

Noise control measures utilized after construction are often barriers or enclosures. The construction materials of the barriers or the enclosures are dictated by the sound level and frequency. In general, the lower the frequency the thicker the wall needs to be. Another factor in noise reduction is distance. Doubling the distance from a source reduces the sound level by 6 dB.

IV. BIBLIOGRAPHY

Gasaway, D. C. (1994). Noise-Induced Hearing Loss. In R.   McCunney (Ed.), A practical Approach to Occupational and Environmental Medicine, 2nd Edition (pp. 230-247). Boston, MA: Little, Brown and Company.

Herring, R. L. (2001). Noise Pollution. In L. Williams, & R. Langley (Eds.), Environmental Health Secrets (pp. 226-229). Philadelphia, PA: Hanley & Belfus, Inc.

Hicks, D. E. (2001). Lightning and Electrical Injuries. In L. Williams, & R. Langley (Eds.), Environmental Health Secrets (pp. 168-171). Philadelphia, PA: Hanley & Belfus, Inc.

Meredith, J. T. (2001). High-Altitude Illness. In L. Williams, & R. Langley (Eds.), Environmental Health Secrets (pp. 148-153). Philadelphia, PA: Hanley & Belfus, Inc.

Moeller, D. W. (1997). Electromagnetic Radiation. Environmental Health (pp.240-269). Cambridge, MA, and London, UK: Harvard University Press.

Moeller, D. W. (1997). Energy. Environmental Health (pp.363-384). Cambridge, MA, and London, UK: Harvard University Press.

Moore, G.S. (1999). Air, Noise, and Radiation. Living with the Earth: Concepts in Environmental Health Science (pp. 10-1 – 10-64). Boca Raton, FL: Lewis Publishers.

Nadakavukaren, A. (2000). Noise Pollution. Our Global Environment: A Health Perspective, 5th Edition (pp. 507-527). Prospective Heights, IL: Waveland Press, Inc.

Nadakavukaren,   A. (2000). Radiation. <u>Our Global Environment: A Health Perspective, 5th Edition</u> (pp. 355-405). Prospective Heights, IL: Waveland Press, Inc.

Sprau, D. D., Emery, R. J. (2001). Radiation. In L. Williams, & R. Langley (Eds.), <u>Environmental Health Secrets</u> (pp. 172-178). Philadelphia, PA: Hanley & Belfus, Inc.

Wagner, T. (1994). Energy Dependence. <u>In Our Backyard: A Guide to Understanding Pollution and Its Effects</u> (pp. 184-234). New York, NY: Van Nostrand Reinhold.

Yassi, A., Kjellström, T., de Kok, T., & Guidotti, T. L. (2001). Nature of Environmental Health Hazards: Physical Hazards. In A. Yassi, [et al](Eds.), <u>Basic Environmental Health</u> (pp. 80-92). New York, NY: Oxford University Press, Inc.

Yassi, A., Kjellström, T., de Kok, T., & Guidotti, T. L. (2001). Health and Energy Use. In A. Yassi, [et al](Eds.), <u>Basic Environmental Health</u> (pp. 311-331). New York, NY: Oxford University Press, Inc.

Yassi, A., Kjellström, T., de Kok, T., & Guidotti, T. L. (2001). Transboundary and Global Health Concerns: UV Radiation. In A. Yassi, [et al](Eds.), <u>Basic Environmental Health</u> (pp. 375-378). New York, NY: Oxford University Press, Inc.

SECTION

III

ENVIRONMENTAL AND OCCUPATIONAL SETTINGS

CHAPTER

11

GLOBAL ISSUES

I. POPULATION BACKGROUND

A. BACKGROUND

1. Introduction

The world is approximately 4 billion years old. It has taken that many years to form the earth, develop its resources, store energy in various forms, and enable living organisms to adapt to the planet. More human-caused environmental degradation has taken place in the last 2,000 years than in all the previous years combined. Hence, we have a need for courses in planet management, ecosystems management, and human environment management. Humans should become the environment's protecting manager rather than its self-serving destroyer.

For almost 300,000 years, human overpopulation was not a problem. Drought, floods, famine, plagues, pestilence, and war kept early populations in check, as did the lack of heating for homes, the inability to preserve food, and the harsh wilderness. Couples had large families to be certain that some children survived these hazards.

When the Europeans discovered America, approximately 250 million people lived on the earth. By 1650, about 150 years later, the population had increased to about 500 million. In 1850, approximately 1.2 billion people lived on the earth. The population increased 70 years later (1920) to just fewer than 2 billion people. In 1950, another one-half billion inhabitants were added to the earth. By 1980, the earth's population had reached approximately 4.5 billion. That is more than a five fold increase in 300 years.

Assuming that the first humans appeared on earth between 1.5 million and 600,000 years ago, we can estimate that somewhere between 60 and 100 billion people have inhabited the planet at some time. Today the earth supports about 6 billion human inhabitants - close to 6% of all who have ever lived. We don't have enough information to estimate accurately what populations were before A.D. 1650. But we can make some educated guesses based on circumstantial evidence (e.g.,number of people who could be supported on X square miles by hunting and gathering, primitive agriculture, and so on). On this basis, it's been calculated that the total human population in 8000 B.C. was about five million people. By the beginning of the Christian era, when agricultural settlements had become widespread, world population is estimated to have risen to about 200-300 million, and increased to about 500 million by 1650. It then doubled to one billion by 1850, to two billion by 1930, and to four billion by 1975. By 1987 world population passed the 5 billion mark, hit 6 billion late in 1999, and continues to climb. Thus not only has world population been increasing steadily (with minor irregularities) for the past million years, but the rate of growth has also increased (Figure 11.1).

2. Demographic Issues

The impact of people on the environment is related to the size of the population and to the level of consumption (Table 11.1). Both expand independently and both lead to increasing pressure on the environment as both a supplier of resources and a repository of waste.

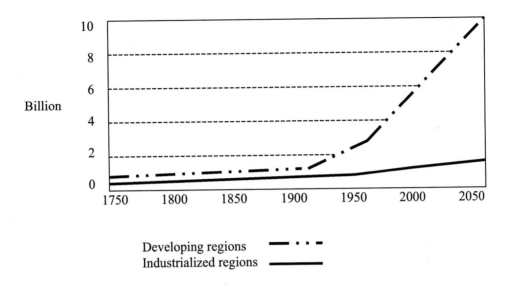

Figure 11.1. Trends and Projections in World Population Growth, 1750-2050. (Source: Nadakavukaren, 2000).

Limited resources have made development in the poorest countries of the world difficult, with increasing demand for water, food, and energy for domestic use being in direct proportion to the number of users. Meanwhile, more people are moving to urban areas where the infrastructures are rarely able to keep up with the influx of new citizens. In temperate and sub-Arctic countries, energy needs may be greater than in other parts of the world because of the climate. Countries in these areas are generally highly developed, and the high level of consumption accompanying their affluence (which until recently, in many countries, was not accompanied by much genuine concern for the environment or the need for conservation of resources) has magnified global problems.

Different areas of the world have different rates of population growth. The global annual increase is thought to have stabilized, with an increase of about 81 million people added each year for 1990-95. Nevertheless, the world population, which was 5.3 billion in 1990, and 5.9 billion in 1999, is expected to be between 7.7 and 11.2 billion by the year 2050.

The size, rate of growth, and age distribution of a population is only part of the demographic problem of a country or region. Movement of populations across borders also constitutes a major component of a demographic pattern. Migrants are usually driven by economic need toward countries where there is a greater potential for employment or the possibility of opening up new land. Increasingly, political refugees have contributed to migratory movements. Ecological change, such as drought, has also forced migration. While the total number of migrants represents a small fraction of the world's population, these people can have a major influence on the resources and structure of the host population, especially when unanticipated environmental or political events cause a large number of people to move to a neighboring country.

Table 11.1. Demographic Indicators of World and Regional Population Development. (Source: Moore, 1999).

	TOTAL POP. 1997	PROJECT POP 2025	AVE. RATE OF NATURAL INCREASE 1995-2000	TOTAL FERTILITY RATE	DOUBLING TIME IN YEARS
WORLD TOTAL	5,848	8,039	1.4	2.79	50
Developed Regions 1	1,178	1,220	0.3	1.59	233
Less Developed Regions 2	4,670	6,819	1.7	3.08	21.2
AFRICA	759	1454	2.6	5.31	26.9
Eastern	234	480	2.9	6.05	24.1
Middle	88	189	2.7	6.01	25.9
Northern	165	257	2	3.67	35
Southern	50	83	2.2	3.92	31.8
Western	222	447	2.8	5.95	25
ASIA	3538	4785	1.4	2.85	50
Eastern	1447	1696	0.9	1.78	77.7
South Eastern	498	692	1.6	2.86	43.7
South Central	1418	2100	1.8	3.42	38.8
Western	175	297	2.2	3.82	31.8
EUROPE	729	701	0	1.45	-
Eastern	309	284	-0.3	1.41	-
Northern	94	96	0.1	1.73	700
Southern	144	137	0.2	1.34	350
Western	182	184	0.3	1.46	233
LATIN AMERICA & CARIBBEAN	492	689	1.5	2.65	46.6
Caribbean	37	48	1.1	2.59	63.6
Central America	128	189	1.9	3.04	36.8
South America	327	452	1.5	3.04	46.6
NORTH AMERICA	302	439	0.8	1.93	87.5
Canada	30	36	9	1.61	77.7
United States	272	333	0.8	1.96	87.5
OCEANIA	29	41	1.3	2.48	53.8
Australia/New Zealand	22	29	1.1	1.91	63.6

1 More developed regions comprise North America, Japan, Europe, Australia and New Zealand.
2 Less developed regions comprise all regions of Africa, Latin America & Caribbean, Asia (excluding Japan), and Melanesia, Micronesia, and Polynesia.

These migrants are often confronted with severe health and environmental problems and seldom have access to basic health services and health insurance coverage. Their living conditions are usually inferior to those of the host population, resulting in a negative effect on their health.

3. Poverty

Poverty has been defined by the World Bank as the inability of an individual or household to attain a minimal standard of living. The level of prosperity in a country and the distribution of resources within it determine the level and nature of poverty. The association between poverty and health is strong and obvious. The poor usually have much lower life expectancy, higher infant mortality, and a higher incidence of disability. They suffer more from communicable diseases and a high proportion of their lives are spent in poor health.

The number of poor people in a given country is estimated from the number of people with incomes below a level defined as the poverty line. The World Bank estimates that in 1985 there were 1115 million people living below the poverty line, defined as $370 U.S. per person per year, or U.S. $1 per person per day. The extreme poverty line is set at $275 U.S. per person per year and there were 634 million people living at that level in the world in 1985.

In the late 1960's and early 1970's ecologists such as Paul Ehrlich, Barry Commoner, and Rachael Carson sensitized the nation to the potential problems caused by human overpopulation, excessive resource consumption, and uncontrolled release of toxic substances. Their contributions gave rise to a strong environmental concern encompassing all age and political groups. Out of this broad based societal concern, emerged governmental regulatory agencies, such as the U.S. Environmental Protection Agency, which were charged with protecting human health and the environment. While federal and state regulatory agencies have "capped' and in some instances reversed some forms of environmental degradation in this nation, on a global basis environmental deterioration has continued, largely due to an ever expanding population placing increased pressures on renewable (i.e., land, water, air, and biota) and non-renewable (i.e., fossil fuels and precious metals) resources. If the world's population continues to increase at the present rate and without the implementation of strong conservation measures, the long-term sustainability of the world's ecosystems and geochemical cycles may be unlikely.

B. OVERPOPULATION

The expected stability of the planet and the population that inhabits the earth has been evaluated in several analyses. One of the more notable and comprehensive appraisals was the Global 2000 Report prepared by 11 separate government agencies in 1980. In the report's executive summary the following conclusion was presented:

"If present trends continue, the world in the year 2000 will be more crowded, more polluted, less stable ecologically, and more vulnerable to disruption than the world we live in now. Despite greater material output the world's people will be poorer in many ways than they are today."

"Prompt and vigorous changes in public policy are needed-to avoid or minimize these problems (i.e., overpopulation, resource depletion and environmental degradation) before they become unmanageable."

Before discussing specifics of the Global 2000 Report, it's important to briefly review how non-human populations grow and compare these possible growth curves to the world's human population. Populations of animals tend to grow exponentially which can be depicted as a percent increase, such as money compounded in a savings account. A percent increase is very slow initially but increases rapidly after some time has passed. The growth curve shown in Figure 11.2 would be typical of an animal population in nature. What is most interesting is that almost without exception the animal population will increase beyond the point where the environment is unable to support the population. This point is called the carrying capacity. Once this carrying capacity is exceeded, the population will most often undergo a decline. The decline may be the result of exhaustion of food supply, increased predation, reduction in suitable breeding areas, and other factors. For some animal species the decline may be very precipitous and in rare cases lead to extinction. Seldom do populations ever stabilize at the carrying capacity. Following a decline, populations will commence an increase in numbers until once again the carrying capacity is exceeded, repeating another growth cycle.

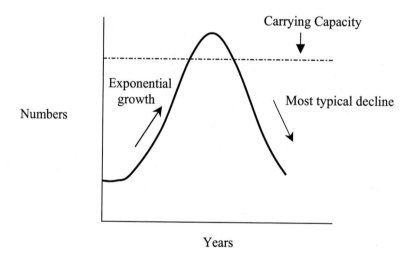

Figure 11.2. Growth Curve of an Animal Population. (Source: Odum, 1971).

The human population has also undergone an exponential growth increase enhanced by application of technology to agriculture, improved sanitation, medicine. Our death rate, therefore, has declined, while our birth rate has remained basically constant. Our growth curve looks like the one shown in Figure 11.3.

As shown by the graph, the world's population has grown rapidly in the past 300 years. It took until 1650 for the world's population to reach about 500 million. By 1800 or 150 years later, it had doubled to about 1 billion. In another 120 years, or in 1920, it doubled again to 2 billion. By 1975, just 55 years, the population had doubled to 4 billion. The time for doubling becomes smaller and smaller, indicative of exponential growth of animal populations. The world's population, now about 5.0 billion people, may double again in 41 years, although the current rate of population increase is only 1.7% per year.

Depending upon their growth rates, individual nations will double their current populations in a few decades to many decades. Sweden's population is growing very slowly at 0.1% per year, so its population will not double for another 700 years, as long as the current growth rate holds. Sweden doesn't have a population growth problem demanding any immediate attention. In contrast, Mexico's growth rate is 3.5%, and its population will double in 20 years, unless its growth rate is sharply reduced. Mexico, which already has immense problems of poverty, sanitation, housing, and unemployment is headed for disaster. Many African nations, too, are projected to double their populations in 20 to 30 years. The United States, with a growth rate of 1.0%, is projected to double its population in about 70 years.

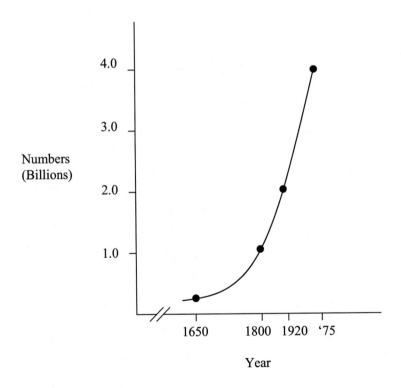

Figure 11.3. Growth Curve of the World's Population. (Source: Miller, 1979).

C. CONCEPT OF DOUBLING TIME AND POPULATION GROWTH

Perhaps the best way to describe growth rate is in terms of doubling time - the time required for a population to double in size. During the period from 8000 B.C. to 1650 A.D., the population doubled about every 1,500 years. The next doubling took 200 years, the next 80 years, and the next, 45 years. Historical evidence indicates that the increase in human numbers did not occur at a steady, even pace but rather that three main surges occurred. The first took place about 600,000 years ago with the evolution of culture (developing and learning techniques of social organization and group and individual survival); the next occurred about 8000 B.C. with the agricultural revolution; and the most recent began about 200 years ago with the onset of the industrial-medical-scientific revolution. Bearing in mind that changes in the size of populations occur when birth and death rates are out of balance, one can reasonably conclude that each of these spurts indicates that the story of human population growth is not primarily a story of changes in birth rates, but of changes in death rates. Let's now take a closer look at some of the demographic facts that help to explain our current population dilemma.

The world population increased more rapidly about 200 years ago with the "Great Awakening," followed quickly by the industrial-medical-scientific revolution. At this time, sanitation, immunization, and other measures of environmental and public health greatly reduced the incidence of childhood and other communicable diseases. As three cases in point:

1. In 1796, Edward Jenner demonstrated that immunizations could prevent smallpox.
2. Walter Reed discovered that the **Aedes** mosquito spread yellow fever.
3. Alexander Fleming later discovered penicillin.

Scientists refined flood control, improved agricultural and food technology, and developed public and environmental health practices. All of this activity served to control plagues and epidemics, which led to fewer children dying and a longer life expectancy. As a result, the world population grew rapidly. At the same time, a culture characterized by large families continued, with few of the children dying. Instead of two of twelve children surviving, now eight, nine, and ten, or more survived.

The doubling time for the world population is decreasing. Table 11.2 highlights this concept. To find the doubling time, we have to know the growth rate. The relationship between growth rate and doubling time is shown in Table 11.3.

Developing nations tend to have greater potential than developed countries for population increase. This is because the potential for population increase becomes greater as more females enter childbearing ages. The women have babies, and the population base and growth potential increase even further. Many developing countries have a "stairstep" or "Christmas tree" graph. In contrast, when the population of developed nations is plotted, it gives a "stovepipe" effect. More babies are born in countries that are less able to provide food and the other requirements of life.

Table 11.2. World Population Doubling Time. (Source: Morgan, 1997).

Year	Estimated World Population	Years to Double
800 B.C	5 million	1,500
AD 1650	500 million	200
AD 1850	1 billion	80
AD 1930	2 billion	45
AD 1975	4 billion	36
AD ??	8 billion	??

Table 11.3. Relationship Between Growth Rate and Doubling Time. (Source: Morgan, 1997).

Growth Rate	Years to Double
0.50%	140
0.80%	87
1.00%	70
2.00%	35
3.00%	24
4.00%	18
5.00%	14
7.00%	10
10.00%	7

The previously discussed and illustrated exponential growth curves can be described by the following equation: $N_t = N_o e^{rt}$

Where: N_t = Population (numbers) after passage of time
           N_o = Initial Population
           r = Growth rate
              = $\dfrac{\text{Birth rate - death rate } \pm \text{migration}}{1000}$
           t = time (in years)

Note that e is equal to 2.718, the base of natural logarithms. The equation can be readily solved because, by definition, the natural log (ln) of e raised to the X power is equal to X ($\ln e^x = X$).

Therefore, the expression $N_t = N_o e^{rt}$ can be simplified to:

$$\ln\left(\frac{N_t}{N_o}\right) = \ln e^{rt}$$

$$\left(\frac{N_t}{N_o}\right) = rt \qquad \text{or}$$

$$\frac{\ln\left(\frac{N_t}{N_o}\right)}{r} = t$$

In working with the expression, the growth rate **r** must be expressed as a decimal. Doubling times of populations can also be calculated as shown below. For doubling of a population, N_t divided by N_o must be equal to two. Therefore:

$$\frac{N_t}{N_o} = e^{rt}$$

$$2 = e^{rt}$$

$$\ln 2 = \ln e^{rt}$$

$$\ln 2 = rt$$

$$\frac{0.693}{r} = t \qquad \text{or} \qquad \frac{69.3}{r\%} = t$$

So if you know the rate of growth (r) of a population, say expressed as a percent growth rate, the doubling time in years can be round by merely dividing it into 69.3.

D. POPULATION RATE MEASURES

1. Birth Rates, Death Rates, and Fertility Rates

Birth rates are generally expressed as the number of babies born per 1,000 people per year. Prior to the Industrial Revolution, birth rates in every society typically were in the 40-50 per thousand range. Today the birth rate gap between nations has widened dramatically, exemplified by Latvia and Bulgaria's 8, the world's lowest, and with a high of 54 in the West African nation of Niger. Indeed, in recent years a nation's birth rate can be looked at as a crude barometer of its level of economic development, since the most prosperous, most technologically advanced countries generally are characterized by low birth rates.

Death rates are calculated in the same way as birth rates, representing the annual number of deaths per 1,000 population. Birth and death rates are frequently referred to as "crude" rates because they don't reflect the wide variations in age distribution within a population, a fact that might result in misleading conclusions when comparing statistics from different countries (Table 11.4). For example, the fact that Jordan has a death rate of 5 per thousand population while the death rate in Germany is 10 might lead one to assume that Jordanians enjoy better health care and a higher standard of living than do

Germans. Such an assumption would be erroneous, however, since the reason for Jordan's apparent advantage is that nearly half the Jordanian population (41%) is under the age of 15, an age cohort everywhere typified by low likelihood of death. Germany, on the other hand, is characterized by an aging population; only 16% of Germans are under 15, while 15% are over age 65 (compared to just 2% in Jordan). Even with excellent medical care, death rates are bound to be higher in a predominantly middle-aged to elderly population than in one primarily composed of the very young.

Total fertility rates (TFR), representing the average number of children each woman within a given population is likely to bear during her reproductive lifetime (assuming that current age-specific birth rates remain constant), perhaps give a clearer picture of reproductive behavior than do crude birth rates. Although world TFR has been gradually falling in recent decades to its present level of 2.9, the wide discrepancies in national fertility rates are illustrated by countries such as Niger, whose total fertility rate of 7.5 is currently the world's highest, and by Hong Kong, whose total fertility rate of 1.1 suggests a preference for one-child families on that crowded island.

Crude birth rates and crude death rates are often used to derive a growth rate. These rates are expressed as numbers per 1000 of the population. Fertility rates provide better estimates of growth rates. There are two types: total and general. The total fertility rate is the average number of children women will have during their entire reproductive years. Reproductive years are considered to range from age 15 through age 49. The general fertility rate is expressed as the number of births per 1000 women per year. Currently the world has a total fertility rate of about 4.7. In order for a women to guarantee their replacement in developing countries a total fertility rate of about 2.7 is needed. In industrialized countries, where infant mortality is lower, a fertility rate of 2.1 is sufficient.

Table 11.4. Calculations of Birth Rate, Death Rate, and Rate of Natural Increase. (Source: Moore, 1999).

Birth rate equals the number of live children born in a year per 1,000 total population
Birth rate in year Y = $\dfrac{\text{Number of live children born in year Y}}{\text{Midyear population in year Y}}$
Birth rate in year 1998 = $\dfrac{4,345,600 \text{ (children born in 1998)}}{271,600,000 \text{ (population in mid-1998)}}$ = 16/1000
Death rate in year Y = $\dfrac{\text{Number of deaths in year Y}}{\text{Midyear population in year Y}}$
Death rate in year 1998 = $\dfrac{2,172,800 \text{ (deaths in 1998)}}{271,600,000 \text{ (population in mid-1998)}}$ = 8 / 1000
Rate of natural increase in year 1998 = (Birth rate – Death rate) = 8/1000 or 0.8%*
* These are approximate numbers for the united states used only for example.

2. Growth Rate

A rate is normally expressed as one quantity in relation to another. Runners like to keep track of the time it takes to run a 10-kilometer course in minutes per mile. This is a rate measurement, and runners can study their progress by decreasing the minutes per mile that it takes to run the course. In a similar way, growth rate can be used to assess additions or deletions to the population. People enter a population by births or immigration and leave a population by deaths or emigration. The rate of births is the ratio of births to the population, and death rates represent the ratio of deaths to the population. Growth rate is then determined by the birth rate minus the death rate. If the growth rate is positive, there will be an increase in population. Even if the rate of growth is slowed (declines), the population will accumulate. Similarly, even if the runner's pace is slowed, he/she will still accumulate miles. Consequently, we are still contributing large numbers of people to the population despite a declining growth rate. This addition becomes exaggerated when the base of people is larger. In 1975, the growth rate was close to 1.75 percent with a global population of four billion people leading to four billion x 0.0175 = 70 million new infants each year. In 2000 there will be nearly 6 billion people with a growth rate of 1.4% leading to 6 billion x 0.014 = 84 million new infants per year.

3. Impacts of Growth on Ecosystems

Certainly the issue of how to feed additional multitudes in the years ahead, when close to a billion of the earth's current inhabitants are malnourished, looms as a monumental task for future world leaders. However, population growth exerts many other socioeconomic and environmental impacts that may be less publicized than famine, yet have a profound influence on human well-being and on the sustainability of planetary life-support systems. In many parts of the world today, evidence is mounting that large and still-growing human and livestock populations have already exceeded the carrying capacity of the land itself. Indeed, at a time when we are trying to produce more and more from a given land area to sustain increasing numbers of people, the activities of those people are damaging natural ecosystems to the extent that they are becoming incapable of supporting their present population, much less future billions.

Giving evidence of the fact that population growth and ecological degradation are inextricably interrelated are the swelling numbers of **"environmental refugees"** - people seeking refuge abroad due to environmental problems at home. Oxford University ecologist Norman Myers estimates that 25 million people have been forced to leave their place of birth due to water scarcity, depleted soils, deforestation, desertification, or other environmental calamities. Regions most affected by this phenomenon include Central America, India, China, the Horn of Africa, and the Sahel.

E. CONSEQUENCES OF OVERPOPULATION

1. Effects Of Overpopulation

In 1791, Thomas Malthus predicted that the population would grow faster than the ability to feed it. This was before automation of farm life, tractors, synthetic fertilizer, mass transport, freeze-drying, and so forth. He suggested that populations grow geometrically while food production increases arithmetically. Malthus' claim may have an unsettling amount of truth.

Despite several decades of agricultural research aimed at increasing the worldwide food supply, one of every three persons living in poor, underdeveloped countries is unable to find enough to eat. These people suffer from starvation and from diseases such as Kwashiorkor, which results from a lack of protein. In many cases large families cannot provide for the children properly and do not receive much-needed health, social, and agriculture services from their government.

Approximately 12 million people die of starvation each year. Thirty million more people each year suffer from diseases made worse by hunger. Areas hit hardest by hunger, the population doubles every 17 to 30 years.

What are the likely consequences of human overpopulation of the planet? To answer this question, in the early 1970's the dynamic computer model of Forester and Meadows was developed. This computer model took information from the years 1900 to 1970 and projected it to the year 2100. The information utilized included rates of population growth, resource utilization, and pollutant releases. Major assumptions incorporated into the model included the premises that the earth had: (1) finite non-renewable resources (2) a finite land area suitable for agriculture and (3) a finite capability of absorbing pollutants. An exponential increase in population, resource consumption, and industrial output were also assumed. The modelers also introduced forms of change such as birth control, recycling, pollution reduction, increased agricultural productivity, and stabilization of industrial output. The results of the Forester-Meadows projections were startling. Even incorporating overly optimistic assumptions, the world's population would undergo rapid declines due to excessive pollution or an inadequate food supply.

Only by using unrealistic assumptions, would the population stabilize and a crisis be averted. As to income distribution, the disparity between the per capita incomes for rich and poor nations will increase. This disparity will be of sufficient magnitude that the Global 2000 Report concluded that it could lead to increased tensions between the rich (industrialized) and poor (developing) nations resulting in resource protection (i.e., oil and precious metals) and price increases in resources required by the industrialized nations. The probability of wars would also be increased under such circumstances. Based upon the Global 2000 Report, the United States should have a strong interest in minimizing the protected income disparities, if nothing more than to insure the availability of needed resources. It is important to note that with only 5% of the world's population, the United States consumes 30 to 60% of the major resources. This disproportionate consumption may not permit the majority of the world's population to reach a standard of living comparable to that of the United States. In fact, as resources decline and their prices increase due to demand placed upon them by wealthy nations, many third world nations will not be able to afford resources, such as oil needed for agricultural and industrial development, and the standard of living will decline.

Several writers such as Barry Commoner have commented on the morality and ethics of nations with few people consuming a disproportionate share of the world's resources. Commoner popularized the concept of "spaceship earth" in his writings in which he posed the following paraphrased question. Is it right for 20% of the world's population to ride in First Class on spaceship earth while generations of the majority (80%) will be required to ride in the cargo holds of the ship? Commoner's analogy to the world situation has always sparked discussion and debate, but it's worth considering if wealthy nations have a responsibility to the poorer nations of the world.

Perhaps the most disturbing consequences of overpopulation is the increase in human suffering and death related to an inadequate food supply. About 5 to 20 million people are believed to die per year from undernutrition or malnutrition and the diseases affected by an inadequate intake of calories or diet. About 50% of these deaths are in children. The World Bank has estimated that 400-600 million people are suffering from nutritional inadequacies and in the year 2000 about 1.3 million people or 20% of the world's population was affected.

2. Food

The dominant forms of nutritional diseases are Kwashiorkor and marasmus. Kwashiorkor is characterized by a diet deficient in protein and sometimes an insufficient intake of calories. It is most often caused by the removal of an infant from a source of mothers milk due to the birth of another child. Kwashiorkor comes from the West African, "displaced child." The disease, characterized by bloat, skin rash, and hair discoloration, can lead to anemia and permanent brain damage. Marasmus comes from the Greek; 'to waste away', and is the result of a diet deficient in both protein and calories. Individuals suffering from marasmus have a haunting appearance - a face of an elderly person, regardless of age. Stomach swelling and shrivelled skin are other external characteristics. Untreated, marasmus can cause dehydration, diarrhea, and permanent brain damage. The majority of people recently observed in Ethiopia as suffering and dying from starvation had contracted marasmus. There is now great promise in treating marasmus victims by the development of an inexpensive and easily administered treatment, called oral rehydration therapy (ORT). By introducing a combination of simple nutrients and salts, dehydration and diarrhea, which were often treated with difficulty, now can be readily reversed.

F. CONTROL OF POPULATION

1. Background

In a given country, there are two ways of controlling the population, which are empowerment or force.

The International Conference on Population Development (ICPD) was held in Cairo, Egypt beginning September 5, 1994. The major topic behind the conference was women's rights. The draft program of action proposed that a full range of reproductive and health-care services, including contraception and sex education should be made available to all. One of the most crucial points of the conference was the need for participation of women in the global work force at different levels. Education and employment were discussed as a tool to make women more powerful. The stabilizing of human population is no longer a mystery. It is best accomplished by improving women's education, providing them with paid employment, and making effective and inexpensive contraception available. Unfortunately, this is not an easy solution in many countries where poverty, cultural traditions, and lack of educational opportunities exist and contribute to the illiteracy of nearly one billion people worldwide. Two thirds of the illiterate population are women formerly young girls who are denied this education. In most of Asia and in Muslim and Catholic countries, a woman's body may not be considered her own, nor is the child in her womb. Collective decisions are often made about a woman and they are accepted because the extended family is the institution that works, the State is often not trusted. Countries attempting to bring population growth under control without first empowering women and providing effective birth control have often resorted to oppressive population control policies.

2. Family Planning Versus Population Control

Those policies established by governments for setting an optimum population size are referred to as **population control**. The policies are directed at reducing population. In a number of developed countries such as in Western Europe, policies may be directed at promoting a higher TFR by providing state financial support for hospital expenses related to childbirth, for monthly support for the parent(s) during the first year or two of the child's life as in Austria, or even tax deductions or special bonuses. Population control is in contrast to **family planning** programs that are directed at assisting couples in having the number of children they desire regardless of how many. Family planning is parent-centered and places the desires of the individual or parent for having children before that of a state or national policy. Some policy makers argue that this style of family planning may not be enough to stem the tide of population growth in these countries where many children are considered an important resource for gathering wood and water, harvesting crops, or performing other forms of manual labor. The simple act of getting water may take several hours a day, and it takes longer and longer as resources diminish. Children are also viewed as a source of security in old age in those countries without a financial support system for the elderly. The persistent desires for large families in many Least Developed Countries is estimated to add nearly 660 million people in the next 50 years.

There is the additional problem of funding needs for family planning services in foreign countries. The ICPD in Cairo (1994) agreed that it would take at least $17 billion annually to provide services for population and reproductive health programs, and the prevention of STDs including HIV. Unfortunately, annual world expenditures are much less than half of this amount with the dollars contributed appearing to have leveled off. Such shortfalls in LDCs is expected to result in as many as 220 million unintended pregnancies. As many as 88 million of these will likely be terminated by abortions. The pregnancies and abortions may cause as many as 117,000 additional maternal deaths with up to 1.5 million women having some form of chronic health problem. This unmet demand for family planning services may likely cause an increase of 1.2 billion in global population. The major elements to offering a better quality of life for the world's billions may depend on: (1) the willingness of governments to set reasonable policies with adequate funding; (2) develop greater motivation for small families through improved economies; and (3) universal access to knowledge and use of family planning services.

G. METHODS OF FERTILITY CONTROL

1. Introduction

The process of conception requires that a viable sperm has access to a healthy egg. When the sperm enters the egg, the tail is released and the ovum secretes a protective chemical barrier that prohibits other sperm from entering. Methods that prevent fertilization of the egg are called contraception, and there are hundreds of different procedures and formulations available today. The enormous variety of contraceptive tools attests to the interest of society in developed countries in preventing unwanted pregnancies. These methods vary in their risks to health, their efficacy in preventing pregnancies, ease of use, acceptance, and cost. Some of the methods and characteristics are described below.

2. Contraceptive Methods that are Reversible

a. Natural Birth Control and Family Planning

This process is sometimes referred to as the rhythm method and relies on voluntary changes in sexual behavior. The method requires that the female predict her fertile periods by examining cervical mucous and/or tracking basal temperature or charting her menstrual cycle and ovulation times on a calendar. She would then abstain from sexual intercourse during times of the month when she is fertile. This method has proven to be very unreliable because menstrual cycles vary, and the narrow window for sexual opportunity is not always observed.

b. Abstinence

The term abstinence has come to mean the exclusion of sexual intimacy including oral-genital kissing and mutual masturbation. These activities are often referred to as "outercourse." Either of these methods can be 100 percent effective in prevention of pregnancies as long as there is not an opportunity for sperm getting near the vagina. The problems with "outercourse" are (STDs) through oral-genital contact, and the motivation and opportunity for intercourse being increased.

c. Hormonal Contraceptives

Oral Contraceptives - Since the introduction of the pill in 1960, it has become widely accepted and is now used by nearly 40 percent of women who wish to avoid pregnancy. The combined effects of the synthetic hormones estrogen and progesterone in the pill prohibits the maturation of ova, prevents the development of the uterine lining, and forms cervical mucous creating a barrier against sperm.

Depo-Provera - This is a long-acting synthetic hormone (progesterone) that is injected into muscles of the arm or buttocks every three months. It has an efficacy of 99 percent and is especially desirable for women who don't want to keep track of taking the daily pill or inserting a device or chemical into the vagina. Most women lose their menstrual period within a year on this hormone. The adverse side effects are minimal and are usually limited to a slight weight gain, occasional dizziness, and headaches.

Norplant - Norplant consists of five or six silicon rubber capsules containing progestin that are inserted under the skin of the upper arm of the female, using minor surgery. Small amounts of progestin are time-released over a five year period and work by suppressing ovulation, thickening the cervical mucous, and inhibiting the growth of the uterine lining. Norplant has been successfully tested in more than 40 countries demonstrating minimal health risks with nearly 100 percent effectiveness in preventing pregnancies. It has been used more frequently in the U.S. since it entered the market in 1991, but the up front costs that may exceed $550 are sometimes a deterrent even though the cost of the pill over the same five year period is more than twice that amount.

d. Spermicides

Chemicals that are designed to kill sperm are called **spermicides**. The substance most commonly used is nonoxynol-9 and it comes in a variety of forms including jellies, creams, foams, and waxy suppositories. These are all meant to be inserted far enough to cover the cervix and so providing a chemical and physical obstacle to sperm. Spermicides are most useful when used together with a barrier method such as a condom. Together they provide 98 percent effectiveness against pregnancy.

e. Barrier Methods of Contraception

Male Condom - Condoms are typically elastic material of latex rubber designed to be rolled onto the erect penis before intercourse. They appear in a variety of colors and textures, with or without lubricants, and with or without reservoir that is designed o capture ejaculate. The effectiveness of condoms to prevent pregnancies is reduced to 88 percent because of improper use or storage which permits sperm to enter the vagina through tears, rips, or spillage. Greater effectiveness can be achieved if the condom is used along with a spermicidal lubricant. Condoms are one of the top three contraceptive methods used in the United States and provide the additional benefit of protecting against the transfer of HIV.

Female Condom, Diaphragms, and Cervical Caps - The female condom is a soft elastic polyurethane conical bag with an elastic ring. The narrow end is inserted into the vagina leaving the wider end to extend over the labia. It has a reported failure rate of around 12 percent based on use in the United States.

The diaphragm is a thin latex rubber cup with a flexible rubber-coated ring intended to cover the cervix. Diaphragms come in a variety of sizes and must be fitted to the female by a trained health professional. Moreover, the user must be familiar with the correct method of inserting and positioning the diaphragm. It is intended to be used with a spermicidal cream or jelly on the concave or inside surface before insertion, and then left in place for up to eight hours after intercourse. This permits sufficient contact time to kill any remaining sperm.

The cervical cap is similar in design but smaller than the diaphragm, and is also fitted by a health professional. It is designed to be used with a spermicide and left in place for several hours after intercourse. Its effectiveness is somewhat less than a diaphragm because it is smaller and more difficult to properly insert.

Intrauterine Devices (IUDs) - IUDs are plastic T-shaped devices that are folded with a special instrument and inserted into the uterus by a trained health professional such that the arms of the "T" open up and cross the uterus where it is braced. Some brands come with a slow releasing synthetic progesterone, while others are copper wrapped. The specific action of IUDs is unknown, but it is believed they interfere with egg fertilization by sperm. The IUDs must be removed or replaced periodically every 1 to 4 years depending on the type used. The effectiveness in preventing pregnancies can reach 95%. Risks include pelvic inflammatory disease, severe cramps, heavy menstrual flow, uterine perforation, tubal infections and infertility. These are among some of the reasons for negative publicity that prompted the manufacturer to remove the Dalkon shield from the market in the 1970s.

3. Contraceptive Methods that are Permanent

a. Vasectomy

Sterilization has become one of the most popular methods for contraception in the United States among married couples who have achieved their desired level of parenthood. Male sterilization by **vasectomy** is usually an outpatient procedure accomplished by making an incision on either side of the scrotum and snipping out a piece of the **vas deferens**. The two ends of the **vas** are then tied off or cauterized. There is some discomfort in this area for about a week, but the risks are minimal and effectiveness in preventing unwanted pregnancies in partners is better than 99 percent.

b. Tubal Ligation

Women may be sterilized by **tubal ligation** which is a slightly more involved surgical procedure requiring small incisions near the navel and just above the pubic area. The abdomen is inflated with a gas so the physician can easily locate the fallopian tubes with the fiber-optic light on the laparoscope and tie off or cauterize the tubes. This procedure blocks the entry of eggs into uterus, and eggs released from the ovaries dissolve and are reabsorbed into the body. Tubal ligations may be reversible while vasectomies have generally not met with similar success at being reversed. However, developments in microsurgical techniques have resulted in a reversal approaching fifty success percent depending on the elapsed time since the vasectomy and the skill of the surgeon.

c. Abortion

Abortion refers to the medical means of terminating a pregnancy. In the United States this is considered to be a decision that a woman and her physician may make within the first trimester without legal restriction. This right was given under the 1973 Roe vs.

Wade Supreme Court decision. However, individual states were given the right under later court actions to impose restrictions on abortions. Despite these restrictions, about 1.6 million abortions have been legally performed each year in the United States since 1980. Nearly 60 million abortions occur annually on a worldwide basis. Three quarters of the world's population live in countries where it is legal to induce abortion medically.

II. COMMUNITY AND URBAN ENVIRONMENTAL HEALTH CONCERNS

A. COMMUNITY LEVEL EXPOSURE

1. Introduction

This is the level at which much environmental epidemiologic research has concentrated, particularly in relation to ambient air pollution, industrial emissions, problems associated with urban transport systems, contamination of local drinking water and local food supplies, and waste management. Difficult methodological choices often confront researchers at this level, particularly whether to attempt to measure exposures and make comparisons at the individual, small-group (microecologic), or community level.

2. Outdoor Air Quality

Urban air pollution has, in recent decades, become a worldwide public health problem. In the industrialized countries, the earlier industrial and household air pollution from coal burning has been replaced by pollutants from motorized transport that form photochemical smog, including ozone (a strong irritant that affects eyes, upper airways, and lungs) in summer and a heavy haze of particulates and nitrogen oxides in winter. Although many industrialized cities do not yet meet annual standards for every pollutant, conditions are generally much better than in the past. Nevertheless, air pollution has become a renewed concern in various industrialized cities where it was believed that the historic problems had been solved. The experience of severe air pollution incidents around midcentury, most famously in London in 1952 when the daily mortality was doubled during a 2-week period, finally led to a political agreement to act against air pollution. During that episode the daily peaks were several thousand ug/m3 for each of the pollutants. Those earlier problems were caused mainly by the industrial and household burning of coal without efficient emission controls, leading especially to high breathing-zone concentrations during temperature inversions. During the subsequent decades the annual average and daily peak levels of particulate matter and sulfur dioxide were decreased tenfold or more in most cities of industrialized countries.

In low- and middle-income countries, urban air pollution has recently attained alarming levels in many cities. In New Delhi, Beijing, and several other Indian and Chinese cities, for example, the annual average concentrations of particulates have been 5-10 times greater than the WHO air quality guideline. In China the main source of pollution is combustion of coal. Industrial, neighborhood, and household sources all contribute, however, and emissions from automobiles are increasing sharply. The estimated morbidity and mortality in Chinese cities due to air pollution is now increasing markedly. Meanwhile, in many cities of central and eastern European countries the mix of industrial emissions and car exhausts has caused increases in air pollution. In eastern Germany and in southern Poland in the late 1980s, winter concentrations of sulfur dioxide from coal burning were even higher than those in London, during the infamous 1952 smog episode.

Asthma, which has been increasing in industrialized countries for 3 decades, has a still unresolved relationship to external air pollution. Although some studies indicate a contributory role of air pollution as trigger, if not as initiator, in this marked rise in asthma rates, other studies are less conclusive. The apparent increasing susceptibility of successive modern generations of children to asthma may well derive from changes in human ecology that have altered early-life immunological experiences-such as reduced exposure to common childhood infections (due to smaller family sizes) or allergenic household exposures (for example, house-dust mites or fungal spores), or to modern vaccination regimes.

3. Traffic and Transport

As cities grow in size, urban transport systems expand and evolve. In particular, private car ownership and travel have increased spectacularly over the past half century, creating new opportunities and freedoms-and new social and public health problems. Currently, there seems to be no agreed vision of an urban future that is not dominated by privately owned vehicles.

Transportation is one of the key polluters in the process of economic development, urbanization, and industrialization. In traditional subsistence agricultural societies, the community's basic needs could be met within a relatively localized distance. Increasing population size and density means that specialized resources for the community, such as firewood, must be acquired from increasingly distant sources, and this creates transportation needs. Modern economic development has accelerated this process, by further specialization of economic tasks and dependence on resources from distant areas. Energy sources, such as coal, have had to be transported from afar to sustain local cottage industries; this was also the case with food items to sustain people in places where little could be grown or gathered for much of the year.

4. Industry and Manufacturing

Industrialization brings many benefits in the form of income and jobs, but, unless regulated in some fashion, can lead to significant occupational and public health hazards. The public hazards may be in the form of releases of toxic or potentially toxic material - as in the notorious cases in postwar Japan. Some industrial facilities carry the risk of large-scale accidental releases of toxic materials. The biggest such release in world history occurred in Bhopal, India, where an explosion at a pesticide manufacturing plant resulted in some 3,000 deaths caused by the chemical methyl-isocyanate and significant health impairment in many tens of thousands. The impact of this accident at the facility was exacerbated by the lack of urban zoning controls, with hundreds of households having been built directly adjacent to the plant. There was also inadequate planning for alerting and evacuating the public once the accident had occurred.

5. Waste Management

Few issues in environmental health have generated such attention and controversy as the management of hazardous wastes, whether chemical or radioactive. This has come about through a strong sense of public outrage about numerous publicized cases in which hazardous materials have been dumped indiscriminately or clandestinely, thus leaving expensive and dirty waste sites for others to handle. Both industry and governments have been responsible for creating such sites, which, in industrialized countries, have become very expensive to clean up. Indeed, in today's dollars the Superfund program of the United States has spent to date at least $50 billion to clean up chemically contaminated industrial sites. The cost of cleaning up the chemical and radioactive contamination left as remnants of a half-century of cold war nuclear weapons development and manufacture will be much higher.

6. Microbiological Contamination of Water and Food

Diarrheal disease from contaminated water and food remains one of the world's great public health problems. Although the hazard is in a sense generated at the household level, failure to initiate community controls can lead to large-scale outbreaks.

An important example is cholera, which spread worldwide during the 1990s. The seventh, and largest ever, cholera pandemic is now causing cases throughout Asia, the Middle East, Europe (occasionally), Africa (where the disease has become endemic for the first time), and Latin America, where it spread widely during the l990s, causing more than 1 million cases and 10,000 deaths. Meanwhile, an apparently new epidemic of cholera was detected in the early 1990s, appearing first in southern India and caused by a new strain (number 0139) of **Vibrio cholerae**. The spread of cholera has been greatly enhanced by the increasing number of slum dwellers in low- and middle-income countries, the speed and distance of modern tourism, and an apparent increase in extreme weather events - such as the massive El Nino-associated floods in Kenya in 1997 that caused epidemics of cholera in two regions of the country.

In the villages and slums of low- and middle- income countries, poor household water quality and sanitation often lead to food contamination. The widespread and unregulated commercial street-food sector in cities offers additional opportunities for exposure. Food contamination remains a concern even in industrialized countries where food is supplied to most of the population via long agriculture, processing, and distribution chains.

7. Chemical Contamination of Water and Food

The sources of chemical contamination are industrial wastes and emissions; household and agricultural chemicals; chemicals that form during storage and handling of food, such as the biotoxin aflatoxin; and natural chemical contaminants. Several major episodes have occurred in Europe over the past 2 decades. In 1981 the toxic Spanish oil episode occurred, in which edible vegetable oil was adulterated with industrial oil, causing several hundred deaths and several thousand severe illnesses. In 1985 batches of Austrian and Italian wine were found adulterated with alcohol-containing antifreeze, a toxic compound. In both those episodes, the hazardous substances were added surreptitiously, for commercial gain, by persons ignorant of or indifferent to the potential risks to public health. In 1999 in Belgium, dioxin-contaminated fats entered the animal feed-manufacturing process, leading to the contamination of pigs, poultry, and dairy cattle on 1,500 Belgian farms and to thousands of tons of contaminated food products. The potential for the rapid globalization of such environmental problems in the modern free-trading world became quickly apparent: countries in the Middle East, the Americas, and Southeast and eastern Asia quickly declared a ban on Belgian food imports.

Similar problems can afflict the quality of drinking water. The widespread problem with arsenic in local drinking water supplies in various communities around the world, particularly in Bangladesh and West Bengal, India, is illustrative.

B. URBANIZATION

1. Concept of Urbanization

There is another dynamic to the world's increasing population. The mass migration of people to the cities is known as **urbanization.** Urbanization, the process by which an increasing proportion of the population comes to live in urban areas, has become a worldwide problem. Urbanization is a reflection of population growth and opportunities in cities. A population can grow, only through increase in births, decrease in deaths (the natural increase); or increased immigration. Decreased emigration may reduce the loss of population if the rate of immigration does not also fall. Urban areas of the world are now experiencing both a natural increase and an increase in net migration to the cities.

Of special concern in this global trend of urbanization is the growth of megacities, or cities with a population of 8 million or more; it is projected that by 2015 there will be 36 megacities.

People migrate from rural to urban areas for a variety of reasons. As life expectancy increases and the birth rate rises, single farms may not be able to support all family members. In addition, rural customs and discriminatory inheritance laws can encourage or force migration from rural areas. Improved survival of children has created a rapid growth in the number of young people without sufficient land to support them.

Globally, urban residents enjoy better health than rural populations. This fact does not take into account, however, the differences within cities between wealthy and poor populations, which can be staggering. In many cities, poverty among urban residents is widespread. In developing countries it can affect the majority of the residents, and in developed countries it is on the rise. Poverty is a major factor in exacerbating the risks. The health situation of the urban poor is often worse than that of people living in rural areas. The urban poor must endure the difficulties of rural life (lack of services, decreased access to health care) along with many urban hazards (crowding, stress, and exposure to industrial hazards).

The process of urbanization has significant requirements, including the provision of water safe for household consumption and sanitation purposes, solid and liquid waste management, and housing and transportation networks.

Air pollution is one of the many problems of modern day experience, no matter what their level of economic development. In the past air pollution was often considered a matter of aesthetics and quality of life, but not of survival or health. Increasing scientific evidence has shown that the effects of air pollution on health are considerable, even in developed countries where the levels of air pollution have been largely controlled. This has led to a reexamination of the need for air quality management. The negative effects of air pollution are now taken much more seriously.

In recent years, it has become obvious that poor communities tend to be more affected by air pollution than those with higher average incomes. This observation has been followed by a number of studies that have shown that exposure to pollution tends to accompany poverty, marginalization from society, and lack of access to social services and health care. The likely explanation for this is that people who have access to personal resources are more likely to live together, avoiding unhealthy or unpleasant neighborhoods. However, there is also evidence that factories, power plants, or other facilities that may be sources of pollution are more likely to be built in or near poor communities in the first place. The problem of equity in environmental risk, called **environmental justice**, is an issue of serious concern in discussions and policies regarding air pollution, contaminated water supplies, and hazardous waste disposal.

The major sources of noise are road and air traffic, construction, industry, and people. These types of noises are generally on the rise as urban centers become denser, industry expands, and the need for transportation increases. Noise is of most direct concern in the workplace, where hearing loss most commonly occurs. Environmental noise, (also called community noise) is often complex.

Motor vehicle usage has increased dramatically around the globe. In 1950, there were approximately 53 million cars on the world's roads; this has increased more than eightfold over the last four decades, with the global automobile fleet now over 430 million. This represents an average growth of approximately 9.5 million automobiles per year. While the growth rate has slowed in the highly developed countries, population growth and increased urbanization and industrialization have accelerated the use of motor vehicles elsewhere.

Globally, two-thirds of motor vehicle-related fatalities involved pedestrians, predominantly children and the elderly. Several factors contribute to this phenomenon.

In 1800, approximately 6% of the U.S. population lived in urban areas. By 1900, 45% resided in cities. Presently, 73% of the U.S. population lives in urban areas. Worldwide, approximately 28% of the population lived in cities in 1950. By A.D. 2020, more than 66% is expected to live in cities. Around the world, as families continue to produce more children than they can support, the children flock to the cities in search of work, where they find that computer-operated machinery and other modern technology reduce the need for manpower. This leads to unemployment, and unemployment leads to problems such as drug addiction, alcoholism, crime, and homelessness. In some cities in developing countries, babies are born in the streets, live there, and die there, with little potential for advancement.

Much of the population growth is the result of unplanned and unwanted pregnancies. Many cities do not provide shantytowns and slums with adequate drinking water, sanitation, food, health care, housing, schools, and jobs because of a lack of money and the fear that improvements will attract even more of the rural poor. In 1994, a report indicated the world's biggest cities were growing by one million a week.

2. Urbanization Population Dynamics

The "**urban explosion**," referring to the tremendous population increase in metropolitan areas, has been one of the most marked phenomena related to the overall growth of human populations during the past century. Urbanization is, of course, one of the oldest of demographic trends, having its roots in the small settled communities made possible by an agricultural way of life. The first true cities are believed to have arisen in Mesopotamia about five or six thousand years ago, but growth of urban areas proceeded rather slowly during the millennia that followed. Increase in urban populations depended almost entirely on an influx of new residents from the surrounding countryside. Due to extremely poor sanitary conditions and crowded living conditions, mortality rates in these urban centers were higher than birth rates, and not until recent times have urban centers become self-sustaining in terms of population growth.

The advent of the Industrial Revolution gave a tremendous impetus to the growth of cities, and the rate of increase has continued to accelerate ever since. As an example of the great population shift that has occurred, consider the change in rural-urban ratios in the United States: in 1800 a mere 6% of all Americans lived in an urban area: the number of city dwellers increased to 15% by 1850 and to 40% by 1900. In 1999, 75% of U.S. population lived in cities. [Note: in the United States, "**urban**" is defined as any community with a population of 2,500 or more]. Different countries use different cutoff points to distinguish "urban" from "rural" populations, complicating the comparison of urbanization statistics from various parts of the world. For example, while American demographers utilize the 2,500 figures, their colleagues in Iceland consider a village of 200 as "urban"; in Italy the corresponding number is 10,000, while in densely populated Japan, a community is considered "urban" only when its population surpasses 50,0001.

In the world as a whole, population increased by a factor of 2.6 during the years between 1800 and 1950; during that same time period the number of people living in cities over 20,000 population grew from 22 million to over half a billion - a factor of 23. In the largest cities (100,000 or more) of the industrialized countries, the growth was even more rapid, increasing by a factor of 35. By 1950, 29% of the world's people lived in cities; by 1999 the percentage of urban dwellers in the world had risen to 45 and is expected to surpass 50% by 2005.

In recent years this urban expansion in the developed world has slowed somewhat, but since 1900 has accelerated at a great rate in the nations of Asia, Africa, and Latin America. While the annual urban growth rate was just 0.7% between 1990 - 1995 in the more developed regions of the world, cities in the developing nations grew by 3.4% each year during the same period. By 2025 the world's urban population is projected to surpass 5 billion - double what it was in the early 1990s. If such forecasts prove accurate, almost two- thirds of humanity will be city dwellers in just 25 years. Of that increase, 90% is taking place in the developing world, particularly in the cities of Asia and Africa (Latin American populations are already 73% urbanized). As of the year 2000, the developing nations boasted 17 of the world's 20 largest cities, each with a population of 10 million or more. Such growth is already having a staggering impact on the ability of those municipalities to provide even the rudiments of a decent standard of living. Much of the population growth in Third World cities occurs in the euphemistically labelled **"uncontrolled settlements"** - slum areas and shantytowns spreading like ugly cancerous growths around the periphery of almost every large city in the developing world. Estimates indicate that between 30-60% of the people in developing world cities currently live in substandard housing. These uncontrolled settlements are growing even faster than the urban areas as a whole, with the consequence that in the years ahead an ever-larger segment of Third World urban populations will be living in the squalor and hopelessness that characterize these shantytowns.

In most cases the trend to the cities seems to be caused by the hope for a better, more comfortable life, and though most migrants continue to live in abject poverty, nearly all seem to prefer to remain there rather than return to the deprivation of their rural home villages. Ironically, recent studies have shown that, contrary to migrant expectations, the quality of life in many Third World cities today is worse than it is in the rural areas they left behind. Throughout the developing world, poverty is increasingly becoming an urban phenomenon. At the beginning of the 21st century, approximately half of the world's poorest people - some 420 million - are living in urban settlements. Historically, urbanization seems to have the universal effect of breaking down the traditional cultures of those who migrate to the cities, where anonymity is the main feature. The overwhelming majority of urban dwellers in the Third World are migrants who have brought their peasant culture with them. They generally lack the specialized education and skills required to penetrate the city's complex social web. Migrants inevitably find that their limited skills make them incapable of contributing to the economy and consequently they are scarcely any better off than before. Many migrants form modified village societies within the city and thus tend to transfer aspects of village culture to the city. This may explain why the reproductive rates and attitudes of these city dwellers closely resemble those of their rural relatives.

The rapid increase in the populations of Third World cities presents a number of very serious problems that government officials are going to find extremely difficult to manage. Two of the most pressing needs, if disease outbreaks are to be prevented, will be the provision of safe drinking water and sewage disposal. During the 1980s impressive gains were made in bringing water and sanitation services to urban residents in the developing nations. By 1990, approximately 500 million more city dwellers worldwide had access to adequate drinking water than was the case in 1980; similarly, those served by sewerage projects increased by close to 300 million. Nevertheless, because of the huge influx of rural migrants into the cities during those years, the number of urban residents *lacking* such services continued to increase. In the mid-1990s, at least 220 million people still had no source of safe drinking water near their homes; many who did have a tap within 100 meters of their house had to share it with as many as 500 other people or had to cope with an intermittent supply, since many communal water taps only function for a few hours daily. In Rajkot, India - a city of 600,000 population - tap water runs for only 20 minutes per day. In general, in the uncontrolled settlements of Third World cities, per capita water availability may be 3-10 times less than in more affluent sections of the same city, a fact which has serious implications for health and sanitation in those areas. Provision of services for disposal of human wastes is lagging even further behind. More than 450 million urban residents of developing countries don't have access even to simple latrines, having to resort to roadside ditches or open spaces. Other families share poorly maintained, often overflowing, privies with 100 or more neighbors. Bombay, the world's third-largest city, needs an estimated half-million public toilets, yet by the mid-1990s had only 200. Exposed, untreated human wastes in the midst of densely populated areas pose a direct public health threat, but on-going efforts to meet the sanitary needs of developing world cities are being overwhelmed by the continually growing number of residents to be served. Municipal officials might be forgiven for wondering if they were on a treadmill - having to run faster and faster just to remain in place.

As urban populations continue to expand, provision of such basic services will undoubtedly lag even further behind, increasing the threat of epidemic disease and worsening already serious problems of water pollution. Air quality, already at critical levels in many Third World cities, will continue to deteriorate as the number of old, poorly maintained automobiles and pollutant-emitting motorbikes, scooters, and motorcycles continue to rise. Pressures on municipal authorities to provide jobs, housing, transportation, and social facilities will mount inexorably within the coming years and will present those societies with economic and environmental challenges which may prove impossible to meet.

Megacities, defined as having a population of more than 10 million, will be commonplace by the year 2015 with 9 of the 10 largest cities being in the developing countries.

3. The Role of Urbanization in the Spread of Disease

Three quarters or 8 million of the 12 million HIV positive people worldwide are located in Africa where the disease is accelerated by war, refugee movements, and uncontrolled settlements linked by improved road systems. Tuberculosis, cholera, and malaria have returned with a vengeance. Substandard housing, inadequate sanitation, and unsafe water in the densely populated cities account for 10 million deaths globally each year, with 4 million infants and children dying from waterborne diseases alone.   Such disease outbreaks produce dramatic economic losses. As an example, a 1994 outbreak of the plague in the Indian city of Surat killing 54 and affecting 5,000 others caused economic damages approaching $1.5 billion in U.S. dollars and caused nearly half a billion people to exodus the country.

4. Violence in Developing Urban Centers

Violence in densely populated urban centers of developing countries is not a certainty. However, there are a number of countries where violence appears to be on the increase, consistent with significant population increases. In some African tribal communities, it is customary and natural to eat at any table with any family. An entire village or community is considered to be the family.

Urban poverty is a socially destabilizing force where hordes of the impoverished people fleeing decaying rural ecosystems for urban centers are threatened by the loss of native customs in expanding cities. Here, their values are undermined, physical necessities are absent, and the spread of diseases is imminent. Many countries in Africa, and others around the world, see the rise of criminal anarchy, unprovoked crime, and the erosion of nation-states and international borders as disease, overpopulation, and disappearing resources become prominent.

5. Environmental Degradation

In countries such as Cote d'Ivoire, Sierra Leone, Guinea, Ghana, and Brazil, the destruction of primary rain forests is proceeding at a blinding speed. Less than 6 percent of the primary rain forest of Sierra Leone remains compared to the 60 percent that was forested 37 years ago. Deforestation has led to soil erosion with more flooding and a proliferation of mosquitoes.

III. GLOBAL ENVIRONMENTAL HEALTH CONCERNS

A. OZONE DEPLETION AND ULTRAVIOLET RADIATION

1. Introduction

In the **stratosphere**, the upper, relatively dense layer of the atmosphere, ozone molecules tend to accumulate through the action of ultraviolet (UV) radiation on oxygen molecules. The energy quanta in UV radiation disrupt the oxygen molecule, which forms ozone (O_3). Ozone has accumulated over time in the stratosphere, where it tends to absorb UV radiation and act as a partial screen that protects the surface of the earth from higher levels of exposure. Reduction of the concentration of ozone in the stratosphere reduces the absorption of UV radiation and allows more to get through. **Ozone depletion** therefore increases exposure to UV radiation at the earth's surface.

2. Stratospheric Ozone Depletion

Stratospheric ozone depletion is not to be confused with **tropospheric** (lower atmospheric) **ozone accumulation**. Although the same molecule is involved, both types of ozone have different health effects. Ozone in the lower troposphere is an air pollutant and throughout the troposphere it is a greenhouse gas, but in the stratosphere it provides *a* vital protective shield against potentially harmful UVB irradiation. Stratospheric ozone is regenerated by splitting and recombination of oxygen when it absorbs energy from UV radiation (a process called **photolysis***)*. Stratospheric ozone is only minimally affected by migration of tropospheric ozone upward into the stratosphere.

3. Human Health Effects of Ozone Depletion

Intracellularly, UV absorption results in breakage of covalent bonds in critical macromolecules and may eventually lead to carcinogenesis, accelerated aging, and cataracts. Those at greatest risk for direct effects of UV exposure on skin are people with fair skin who sunburn easily. The human health effects of increased UV irradiation due to ozone depletion include higher risks of **non-melanoma skin cancer**, particularly squamous cell carcinoma and actinic keratitis, a premalignant condition; **malignant melanoma, cataract**, and **retinal degeneration**; and possibly impaired **immunological** responses. Relatively minor but cosmetically significant effects may include **accelerated aging** of skin and perhaps increased frequency of **pterygia**, small wedge-shaped tissue webs on the whites of the eye. Of these conditions, the effects on immune status and the propensity for inducing skin cancer are potentially the most serious.

B. CLIMATE CHANGE AND THE GREENHOUSE EFFECT

1. Introduction

Global climate change will occur as a result of changes in the balance of heat taken on and retained by the planet. An increase in heat may lead to global warming and chaotic weather conditions, and a decrease in heat may lead to cooling, longer winters, and an increase in water trapped in the polar ice caps. Human activity, primarily reflecting changes in industry and agriculture, causes an increase in the amount of heat retained by the planet. This leads to an average warming of the earth's surface but with a great deal of local variation, which makes it difficult to predict changes for local areas. Changes in climate of the magnitude that is predicted may lead to many health problems related to heat stress, natural weather disasters, changes in the distribution of vectors causing human and animal diseases, new infectious disease patterns, unreliable crop production, local food shortages, and flooding. Many of the health problems are likely to be indirect, resulting from the social and economic consequences of these effects. The **Intergovernmental Panel on Climate Change** (IPCC), which represents the consensus of the international scientific community, estimates that current emission patterns are likely to increase the average temperature to 3.5^0C by 2100, and raise sea levels 15-19 centimeters. The effects could be devastating.

The term **greenhouse effect** is used to describe how the earth's atmosphere acts like the panes of glass in a greenhouse where plants are grown. Carbon dioxide, water vapor, and other gases in the atmosphere act like the glass in the greenhouse. The glass in the windowpane is transparent to infrared radiation in sunlight, so the radiation passes through and warms the plants and interior of the greenhouse. However, the glass also insulates the greenhouse, trapping the heat that is created when the infrared radiation is absorbed. Likewise, infrared radiation from the sun passes through the earth's atmosphere, but the carbon dioxide and some other gases in the atmosphere tend to insulate the earth, trapping heat. The greenhouse effect normally contributes to stability of the world's temperature and maintains the biosphere within a temperature range conducive to life - the earth absorbs a certain amount of heat and loses the same amount by radiation; the carbon dioxide and water vapor in the atmosphere keep the average temperature higher than it otherwise would have been.

2. Global Warming

Global warming is likely to produce exaggerations in existing trends in weather and to make extreme weather conditions more frequent. There is no simple prediction as to what effect atmospheric changes will have on climate, except that there will not be a uniform, stable trend of rising temperature. No one weather pattern will predominate or envelop the planet.

Changes in climate of the magnitude that is anticipated are likely to lead to certain important outcomes: health problems related to heat stress, natural weather disasters, changes in vector distribution and, consequently, infectious disease patterns, unreliable crop production, and flooding. Many of the health problems are likely to be indirect. Unlike previous periods of rapid change in climate, humankind is now dependent on an intricate system of agriculture, trade, and communication that threatens to be disrupted. Social disruptions leading to violent behavior may also be a factor in situations of food shortage or prolonged heat stress. Violent behavior has been shown to increase in frequency in hot weather, leading to the possibility of increased incidents of civil disturbance.

The reasons for this projected change in climate are complex, but all relate to the release of increasing amounts of greenhouse gases, such as carbon dioxide and water vapor, into the earth's atmosphere. The increase in the release of these gases exaggerates the greenhouse effect, but the underlying reason for this increase is intensive industrial and agricultural development and increasing consumption of fossil fuels. The rapid rise in concentration of these greenhouse gases is occurring in the troposphere. Carbon dioxide is increasing at 0.4% per year, methane at about 1% per year, CFCs until recently at about 5% per year, and oxides of nitrogen at 0.3% per year; the concentration of ozone and a miscellaneous group of other gases is also on the rise. This increase is mostly the result of industrial and transport development, especially the use of internal combustion engines and coal-burning electric power generators. Methane also comes from agriculture, landfills, and other sources, such as the decomposition of rotting vegetation and from the digestive tracts of plant-eating animals like cattle. Water vapor, another important greenhouse gas, has not been increased as much by human activity and does not seem to be rising.

3. Solutions to the Problem

The solution to the problem of climatic change is deceptively simple but difficult to achieve: reduce the generation of greenhouse gases, particularly of carbon dioxide, and increase the capacity of the sink for carbon dioxide by stopping deforestation and increasing forest growth. Although what needs to be done may seem obvious, it is very difficult in practice to reduce the combustion of fossil fuels and to increase forest growth.

C. DEFORESTATION AND DESERTIFICATION

1. Introduction

Human activity has changed the face of the earth considerably. Only remnants now remain of the huge forests that once covered Europe, the Middle East, and China. Central Europe was once a dense forest and in Roman times the cedar groves of Lebanon were famous. North America used to be much more heavily forested along the East Coast than it is today, although the forest is coming back in many areas of the East Coast. Large tracts of forest remain in protected areas in North America, in the mountains of the West, along the Pacific Northwest, and in the far North. Southeast Asia, South America, and Africa still have vast expanses of rain forest but through the clearing of huge areas for agriculture and industrial development, the total area of forest coverage has been rapidly reduced.

2. Forest Ecosystem Changes

Woodlands protect the soil on which they stand in many ways. Root systems and ground cover slow down the passage of water through the ground and keep soil in place. Forest debris and ground cover recycle nutrients and provide food for wildlife. Trees and fallen trees provide shelter and habitat for wildlife and reduce the impact of strong winds.

Forests also play a critical role in the removal, storage, and release of carbon dioxide from the atmosphere. Throughout history, at least since the last Ice Age, it would appear that the global sinks for carbon dioxide have had sufficient capacity to absorb any excess caused by volcanic eruption or forest fires. As a result, the content of carbon dioxide in the atmosphere remained relatively stable. Today, however, production of carbon dioxide exceeds the capacity of the global sinks, and the concentration of the gas in the atmosphere is steadily increasing, leading ultimately to the exaggerated greenhouse effect described above.

D. BIODIVERSITY

1. Introduction

Biodiversity refers to the multiplicity of species of plants and animals in a biological community and the many ecological niches that they may occupy. It is a fundamental principle of ecology that diversity in animal and plant species leads to greater stability of the ecosystem. The ecosystem functions more efficiently, with different species occupying more niches and extracting full benefit from the energy and nutrients available. More complicated systems have greater adaptability in the face of environmental changes and the ecological niches occupied by different species may partly overlap and allow substitutions if one or more are lost. Loss of biodiversity therefore means a less stable, less adaptable, and less self-restoring ecosystem.

2. Biological Significance of Biodiversity

Biodiversity is also a means of preserving genetic diversity. Each species and subspecies contains within their genes the result of hundreds of thousands, even millions of years of evolution. This genetic constitution is written onto DNA, the molecule that conserves the genetic code. It constitutes a library of 'blueprints' for living beings and for biological adaptation.

3. Economic Aspects of Biodiversity

Much of the diversity among species and subspecies and many of the variations among individuals within a species have direct practical uses to human society. They have been the basis for developing all agricultural crops and breeding all livestock, for example. Biodiversity is reduced in agriculture in the long run as certain strains are chosen for their greater productivity, resistance to pests, or ability to grow with less water, for example, and these strains are selected or hybridized to existing strains.

4. Biodiversity: Losses and Invasions

Ecosystems can lose biodiversity in many ways. Individual species may become extinct through hunting, habitat loss, or reduction in the species that they depend on for food. Entire ecosystems or large areas of larger ecosystems may be changed or lost by urbanization and agricultural clearance. Particular habitats of individual species with limited ranges may be lost in the same way: the essential area lost might relate to feeding requirements, territoriality, or breeding. Sometimes foreign species are introduced into a stable ecosystem, preying on and reducing the numbers of the local species that give the ecosystem stability. Often all of these mechanisms occur at the same time.

Through humankind's spectacular reproductive and technological "success," the natural habitats of many other species have been occupied, damaged, or eliminated. Biologists estimate that this fastest mass extinction may cause around one-third of all species alive in the 1800s to be gone before the end of this century. The loss of various key species would weaken whole ecosystems, with consequences that would often be adverse to human interests, such as disturbing the ecology of vector-borne infections and food-producing systems that depend on pollinators and the predation of pests, and impairing the cleansing of water and the circulation of nutrients that normally pass through ecosystems. A rich repertoire of genetic and phenotypic material would also be lost. To maintain the hybrid vigor and environmental resilience of "food" species, a diversity of wild species needs to be preserved as a source of genetic additives. Similarly, a high proportion of modern medicinal drugs in western medicine have natural origins, and many defy synthesis in the laboratory. Scientists test thousands of novel natural chemicals each year, seeking new drugs to treat HIV, malaria, drug-resistant tuberculosis, and cancers.

The other side of this coin is the accelerating spread of "invasive" species, as long-distance trade, tourism, and migration increase in intensity. Several examples with public health consequences are given in "**Environmental Hazards Resulting from Forms of Globalization**". There are many others: the vast proliferation of water hyacinth (a decorative plant from Brazil) in Lake Victoria, eastern Africa, has extended the breeding grounds for the water snail that transmits schistosomiasis. The planting of **Lantana camerata** as a garden border shrub, with subsequent dispersed spread within Uganda, has increased the habitat for the tsetse fly that transmits African sleeping sickness.

E. Acid Precipitation

Acid precipitation (acid rain) occurs when rainwater, snow, and other forms of precipitation have a lower than natural pH as a result of dissolved acidic chemicals that occur from air pollution. This is caused by increased production of acidifying emissions from industrial sources, principally sulfates and nitrates, and airborne transport of these pollutants. Often, these pollutants are carried very long distances and fall as acid precipitation hundreds or even thousands of kilometers away from the original site of production. When the precipitation reaches the ground, it can change the pH of small lakes and the soil, causing ecological damage. This is particularly a problem in areas where there is little natural buffering capacity in the soil or water.

F. PEST CONTROL

1. Early Attempts

Pests compete with humans for food, serve as vectors of disease, destroy crops or depress their market quality, cause structural damage to buildings and homes, and attack people directly causing annoyance, injury, or even death. Prior to the 1800s, there was very little most people could do but suffer the consequences of pest invasions and co-habitation. In the middle to late 1800s, copper arsenate compounds (Paris Green) and lead arsenate (Bordeaux mixture) were introduced as fungicides and pesticides. These substances remain indefinitely in the environment and are toxic to insects and humans while contaminating soils and water. Compounds made from copper, chromium, and zinc were used to control insects while hydrogen cyanide was used to control red scale on plants.

All of these compounds are highly toxic, most are long-lived in the environment, and resistant species developed against many of them. All arsenicals were banned following the introduction of better alternatives. The advent of the chemical revolution in pesticides probably began in 1939 with the discovery of dichlorophenyltrichloroethane (DDT) by Paul Muller of the Geigy Corporation. DDT was found to be highly toxic to most insects but not to humans. The use of DDT became critical to the effort of the allied troops in WWII who were combating malaria, yellow fever, and a host of mosquito-borne, louse-borne, and other vector-borne diseases. Within the next 15 years, more than 25 new pesticides were synthesized including many chlorinated organics (chlordane, heptachlor, dieldrin, endrin, and iodrin) and the toxic organophosphate, parathion. These compounds were credited with saving millions of lives by suppressing insect vectors of malaria, filariasis, dengue fever, and typhus.

These pesticides were widely used in the United States since their introduction after WWII until the 1970s when it became evident that many of the chlorinated organics produce significant effects on ecology and human health. Consequently, the use of most organochlorine insecticides was canceled for use in the United States although DDT and a few other of the organochlorines introduced about the same time continue to be used in other parts of the world. Such uses occur in LDCs where vector-borne diseases remain a major threat and the need for low cost insecticides is great. Nevertheless, the promise of a world free of vector-borne disease and unmarred crops free of insects and fungi has vanished in the avalanche of unforeseen events over the last 40 years. These problems include: (1) the resistance of vectors to pesticides; (2) the adverse health and ecological effects of pesticides; and (3) the proliferation of pesticides globally.

Human efforts to control pest outbreaks date back to the development of agriculture approximately 10,000 years ago, when relatively large expanses of a single crop and sizeable numbers of people living close together in none-too-sanitary conditions favored an increase in pest populations which wouldn't have been possible among small, scattered societies living a nomadic, hunter-gatherer type of lifestyle. Early attempts to reduce pest damage included purely physical efforts - stomping, flailing, burning - as well as the offering of prayers, sacrifices, and ritual dances to the local gods. A few effective measures were discovered even at such early dates, however. The Sumerians, in what now is Iraq, successfully employed sulfur compounds against insects and mites more than 5,000 years ago; over 3,000 years ago the Chinese were treating seeds with insecticides derived from plant extracts, using wood ashes and chalk to ward off insect pests in the home, and applying mercury and arsenic compounds to their bodies to control lice. Among the Chinese is found the earliest example of using a pest's natural enemies to control it: by A.D. 300, the Chinese were introducing colonies of predatory ants into their citrus groves to control caterpillars and certain beetles.

During the peak of Greek civilization, records indicate that some of the wealthier citizens used mosquito nets and built high sleeping towers to evade mosquitoes. They also used oil sprays and sulfur bitumen ointments to deter insects. The Romans designed rat-proof granaries, but relied largely on superstitious practices such as nailing up crayfish in different parts of the garden to keep away caterpillars. In medieval Europe people increasingly relied on religious faith to protect them from pest depredations; as late as 1476, during an outbreak of cutworms in Switzerland, several of the offending insects were hauled into court, proclaimed guilty, excommunicated by the archbishop, and banished from the land!

Not until the 18th and 19th centuries did efforts at pest control make any meaningful progress. This was a time, when European farming practices were becoming more productive and scientific, and help in combating agricultural pests was eagerly sought. Botanical insecticides such as pyrethrum, derris (rotenone), and nicotine were introduced at this time. Heightened interest in improved pest control methods was generated during the mid-19th century by several of the worst agricultural disasters ever recorded - the potato blight in Ireland, England, and Belgium in 1848, caused by a fungal disease; the fungus leaf spot disease of coffee in Ceylon which completely wiped out coffee cultivation on the island; and the outbreak of both powdery mildew and an insect pest, grape phylloxera, which nearly destroyed the wine industry in Europe. Such problems led to the development of new chemical pesticides and ushered in a whole new era of pest control. Two of the first such compounds, Bordeaux mixture (copper sulfate and lime) and Paris Green (copper acetoarsenite), were originally employed as fungicides but were subsequently found to be effective insecticides as well. Paris Green became one of the most widely used insecticides in the late 19th century and Bordeaux mixture even today is the most widely used fungicide in the world. Early in the 1900s arsenic-containing compounds such as lead arsenate, highly toxic to both insects and humans, became the most widely sold insecticides in the United States and retained their leading position until the advent of DDT after World War II.

In 1939, Paul Muller, a Swiss chemist working for the Geigy Corporation, discovered that the synthetic compound dichlorodiphenyltrichloroethane (referred to as DDT) was extremely effective in killing insects on contact and retained its lethal character for a long time after application. Muller had simply been looking for a better product to be used against clothes moths, but the outbreak of war in Europe gave far wider significance to the new chemical. Military authorities, recognizing that extensive campaigns would be carried out in the tropics where insect-borne disease threatened high troop losses, made the search for better insecticides a top priority. DDT, highly lethal to every kind of insect yet harmless to humans when applied as a powder, was just what the military needed. Initially, production of DDT was exclusively for use in the armed forces where it was employed first as a louse powder and later for mosquito control. At the end of the war DDT was released for civilian use, both in agriculture and for public health purposes. Its use quickly spread worldwide, amidst high expectations of complete eradication of many diseases and greatly reduced crop losses due to insects.

Muller was awarded the 1948 Nobel Prize in Physiology and Medicine in recognition of his contribution. The enthusiastic reception given to DDT encouraged chemical companies in their search for new and even more effective synthetic pesticides. By the mid-1950s at least 25 new products which would revolutionize insect control practices were put on the market, among the more important of which were chlordane, heptachlor, toxaphene, aldrin, endrin, dieldrin, and parathion. The age of chemical warfare against pests had begun.

2. Pesticides: The Double-Edged Sword

Pesticides are natural or synthetic substances developed primarily to kill, repel, or control living organisms that are considered pests - species deemed undesirable by humans. These include plants, animals, insects, or other organisms, determined to be undesirable for some economic, medical, or aesthetic reason.

America's use of pesticides, the one class of chemicals intentionally designed to be toxic, has been questioned since 1962, when Rachel Carson's monumental book, **Silent Spring**, attacked our reliance on them in light of their hazardous effects on human health and the environment. In her book, Carson said: If we are going to live so intimately with these chemicals - eating and drinking them, taking them into the very marrow of our bones - we had better know something about their nature and their power.

Silent Spring focused on the highly controversial pesticides of the time, such as DDT. Since then, the use of pesticides and their health and environmental effects have been more thoroughly scrutinized and controlled.

Although pesticides such as arsenic had been used for centuries, DDT and other synthetic pest control chemicals were not discovered until World War II. These pesticides were credited with saving many lives through the control of mosquitoes and malaria. Following the war, they were used domestically on a massive scale, catapulting America into an agricultural revolution. These pesticides brought many new benefits to society, including reduction of disease and more plentiful food, cheaper prices, and longer shelf-life, but their potential environmental impacts were then unknown.

The public soon became dependent on chemical pesticides to control nearly any type of ecological "nuisance," without understanding their potential effects to the environment or to themselves. There is considerable evidence that the overuse of pesticides can lead to a decrease in crop yields and a resurgence in the diseases and pests they are supposed to control. The near extinction of prominent wildlife species, along with industrial accidents and groundwater contamination, led society to question the degree to which we use and test chemical pesticides.

Pesticide uses range from controlling fleas on pets to hospital sterilization to fire ant control; however, the discussion here is on the agricultural pesticides, insecticides and herbicides, which account for 75 percent (by weight) of all pesticides used in the United States.

3. Primary Uses of Pesticides

The majority of pesticide products (approximately 75 percent by weight) are used in agriculture to control pests that attack food, animal feed, and forest products (Table 11.5). Other nonagricultural pesticides are used for a variety of institutional, industrial, and household purposes, including:

1. Pet care
2. Health care
3. Milk-handling equipment
4. Disposable diapers
5. Lawn care
6. Household cleaners
7. Personal hygiene products
8. Swimming pools
9. Golf courses
10. Wood preservatives
11. Oil wells
12. Airports
13. Highway medians
14. Hospital equipment
15. Tobacco
16. Beauty and barber shops

4. Cases of Major Pesticide Poisoning

Each year, there are an estimated 3,000 pesticide-poisoning cases admitted to hospitals, with 200 fatalities. For example, the EPA has reported that each year there are some 350 cases of poisoning to farm workers from the pesticide ethyl parathion alone. Most of these cases affect people working at farms or pesticide manufacturers or unsuspecting individuals (those that unknowingly enter a recently treated area). There also have been some dramatic but rare cases of serious poisoning events, such as Bhopal, India, where 2,800 people were killed and 20,000 injured as a result of a release of a pesticide component (methyl isocyanate) from an adjacent pesticide manufacturing plant.

5. Human Exposure to Pesticides Already in the Environment

Besides direct consumption through allowable residues in commercial foods, humans also can consume pesticides in contaminated wildlife and, even more likely, in fish. The potential for consuming contaminated fish is higher in agricultural areas and near pesticide manufacturers. Although government warnings and advisories may alert individuals to the concerns in these areas, there also can be unsuspecting consumption.

Table 11.5. Major Types of Insecticides. (Source: Wagner, 1994).

Type	Examples	Mode of action	Effects	Current uses
Chlorinated Hydrocarbon or Organochlorine	DDT, Aldrin, Heptachlor, Toxaphene, Lindane, Chlordane	Contact (kills upon contact; ingestion not required) and systemic (translocated to other parts of the organism other than what it was applied to)	Very persistent in the environment, affects the nervous system, leading to paralysis	Most uses are cancelled, but some formulations are still used
Organophosphate	Malathion, Parathion, Azodrin, Phosdrin, Methyl parathion, Diazinon, TEPP, DDVP	Contact and systemic	Ties or inhibits certain important enzymes of the nervous system (cholinesterases) at synapses, leading to paralysis; highly toxic, but low persistence	Control of aphids, spider mites, and other sucking and chewing insects that attack fruit, vegetables, ornamentals, and stored products
Carbamate	Carbaryl (Sevin), Zineb, Maneb, Baygon, Zectran, Temik, Matacil	Contact and systemic	Ties or inhibits certain important enzymes of the nervous system (cholinesterases) at synapses, leading to paralysis; highly toxic, but low persistence	Control of insects, mites, and nematodes on citrus, cotton, tobacco, beans, wheat, corn, and forests
Pyrethoid	Pyrethium, Cypermethrin, Resmethrin, Bioresmethrin	Contact	Affects the nervous system, leading to paralysis	Control of insects on pets, livestock, households, and gardens.

6. Environmental Effects of Pesticides

In large part, pesticides enter and are distributed throughout the environment through their legal application, as shown in Figure 11.4. However, the small size and mobility of many pests require large "blanket" applications of pesticides. Except for the direct spraying of weeds and trees, most pesticides do not directly reach target pests, particularly flying insects. Given their small size, it is nearly impossible to control insect pests on crops by attempting to apply pesticides directly to them. As a result, pest control is more effective when a protective cover is sprayed on the vegetation, thereby ensuring pest exposure to the pesticide. However, such a blanket spraying increases the opportunity for pesticides to reach the environment and contaminate the atmosphere, soil, surface water, and groundwater, where they are likely to accumulate in the food web and impact wildlife, fisheries, and nontarget organisms.

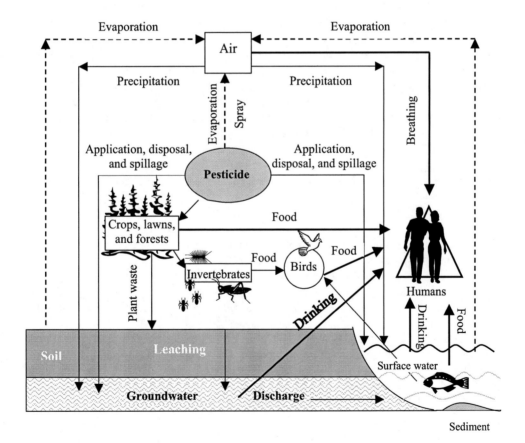

Figure 11.4. Pesticide Distribution in the Environment. (Source: Wagner, 1994).

G. ENVIRONMENTAL JUSTICE

1. Environmental Justice Movement

At the beginning of the 21st century, **"environmental justice"** is both a nationally prominent public policy issue and a catalyst in the ongoing debate about societal values. Although environmental justice remains an emotionally charged and ill-defined concept, virtually everyone agrees it is an appropriate societal goal. This consensus quickly erodes, however, when the discussion turns to practical questions. Our society finds itself in the awkward position of trying to put environmental justice principles into practice while at the same time debating the meaning of the term and its implications for decision making. "Environmental Justice" is a movement comprising Civil Rights activists and environmentalists working to ensure the rights of low-income and minority communities to clean and healthy environments. Movements, often comprised of an aggregate of issues and events, are usually defined in singular moments - catalysts for momentum towards comprehensive, cohesive action and response.

As is the case with many social and political conflicts, environmental health issues in U.S. minority communities are determined in large part by basic economic disparities and historical discriminatory practices in housing, education, employment opportunities, health care access and availability, legal representation, and voting rights. More affluent communities are able to wield greater influence and power through community organizations and political representation because of established social, political, and economic advantages. Their communities are able to exclude proximal development of enterprises or projects that carry environmental risk such as waste incinerators, dumps, and handling of radioactive minerals and waste.

In general, more affluent communities develop in areas away from toxic-waste sites and industrial pollutants and thus insulate themselves from most forms of environmental contamination. In some wealthy urban core enclaves, smog, primarily from vehicle emissions, may be unavoidable. Overall, however, the wealthy can afford homes at a comfortable distance from the urban core and other economically depressed areas in peripheral urban quadrants. In areas where city or groundwater is considered contaminated, the affluent are able to afford water purification systems or bottled water. These trends may seem obvious, but have been poorly studied.

Historical, social, and economic discrimination, based primarily on ethnicity and physical appearance, has led to varying degrees of poverty among some ethnic minority groups. Poverty and social stressors play a role with regard to disease engenderment and susceptibility.

Health care access and poverty have been associated with racial and ethnic discrimination. Health services research indicates that minority groups and the poor have a higher risk for occupational illnesses. In a landmark study the U.S. Department of Health and Human Services' 1985 "Report of the Secretary's Task Force on Black and Minority Health" linked discrimination, race, and ethnicity with disease.

2. Challenges

Americans overwhelmingly deplore both racial discrimination and environmental degradation, but until recently these concerns seldom directly intersected in public policy discourse. Throughout the 1960s and 1970s environmentalists attended to an agenda far removed from racial minorities and the poor. Although environmentalists as individuals often sympathized with, and even actively supported, the political struggles of ethnic minorities (and African Americans in particular), environmentalism and civil rights/social welfare evolved as distinct issue spheres, each with its own statutory framework, institutions, and audiences. Environmentalism, especially at the national level, had little racial aspect as such.

Today the environmental decisions of business and government alike are widely recognized as having potentially serious equity implications, especially for minority and low-income communities. Environmentalists, community representatives, and policymakers address this new blend of concerns under three labels: environmental racism; environmental equity; and, most recently, environmental justice. The core claim of the environmental justice movement is that a variety of environmental burdens (for example, toxic waste sites, polluted air and water, dirty jobs, underenforcement of environmental laws) have fallen disproportionately on low-income persons and communities of color. A related claim, or frequent presumption, is that health risks associated with pollution have likewise been borne disproportionately by such persons and communities.

Most writing about environmental justice has had at least one of two aims, and sometimes both. One purpose is political agenda-setting. Activists and journalists have tried to dramatize and legitimize environmental justice as a problem by drawing attention to examples of local environments that have received short shrift from the political and economic system. This activist literature approvingly recounts tales of communities mobilizing against an array of hazardous conditions and unwanted facilities. Community energies are driven largely by residents' belief that adverse health effects either have already appeared (due to past or present pollution) or could appear in the future (if new pollution sources are created or if existing ones are either enhanced or ignored). A second focus in the literature is empirical enlightenment. Some analysts - including both activists and more dispassionate observers, often employing quantitative techniques - have attempted to ask: How much environmental injustice or inequity is there? Some commentators, perhaps most notably sociologist Robert Bullard, have played interchangeable advocacy and analytic roles. In a substantial series of publications since the 1980s Bullard argues that significant (and especially race-based) inequity has often prevailed in the distribution of environmental burdens and benefits. This state of affairs, according to Bullard, justifies fundamental policy **reform** grounded in what he calls an **"environmental justice"**.

3. Disparities in Health Status in the United States

a. Introduction

An extensive body of literature documents the fact that not all segments of the U.S. population have experienced the same advances in health status and gains in life expectancy. Racial and ethnic minority groups, individuals of low socioeconomic status, and medically underserved populations, among others, face lower life expectancies and greater health problems than the middle- and upper-class U.S. white population. Some of the disparities in health status are associated with socioeconomic status. For example, at age 45, individuals with family incomes above $25,000 can expect to live from 3 to 7 years longer than those with family incomes below $10,000. Also, the death rate from chronic disease for individuals ages 23 to 64 with less than 12 years of education is more than twice as high as that for comparable individuals with more than 12 years of education. Nonelderly adults living in poverty-stricken areas experience a significantly higher risk of mortality from all causes.

Rates of disease and death in the United States vary substantially by social class and ethnicity/ race. Both are predictors of health status, and both are associated with susceptibility factors, such as access to health-promoting and health-protecting resources (e.g., healthy diet and sanitation) and preventative medical practices (e.g., prenatal care and childhood immunization), as well as lifestyle choices about alcohol and tobacco use, sexual behavior, and occupation. Socioeconomic status (SES) is known to be a critical risk factor affecting morbidity and mortality. Yet despite its apparent importance, the mechanisms by which SES exerts its influence are largely a matter of conjecture. Similarly, the influence of ethnicity/race on health status is also well known and, as with SES, the causal relationships are poorly understood. The situation is complicated by the fact that ethnicity/race is associated with both absolute and relative poverty. Consequently, it is often difficult to distinguish the separate effects of class and race on health.

Health status is clearly a product of multiple variables, many of which are poorly understood. There is substantial evidence suggesting that large-scale social factors are the primary determinants of health - determining not only individuals' social class but also their access to resources and exposure to risk factors. However, the precise mechanisms by which position in the social structure is causally related to health status are not well elucidated. Currently, there is mounting evidence that disparities in health status between higher and lower SES strata are increasing, and that the health of some racial groups is steadily deteriorating. These realities moved Williams and Collins in 1995 to observe that "Racial and socioeconomic inequality in health is arguably the single most important public health issue in the United States."

Although the health status of all U.S. racial and ethnic groups has improved steadily, disparities in major health indicators between white and non-white groups are growing. In general, African Americans, American Indians, and Hispanics are dramatically disadvantaged relative to whites in terms of most health indices, whereas Asian Americans appear to be as healthy, if not healthier, than whites in terms of some indices. These overall group differences, however, mask important differences in the health statuses of subgroups. Americans of Southeast Asian descent, for example, suffer from among the highest rates of cervical and stomach cancers of all U.S. population groups and experience poorer health overall than U.S. whites. Socioeconomic status appears to operate in complex ways with race and ethnicity to account for the observed differences in health status. In general, white Americans enjoy higher incomes and education attainment levels than any other U.S. racial and ethnic group and therefore are more likely to have health insurance and to be better educated with regard to healthy behaviors and diets, are more likely to seek routine medical care, and are more likely to have better access to preventive medical services.

Socioeconomic factors, however, do not completely account for racial and ethnic differences in health status. Several studies indicate that racial disparities in health status persist even when controlling for socioeconomic status. Mounting evidence indicates that in addition to resource inequities, other factors, including discrimination in the health care system, racism-related stresses, migration, and differences in levels of acculturation may also lead to poor health among members of racial minority groups. Disparities in exposure to environmental hazards are also suspected as a factor in the relatively poorer health of individuals in minority and lower-income communities in the United States.

b. Examples of Health Disparities

The following examples show that significant disparities exist between U.S. racial and ethnic groups in terms of several key health indicators, even when socioeconomic differences are taken into account.

(1) Low Birth Weight

During the period from 1989 to 1996, among women with 13 or more years of education, African American women were twice as likely as white women to give birth to low-birth-weight infants (infants weighing less than 2,500 grams [5.5 pounds]) (11.9 versus 5.5 percent). This occurred even though African American women are less likely than white women to smoke during pregnancy, which is considered an important factor in causing low birth weight. Similarly, the percentage of low-birth-weight infants was higher among American Indian women (6.0 percent), Asian or Pacific Islander women (6.8 percent), and Hispanic women (6.0 percent) than white women with similar levels of educational attainment.

(2) Infant Mortality

From 1989 to 1991 African American women experienced an infant mortality rate over two and a half times higher than that experienced by white women with the same levels of education (13.7 versus 5.1 per 1,000 births). The infant mortality rates among American Indian women and Hispanic women with similar levels of education were 8.1 and 5.8 per 1,000 births, respectively.

(3) Death Rates

African Americans experience higher mortality rates than whites even in areas with equivalent levels of urbanization. In large, core metropolitan areas, the mortality rate among African Americans between 1993 and 1999 was 810.5 deaths per 100,000 population, compared with a rate of 491.9 per 100,000 among the white population. This disparity in mortality is also pronounced in other geographic areas: the modality rates among African Americans in rural and urban, nonmetropolitan areas were 737.1 and 761.9 per 100,000 population, respectively, compared with rates of 503.9 and 499.4 per 100,000 population, respectively, among whites.

(4) Cancer

In general, African American males experience cancer approximately 15 percent more frequently than white males, with incidence rates of 560 and 469 per 100,000 population, respectively. The pattern of cancer incidence rates among males in other racial and ethnic groups is more varied, but disparities are exhibited in specific cancer sites. For example, colon and rectal cancers are more common among Alaskan Native men (79.7 per 100,000 population) and Japanese American men (64.1 per 100,000 population) than white men (57.5 per 100,000). Racial and ethnic minorities also experience higher rates of mortality from cancer than whites.

Many communities contain environmental hazards that represent potential sources of health risks. Although these can affect all racial, ethnic, and socioeconomic groups, there is evidence that minorities and lower-income groups face higher levels of exposure to these hazards and, therefore, potentially higher rates of adverse health outcomes. It has been shown, for example, that non-whites are disproportionately exposed to ambient air pollutants associated with respiratory symptoms and exacerbation of other ailments.

Despite the absence of systematically collected data, there is strong presumptive evidence that low-income communities are routinely both more exposed to environmental hazards and more susceptible to their effects than the general population. Although the ramifications of these disparities for environmental health risks are unclear, there is legitimate reason for concern and ample justification to begin targeted research aimed at answering important risk-related questions.

Most of the published literature consists of anecdotal case studies or observational studies that have tended to find positive statistical correlations between sociodemographic characteristics of populations (i.e., lower socioeconomic status and ethnicity/race) and residential proximity to pollution sources, such as waste sites and industrial plants. A few studies have also found similar positive correlations for estimated industrial air pollution emissions and measured ambient air pollution concentrations.

The levels of lead are higher in the older homes with the mean and median progressively increasing from 256/113 (mean/median) μ/g in homes built since 1980, to 2115/685 μg/g in homes built before 1940. House dust contaminated with lead can be traced to the common use of lead-based paints and leaded gasoline for decades until the 1970s when their use was phased out. Older homes painted with lead-based paint can continue to be a source of lead exposure as the paint weathers and sloughs from surfaces. Outdoor air particulates that were enriched in lead from automobile combustion eventually penetrated into homes as lead-contaminated house dust. A similar stepwise trend was observed for lead in surface dust, or dust that was collected on a smooth surface in the living area. The progression of lead levels went from 128/93 (mean/median) μg/g to 1075/236 μg/g in homes built before 1940.

Although scientific evidence is scarce and uneven, there are mounting concern that environmental health risks are borne disproportionately by members of the population who are poor and nonwhite. From an environmental health perspective, research to reduce critical uncertainties in health risk assessment must necessarily be at the heart of efforts to evaluate and resolve issues of environmental justice - helping to define the dimensions of the problem, understand its causes, and identify effective and efficient solutions. The full range of environmental health sciences, including exposure analysis, epidemiology, toxicology, biostatistics, and surveillance monitoring, is needed to build a strong scientific foundation for informed decision making. This is the best and surest way to promote health and safety for all members of our society, regardless of age, ethnicity, gender, health condition, race, or socioeconomic status.

In the occupational setting, the disproportionately increased risk of minority and poor workers for adverse health effects due to increased exposure to occupational hazards has been well established. Although a recently identified issue, Environmental Justice describes the disproportionate distribution of environmental risks in poor and minority communities, present for centuries in these communities and their workplaces due to lack of political and economic power. Examples in the scientific literature have focused on the increased location of hazardous waste sites in such communities. However, more basic deficiencies in environmental health are the lot of many poor and minority communities, even in the United States.

These problems include poor sewage, inadequate access to potable water, waste disposal, housing and vermin. Possible secondarily associated issues are increased injury rates (especially in children) due to inadequate housing and waste disposal; the spread of infectious diseases due to poor sewage, vermin and lack of potable water; and, increased stress and violence associated with over-crowding and poor housing. All of these are issues of basic public health which would be unacceptable and unthinkable in more wealthy communities in both the United States and other developed nations. And yet, these basic public health problems continue to exist today, even within such relatively wealthy areas as Broward County, Florida.

c. Historical Struggle

By the 1980s, hundreds of community groups had organized around issues of differential exposure to environmental risks. In 1982, North Carolina's impoverished Warren County community, largely African American, gained national attention by protesting a proposed hazardous-waste site to dump soil contaminated with polychlorinated biphenyls in a landfill that would be 10 ft above the water table. Then, in 1983, the U.S. General Accounting Office (GAO) published a study of southeastern U.S. communities surrounding four large commercial hazardous-waste landfills. The GAO found that three of four sites were located in predominantly African-American communities. Bullard, also in 1983, showed that in Houston, 21 of 25 solid-waste facilities were located in its African-American communities.

Warren County became a rallying point for those eager to see national attention focused on the inequities clearly present in the siting of unwanted land uses. At the behest of Congressman Walter Fauntroy, the U.S. General Accounting Office (GAO) conducted a study of the states comprising Region IV (Alabama, Florida, Georgia,

Kentucky, Mississippi, North Carolina, South Carolina, and Tennessee) "to determine the correlation between the location of hazardous waste landfills and the racial and economic status of the surrounding communities."

The study's conclusions, while not surprising, were disheartening. The report found that three out of every four landfills, in the EPA's Region IV, were located near predominately minority communities.

In 1987, a landmark study by the United Church of Christ's Commission for Racial Justice described the extent of inequitable environmental risks and the consequences for those who are victims of polluted environments. Their study revealed that race was the most significant variable associated with the location of hazardous-waste sites, even after controlling for urban and regional differences in socioeconomic status. The greatest number of commercial hazardous-waste facilities were located in communities with the highest proportions of racial and ethnic minorities. Another important finding was that the average minority population in communities with one commercial hazardous-waste facility was twice the average minority percentage in communities without such facilities.

The United Church of Christ report also showed that three out of every five African and Hispanic Americans lived in communities with one or more toxic-waste sites. More than 15 million African Americans, more than 8 million Hispanics, and approximately one-half of all Asian/Pacific Islanders and Native Americans were living in communities with one or more abandoned or uncontrolled hazardous-waste sites.

Studies since then have shown a relationship between race or ethnicity and the location or attempted location of hazardous-waste sites. This relationship appears to be independent of social class. Additionally, other studies have shown that race or ethnicity and income are associated risk factors for a variety of environmental exposures and susceptibility.

Countering this picture of environmental racism, a GAO report in 1995 showed that neither minorities nor low-income people were overrepresented in any consistent manner within a 1-mile radius of municipal landfills. However, this conclusion only referred to municipal solid-waste facilities (i.e., city dumps) and compared groups overall at the national level. It did not examine variations on the regional level, and population densities were not taken into account. The relationship between an arbitrary 1-mile radius and effects on the local water supply or air quality within a larger area was not specified. The report only cited existing sites and did not address, for example, the numerous attempts by hazardous-waste disposal firms to locate waste facilities on Native American lands and other impoverished communities.

Aside from the siting of hazardous-waste sites, minorities and the poor face a concentration of toxin-producing industries within their communities. One obvious reason for the disproportionate siting of potentially hazardous industries and waste sites is that land and labor costs tend to be less in many of these communities. Another explanation is the dire need for employment and a perception by business and community leaders that impoverished minorities prefer to have jobs, even those that expose themselves and their communities to hazardous conditions. The location of these industries has been termed **LULU**, for **l**ocally **u**ndesirable **l**and **u**se. After one LULU has taken hold within a community, there seems to be a decreased barrier to establishing subsequent LULUs. This phenomenon of concentrated industrialization may contribute greatly to the exposure of a community to multiple potential toxins.

Lead exposure, particularly in children, has been a particular concern of poor communities living close to industries. Long-term negative health impacts include neurobehavioral and hematopoietic abnormalities in children and hypertension in adults. Children living in substandard housing, especially those with poor nutritional status, are particularly at risk for lead toxicity. Sources of lead exposure in children include paint chips, contaminated soil and air from industry, and, in some communities, ceramic glazes and Cosmetics. Repeated studies have shown that the poor, particularly African-American and Latino children, are disproportionately exposed to toxic levels of lead.

The health effects of industrial pollutants on a particular population can be difficult to assess owing to multiple confounding variables. These variables include nutritional status, health status, age, genetic susceptibility, degrees and quality of exposure (i.e., route, dose, duration, repetitive, additive, synergistic), or exposure to complex mixtures of toxins, latency, prior exposure to other toxins, the quality and accuracy of methods used to determine the degree of exposure, and the ability of testing to detect subtle health effects.

Today, environmental justice is at the forefront of the nation's environmental policy agenda, and related policies and programs are being implemented at federal, state, and local levels. Through actions by the courts, the executive branch, the Congress, and the states, environmental justice concerns are gradually being incorporated into the fabric and structure of everyday environmental decisions. But environmental justice remains a conspicuously political and increasingly litigious topic, raising the question of whether science can make a difference in such a politicized, value-laden debate.

In 1990, the Environmental Equity Workgroup established by William K. Reilly then administrator of the Environmental Protection Agency found that minority and low-income populations experience higher than average exposure to environmental hazards and also there is a need to improve procedures for risk assessment and risk management. The National Law Journal issued its study in 1992 which revealed that penalties assessed to violators in minority communities were not as great as those in white communities. This study also uncovered that Superfund site evaluations and cleanup were conducted slower in minority communities.

On February 11, 1994, President Bill Clinton issued Executive Order 12898, committing the Federal government to EJ principles. The Order directs Federal Agencies to incorporate environmental justice as part of their overall mission by identifying and addressing, disproportionately high and adverse human health and environmental effects of programs, policies, and activities on minority populations and low-income populations. The Order also establishes an Interagency Working Group to: 1) provide guidance to the Agencies on identifying EJ problems; 2) work with the Agencies to develop EJ strategies; 3) coordinate EJ health research, data collection, and analysis; 4) develop interagency model EJ projects; and hold public meetings. During that same year, the Florida Legislature adopted joint Senate-House Bill 1369 to address environmental equity issues through creation of the Florida Environmental Equity and Justice Commission with a mandate to seek the equal protection of all citizens from environmental hazards.

There is evidence that there is a disproportionate number of environmentally-overburdened minority and socioeconomically disadvantaged communities in the Florida. Contamination in Florida resulted in a bill (House Bill 1369), which became law in 1994 and created the Florida Environmental Equity and Justice Commission. The Commission was appointed by the Governor. The Commission was directed to scientifically study whether low-income and minority communities are more at risk from environmental hazards than the general population. The Florida Environmental Equity and Justice Commission, in its review of environmental hazardous wastes sites in Florida, found that these sites am disproportionately located in minority and low-income communities. These communities were also impacted by the location of multiple sites. The Commission also found significant date gaps: environmental factors, influencing health effects, minority and low-income vulnerabilities, socioeconomic considerations and health implications and availability to government officials in assessing the health effects associated with exposure to environmental hazards. The Commission recommended to the Florida Legislature the need for funding and requisite implementation of retrospective and prospective cohort analyses and exposure assessments, including synergistic effects and cumulative exposures to develop a better understanding of the impact of pollution on population by race and income.

Environmental justice is the fair treatment and meaningful involvement of all people regardless of race, color, national origin, or income with respect to the development, implementation and enforcement of laws, regulations, and policies. Fair treatment means that no group of people, including racial, ethnic, or socioeconomic group should bear a disproportionate share of the negative environmental consequences resulting from industrial, municipal, and commercial operations or the execution of federal, state, local, and tribal programs and policies.

IV. **BIBLIOGRAPHY**

Fernandez, M.C., Ortega, H.H. (2001). Environmental Contamination and Minority Communities. In Sullivan Jr, J.B., Krieger, G.R. (Eds). Clinical Environmental Health and Toxic Exposures (pp. 129-131). Philadelphia, PA: Lippincott Williams & Wilkins.

Foreman Jr, C.H. (1998). Challenges. The Promise and Peril of Environmental Justice (1-3). Washington, D.C.: Brookings Institution Press.

Institute of Medicine. (1999). Establishing A Baseline. Toward Environmental Justice Research, Education, and Health Policy Needs (pp. 11-16). Washington, D.C.: National Academy Press.

McMichael, A.J., Kjellstrom,T., & Smith, K.R. (2001). In M. Merson, R. Black, & A. Mills (Eds). International Public Health Diseases, Program Systems, and Policies (pp. 413-422). Gaitherburg, MD: Aspen Publishers, Inc.

Meggs, W.J. (2001). Global Warming. In L. Williams, & R. Langley (Eds.), Environmental Health Secrets (pp. 63-66). Philadelphia, PA: Hanley & Belfus, Inc.

Miller, G.T. (1979). Living in the Environment. 2nd Edition. Wadsworth, Belmont, CA.

Moore, G.S. (1999). Human Population. Living with the Earth: Concepts in Environmental Health Science (pp. 2-21 – 2-43). Boca Raton, FL: Lewis Publishers.

Morgan, M.T., et al. (1997). World Population. Environmental Health. 2nd Edition. (pp. 1-12). Englewood, CO: Morton Publishing Company.

Nadakavukaren,   A. (2000). Impacts of growth on Ecosystems. <u>Our Global Environment: A Health Perspective, 5th Edition</u> (pp. 143-181). Prospective Heights, IL: Waveland Press, Inc.

Nadakavukaren, A. (2000). Population Control. <u>Our Global Environment: A Health Perspective, 5th Edition</u> (pp. 83-109). Prospective Heights, IL: Waveland Press, Inc.

Nadakavukaren, A. (2000). Population Dynamics. <u>Our Global Environment: A Health Perspective, 5th Edition</u> (pp. 45-81). Prospective Heights, IL: Waveland Press, Inc.

Nadakavukaren, A. (2000). The People-Food Predicament. <u>Our Global Environment: A Health Perspective, 5th Edition</u> (pp. 111-141). Prospective Heights, IL: Waveland Press, Inc.

Odum, E.P., (1971). <u>Fundamentals of Ecology 3rd Edition</u>. Sanders, Philadelphia.

Parker, C.M. (2001). Indoor and Outdoor Shooting Ranges. In L. Williams, & R. Langley (Eds.), <u>Environmental Health Secrets</u> (pp. 145-147). Philadelphia, PA: Hanley & Belfus, Inc.

Payne, Melisssa., Rubenstein, R. (2001). Ozone Depletion and Chlorofluorocarbons. In L. Williams, & R. Langley (Eds.), <u>Environmental Health Secrets</u> (pp. 30-32). Philadelphia, PA: Hanley & Belfus, Inc.

Shear, T.H. (2001). Desertification. In L. Williams, & R. Langley (Eds.), <u>Environmental Health Secrets</u> (pp. 58-62). Philadelphia, PA: Hanley & Belfus, Inc.Payne.

Wagner, T. (1994). Pesticides: The Double-Edged Sword. In T. Wagner (Ed.), <u>In our Backyard: A Guide to Understanding Pollution and Its Effects</u> (pp 235-269). New York, NY: Van Nostrand Reinhold.

Yassi, A., Kjellström, T., de Kok, T., & Guidotti, T. L. (2001). Demographic Issues. In A. Yassi, [et al](Eds.), <u>Basic Environmental Health</u> (pp. 41-44). New York, NY: Oxford University Press, Inc.

Yassi, A., Kjellström, T., de Kok, T., & Guidotti, T. L. (2001). Transboundary and Global Health Concerns. In A. Yassi, [et al](Eds.), <u>Basic Environmental Health</u> (pp. 375-393). New York, NY: Oxford University Press, Inc.

CHAPTER

12

LOCAL ISSUES

I. <u>HOUSING AND HEALTH</u>

A. <u>INTRODUCTION</u>

All humans need shelter: protection against the elements, somewhere to store food and prepare meals, and a secure place to raise offspring. The effects of housing conditions on health have been known since antiquity. Deplorable living conditions in urban slums became a political issue in the nineteenth century when vivid descriptions by journalists, novelists, and social reformers aroused public opinion. Osler's **Principles and Practice of Medicine** (1892) and Rosenau's **Preventive Medicine and Hygiene** (1913) noted the association between overcrowding and common serious diseases such as tuberculosis and rheumatic fever.

B. <u>HOUSING CONDITIONS</u>

Housing conditions have greatly improved in the affluent industrial nations throughout the second half of the twentieth century, but more than two-thirds of the households in the world are in developing countries, the great majority of them in rural areas; the most prevalent indoor environment in the world is the same now as throughout history - huts in rural communities. But this is changing. Urbanization is rapidly transforming the distribution of populations in the developing world, where the proportion living in urban areas rose from less than 25 percent to over 33 percent between 1970 and 1985; in this new millennium, the proportion living in urban areas in the world has exceeded 50 percent, and in the world as a whole the urban population will compose 65 percent or more by 2025. Many cities will be very large.

Many of these new urban dwellers have terrible living conditions. In the last 30 years there has been a great increase in the numbers of people living in periurban slums in developing countries. They often lack sanitation, clean water supplies, access to health care, and other basic services such as elementary education. The proportion of people in such circumstances ranges between 20 to more than 80 percent in most cities throughout Africa, Latin America, and South, Southeast, and Southwest Asia. The plight of children is especially deplorable; infant mortality rates exceed 100 in many places. Children are often abandoned by parents who cannot provide for them and must fend for themselves from ages as young as 5 years; many turn to crime and child prostitution to survive.

These shantytowns and periurban slums endanger the health and security of many millions in Latin America, Africa, and many parts of Asia. They are ideal breeding places for disease and social unrest. Accurate numbers are impossible to obtain because the missing services include enumeration by census-takers and because situations change so rapidly, but in Mexico City, Lima, Santiago, Rio de Janeiro, São Paulo, and Bogotá, well over half the total population live in the periurban slums. In the mid-1990s, there were as many as 40 million periurban slum-dwellers in these six cities alone. Others are even worse off; worldwide, an estimated 100 million people are entirely homeless, living on the streets without possessions, often from infancy onward. Although this is a problem mainly in developing countries, homeless people have increased in numbers in the most affluent industrial nations in the last decade, often forced out of their homes by hard economic times. Public health departments in large cities such as New York and London have been obliged to spend increasing proportions of their budgets on emergency shelter for growing numbers of homeless destitute families.

Increasing numbers, an estimated 22 million in 1995, live in refugee communities in Africa and the Middle and Far East where housing conditions are equally deplorable, sometimes worse than in periurban slums. Refugee communities may have health services, but these are seldom adequate; supplies and continuity of services are often precarious; the safety and security of the inhabitants is often threatened by hostilities, and their long-term prospects for a better life are poor.

Most urban centers in Africa and Asia have no sewage system at all, including many cities with a million or more inhabitants. In 1994, at least 220 million people still lacked an easily accessible source of potable water. Figures for water supply and sanitation often understate the problem because they do not take into account the quantity of water needed by a household for proper hygienic practices. Moreover, figures given for clean water sources or adequate sanitation facilities in a community may also conceal some problems. If people have to wait in long lines for their water, they often reduce their water consumption below what is needed for good health. People who have to walk long distances to use a latrine may end up defecating where it is most convenient to save effort. Improving sanitation will only work if other factors such as personal hygiene and adequate water supply are addressed simultaneously. Improving access to water and sanitation facilities alone can reduce the incidence of diarrheal disease by at least 20%.

Industrially developed nations are experiencing other challenging new health problems related to housing conditions. Rising land values and the need to provide cheap housing for expanding populations have led to proliferation of high-rise, high-density apartment housing. Publicly supported housing projects economize by restricting living space and providing few amenities. This kind of dwelling creates new sets of problems: emotional tensions attributable to living too close to the neighbors, inadequate play areas for children, poor services, and defective elevators and communal washing machines. Only a small minority of people, predominantly the educated professional classes, enjoy comfortable, aesthetically pleasing, healthy living conditions.

In the 1970s, international agencies began to look at alternative low-cost sanitation technologies for rural and low to medium-density urban settlements. There are now over 20 different excreta disposal systems that offer varying degrees of convenience and protection. One such system is the ventilated improved pit (VIP) latrine. Concerted efforts during the 1980s brought improved water and sanitation services to many of the world's poorest people. Although the target of the International Drinking Water Supply and Sanitation Decade (IDWSSD) was to provide safe drinking water and sanitation to underserved urban and rural communities by 1990, the progress of the decade was not enough.

C. Housing, Communicable Diseases, and Infections

Housing conditions play a crucial role in the control of many diseases, especially in the transmission of communicable diseases. The home can both protect from disease and facilitate disease. Of all the factors, water supply and sanitation facilities often appear to be the most important in determining a community's health. Efficient drainage of surface water helps to control communicable and vector-borne diseases and reduces safety hazards and property damage. Lack of, or a breakdown in, drainage systems can result in vector-breeding sites. Flooding can result in similar problems. Appropriate solid waste disposal and storage can discourage insect and rodent vectors of disease and reduce population exposure to urban conditions likely to cause problems. Solid waste management is even more crucial when excreta are among the waste products. Waste disposal problems tend to exist predominantly in urban settings, where there are space constrictions, crowding, and greater consumption. The urban poor are especially at risk because of their dependency on scavenging for their livelihood, placing them in direct contact with all types of waste materials.

Personal and domestic hygiene is crucial to the reduction of numerous infections, including skin complaints such as sepsis, dermatitis, and eczema, or eye disease such as trachoma and conjunctivitis, or contagious diseases such as **tuberculosis (TB)** and meningitis. Good hygiene is impossible to maintain without adequate water supply.

Communicable Diseases - If there are not sufficient rooms in a house to allow for separation of sick people from healthy inhabitants, contagious diseases are more readily transmitted. Overcrowding is therefore an important factor in the spread of a number of communicable diseases. Additionally, housing with no adequate sunlight and ventilation facilitates the spread of disease by increasing available breeding sites of vectors. This is especially true for TB, one of the more common killers globally. Tuberculosis is a contagious disease that flourishes in crowded, unhygienic environments, and it is caused by bacteria that produce lung lesions, which eventually impair lung function sufficiently to cause death. Once in place in the human body, the bacteria are very resilient to treatment with antibiotics, making the cure of patients with TB difficult and expensive. Elimination of the spread of the disease, however, may be as simple as placing the sick person in a space with adequate ultraviolet (UV) light and ventilation. As TB makes its way into poor urban environments, it has the potential to have disastrous effects on many inhabitants in both the developed and developing world because of overcrowding.

Meningitis is a communicable disease that kills many people worldwide. Like TB, it is spread by airborne transmission and is linked to overcrowding and poor-quality housing. Meningitis can be caused by many different viruses and bacteria when they are able to penetrate the blood-brain barrier, which is normally impenetrable. There is no external cure for the viral form of the disease, meaning that patients' chances of surviving depend on the state of their immune systems. The bacterial forms can be treated by antibiotics, but the disease is fatal and may develop rapidly, and it requires rapid and extensive treatment that is not always successful. Other diseases, such as influenza, may also be transmitted more readily if housing is inadequate.

Poorly maintained, unhygienic buildings also provide excellent breeding grounds for many insect vectors, particularly in tropical regions. For example, Chagas' disease is caused by a parasite transmitted by the Vinchuca bug, which lives in the dark cracks and crevices of poorly built and maintained homes in certain parts of South America. Its bite leads to a specific type of heart disease that is usually fatal within 10 years for adults and in much less time in children.

The poor are especially vulnerable to inadequate housing conditions. Just as they cannot afford adequate housing, they also are generally not able to afford proper nutrition, education, and health services. They are also more likely to be exposed to dust, pollution, noise, and the hazards of climatic extremes because of the nature of their economy and often flimsy housing.

D. HOME ACCIDENTS AND TOXIC EXPOSURES

Housing should also protect its inhabitants against physical hazards and toxic exposures: this depends on both the structure of the facility and the behavior of the people using it. In the planning of housing, many factors must be taken into consideration to protect residents against these hazards, including structural features and furnishings. Poorly designed or inadequately built homes increase the risk of accidents and injuries, particularly for children.

A variety of injuries can be due to poorly designed or maintained housing. Makeshift buildings that collapse on top of their inhabitants in earthquakes, heavy rains, storms, or mudslides are common in the poorest areas of many countries. Even under "normal conditions, makeshift buildings made of poor materials result in a high number of injuries in or around the home. In more affluent countries, elderly people and young children tend to suffer more severe injuries from falling down the stairs, particularly if proper safety precautions are not incorporated in housing. Elderly people often stumble on thresholds, carpets, or other flooring hazards, causing hip fractures, one of the more common and costly injuries among elderly people. Other injuries related to unsafe housing include burns from contact with unprotected fireplaces or stoves or from house fires when occupants cannot escape in time. Fires in factories, hotels, and other buildings where large groups of people congregate can have disastrous consequences if buildings are not suitably designed, lack fire protection or fire-fighting equipment such as extinguishers or sprinklers, or have insufficient emergency exits and evacuation planning.

In many communities, indoor air pollution presently poses a much greater health risk than outdoor air pollution. Residents dependent on open fireplaces or unventilated stoves in their homes are most vulnerable, and the resulting respiratory diseases in children are responsible for as many fatalities globally as diarrhea diseases. Biomass fuels are used extensively for domestic purposes; in some settings the associated health risks are severe. Fossil fuels are also commonly burned domestically and poor combustion technologies expose people to harmful emissions of carbon monoxide (CO), nitric oxides (NO_x), dust (suspended particles), and volatile organic compounds (VOCS). Lack of ventilation, proper stoves, and chimneys greatly compounds the risks associated with both fuel types. Additionally, construction materials and furnishings are often a source of indoor pollutants, releasing a wide variety of airborne contaminants (e.g., formaldehyde, asbestos). Cigarette smoking also contributes to air pollution, and the effects of environmental tobacco smoke (ETS) can be severe.

Pollutants from the environment surrounding dwellings can also become a problem. In a number of countries the natural leakage of radon and radioactive gas has caused high levels of exposure inside dwellings and thus an increased risk of lung cancer. Air pollution builds up in urban areas from the concentration of population and industry. The heating of houses with wood or coal fires is a major source of outdoor urban air pollution in some countries.

Lead-based paints are a source of lead poisoning, especially in children. Aging water pipes made of lead or which have lead soldering in them are still in use in some parts of the world.

Cottage industries, where the home is used as a workplace, carry an associated risk of contaminant exposure. Home industries often involve the use of hazardous materials and produce noise and/or waste contaminants (either solid or airborne). These risks are compounded in an urban setting, where, in areas of high-population density, accidents such as fires can affect an entire community.

In some industrialized countries, the problem of **sick building syndrome (SBS)** - or **building-related illness**, as it is sometimes called - is common. The fact that most people spend 80% to 90% of their time indoors underscores the importance of dealing with this problem. When the oil crisis in the early 1970s sent the price of energy skyrocketing, industrialized countries put a priority on making new buildings as airtight as possible. It was soon noted that gases given off by construction materials and other pollutants could become trapped inside these airtight environments, resulting in a range of health problems among those living or working inside. Throughout the next two decades, the incidence of complaints regarding air quality in homes, schools, office buildings, and other workplaces increased dramatically. The term **tight building syndrome** was originally coined to describe this phenomenon.

Often SBS-related complaints are general and nonspecific. Causes of SBS include inadequate ventilation (estimated in the United States in the mid-1980s to be responsible for 50% of cases); some source of environmental contamination, from either inside or outside the building (30%); and unknown causes (10%). Building materials, humidity, molds, cigarette smoke, noise, and illumination account for the rest (10%). In addition, inadequate humidification can cause dry air (a known cause of irritation to eyes, skin, and throat), static electricity, and temperature fluctuations.

Sources of environmental contamination include off gassing from new furniture or carpeting, cleaning materials, chemicals from adjacent offices, unclean ducts, fiberglass, and cigarette smoke. Virtually all dusts, vapors and aerosols that can react with proteins can cause an allergic reaction. Generally considerable exposure is required to become sensitized. However, once the individual has become sensitized to any of these, allergic reactions may be elicited after only a brief and low-concentration exposure.

E. INDOOR ENVIRONMENT

Indoor climate and indoor air pollution, biological exposure factors, and various physical hazards encountered inside the home are encompassed by the term **indoor environment**. The indoor climate may be the same as that out of doors, or it may be modified by heating, cooling, or adjustment of humidity levels, and often in sealed modern buildings, by all of these.

1. Physical Hazards

Physical hazards in the indoor environment include toxic gases, respirable suspended particulates, asbestos fibers, ionizing radiation, notably radon and "daughters," nonionizing radiation, and tobacco smoke. Indoor air may be contaminated with dusts, fumes, pollen, and microorganisms. Many of the pollutants are harmful to health. Some occur mainly in sealed office buildings, and others, such as tobacco smoke, in private dwellings.

In developing countries, indoor air pollution with products of biomass fuel combustion is a pervasive problem. The fumes from cooking fires include high concentrations of respiratory irritants that cause **chronic obstructive pulmonary disease (COPD)** and that sometimes contain carcinogens too. Premature death from COPD is common among women who from their childhood have spent many hours every day close to primitive cooking stoves, inhaling large quantities of toxic fumes.

The toxic gases come from many sources. Formaldehyde is emitted as an off-gas from particleboard, carpet adhesives, and urea-formaldehyde foam insulation; it is a respiratory and conjunctival irritant and sometimes causes asthma. It is not emitted in sufficient concentrations to constitute a significant cancer risk. Although rats exposed to formaldehyde do demonstrate increased incidence of nasopharyngeal cancer, there is only weak evidence of elevated cancer incidence or mortality rates even among persons occupationally exposed to far higher concentrations than occur in domestic settings. Nonetheless, urea-formaldehyde foam insulation has been banned in many jurisdictions on the basis of the evidence for carcinogenicity in rats. Gases and vapors from volatile solvents, such as cleaning fluids, have diverse origins. There is a wide range of other pollutants, such as many organic substances, oxides of nitrogen, sulfur, carbon, ozone, benzene, and terpenes. All such toxic substances can be troublesome, especially in sealed air-conditioned buildings and most of all when the air is recirculated to conserve energy used to heat or cool the building. In combination with fluorescent lighting, these gases and suspended particulate matter can produce an irritating photochemical smog that may cause chronic conjunctivitis and nasal congestion.

Imperfect ventilation can become a serious hazard if it leads to accumulation or recirculation of highly toxic gas such as carbon monoxide; this is especially likely when coal or coke is used as cooking or heating fuel in cold weather, and vents to the outside are closed to conserve heat.

Asbestos was used for many years as a fire retardant and insulating substance in both domestic and commercial buildings. Its dangers to health have led to restriction or banning of its use and to expensive renovations aimed at removing it. Fibrous glass insulation may present hazards similar to those of asbestos but less severe.

Ionizing radiation, in particular radon and "daughters," can be a health hazard, especially if houses are sealed and air recirculated, in which case there is greater opportunity for higher concentrations to accumulate. Sources of radon include trace amounts of radioactive material incorporated in cement used to construct basements. Radon can also be emitted from soil or rocks in the environment where the houses are built.

Extremely low frequency electromagnetic radiation (ELF) has attracted much attention since the observation of cancer incidence at higher rates than expected among children living close to high voltage power lines. No convincing relationship has been demonstrated between childhood cancer and exposure to ELF from domestic appliances, with the possible exception of electric blankets. Microwave ovens and television screens are safe. The nature of the relationship, if any, between ELF and cancer remains controversial, however.

Tobacco smoke is often the greatest health hazard attributable to physical factors in the indoor environment. Infants and children are significantly more prone to respiratory infections, and nonsmoking spouses are more prone to chronic respiratory illnesses and to tobacco-related respiratory cancer when living in the same house as a habitual cigarette smoker. Cigarette smoking is a hazard in another way as well: about 20 to 25 percent of deaths in domestic fires are a result of smoking.

2. Biological Hazards

Biological hazards in the indoor environment include many varieties of pathogenic microorganisms. **Mycobacterium tuberculosis** survives for long periods in dark and dusty corners, **Legionella** lives in air conditioners, water-cooled air conditioning systems, stagnant water pipes, and shower stalls, for example. Mites that live on mattresses, cushions, and infrequently swept floors cause asthma, as may many organic dusts and pollens. Many other infections, especially those spread by the fecal-oral route, occur most often when homes are dirty, verminous, or rat infested. Food storage and cooking facilities should be kept scrupulously clean at all times because many varieties of disease-carrying vermin are attracted by filth and because food scraps can be an excellent culture medium for many pathogens that cause food poisoning or other diseases.

3. Socioeconomic Conditions

Socioeconomic conditions are related to the quality of housing in many ways, some already alluded to. Crowding always is greater among the poor than among the rich; this increases risks of transmitting communicable diseases and often imposes additional emotional stress that probably contributes to domestic violence. Street accidents involving children are more common in poor than in wealthy neighborhoods because the children often have no other place than the street to play. Poor people generally live in poorly equipped and maintained homes, adding to the risk of domestic accidents ranging from falls down poorly lit stairwells to electrocution. Lead poisoning is a particular hazard for children in dilapidated houses where they are likely to ingest dried-out flakes of lead-based paint. Emissions from factory smelter stacks contribute to environmental lead and other toxic metal contamination and are more often present in poor than in well-to-do neighborhoods because the former are more often located in or close to heavily industrialized areas.

F. Housing Conditions And Mental Health

Many descriptive studies by social epidemiologists and psychiatrists have demonstrated a consistent association between mental disorders and urban living conditions. There is also a close relationship between mental health and social class. Those who cannot cope with the competitive pressures of industrial and commercial civilization because they suffer from such disorders as schizophrenia, alcoholism, or mental retardation and have inadequate family and social support systems drift downward to the lowest depths of the slums or become homeless street people. There are estimated to be between 500,000 and 2 million homeless mentally ill persons in the United States. Schizophrenia and alcoholism have maximum prevalence in slums and "skid row" districts, and depression, manifested by attempted and accomplished suicide, is clustered in neighborhoods where a high proportion of the people live in single-room rented apartments. Adolescent delinquency, vandalism, and underachievement at school have high prevalence in dormitory suburbs occupied mainly by low-paid workers where recreational facilities for young people are often inadequate and schools are often of inferior quality. Bad housing does not cause these problems; they are usually symptoms of more complex social pathology. A different set of factors contribute to the syndrome called "**suburban neurosis**," which occurs among women who remain housebound for much of the time while their husbands are at work and their children are at school; this condition has been alleviated by television, which by bringing faces and voices into the house relieves loneliness. It has also been alleviated by changing work patterns, with increasing proportions of married women joining the workforce.

G. HOUSING STANDARDS

Public health workers are directly concerned about the quality of housing because of the many ways it can affect health. Local health officials have special powers to intervene when health is threatened by inadequate housing conditions. A handbook frequently revised by the Centers for Disease Control and Prevention and the American Public Health Association, **Housing and Health; APHA-CDC Recommended Minimum Housing Standards**, sets out specific details on basic equipment and facilities, fire safety, lighting, ventilation, thermal requirements, sanitation, space requirements (occupancy standards), and the special requirements for rooming houses. This valuable reference spells out general guidelines that can be used by local authorities as the basis for regulations, but there are no universal legally enforceable standards until local jurisdictions introduce them. **Health Principles of Housing**, a WHO manual, gives guidance on a wide range of behavioral factors that can influence health in relation to housing conditions, for example, by providing guidelines on ways to reduce psychological and social stresses by ensuring privacy and comfort and on the housing needs of populations at special risk such as pregnant women, the handicapped, and the elderly infirm. Both booklets should be part of the library of every local health officer.

H. STATISTICAL INDICATORS OF HOUSING CONDITIONS

Health planning requires every type of information pertinent to community health, including statistics on housing conditions. Useful information is routinely collected at the decennial census on density of occupancy (persons per bedroom), cooking and refrigerating facilities, and sanitary conditions. Perusal of tables showing these and other housing statistics enables health planners to identify neighborhoods at high risk of diseases associated with crowding and poor sanitation.

Census tables also enable health planners to identify less obtrusive health hazards, such as proportions of elderly persons living alone, whether in small apartments or multiple-room dwellings that perhaps were once the family home before all the others in the family moved away or died, leaving an elderly person as sole resident. Once such neighborhoods are identified, public health nurses and other community health workers can more easily locate the individuals at risk, who may need but have not yet asked for help.

In addition to census tables, there are other useful sources of information on neighborhoods with a high incidence of social pathology. Fire departments record false alarms and fires deliberately lit; police departments record details of vandalism and calls to settle domestic disturbances; and schools record absenteeism and truancy. All can be analyzed by area, thus pinpointing high-risk neighborhoods; this method has been used as part of a program aimed at improving the chances of getting a good start in life for children from disadvantaged homes. There is a high correlation between these indicators of social pathology in a neighborhood, such as a high-rise, high-density apartment complex for low-income families, and the incidence of emotional disturbances and similar behavioral upsets among young and teenaged children.

I. HEALTHY COMMUNITIES AND HEALTHY CITIES

As part of the initiative for "Health for all by the year 2000" that followed resolutions passed at the World Health Assembly in 1977," health planners in many nations, notably in the European region of the World Health Organization (WHO), began active planning for health promotion (to be distinguished from disease prevention). Health promotion requires action by many individuals and groups not usually identified with care of the sick or prevention of disease. The definition of health promotion, "the process of enabling people to increase control over and improve their health" implies that people may often have to take action aimed at improving their living conditions. The Healthy Cities movement is a coordinated program involving community health workers, local elected officials in urban affairs, and a wide variety of community groups who collectively seek to upgrade living conditions. Initially, some of the participating cities were relatively healthy places to live (e.g., Toronto, Canada) while others, (e.g., Liverpool, England) were not. The Healthy Cities initiative emphasizes activities that could be expected to enhance good health, such as provision of improved recreational facilities, services for children and their mothers (including basic education for the mothers as well as the children), and aggressive action to eradicate urban wasteland, industrial pollution, toxic dump sites, and other forms of urban blight. From modest beginnings the Healthy Cities movement has spread all over the world and in some places has extended beyond cities to embrace rural communities. Since the environment in which people live, grow, work, and play so manifestly influences their health and happiness, the Healthy Cities initiative is potentially among the most valuable means at our disposal to make this environment healthful.

J. SPECIAL HOUSING NEEDS

Elderly and disabled people require accommodation that has been adapted to enable easier access (ramps, handrails, wide doors to permit passage of wheelchairs), to facilitate storage and preparation of food (low-placed cupboards and stoves with front-fitted switches, which are inadvisable in homes where there are small children), and with special equipment for bathing and toileting (strong handrails, wheelchair access). Special accommodation of this type is often segregated, which tends to set the occupants apart in an urban ghetto for the elderly and disabled. Integrated special housing is preferable, as examples in Denmark, Sweden, and the United Kingdom have demonstrated; in this setting, elderly, infirm, and younger disabled persons live among nondisabled people, a situation that many of them prefer and that helps to accustom nondisabled people to making allowances for their disabled fellow-citizens.

K. HOUSEHOLD EXPOSURES

Because it is where much human activity takes place, the potential for damaging exposures in households is high if pollutants are present. Unfortunately, two of the most fundamental and mundane human household activities-defecation and cooking- produce significant volumes of health-damaging waste products. When human waste is not removed completely from the household environment and isolated from drinking water supplies, it leads to outbreaks of diarrhea and other waterborne diseases. When the smoke from cooking fires fueled with wood, coal, and other low-quality fuels is released into households, it leads to respiratory diseases and other health impacts. Indeed, together, these two environmental health impacts account for the largest environmental burden of ill health globally and probably account for a larger burden than any other major risk factor, environmental or not, except malnutrition.

1. Sanitation and Clean Drinking Water

Ever since hunter-gatherers turned to cultivation and settled living, sanitation has been a public health problem for human societies. Further, as urban populations have increased in size, the pressure on local sources of fresh drinking water has increased. Today, these two perennial difficulties remain widespread health hazards in the world, particularly in low- and middle-income countries in semiarid regions. Approximately 40% of the world's population does not have ready access to clean safe drinking water and approximately 60% does not have satisfactory facilities for the safe disposal of human excreta.

Water shortage amplifies the risk of many "water-washed" infectious diseases, such as chlamydia and scabies. Water shortage in combination with local fecal contamination increases the likelihood of transmission of waterborne diarrheal diseases, cholera, campylobacter, and other infections. Every year, several million children die from diarrheal diseases, contracted from infectious agents in drinking water and on food.

2. Solid Household Fuels

The oldest of human energy technologies, the home cooking, fire using, wood or other biomass remains the most prevalent fuel-using technology in the world today. Indeed, in more than 100 countries household fuel demand makes up more than half of total energy demand.

A useful framework for examining the trends and impacts of household fuel use is the "energy ladder." It ranks household fuels along a spectrum running from the simple biomass fuels (dung, crop residues, and wood), through the fossil fuels (kerosene and gas), to the most modern form, electricity. In moving up the ladder, the fuel-stove combinations that represent the higher rungs increase the desirable characteristics of cleanliness, efficiency, storability, and controllability. On the other hand, capital cost and dependence on centralized fuel cycles also tend to increase with upward movement. Although there are local exceptions, history has generally shown that when alternatives are affordable and available, populations tend to naturally move up the ladder to higher quality fuel-stove combinations. Although all of humanity had its start a quarter of a million years ago at what was then the top of the energy ladder, wood, only about half has moved to higher quality rungs. The remaining half is either still using wood or has been forced down the ladder by local wood shortages to crop residues, animal dung, or, in some severe situations, to the poorest quality fuels, such as shrubs and grass.

Throughout history, in places where it was easily available, shortage of local wood supplies led some populations to move to coal for household use. This occurred in the early 1800s in the United Kingdom, for example, although it is relatively uncommon there today. In the past 150 years, such transitions occurred in Eastern Europe and China, where household coal use still persists in millions of households. In terms of the energy ladder, coal represents an upward movement in terms of efficiency and storability. Because of these characteristics and its higher energy densities, coal can be shipped economically over longer distances than wood and efficiently supply urban markets. In this regard, it is like other household fossil fuels. Unlike kerosene and gas, however, coal often represents a decrease in cleanliness as compared to wood.

3. Housing Quality

General housing quality involves such factors as ventilation, drainage, crowding, dustiness, materials that resist pests, and insulation from sun, wind, and cold. All these factors have a significant influence on health. Indeed, much of the improvement in health that occurred in western Europe and North America during the latter part of the nineteenth and early part of the twentieth centuries is attributable to improved housing-although it is difficult to separate the relative benefits of improved housing from those due to concurrent changes in nutrition and personal hygiene behavior. Studies in some communities in low- and middle-income countries, however, indicate that health gains require improvements in a mix of factors, including general "housing" quality, rather than in just one factor at a time.

Good quality housing for low- and middle- income communities can protect health in various ways. It provides shelter from cold, hot, or wet weather conditions. Incremental improvements of traditional designs that are basically adapted to the local conditions would be the most cost-effective means of improving shelter. A factor of importance is the structural integrity of the housing in the face of typhoons, floods, or earthquakes. The location of the house is also of importance. The houses of many persons injured or killed in floods are in low-lying areas prone to flooding.

The risk of physical injuries is another important aspect of housing quality. Children and elderly need to be protected from falls. Animals, machinery, vehicles, and cooking stoves and heaters need to be separated from areas to which small children have access.

Another factor of importance in tropical countries is the avoidance of breeding sites for insect vectors of disease. Good drainage around the home and elimination of any sites where water can stagnate and mosquitoes can breed are of great importance to prevent malaria and dengue fever. In parts of Latin America the prevention of Chagas disease (South American sleeping sickness) and the elimination of its vector, the triatomine bug, depends on the use of solid ceiling and wall materials without cracks.

L. MIGRANT HOUSING

Approved migrant housing may be a mobile home, a small tenant house, a large barracks-style camp, or, in some states a canvas tent. Unapproved migrant sleeping quarters may include substandard rental housing, cardboard structures, and hotels and motels with room occupancy exceeding capacity limits.

Inspections of migrant housing varies from state to state. Several agencies are empowered by state and federal regulations to conduct migrant farm labor housing inspections. The US Department of Labor, Wage and Hour Division, and the staff of the local Job Service Office have this authority, along with the federal or state Occupational Safety and Health Administration (OSHA), or state health departments. These agencies generally coordinate inspection activity.

A special provision in the annual appropriations bill funding US DOL prohibits OSHA from conducting enforcement inspections on the farm of any farm employer who employs fewer than 11 full and part-time workers in a calendar year. However, an agricultural establishment that operates a "temporary labor camp" is subject to OSHA regardless of workforce size. OSHA is obligated to investigate in the event of a death on the job, without regard to industry or the number of workers involved. Federal OSHA has approved state-run programs in approximately 24 states. These states must have rules that "are at least as effective as" the federal OSHA regulations.

The OSHA regulations governing temporary labor camps include standards relating to first aid, drinking water, washing and bating facilities, square footage required in sleeping rooms, hot water requirements, and refuse disposal, among others.

The 1910.142 standards for Temporary Housing found in the Code of Federal Regulations (CFR) 29, Parts 1900.10 1910 (Sections 1901.1 to 1910.999), are minimum requirements. Specific examples include the following requirements:

1. One toilet for each 15 residents,
2. One shower bead for each 10 residents, and
3. 50 square feet of space per resident in sleeping areas.

If the housing does not pass inspection, it cannot be certified. If the housing is occupied without certification, citations and penalties may result for failure to register the housing and have it inspected. In addition, penalties and citations may result for items not in compliance.

In order to receive a permit, the drinking water must pass inspection at the time of the facility inspection. Tests are typically conducted by the local health department. No provisions are made in the standards to test the water multiple times throughout the season.

Many sites are on public water supplies, and this water is tested on a regular basis. Water from private sources, such as well water, is not tested throughout the season.

Water tests typically target total and fecal coliform bacteria. Tests for pesticides are made on request of the owner/operator or the housing inspector.

Acceptable toilet facilities include both indoor and outdoor plumbing. Local health departments often have jurisdiction over the examination and testing of both water and septic systems.

The regulations governing field sanitation stipulate that the following items must be provided without cost to the employee:

1. One toilet facility for every 20 persons,
2. Potable drinking water and disposable cups,
3. Hand-washing facilities with soap, water, and disposable towels,
4. Toilet and hand-washing facilities shall be located within a quarter-mile walk of each employee's place of work in the field, and
5. The toilets and hand-washing facilities are not required if employees remain in the field 3 hours or less.

Waterborne disease outbreaks in the United States in the 1980s included viral gastroenteritis, giardiasis, chemical poisoning, shigellosis, and hepatitis A.

Diseases related to substandard housing may include those caused by improper storage of food, those caused by poor hygiene due to the lack of hot water and adequate sewage systems, and those caused by the proximity to fields sprayed by toxic chemicals. For example, diseases caused by improper food storage, if refrigeration is not available or is inadequate, include gastroenteritis, which may be due to Salmonella sp. and other microbial foodborne pathogens.

Diseases related to poor hygiene and inadequate waste disposal systems include gastrointestinal illnesses and rarely septicemia. Residents may be exposed to pesticides when the housing is located within a field of crops that is routinely sprayed.

Diseases related to substandard materials present in the housing structure may occur. For instance, if the housing is old and paint is chipped, lead poisoning may be a problem. Asbestos exposure from damaged ceilings, old flooring, and insulation may occur and pulmonary illness may develop years later.

Health risks depend on the crop cultivated and harvested. Below is a grouping of illnesses or hazards farm workers may develop or encounter based on the type of agriculture involved.

Respiratory Illnesses - Organic dust toxic syndrome (ODTS) from exposure to dusts from decayed grain, hay, and silage; hypersensitivity pneumonitis from exposure to dusts from grains, hay, or animals.

Chemical Hazards - Acute and chronic pesticide poisoning, especially from organophosphates and carbamates; respiratory effects from fumigant inhalation such as methyl bromide; hematologic cancers, such as leukemia, multiple myeloma, and non-Hodgkin's lymphoma from solvents and pesticides; irritant or allergic contact dermatitis from pesticides, solvents, and plants; infertility from pesticide exposure.

Infectious Diseases - Histoplasmosis, ornithosis, Q fever, bovine tuberculosis, tuberculosis, hydatidosis, Newcastle disease, swine influenza, tularemia, Rocky Mountain spotted fever, and Lyme disease.

Occupational Illnesses/Injuries - Green tobacco sickness, insect stings/bites, heat stress/heat stroke, dehydration, frostbite, rashes from toxic plants such as poison ivy/poison oak, skin cancer from sun exposure, electrocutions, animal bites/kicks, injuries from farm equipment – Crushing/laceration/abrasion, puncture, sprain/strain, fracture /contusion, burns, and hearing loss are just examples of occupational illnesses/ injuries.

Migrant workers may seek medical treatment, but barriers to this are many. Barriers to medical treatment include distance to health clinics, lack of transportation, lack of support from the employer or crew leader, language barriers, lack of knowledge of the existence and hours of clinic operation, and reliance on traditional medicinal practices.

Health centers receiving grants under subsection (g) of public law 104-299, the Health Centers Consolidation Act, may offer special occupation-related health services for migratory and seasonal agricultural workers.

The Migrant Health Program, sponsored by the U.S. DUBS finances migrant health services of community and migrant health centers located across the U. S. These centers, approximately 150 nationwide, provide medical services to farm workers, include screenings for infectious diseases and injury prevention programs and may include outreach programs as part of their medical service to the farm worker community.

There is no national database of migrant housing locations. State agencies responsible for conducting inspections may have data base information noting camp locations characteristics. A comprehensive national database would be helpful to health agencies. Such a database would need to be updated on a regular basis in order to provide accurate information.

The U.S. DOL conducts a survey that covers field workers in seasonal agricultural services (SAS) as defined by the U.S. DOA. These field workers, by definition, are not migratory. The Centers for Disease Control and Prevention in Atlanta maintains a database of communicable diseases.

All states report the existence of specific infectious diseases to the Centers for Disease Control and Prevention (CDC) on a weekly basis. Each state determines its own list of reportable infectious diseases. Either local health departments or state health departments have an investigative and reporting process. Specific diseases are reported to the CDC on a nationwide basis. Examples of these diseases include tuberculosis, hepatitis, Rocky Mountain spotted fever, Lyme disease, botulism, Escherichia coli 0157:H7 illness, and other foodborne illnesses.

According to a study conducted by North Carolina State University's School of Design, families who engage in farm work would like a place to live that "looks like a home." Adequate hot water, privacy, ample kitchen facilities, outdoor areas ("green space"), access to a telephone, and shopping areas were also priorities.

In regions where tobacco is a cash crop, farm workers would benefit from a clear understanding of the symptomatic differences between green tobacco sickness and pesticide exposure. Green tobacco sickness is often diagnosed when the actual condition may be related to pesticide exposure.

Other diagnostic problems may be due to language and cultural problems and could be resolved through the use of medical personnel who are familiar with the language and the culture of the client. The physician has the obligation to notify the proper authorities, which will send trained personnel to conduct an investigation of residential and/or field sanitation.

Cysticercosis, giardiasis, typhoid fever, intestinal infections, tuberculosis, and cholera have all been listed as endemic illnesses among migrant workers.

II. ENVIRONMENTAL SAFETY

A. INTRODUCTION

Injuries continue to constitute a significant public health problem in the USA. Injuries are just as predictable and preventable as illnesses such as mumps, heart attacks, and lung cancer. Injuries may be intentional or unintentional.

Intentional injuries include homicide, assault, suicide, child abuse, rape, and other acts of violence.

Unintentional injuries are those that frequently are referred to as accidental injuries because they do not involve someone attempting to inflict harm on another person. Another way to consider the magnitude of injury mortality is to review data pertaining to **years of potential life lost (YPLL)** published by CDC National Center for Health Statistics.

B. SAFETY CONCEPTS

Forms of physical energy:

1. Kinetic or mechanical energy,
2. Chemical energy,
3. Electricity,
4. Radiation, and
5. Thermal energy.

Injury is physical damage to the body that results when energy is transferred to the body in amount greater than it can withstand, such as fires or poisons or when the body is deprived of sufficient energy, such as oxygen or heat.

C. CONSUMER PRODUCT SAFETY COMMISSION

In 1972 U.S. Congress passed the Consumer Product Safety Act, which created the Consumer Product Safety Commission (CPSC) because "An unacceptable number consumer products which present an unreasonable risk of injury were distributed in commerce".

CPSA authorizes CPSC to ban hazardous consumer products, to initiate recalls for products that pose imminent or substantial hazards to the public, and to establish mandatory performance standards and warning and instruction requirements for consumer products.

D. HOME SAFETY

Someone once wrote, **"Your home may be your castle, but the enemy is not entirely outside the wall"**, a thought-provoking statement, as more accidents occur in and around the home than in any other place.

Falls are the leading cause of accidental death in the home, outpacing burns and all other causes combined. In **children**, falls occur under a wide variety of circumstances, but the risk of death or permanent impairment is related to the height of the fall and the nature of the material struck. Many falls from children's furniture occur. Many of the serious childhood injuries occurring on stairs are related to walkers. Unlike fall victims who are children, **older** fall victims are much more likely to die from falls. Stairways are the site of more than 750,000 fall injuries each year. Falls also occur on floors and walkways and in bathtubs and showers.

E. FIRE AND BURN INJURIES

Despite continuing efforts to prevent injuries and deaths from fires and burns, fire still kills about 5,000 people in the United States annually - an average of 13 per day. This is one of the highest rates in industrialized world.

Ten years ago, 48% of fire deaths occurred during January, February, and December and the 3 leading causes of death of children younger than 5 years, were:

1. Children playing with fire-ignition sources such as matches (37%),
2. Faulty or misused heating devices (19%), and
3. Faulty or misused electrical distribution sources (11%).

For persons older than 70 years, the 3 leading causes were:

1. Careless smoking,
2. Faulty or misused heating devices (19%), and
3. Faulty or misused electrical distribution sources (12%).

The increased occurrence of fire-related deaths during winter months reflects the seasonal use of portable heaters, fireplaces, and chimneys, and Christmas trees.

F. POISONING

In 1961, poisoning claimed the lives of 450 children under the age of 5. By 1989, it had dropped to 42. The substances that children ingest most commonly are aspirin, solvents and petroleum products, tranquilizers, and iron compounds. The highest rates are seen in children about 1-2 years of age; boys are at slightly higher risk than girls.

The American Academy of Pediatrics offers the following recommendations:

1. First and foremost, store household products and medicines out of reach of children, and use safety latches on all drawers and cupboards that contain potentially harmful substances.

2. Keep products in their original containers, never put products that can be poisonous in old food or beverage containers.
3. Never call medicine "candy".
4. Have syrup of ipecac available at home, and use it to induce vomiting if a child ingests a poisonous substance.
5. Keep poison control and other emergency phone numbers near the phone, and call immediately in an emergency.
6. Leave original labels on all products.
7. Clean out medicine cabinets periodically and discard unneeded and dated medication in safe manner.

G. FIREARM INJURIES

From 1968 through 1991, firearm-related deaths increased by 60% (from 23,875 to 38,317). Based on these trends, by the year 2003 the number of firearm-related deaths will surpass the number of motor vehicle-related deaths and firearms will become the leading cause of injury-related death.

A multifaceted approach to reduce firearm-related injuries should include at least three elements:

1. Foster changes in behavior through campaigns to educate and inform persons about the risks and benefits of possessing firearms and the safe use and storage of firearms.
2. Direct legislative efforts towards preventing access to or acquiring firearms by specific groups that should not have firearms (e.g. felons and children) and towards regulating the storage, transport, and use of firearms.
3. Make technologic changes to modify firearms and ammunition so as to render them less lethal (e.g. a requirement for childproof safety devices such as trigger locks).

Non powder firearms (those using gas, air, or a spring propel ammunition, including BE guns) cause more than 14,000 injuries annually among children younger than age 15, with boys accounting for over 80% of the injuries.

H. POWER LAWNMOWER INJURIES

Power lawnmowers (walk-behind and ride-on) continue to be responsible for hundreds of injuries each year, in spite of CPSC's long-time effort to reduce injuries associated with these labor-saving machines.

I. RECREATIONAL SAFETY

Millions of Americans participate in leisure activities each year.

Swimming - Swimming is one of the most popular recreational activities in U.S., and one of the most dangerous. Drowning, the fourth leading cause of childhood fatal injuries is most common in children 4 years of age and males aged 15-19 years.

Recreational Boating - Recreational boating continues to grow in popularity each year, and with it comes a corresponding increase in risk. Recreational boats include canoes, rowboats, duck boats, sailboats, motorboats, yachts, jet skis, and kayaks. Boaters should take the following precautions to reduce the risk of an accident:

1. Be totally familiar with the boat's operation. This means that young inexperienced operators should be supervised until they acquire skills necessary to be safe operators.
2. Equip boats with approved personal floatation devices for each person, and with fire extinguishers and other safety equipment.
3. Be familiar with all of the rules of safe boating.
4. Avoid the use of alcoholic beverages. Studies conducted by the U.S. Coast Guard suggest that alcohol may be involved in as many as 60% of recreational boating facilities.

Ride horses - Each year in the U.S. an estimated 30 million persons ride horses. The rate of serious injuries per number of riding hours is estimated to be higher for horseback riders than for motorcyclist and automobile racers. Horseback riders sometimes are injured when they collide with fixed objects, are dragged along the ground with a foot caught in a stirrup, are crushed between the horse and ground, or are trampled, kicked, or bitten.

All terrain vehicles (ATVs) - Recreational use of snowmobiles is extremely popular in many regions of the country. One study suggest that most fatal snowmobile incidents involve male operators in their 20s, use of alcohol, or excessive speed, and that half the persons killed sustained head injuries. All terrain vehicles (ATVs) are three or four-wheeled vehicles designed mainly for recreational or agricultural off-road use. Licensing is not required in most states. ATVs overturn easily, especially on rough terrain.

J. TRANSPORTATION SAFETY

1. Introduction

Over the past 4 decades, numerous interventions in motor vehicle and highway safety have contributed to reducing transportation injuries and death in the U.S.

The impact of motor-vehicle injuries on certain groups is illustrated by the following:

1. Motor-vehicle crash injuries claim the lives of more than 5,500 teenagers each year,
2. More than over 2,200 children ages 0-12, die in motor-vehicle crashes annually,
3. More than 40% of the deaths of 16 to 19 year olds from the causes result from motor vehicle accidents,
4. More vehicle accidents are the cause of about half of all child deaths from injury,
5. Alcohol is involved in about half of all deaths from motor vehicle crashes,
6. Motor-vehicle crashes cause the death of more than 5,500 pedestrians each year,
7. Motor-vehicle crashes cause 23% of all occupational injury deaths, and

8. Annually, motor-vehicle crashes are the cause of fatal injuries of more than 6,000 elderly people (65 years of age and older); *65%* are passenger car occupants and 20% are pedestrians.

The increase in child safety seat use has saved lives of and prevented injuries to infants (children 1 year old and younger) and toddlers (children aged 1-4 years). The leading cause of death in children ages 1-4 years continues to be injuries to motor-vehicle occupants.

2. Pedestrian Safety

Pedestrian injuries are a leading cause of death in children aged 4-8, with the peak at age 6. Each year approximately 1,100 pedestrians ages 0-14 years are killed in traffic accidents.

3. Motor Vehicles

Human error accounts for more than 80% of all accidents, including motor vehicle accidents. "Improper Driving" includes actions such as speeding, failure to yield right-of-way, driving left of center, incorrect passing, and following too closely.

Law enforcement personnel and organization such as Mothers Against Drunk Driving (MADD) have worked closely with legislators and citizens to develop better ways to educate the public about the hazard of drinking and driving. Environmental factors, both natural and manmade, account for less than 5% of vehicle accidents. Another factor that must be considered in motor vehicle crashes is the vehicle design.

III. SWIMMING POOLS AND SPAS

A. SWIMMING POOL SAFETY

Drowning is the most deadly risk, but head and neck injuries from diving into shallow water are all too common. Swimming pools and particularly spas may also serve as a source of infections, which can be life threatening. Some common infections associated with pools include skin or ear infections caused by Pseudomonas and staphylococcus bacteria. Respiratory infections caused by Legionella bacteria, and a variety of gastrointestinal diseases including cryptosporidiosis, can also be spread in pool water.

Drowning is one of the leading causes of death for children 3-5 years old. Older children who are not properly supervised around the pool and adults who swim alone, particularly after drinking alcoholic beverages, are at an increased risk.

Provide proper barriers to prevent small children from wandering into the pool area, properly supervise children in the pool area, and do not allow anyone to swim alone. It is also helpful to have safety equipment such as a life hook, floating ring buoy, and telephone handy and to discontinue use of the pool if the water gets too cloudy to see the bottom of the pool. Covering pools and spas when not in use can help protect small children.

Both the U.S. CPSC and the National Spa and Pool Institute have recommended standards for pool fences. Standards call for a fence or barrier at least 4 feet tall and constructed so there are no handholds or footholds that can be used for climbing.

Gates or doors should be self-closing and self-latching and should have latches out of reach of small children. Doors and windows entering the pool area from a dwelling should have alarms, screens, or some other form of child protection.

Additionally, the following precautions should be taken to ensure pool safety:

1. Clearly mark the depth of water on the edge of the pool and do not allow anyone to jump or dive into less than 5 feet of water.
2. Remove diving boards from pools that do not have a diving area larger than the minimum diving area standards established by the National Spa and Pool Institute.
3. Make sure people are familiar with the pool before diving into it and discourage drinking and diving.

B. SWIMMING POOL WATER QUALITY

Circulation pumps and pipes move water through filters and mix chemicals uniformly throughout the pool. Filtration is essential to keep water clear, and chemicals are necessary to prevent bacteria, algae, and other organisms from growing in the pool or spa.

Pool water clouds up when suspended solids build up in the pool faster than the filter can remove them. Sometimes a faulty pump does not circulate enough water through the filter or the filter does not filter properly, but most water clouding is related to water chemistry problems. Bather wastes such as sweat and urine can raise the pH of pool water and cause water to appear cloudy. Algae growing in a pool can also cause the water to appear cloudy or green.

In this case, certain investigatory steps should be taken. For example:

1. Close the pool to bathers and check to see if the pump is moving water and if the filter is working.
2. Test the water chemistry to see if the pH of the water is too high (above 7.8).
3. If the pH is high, adding muriatic acid or sodium bisulfate to the pool will lower the pH and help clear the water.
4. Both of those chemicals are readily available at most pool supply stores.
5. If the pH is not high, adding one of the pool clarifiers available from pool suppliers should help.

Free chlorine residual and pH should be checked daily. Total alkalinity, which affects the pH, should be tested about once a week or whenever maintaining proper pH becomes difficult. The strong chlorine odor in some pools is usually caused by chloramines, which are created when chlorine combines with ammonia from bathers and other organic material in the pool. Chloramines are destroyed by high doses of chlorine, so adding 1 ¼ pounds of granular calcium hypochlorite per 10,000 gallons of pool water should help.

One cause is improper pool water pH. If the pH is too low (below 7.2) or too high (above 7.8) eye irritation can occur. Eyes are most comfortable at a pH of 7.4 to 7.6. Chloramines are also a major source of eye irritation. The free chlorine residual for a swimming pool should be between 1 and 3 parts per million. Spa water should have from 2 to 10 parts per million and ideally 3 to 5 parts per million of free chlorine.

In swimming pools where people are active, it is possible for a swimmer to overheat if the pool temperature gets above 90°F. In spas, where people are sitting still, the temperature should not exceed 104°F and bathers should limit their exposure to short (15-minute) stays.

IV. ENVIRONMENTAL INFECTIONS

The environment is what we live in; it surrounds us-urban, suburban, or rural. Air, water, inanimate materials, and living organisms big and small can harbor, transmit, or be a potential pathogen. Humans are often a host for pathogens more by accident than by intent, even serving as a reservoir and possibly even as a vector for the spread and propagation of disease.

Many of the sources for pathogenic organisms are readily apparent (visible sewage, spoiled food, turbid water, insects, and wild animals, for example), or not readily obvious and easily perceivable as safe (mountain stream water, fruit and other edibles found in the wild, contact with seemingly healthy domesticated animals).

One of the triumphs in public health is the systematic interruption of the chain of infection. This has been achieved by the successful identification, tracking, containment, eradication, and prevention of diseases in populations and geographic areas of the world. This is in addition to advances in medicine in the diagnosis and treatment of diseases. Examples include vaccinations to promote immunity to pathogens, sanitary practices such as garbage removal as a matter of vector control and to limit the presence of animal reservoirs, food preparation and storage techniques to nullify the risk of infection from contaminants, and water treatment to cut down the risk of waterborne infectious pathogens in seemingly clear water. However, the war against infectious diseases is far from won.

There are four underlying forces at work: the global population continues to grow, encroaching on and impacting undeveloped lands; the emergence of new and previously undescribed pathogens, such as hantavirus; the reemergence or persistence of old pathogens with new characteristics (e.g., resistance to standard antibiotic therapy), such as Salmonella and Plasmodium falciparum; and the periodic lapses and gaps in surveillance and other public health strategies for various reasons.

Collectively there will continue to be new and recurring problems from exposures to pathogens that are ever present in the environment. It should be noted that much of this discussion is aimed at a North American- based audience. U. S. has a well-established public health system of surveillance, prevention, and eradication: infectious diseases that continue to be scourges around the world, such as tuberculosis, measles, polio, diphtheria, and malaria, are now rarely seen in the U. S.

Unfortunately, we can be victims of our own success, for many in health care today are unfamiliar with the plagues that their predecessors dealt with routinely. Outbreaks of such diseases can infect and spread among those at risk until a diagnosis is made. Thus, the key consideration in an outbreak or situation is to still consider either a new disease or even an old pathogen when the common causes are quickly eliminated.

A. TICKBORNE DISEASES

Some of the tickborne diseases are historically well known, such as Rocky Mountain spotted fever (RMSF: the pathogen is Rickettsia rickettsii); the new and emerging tick-borne infectious diseases described within the past 25 years include Lyme disease (LD; Borellia burgdorferi), human monocytic ehrlichiosis (HME; Ehrlichia chaffeensis-occasionally referred to as "Rocky Mountain spotless fever"), and human granulocytic ehrlichiosis (HOE; an F. equi-related ehrlichia species).

In the United States, tick activity is generally between late spring and early fall (April- October; this may be extended in warmer regions of the country). During this time people are more apt to be outdoors and wearing less clothing, and the ticks are more active, feeding and breeding. The major ticks are the Ixodes species, Ixodes scapularis (formerly L. damnini) in the eastern United States, and I. Pacificus in the western United States; dermacentor species (principally D. variabilis; D. andersoni is prevalent in the Rocky Mountain States); and Amblyomma americanum.

B. LYME DISEASE

Lyme disease was first described around Old Lyme, Connecticut in the mid-1970s. It tends to be a seasonal disease, occurring mostly from the late spring to the early fall. The number of cases of Lyme disease in the U.S. has been steadily increasing since 1982; in 1998 just over 16,000 cases were reported to the Centers for Disease Control (CDC). The geographic areas of the US where Lyme disease is most prevalent are the northeastern U.S., the upper midwest, and California.

The vectors are ticks: Ixodes scapularis (formerly I. dammini) is prevalent in the eastern U.S., and I. pacificus in die western U.S. Both the adult tick and the nymph form can harbor and transmit the organism B. burgdorferi, but most cases are due to the smaller nymph. The primary reservoirs are field mice [the white-footed mouse (Peromyscus leucopus) is usually the reservoir for nymphs; the white-tailed deer (Odocoileus virginianus) is the preferred host for adult ticks). Less than 1% of ticks collected and studied in endemic areas have the organism.

C. NEWLY DESCRIBED TICK-BORNE DISEASES. THE EHRLICHIOSES

Ehrlichiosis is a relatively new disease. Human monocytic ehrlichiosis was first described around 1986 in humans, although it was well known as a veterinary disease for most of the century. The Ehrlichia species are closely related to the rickettsial class of bacterium.

Unlike Lyme disease, the ebrlichioses are not well known to the public or to many practicing physicians, although awareness is improving.

D. ROCKY MOUNTAIN SPOTTED FEVER

Through 1995, around 600 cases of RMSE were reported to the CDC on average annually. Despite the misnomer of the name, more cases are reported from the southern and southeastern U.S. than elsewhere around the country. The causative organism is Rickettsia rickettsii and it does not have an animal reservoir, rather the Dermacentor ticks maintain and pass the organism to their offspring.

E. BABESIOSIS (TICK-BORNE DISEASE)

The causative agent of this malaria-like illness in humans is Babesia microti. This organism is a protozoan parasite rather than a bacterium. Related Babesia spp. are well-known veterinary parasites that are responsible for Texas cattle fever, which is thought to be one of the biblical plagues mentioned in Exodus. The 1st U.S. case was reported in 1969 and approximately 100 cases total have since been tallied in the U.S. Babesia microti is a parasite on red blood cells (RBCs). The northeastern U.S. is the common area where babesiosis is diagnosed, but it has been found in other areas of the country (rarely) and throughout the world (infrequently).

F. Q FEVER

Q (for query) fever was first suspected in 1935 in an Australian meat works; eventually the causative organism defined was Coxiella burneti, which was thought to be related to the rickettsial species but is in fact most closely related to the Legionella group. Animals that serve as reservoirs are dogs, cats, birds, and even ticks, but it is mostly associated with domesticated ungulates, such as sheep or cattle. It is an obligate intracellular pathogen, but also has a spore stage that makes it unusually resistant to harsh environments. It is considered an occupational disease for people who work with animals; at this time there is an investigational vaccine available for human use.

G. RABIES

Rabies is one of the great success models in surveillance, prevention, and control. Awareness about rabies in the United States remains high. In the industrialized world it is confined mostly to feral animal populations.

In the United States it is associated with raccoons (the majority of animal rabies discovered), skunks, bats, and foxes; approximately 93% of 11 animal rabies cases in 1997 were from wild animals. By law in the United States, canines are required to be vaccinated against rabies, and owners of other domestic animals such as cats are encouraged to have their pets vaccinated.

Due to the high mortality rate of rabies and the lack of an objective marker of exposure to the rabies virus, health care providers tend to have an extremely low threshold to administering post exposure prophylaxis (PEP), thus hundreds of doses are given each year whether warranted or not. Persons who are at high risk for rabies exposure, such as veterinarians and animal handlers, are encouraged to be vaccinated as a prophylactic measure.

H. BRUCELLOSIS

Brucellosis is a worldwide infection of animals. There are several species of the genus Brucella and each tends to have a host preference. Only four Brucella spp. are known to be pathogenic for humans: Brucella abortus (typically associated with cattle; it is known as Bang's disease), B. melitensis, B. suis, and B. cams. Brucellosis is considered an occupational disease in the livestock industry from exposure to sick animals and animal debris or birth products, although it can be a food-borne illness from unpasteurized food products (camel milk, goat cheese).

I. PLAGUE

Plague is a historically significant disease dating back to antiquity, and is held responsible for the Black Death across Europe in the mid-1300s. It continues to have a worldwide distribution, particularly in countries where wild rodent populations are large. Today in the United States it is a rarely seen disease. According to the CDC there have been 13 cases/year on average in the U.S. (1970-1995), largely confined to the southwest United States, where plague is a zoonotic infection among indigenous wild rats.

The organism is a small gram-negative bacillus. The vector is the rat flea [in the U.S. the oriental rat flea (Xenopsylla cheopis) is the most commonly implicated arthropod] and the hosts and reservoirs are usually wild rats; other hosts can include rodents (ground squirrels and prairie dogs) and occasionally domestic animals such as cats. The most common exposure risk is a flea bite, but infection can occur directly from exposure to animals that are ill from Yersinia pestis via inhalation of aerosolized respiratory secretions.

J. COMMON FUNGAL DISEASES

Fungi are microscopic organisms that are usually ubiquitous in the environment. Unlike most of the diseases so far, these are not considered zoonotic infections, do not have an animal host or a vector of some sort implicated, and are not associated with food or waterborne disease syndromes. Their habitat is soil, although in some instances the organism can be in the guano of birds.

In the United States, there are four fungi in particular: Histoplasma capsulatum, blastomyces dermatitidis, Cryptococcus neoformans and Coccidioides immitis. Histoplasma capsulatum and C. neoformans are associated with the disturbance and aerosolization of bird droppings, particularly pigeons; C. neoformans has a worldwide distribution and H. capsulatum and B. dermatidis have a distribution in the United States mostly along the Mississippi and Ohio River valleys. Coccidioides immitis is limited to the southwestern U.S. and cases tend to appear in clusters after a natural disturbance that agitates the soil, such as windstorms and earthquakes.

K. HANTAVIRUS

In 1993 a new clinical syndrome with a novel infectious agent was described among the indigenous population in the Four-Corners area of the southwestern United States (the only point in the U.S. that four states touch at a single point). This syndrome is known as hantavirus pulmonary syndrome (HPS) and the infectious agent is known as Sin Nombre ("without name") virus (SNV). Hantaviral syndromes are a zoonotic viral syndrome found among rodents, and humans are considered an accidental host. The most common reservoir is the deer mouse (Peromyscus maculatus), but unlike other diseases, the hantavirus is not spread by an arthropod vector, but rather by the aerosolization of rodent excrement, urine, or saliva and subsequent exposure of humans by inhalation.

L. GIARDIA LAMBLIA

Giardia lamblia is a protozoan typically associated with intestinal infections causing diarrhea, and sometimes leading to chronic states of weight loss and malabsorption. Giardia is considered the most common protozoan cause of diarrheal disease. The most common route for exposure is fecal/oral, and is associated with water contamination. Raw foods such as vegetables and fruit may be contaminated with Giardia oocysts, thus washing foods prior to eating or preparation is warranted.

M. PARASITES IN DRINKING WATER

Though there are several protozoans in the environment, there are two worth noting: Cryptosporidium parvum and Cyclospora cayetanensis.

Cryptosporidiosis is a relatively newly recognized protozoan that causes human diarrheal disease (it was first described in 1976); it is usually associated with animal waste and water-borne epidemics. Interestingly, this protozoan is highly resistant to chlorination, which led to the Milwaukee (WI) outbreak in 1993 from municipal water contamination. However, in municipal water treatment it is easily filtered out or killed by ozone flocculation. Outbreaks of cryptosporidiosis have been linked to swimming pools that were adequately chlorinated. For healthy people with intact immune systems, cryptosporidiosis is a self-limited intestinal disease (the protozoan is cleared from the intestines). For people with cell-mediated immune deficits, particular those with advanced HIV disease, cryptosporidiosis can become a chronic and debilitating condition because they are unable to clear the organism from the GI tract, leading to prolonged bouts of diarrhea, dehydration, and death. At present there is no reliable antiprotozoan medication against C. parvum.

Another relatively new protozoan implicated in human diarrheal disease is Cyclospora cayetanensis. It was first reported in U.S.A. in 1985 but became more prominent after an outbreak in a Chicago area hospital in 1990; it is best known as the organism that caused several epidemics in 1996 across the U.S. that was traced to imported raspberries from Guatemala.

The low incidence of Entamoeba histolytica infection is an example of the success of good water treatment and surveillance: this protozoan scourge of the world, the cause of amoebic dysentery, is now seen in the U.S. usually only in people returning from travels in the developing world.

N. MALARIA

Malaria ("bad air") continues to be a worldwide leader in causing morbidity and mortality in the developing world.

The disease is caused by four Plasmodium spp., the most serious being P. falciparum, and is of great historical significance (for instance, Alexander the Great supposedly died from complications of malaria when conquering the subcontinent of India in 323 B.C.).

In the industrial nations, it is less of a problem thanks to surveillance, sanitation, and control of its vector, the Anopheles species of mosquito. Malaria continues to be a problem in large part because of the failure to create an effective vaccine, inconsistent results in vector control, the incomplete application of prophylaxis in vulnerable persons, and the emergence of drug resistance to established antimalarials to Plasmodium in endemic areas of the world.

O. ANTHRAX

Anthrax is an ancient disease [the Fifth Plague described in the Holy Bible (Exodus)] may have been anthrax) and continues to have a worldwide distribution. In most instances it is an occupational disease in people working with herbivores, notably cattle and sheep.

Recently it has come to the attention of the media, government, military and public health officials, and the citizenry at large because of the increasing awareness or small organized groups of people intent on causing harm in order to draw attention to their cause. Anthrax has been used as a threat because it is easily transmissible and can cause morbidity and mortality in a short amount of time.

P. LEPTOSPIROSIS

Leptospirosis is another zoonotic disease that was primarily an occupational hazard of working with livestock and other animals, but now is more commonly seen in recreational and home settings. Though associated with mammals (farm animals and vermin), it has been isolated from reptiles, fish, and birds.

Humans are infrequently infected in the United States approximately 40-120 cases are reported to the CDC each year, mostly sporadic and occasionally in small outbreaks (for example, there were two outbreaks in 1998 among competitive triathletes swimming in lake water).

V. CHILDHOOD LEAD POISONING

A. INTRODUCTION

In the United States, elevated blood lead levels (BLLs) ($\geq$10 μg/dL) are a major health risk for children. This risk is totally preventable. Lead exposure has been dramatically reduced over the last two decades because of the phase-out of lead from gasoline, food, beverage cans, house paint, as well as limitations of its use in industrial emissions, drinking water, consumer goods, hazardous waste sites, and other sources.

Nevertheless, it remains a primary public health problem that needs to be addressed especially in old major U.S. metropolitan areas. In fact, as part of EPA's ongoing efforts in preventing and reducing lead poisoning among children, it has set new lower standards of exposure. Recent data from the Centers for Disease Control and Prevention (CDC) show that nearly one million children are lead poisoned. A large body of evidence shows that the most common source of lead exposure for children today is lead paint in older housing and the contaminated dust and soil it generates. Poisoning from lead paint has affected millions of children ever since this problem was first recognized more than 100 years ago and it persists today despite a 1978 ban on the use of lead in new paint.

Older housing, especially pre-1950, poses greater risk for children. A vast majority of these children are of minority, non-white groups. Several reports and studies show that these children are at the highest risk of lead poisoning, because they are most likely to live in old dilapidated homes built before 1950. A report from the Urban League stated that nearly, 1 in 10 Latino, Native American and African American children in Oregon have too much lead in their blood. An estimated 890,000 U.S. children age 1-5 have elevated blood lead levels (BLLs) ($\geq$10 μg /dL, which is the CDC Level of Concern), and more than one fifth of African American children living in housing built before 1946 have elevated BLLs.

Lead poisoning can cause brain damage and can have a permanent effect on the central nervous system. Even low levels of exposure have been associated with learning disabilities, including decreased intelligence quotient (IQ) and other behavioral problems.

B. MAJOR HEALTH ENDPOINTS

Lead is highly toxic, especially to children under 2 years of age. In the second year of life, the still unfinished maturation of the brain coincides with peak blood lead concentration as children explore their environments with increasing ambulatory and oral intensity. In addition, lead can harm a child's kidneys, bone marrow, and other body systems. At higher levels, lead can cause coma, convulsions, and death. The National Academy of Sciences has reported that comparatively low levels of lead exposure are harmful. Levels as low as 10 μg /dL of blood in infants, children, and pregnant women are associated with impaired cognitive function, behavior difficulties, fetal organ development, and other problems. In addition, low levels of lead in children's blood can cause reduced intelligence, impaired hearing and reduced stature.

Lead toxicity has been well-established, with evidence of harmful effects found in children whose blood lead levels exceed 10 μg /dL. Once in the body, children's health effects vary. With severe lead poisoning, problems range from permanent mental retardation to death. At different child's blood lead levels, the health effects include IQ levels decrease, verbal function / linguistic deficits, decreased educational performance, cognitive function deficits, learning difficulties, autism, aggression, violence, hostility, anti-social or delinquent behavior, externalizing and internalizing behaviors, inappropriate / uncontrolled behaviors similar to attention deficit disorder (ADD) behaviors with increased frequency, lethargy, hearing impairment, decrease of auditory sensitivity, auditory processing altered, attention problems, distractibility, restlessness, hyperactive behaviors difficult to manage, irritability, increased school absenteeism, auditory evoked response patterns altered, retinal degeneration, perceptual function deficits, depressed sensitivity of rod photoreceptors, and visuo-spatial skills deficit. In recent years, many studies have confirmed that lead not only diminishes intellectual capacity, but it also causes loss of hearing, reduces hand-eye coordination, impairs the ability to pay attention, and creates a propensity toward violence. Children who have been poisoned by lead are less able to handle stress and are more prone to violent outbursts.

The American Academy of Pediatrics reviewed 18 scientific studies showing that lead diminishes a child's mental abilities and found that the relationship between lead levels and IQ deficits was remarkably consistent. A number of studies have found that for every 10 μg /dL increase in blood lead levels, there was a lowering of mean [average] IQ in children by 4 to 7 points. This may not sound like a major loss, but an average IQ loss of 5 points puts 50% more children into the IQ 80 category, which is borderline for normal intelligence. It also reduces the number of high IQs; for example, one small group that should have contained 5 children with IQs of 125, contained none. The American Academy of Pediatrics says such losses are permanent and they translate into reduced educational attainment, diminished job prospects, and reduced earning power. A small drop in the average IQ would have staggering implications. In **"Our Stolen Future"**, Theo Coburn is reminding us that, if the average were to drop just five points ... this society would have lost more than half its high-powered minds with the capacity to become the most gifted doctors, scientists, college professors, inventors, or writers.

Numerous studies have shown that there is no "safe" dose of lead in children's blood. According to the 1993 National Research Council report, there is growing evidence that even very small exposures to lead can produce subtle effects in humans. Therefore, safety guidelines should drop below 10 μg /dL as the mechanisms of lead toxicity are now better understood. The NRC offered evidence that lead at 5 μg /dL (half the official "safe" level) can cause attention deficit in children and in monkeys, reduced birth weight in children, and hearing loss in children. According to the 1993 NRC summary of a series of recent studies, there is growing evidence that there is no effective threshold for some of the adverse effects of lead. At the recent Joint Meeting of the Pediatric Academic Societies and American Academy of Pediatrics in Boston, Lanphear and his colleagues reported that the current limit of 10 μg/dL is inadequate to protect the children, and should be at least half that amount. Inverse associations were observed between blood lead concentration and deficits in cognitive functioning and academic achievement in children at levels below 5.0 μg /dL.

The National Research Council says modern humans are estimated to have total body burdens of lead approximately 300-500 times those of our prehistoric ancestors. According to careful measurements of human bones, pre-Colombian inhabitants of North America had average blood lead levels of 0.016 μg /dL – some 625 times lower than 10 μg /dL now established as "safe" for our children. On the face of it, it seems unlikely that levels of a potent nerve poison 625 times natural background can be "safe" in children.

C. LEAD IN THE ENVIRONMENT

Now that lead additives in motor fuels for highway use are banned, emissions of lead from its source have diminished to very low levels. Nevertheless, the deposited organolead compounds and their transformation products are still in the soil. The natural lead content of soil derived from crust rock, mostly as galena (PbS), typically ranges from <10 to 30 µg /g soil. However, the concentration of lead in the top layers of soil varies widely due to deposition and accumulation of atmospheric particulates from anthropogenic sources. Soils contaminated with lead are the legacy of decades of use of lead additives in gasoline and paints. According to the 1999 report by Mielke, in many of America's inner cities, soil-lead is most concentrated where children are apt to play - in the yards and play areas around their houses, particularly if these houses are near heavy automobile traffic. The soil-lead concentration in old communities of large cities is 10 to 100 times greater than comparable neighborhoods of smaller cities. In addition, soil-lead concentrations diminish with distance from a city center. Statistics suggest that lead-contaminated soil is a major source of lead exposure in urban areas.

The estimated lead levels in the upper layer of soil beside roadways are typically 30-2,000 µg/g higher than natural levels, although these levels drop exponentially up to 25 meters from the roadway. Soil adjacent to a smelter in Missouri had lead levels in excess of 60,000 µg/g. Soils adjacent to houses with exterior lead-based paints may have lead levels of > 10,000 µg/g. Soil collected by scraping the top 2.5 cm of soil surface near homes and streetsides in Louisiana and Minnesota contained median lead concentrations of greater than 840 µg/g in New Orleans and 265 µg/g in Minneapolis. In contrast, the small towns of Natchitoches, Louisiana, and Rochester, Minnesota, had soil-lead concentrations of less than 50 µg/g and 58 µg/g, respectively. Studies carried out in Maryland and Minnesota indicate that within large light-industrial urban settings such as Baltimore, the highest soil lead levels generally occur in inner-city areas, especially where high traffic flows have long prevailed and that the amount of lead in the soil is correlated with the size of the city. It has been suggested that the higher lead levels associated with soils taken from around painted homes in the inner city are the result of greater atmospheric lead content, resulting from the burning of leaded gasoline in cars and the washdown of building surfaces to which the small lead particles adhere by rain.

D. LEAD IN THE PAINT

1. Background

Lead-based paint hazards in homes remain the most important source of lead exposure in U.S. children. About four out of five homes built in the United States before 1978 still contain some lead-based paint at a concentration of at least one mg/cm^2. Flaking paint, paint chips, and weathered powdered paint, which are most commonly associated with deteriorated housing stock in urban areas, are major sources of lead exposure for young children residing in these houses, particularly for children with pica (a compulsive, habitual consumption of nonfood items). Lead concentrations of 1-5 mg/cm^2 have been found in chips of lead-based paint, suggesting that consumption of a single chip of paint would provide greater short-term exposure than any other source of lead. An estimated 40-50% of currently occupied housing in the United States may contain lead-based paint on exposed surfaces.

The EPA sponsored a comprehensive technical report on a HUD-sponsored survey to provide estimates of the extent of lead-based paint in housing. The EPA report estimated that 64 million ($\pm$7 million) homes, or 83% ($\pm$9%) of privately-owned housing units built before 1980, have lead-based paint somewhere in the building (defined as a concentration of 1.0 mg/cm^2 or greater. Approximately 12 million ($\pm$5 million) of these homes are occupied by families that have children under the age of 7 years. Approximately 49 million ($\pm$7 million) privately owned homes have lead-based paint in their interiors. By contrast, approximately 86% ($\pm$8%) of all pre-1980 public housing family units have lead-based paint somewhere in the building. The lead levels in older private deteriorating or dilapidated housing were higher than the levels in newer public and rehabilitated housing. Releases from lead-based paints are frequently confined to the area in the immediate vicinity of painted surfaces; deterioration or removal of the paint can result in high localized concentrations of lead in indoor air (from sanding and sandblasting) and on exposed surfaces. Findings from the Third National Health and Nutrition Examination Survey (NHANES III), conducted in 1988 to 1994, show that of the multiple sources of exposure, lead-based paint is the principal high-dose source of lead. Exposure occurs not only through the direct ingestion of flaking and chalking paint but also through the inhalation of dust and soil contaminated with paint.

The U.S. Consumer Product Safety Commission banned the residential use of lead-based paint in 1978. However, lead-based paint is still manufactured for many other uses (e.g., automotive paints). An estimated 25-30 million homes were painted with lead-based paint in the United States. In general, the older a home is, the more likely it is to contain lead-based paint (particularly homes built prior to World War II).

Residential paints produced prior to 1978 frequently contained lead as an additive to improve durability. In many homes, old layers of lead-based paint are safely hidden under layers of lead-free paint. However, many homeowners are not aware that even simple remodeling and renovation projects that can disturb paint can result in spreading an almost invisible layer of lead-contaminated dust throughout the house. Exposure to lead-contaminated dust is the most common route of exposure for young children. Lead can affect anyone, but children under 6 years of age, because of their normal hand-to-mouth behavior, are especially vulnerable to lead. For example, children are easily exposed to lead-contaminated household dust by crawling around on the floor and then putting their fingers and toys in their mouths. Also, many children will chew on easy-to-mouth surfaces that may contain lead-based paint, such as old crib railings, window sills, and trim molding.

Lead poisoning in young children is difficult to detect without a blood test. Frequently there are no observable symptoms, and if there are, symptoms may mimic common childhood illnesses such as a cold or the flu. The only way to determine if your child has lead poisoning is to get a blood lead test from your medical provider. It is a simple fingerstick procedure and all children are encouraged to be tested, especially those who live in homes built prior to 1978 that have chipping or peeling paint, or that have been recently remodeled or renovated.

Before beginning a remodeling project, in order to take appropriate precautions, you should assess whether you will be disturbing lead-based paint. A certified lead risk assessor can evaluate painted surfaces in your home and recommend appropriate control measures. Usually, the inspector will use a portable electronic device, called an x-ray fluorescence (XRF) analyzer, to determine the lead content of painted surfaces. Depending on the size of the residence, a typical inspection may cost $300 not including laboratory fees. Alternatively, you may collect samples for analysis by a certified laboratory. Prices typically range from $15 to $20 per sample analyzed. Contact your local or state health department or environmental agency for a listing of certified laboratories.

Lead-based paint that is stable, undisturbed, and covered by layers of lead-free paint is not a hazard if properly maintained. However, painted surfaces that are flaking, chipping, or peeling or are areas of friction and impact can generate harmful levels of lead-contaminated dust, windows, doors, and porches should be inspected for accumulated lead-contaminated dust and deteriorated paint.

If you know or suspect that your home has lead hazards, you can reduce your family's risk of exposure by implementing interim control measures, and not conducting renovation, remodeling, or abatement work by yourself. Instead, hire a trained contractor who knows how to work safely with lead and how to protect your family from exposure to lead-contaminated dust.

If you choose to do your own work, you should follow the lead-safe work practices and safety guidelines available from the Environmental Protection Agency as well as from state and local public health agencies.

2. Interim Controls and Abatement

Interim controls are treatments designed to reduce the risk of exposure to lead hazards temporarily, whereas abatement methods permanently eliminate or control lead hazards. Examples of interim controls include planting grass in areas of bare soil near the house foundation to cover contaminated soil and carefully repairing and repainting deteriorated surfaces (paint film stabilization). Sometimes the temporary fix may solve the problem; however, routine monitoring is needed to know when conditions worsen.

Many families successfully manage lead-based paint in their homes by using a combination of lead-safe maintenance practices and, most importantly, specialized cleaning methods designed to remove lead-contaminated dust. There are four methods of lead-based paint abatement:

a. **Replacement**: Removal of items covered with lead-based paint, such as doors, windows, and trim, followed by the installation of lead-free components,

b. **Encapsulation**: Surfaces covered with lead-based paint are contained by specialized coatings (When these coatings dry they provide a hard, durable surface that prevents contact with the underlying lead-based paint and prevents the spread of lead-contaminated dust),

c. **Enclosure**: Surfaces covered with lead-based paint are enclosed behind durable materials such as sheetrock, paneling, or siding. Enclosure systems prevent contact with the underlying lead-painted surfaces and prevent the spread of lead-contaminated dust,

d. **Paint removal**: Paint is stripped using heat or chemicals either on-site or at an off-site facility. Paint removal methods also include wet scraping wet planing, and wet sanding.

The advantages of interim controls over abatement are the lower initial cost and the timeliness of intervention.

The disadvantages are that lead-based paint remains and ongoing monitoring is required. Some health departments target landlords and tenants with programs that incorporate interim control measures and specialized cleaning for lead-contaminated dust.

In NC, the Lead-Based Paint Preventive Maintenance Program rewards owners of pre-1978 rental housing with liability relief from potential lead poisoning litigation if they can demonstrate compliance with lead-safe work practices and specialized cleaning protocols.

There is need to remove lead-contaminated dust by high-efficiency particulate air (HEPA) filter vacuuming and wet cleaning areas where children spend time, especially floors. Most household vacuum cleaners do not adequately capture microscopic lead particles and should not be used to clean up lead-contaminated dust. A HEPA vacuum with a specialized filter for removing very fine dust particles is needed.

The cleaning method most frequently followed is to thoroughly vacuum all exposed interior surfaces with a HEPA filter-equipped vacuum. Next, all horizontal surfaces such as floors and window sills and troughs are washed with a cleaning solution made from water and an all-purpose detergent or a cleaner made specifically to remove lead-contaminated dust, maintaining all painted surfaces intact, adjusting doors and windows to minimize friction that may generate lead-contaminated dust, keeping children and pets away from areas of bare soil near the house.

The major disadvantages of abatement are the higher initial cost and the difficulty in finding properly trained and certified contractors to perform the work. Do not try to abate lead hazards yourself because, if not properly conducted, abatement and well-intentioned maintenance activities can, and usually do, increase the risk of lead exposure.

In many cases, complete abatement may not be the most cost-effective option. Interim controls, such as paint film stabilization, window treatments, and the elimination of friction and impact surfaces that create lead-contaminated dust, will in many situations provide effective control of lead-based paint hazards.

VI. **DISASTERS**

A. Natural and Technological Disasters

Disasters have been defined as 'any disruption of the human ecology that exceeds the capacity of the community to function normally. An event that is a disaster in one community may not be so in another, since disaster occurs only when a community is unable to absorb the impact of a physical event upon its people.

Other definitions for disasters reflect the particular perspective of different organizations. The Pan American Health Organization has defined a disaster or major emergency as "a natural or man-made occurrence that produces a massive disruption in the normal delivery of health services, and that poses such a great and immediate threat to public health that the affected country requires external assistance to respond to the situation". The World Bank defines a disaster as "an extraordinary event of limited duration, such as war or civil disturbance, or a natural disaster that seriously dislocates a country's economy."

Each disaster usually captures worldwide attention and causes widespread devastation. Viewed over a span of time, natural disasters are not a major cause of injury mortality in most developing countries but do cause considerable losses in certain individual countries. Nevertheless, disasters occur more often and have a proportionately greater impact on poor countries than on rich ones. Development projects sometimes increase susceptibility to disasters and earn result in severe economic and human losses when a disaster does occur.

Disasters are of two general types (either **natural** or **man-made**), and the responses of communities tend to differ with each type. Upon close examination, however, few disasters are either totally "natural" or totally "man-made." For example, the consequences of geological and climatological disasters are often exacerbated by inadequacies on the part of humans - witness the failure to design a building to resist an earthquake or a ferry to resist heavy seas. Even events such as droughts may be influenced by human destruction of forests. **Natural disasters** occur as a result of the action of natural forces and tend to be accepted as unfortunate but inevitable.

The human impact of natural disasters is often greatly exacerbated by technical factors, such as the design and construction of housing. Natural disasters include earthquakes, floods, cyclones, typhoons, hurricanes, volcanic eruptions, droughts, desertification, wildfires, and infestations of grasshoppers and locusts. The most common disasters today are droughts and flooding, and both appear to be increasing. Environmental degradation because of overpopulation has been a critical factor in some countries, while in others, disasters have resulted from short-sighted destruction of the natural environment for farming or other uses.

Many disasters are acute events, while others, such as drought, are chronic. Nevertheless, even though many disasters occur suddenly, they are often precipitated or exacerbated by long-term predisposing factors in the manmade infrastructure or by anthropogenic damage to the natural environment. Many disasters have a long-term impact on populations that persists for a generation or much longer, and some disasters are significant determinants of political violence.

Technological disasters occur as the result of some human activity and tend to be deeply disturbing to a community, leading to the blaming of culprits and a sense of shame in the community.

Natural disasters result from natural forces of climate and geology. In terms of the numbers of people affected, the natural disasters having the largest impact are hurricanes and floods (that is, events related to climatological factors), as contrasted to earthquakes, volcanic eruptions, and tsunamis (events related to geological factors). Climatological disasters also occur more frequently than geological disasters. In terms of deaths, however, geological disasters, particularly earthquakes, have the largest impacts. Because their homes are less sturdy and their resources more limited, people in the less-developed countries suffer far more devastation from natural disasters than those in the developed countries. Ninety-five percent of deaths from natural disasters occur in the developing countries of the world, and the economic losses, computed as a percentage of gross national product, are almost 20 times higher than in the developed countries. On a geographical basis, Asia is most prone to natural disasters; Latin America and Africa are intermediate; North America, Europe, and Australia are least prone. For each major natural disaster in Europe and Australia, 10 occur in Latin America and Africa and 15 in Asia. In the United States, there was an average of 323 deaths per year from natural disasters from 1945 to 1989. Floods are the most frequent natural disaster. From 1980 to 1990 floods accounted for one-third of all natural disasters globally. Windstorms (hurricanes and tornadoes) were the next most frequent, but earthquakes caused the greatest number of deaths.

Throughout the world, natural disasters -floods, tornadoes, hurricanes, earthquakes, volcanic eruptions- and accidents involving industrial and technological facilities -oil spills and accidents at chemical and nuclear power plants- are having a significant impact on both people and the environment. Natural disasters alone have caused an estimated 3 million deaths worldwide over the past two decades. Table 12.1 summarizes the impacts of some of these events. The economic and human costs vary widely, depending on the concentration of population, the existence of emergency response capabilities, the area's accessibility to outside assistance, the efficiency of rescue operations, building design and construction practices, and soil conditions.

By definition, disasters involve many casualties occurring in a short period of time, following an unusual event. They may be natural or the result of human activity. The emphasis in modern times in responding to disasters is on disaster planning and preparation. Although there is often a history of such disasters in a given area, natural disasters are usually unpredictable in the short term. The circumstances preceding the actual event may make the disaster much worse than it had to be. For example, extensive building on an earthquake fault or on an exposed shoreline subject to storms may greatly increase the casualty rate from an otherwise moderate event. Building with inadequate materials and failing to provide access to evacuation or emergency services routes may greatly complicate the rescue effort. The rescue effort may be inadequate or poorly organized; if it is delayed by more than a few hours in a major disaster, the responsible agency often comes under heavy criticism. The reconstruction effort may be prolonged, poorly coordinated, and complicated by bureaucracy, often leading to great public dissatisfaction, even if the immediate response to the disaster was received with gratitude. Natural disasters that result from climate, such as hurricanes, tornadoes, and flooding due to prolonged rains, tend to cause more property damage than deaths. They are profoundly demoralizing to the people displaced from their homes, but the community affected tends to respond quickly, and the long-term consequences are often less than one would expect. These are relatively familiar hazards, are easily understood, and are often common enough in the area affected to be thought of as a fact of life. Disruption of sanitary facilities and transportation tends to be less severe than in other types of natural disasters, except in the case of flooding. A severe storm is clearly terrifying and threatening, but communities tend to handle this type of disaster more easily than other types.

Table 12.1 Examples of Major Natural and Man-Made Disasters 1985 and Later (Source: Moeller, 1997).

EVENT	LOCATION	DATE	IMPACT
Natural Disasters			
Volcanic eruption	Nevado del Ruiz, Colombia	13 November 1985	25,000 deaths, thousands homeless
	Mount Pinatubo, Philippines	June-July 1991	700 deaths, 300,000 homeless
Gas release	Lake Nyos, Cameroon	21 August 1986	1700 deaths
Earthquakes	Mexico City, Mexico	19 September 1985	9,000 deaths, 30,000 injured, 95,000 homeless
	Armenia, former USSR	7 December 1988	>55,000 deaths, 250,000 homeless
	Erizincan, eastern Turkey	13 March 1992	4,000 deaths, 180,000 homeless
	Northwestern Iran	21 June 1990	>40,000 deaths
	Latur District, India	30 September 1993	11,000 deaths, 80 villages destroyed
	Los Angeles, California	17 January 1994	60 deaths, 8,500 injured, $40 billion damage
	Kobe, Japan	17 January 1995	>5,000 deaths, 25,000 injured , >300,000 homeless
	Sakhalin Island, Russia	June 1995	>3,000 deaths
Hurricane	Gilbert: Jamaica, Yucatan Peninsula, northeast Mexico	September 1988	300 deaths, widespread destruction
	Andrew: Florida, Louisiana, Bahamas	August 1992	51 deaths, 250,000 homeless, $25 billion damage
	Bertha: Caribbean, coastal North Carolina	July 1996	>$300 million in crop and property damage
Cyclone	Bangladesh	30 April 1991	138,000 deaths, 9 Million homeless;
	Southeast India	6 November 1996	2,000 deaths, 500,000 homeless
Landslide	Leyte and Negros Island, Philippines	6 November 1991	3,000 deaths
Flood	Pakistan and India	September 1991	2,000 deaths, thousands missing, millions homeless
	Midwestern United States	July 1993	46 deaths, 2 million acres affected, $25 billion damage
Sinking of passenger ferry	Baltic Sea	28 September 1994	>900 deaths
Sinking of passenger ferry	Tanzania	21 May 1996	615 deaths
Man-Made Disasters			
Nuclear power plant accident	Chernobyl, former USSR	26 April 1986	42 immediate deaths, many latent cancers
Fuel storage fire	Dronka, Egypt	2 November 1994	>470 deaths, thousands of homes destroyed
Forest fire	Oakland and Berkeley, California	October 1991	16 deaths, 49 missing, 3,000 homes destroyed, $5 billion damage
Gasoline pipeline explosion	Guadalajara, Mexico	22 April 1992	190 deaths, 1400 injured, thousands homeless
Oil tanker spill	*Exxon Valdez*, Prince William Sound, Alaska	March 1989	11 million gallons, heavy contamination
	Braer, off Garths Ness, near Scotland	January 1993	26 million gallons
	Maersk Navigator, Indian Ocean off Indonesia	January 1993	78 million gallons
	Sea Empress, Milford Haven, Wales	February 1996	19 million gallons
Oil spill (not tanker related)	Three major spills into Persian Gulf from refineries	January 1991	250-350 million gallons, heavy contamination
Oil spill (from pipeline)	Komi Republic in Arctic	October 1994	100 million gallons spilled, contamination and fires
Oil well fires	Kuwait	Feb.-Nov. 1991	>700 burning wells, initially widespread air pollution
Rioting	Los Angeles, California	April 1992	> 60 deaths, 2,400 injuries, billions of dollars damage
Terrorism	Oklahoma City, Oklahoma	19 April 1995	169 deaths, federal building destroyed

Natural disasters that result from geological activity, such as earthquakes, volcano eruptions, mud slides, **tsunamis** (seismic tidal waves), and flash floods (involving sudden rainfall in terrain that funnels it into swiftly flowing channels), tend to result. In more casualties than those due to climate and may severely disrupt the ability of the community to take care of its own needs in the hours and days following the event. Forest fires share many of these characteristics. In both kinds of disasters, there are often many missing persons and trapped victims who require rescue. The type of injury is usually more severe, reflecting the risk of collapsing buildings and the massive forces involved, and may lead to serious public health problems even when adequately treated. Psychological stresses associated with the event appear to be greater than for disasters related to climate, and affect both victims and rescuers.

Natural disasters can be classified as being of acute onset or of chronic onset:

1. Acute or sudden-impact natural disasters include earthquakes, tornadoes, floods, tsunamis, tropical storms, hurricanes, cyclones, typhoons, volcanic eruptions, landslides, avalanches, and wildfires. Epidemics of water-, food-, or vector-borne diseases often accompany these disasters.
2. Slow or chronic-onset natural disasters include drought, famine, environmental degradation, desertification, deforestation, and pest infestation.

Technological (or man-made) disasters result from some human activity such as explosions, the release of toxic chemicals or radioactive material, bridge or building collapse, fires, and crashes. Man-made disasters also cover a wide range. Examples of those that can cause immediate and widespread effects are the release of toxic chemicals from an industrial plant, as occurred in Bhopal, India, in 1984, and the widespread distribution of radioactive materials as the result of a nuclear power plant accident, as occurred at Chernobyl in 1986. Estimates of the number of people killed in the Bhopal accident range from 2,500 to 7,000. Although immediate deaths due to acute exposures from the Chernobyl accident were less than 50, the long-term effects, particularly the development of latent cancers due to chronic exposures, may lead to many more deaths. In terms of potential direct effects on the environment, few disasters are more dramatic than those involving major oil spills, which unfortunately continue to occur on a regular basis (Table 12.2). Other man-made disasters that may have equal or even more far-reaching effects are not so readily apparent. If the predictions of global warming due to the release of carbon dioxide into the atmosphere prove true, the worldwide impacts could be catastrophic. Consequences of comparable magnitude could occur as a result of the depletion of the ozone layer due to the use and release of chlorofluorocarbons.

Technological disasters tend to involve many more casualties than natural disasters of the same magnitude of energy release. They are also much more difficult for the community to deal with and for victims to accept. The psychological factors that influence perception of technological disasters are very different from those for natural disasters in technological disasters, there are issues of blame involved and the community spends much time discussing who was responsible and what mistakes were made. Often there are complicated lawsuits, investigations and claims for disability involved. If there was previously a feeling that the owners of the facility responsible were abusing the community or making excessive profits, this adds to the fury of the community's response. Sometimes victims are shunned by their neighbors, who feel that they are exploiting the situation for personal gain or who are fearful that the response to the incident will cause economic loss to the community. As a result, technological disasters tend to divide the community and to cause long-lasting psychological trauma to local residents as well as to victims. Examples of major technological disasters in recent times include the release of toxic methyl isocyanate gas in Bhopal, India in 1984 and the explosion and release of radiation from the Chernobyl nuclear reactor in the Ukraine in 1986. Incidents on a much smaller scale are not rare but do not get as much attention.

Table 12.2. Health Effects of Natural Disasters (Source: Moeller, 1997).

Health effect	Earthquake	Hurricane, high wind	Volcanic eruption	Flood	Tidal wave, flash flood
Deaths	Many	Few	Varies	Few	Many
Severe injuries (requiring extensive medical care)	Overwhelming	Moderate	Variable	Few	Few
Increased risk of infectious disease	A potential problem in all major disasters; probability increases with overcrowding and deteriorating sanitation				
Food scarcity	Rare (may occur as a result of factors other than food shortages)	Rare	Common	Common	Common
Major population movements	Rare (may occur in heavily damaged urban areas)	Rare	Common	Common	Common

B. EARTHQUAKE

An earthquake is a shaking of the ground, usually caused by rocks rupturing under stress. Energy is released from the ruptured rocks and travels in the form of waves. The place within the Earth where the rock breaks is the hypocenter of the earthquake and the point on the Earth's surface directly above this focus is called the epicenter. Damage is usually the most severe at the epicenter.

Fault - A fault is a fracture, a crack in the Earth along which the rocks on each side move past each other. Fault movement can be vertical, horizontal, or a combination.

Strength of an Earthquake - Intensity and magnitude are the two ways earthquakes are measured. The intensity perceived by humans is measured by the Mercalli scale whereas the magnitude, the actual physical energy released at its source, is measured by instruments using the Richter scale.

C. VOLCANOES

A volcano is a mountain formed by the accumulation of erupted lava and/or volcanic ash.
Active Volcanoes Worldwide - There are approximately 600 active volcanoes. On average, about 50 volcanoes erupt yearly.
Volcanic Explosivity Index (VEI) - The VEI is a method to compare energy released from different volcanoes. The VEI is based on the volume of material ejected, height of the ash plume, and duration of continuous blast.
Hazards and Factors Influencing Morbidity & Mortality - The hazards and factors influencing morbidity and mortality are the following:

1. Blast and projectiles
2. Pyroclastic flows and surges
3. Floods and mud flows
4. Ashfalls and tephra (airborne lava fragments)
5. Lava flows
6. Poisonous gases
7. Building collapse due to accumulated roof ash
8. Possible ionizing radiation risk from radon daughter particles attached to ash
9. Problems with public utilities functioning (clogging of pipes from ashfalls, short circuiting of equipment)
10. Lightning frequently accompanies ash plumes, posing a potential risk

Toxic Gases - Although the major component of volcanic gas is water vapor, various amounts of carbon dioxide, sulfur dioxide, carbon monoxide, hydrogen sulfide, sulfuric acid, hydrochloric acid, and hydrofluoric acid maybe present.
Health Effects After Mount St. Helens Eruption In 1980 - An increase in the number of patients seeking treatment for asthma and bronchitis was seen in the region surrounding Mount St. Helens. People with chronic lung illness also reported a marked exacerbation of their respiratory symptoms.

D. TORNADOS

A tornado is a violently rotating column of air in contact with the ground. It is pendant from a parent cumulonimbus cloud. Tornados usually rotate counterclockwise, have very low pressure interiorly, and have very high velocities in their walls. Tornado Classification is done using Fujita Scale.
Annual Number Of Tornadoes - From 1953 to 1991, the United States averaged 768 tornadoes per year, with an average of 93 people killed yearly.
Destructive Actions Of Tornadoes - There are three main destructive actions:

1. High wind speeds that blow away buildings and trees
2. Winds that rush up the funnel with a lifting force in the updraft
3. And a pressure difference between the inside and outside of the funnel that creates an explosive environment.

Factors Influencing Morbidity and Mortality - Natural factors contributing to morbidity and mortality include tornadic strength and path length, time of day the tornado strikes, and other adverse weather conditions occurring at that time that may interfere with detection by weather spotters.

Human factors include residing in mobile homes, age >60 years old, remaining in a vehicle, failing to seek shelter after a tornado warning, and being unfamiliar with tornado warning terminology.

E. HURRICANES

Tropical Cyclone - Tropical cyclones are meteorological depressions, or low-pressure systems, that originally develop over open waters in the tropics, usually between 30 °N and 30 °S latitude. Tropical cyclones vary in size and strength and are classified by peak wind speeds.

Tropical Cyclone Circulations - A hurricane watch means that hurricane conditions are possible in the specified area usually within 36 hours. A hurricane warning means hurricane conditions are expected usually within 24 hours. Measure of hurricanes is done using Saffir-Simpson Scale.

Annual Number Of Tropical Storms - Worldwide, in an average year 84 tropical storms develop, of which 45 have peak sustained winds of 75 mph or more.

Names of Hurricanes – The names are the following:

1. In the Atlantic and eastern Pacific (east of the international dateline), storms with sustained winds of 74+ mph are called hurricanes.
2. In the Western Pacific, these storms are known as typhoons.
3. In the Indian Ocean and Bay of Bengal the storm is called a cyclone, and
4. In Australia hurricanes are referred to as Willy Willys.

Eye And Eye Wall Of A Hurricane - In the center of the hurricane is an area of calm known as the eye. The eye is usually 5-15 miles across and may have sunny skies and minimal wind. The eye wall is the tall circular ring of thunderstorm-like clouds surrounding the eye. The eyewall often contains the most severe wind and rain. The more violent the storm, the smaller the eye.

Public Health Problems - Hurricane-related morbidity and mortality generally include drowning from the storm surge, trauma from structural collapse or during cleanup, gastrointestinal and respiratory illnesses, and dermal conditions. An increase in animal bites and stings and an increase in mosquito vectors have been noted. Mental health effects, both short and long term, may occur.

Risk Factors Affecting Morbidity and Mortality - Natural factors contributing to morbidity and mortality include the storm surge, violent winds, and rain. About 90% of all cyclone-related deaths are due to drowning associated with the storm surge. Tornadoes are also often spawned from a hurricane and can cause injury and death. Human factors include poor building construction, insufficient lead time for warning and evacuation, noncompliance with evacuation notices, and the use of inadequate shelter. Fatalities during cleanup are due to electrocution from improper use of generators, chain saw injuries, and trauma from weakened structures and trees. Burns and smoke inhalation from fires due to unattended open flames were treated after Hurricane Hugo.

F. FLOODS

Definition - Floods are overflows of areas that are not normally submerged with water. Causes include streams that have broken normal confines or water accumulation due to lack of drainage.

Floods - Of all natural disasters, floods occur most often and are the most widespread in scope and severity. Of all natural disasters in the United States, floods are the main cause of deaths.

Factors Causing Or Contributing To Flooding - Heavy rains, rapid snowmelts, steep slopes, dam failure, storm surges, and human manipulation of the land, such as deforestation.

Flood Severity - Flood severity depends on both natural and man-made conditions, such as the rate of rainfall, infiltration capacity of the ground, slope of the terrain, presence of vegetation, climate, season, urbanization, agriculture, and timbering. Flood control using floodways, floodwalls, dams, and levees is also a factor.

Public Health Concerns - Disruption of water purification systems and sewage treatment plants may put the community at risk of infections from contaminated food and water. Although the potential for an outbreak is present after flooding, in reality such outbreaks rarely occur. Surveillance for water- and vector-borne diseases, endemic illnesses, and cleanup-related injuries is recommended, however. There is the potential for exposure to hazardous materials due to the rupture of underground tanks and pipelines, as well as overflow from toxic waste sites or chemical and pesticide storage facilities. Stings and bites from displaced animals have been noted after a hurricane. Electrical injuries from downed power lines and chain saw injuries from tree removal are not uncommon. Psychological distress is common after a flood but severe long-term distress is rare. Mold and mildew growth in flooded residences and offices may exacerbate allergic and asthmatic symptoms. When cleaning up homes after a flood to remove mold and mildew, occupants must not mix bleach and ammonia because toxic gases may form and, if inhaled, can lead to pulmonary edema.

G. PUBLIC HEALTH CONSEQUENCES OF DISASTERS

1. Introduction

What is identified, as a "disaster" is often better understood as a trigger event that exposes and exacerbates underlying societal problems and weaknesses. For example, in virtually every famine of the last 20 years, drought has been an important contributing factor, but food shortages have been primarily the result of armed conflict, inadequate economic and social systems, failed governments, and other human-made factors. The famine in Somalia in 1992-1993 highlights the dramatic amplification of drought by internecine clan warfare. Understanding the consequences of disasters, and effectively coping with them, requires looking well beyond the event itself.

The increase in unexpected injuries, illnesses, and deaths caused by a natural disaster may exceed the capacity of local health care agencies. Disasters may destroy the local health infrastructure, which will therefore not be able to respond to the emergency. Some disasters may increase the potential risk for communicable diseases and environmental hazards. Disasters may affect the social and mental health of the citizens of the affected community. A shortage of food may lead to nutritional deficiencies or even starvation. Large population movements may be necessary, often to areas that do not have the facilities to cope with the new situation.

Psychological symptoms following disasters tend to be similar among children, but among adults they are somewhat more complicated and variable. Children are often fearful and show disproportionate anxiety over separation from their friends or parents. They may lose motivation, act in rebellious ways, and begin to do poorly in school. Children often respond well to immediate mental health interventions aimed at helping them to express their feelings and fears about the event. Adults are often able to cope reasonably well during the event but may fall apart afterward: a small minority will become incapable of acting during the stress of a crisis and will have to be forced to move. Adults who survive a disaster may experience a range of adverse effects, such as nightmares, uncontrollable thoughts that involve reliving the events, trouble sleeping, no emotion, and a sense of detachment from the other people in their lives and the world in general. In adults these symptoms are characteristic of post-traumatic stress syndrome. Adults may also be helped by mental health professionals who discuss with them as a group what happened and what their reactions are, a process known as **critical incident debriefing**. Part of what is helpful about this process is the reassurance that these feelings are natural and that those affected are not mentally ill. Rescue personnel often have the same symptoms and feelings as survivors and victims, and may also benefit from critical incident debriefing. While there is some questioning of the value of psychological debriefings in preventing post-traumatic stress disorder, most authorities do recommend it when appropriate.

Mutual assistance and disaster intervention programs may significantly limit the impact of a disaster on the community. International assistance is difficult to manage and coordinate but may make a decisive difference in the outcome, especially in countries and areas with very limited resources. Emergency management of water resources, food preparation and distribution, provision of shelter, proper disposal of human and solid waste, injury prevention, vector control, and personal hygiene are areas that will need immediate attention following a disaster. Outbreaks of disease after a disaster are more likely in developing countries where poverty, lack of access to potable water, poor sanitation, and low immunization rates are found.

Disasters may increase the number of various disease vectors by increasing breeding sites. Damage to power systems, sewage systems, and public water facilities may contribute to disease transmission. Additionally, disruption in public health services will have an adverse impact on methods to control disease propagation in the affected community. Diseases that have been reported in disaster settings include measles, meningococcal meningitis, cholera, malaria, hepatitis E, dysentery, and acute respiratory conditions. Although usually not associated with acute disasters, when health care facilities are inadequate or destroyed, an increase in the transmission of tuberculosis and, possibly, sexually transmitted diseases has been noted.

2. **Natural Disasters**

In the past 20 years, natural disasters have affected at least 800 million people and caused more than 3 million deaths. Each week there is at least one natural disaster of sufficient magnitude to require external assistance from the international community. The incidence of natural disasters appears to be increasing, and the number of highly vulnerable persons in disaster-prone areas, particularly in the developing world, is at least 70 million peoples and growing. The devastating tropical cyclone in Bangladesh in 1991, in which more than 100,000 persons were killed, illustrates the potential impact of a natural disaster on a population residing in a hazardous coastal region.

Natural disasters may be associated with a wide variety of acute and long-term health effects. For example, volcanic eruptions may result in injury or death due to lava flow, falling debris, asphyxiating gases, mudflows, and blast injury from violent explosions. Ash and other particulate matter vented from an active volcano may exacerbate respiratory illness in persons within the downwind population for many months following the eruption. Volcanic ash may contaminate the soil or water, resulting in long-term toxic exposures to the population. One of the most unusual gas releases associated with volcanic activity occurred in 1986 in Cameroon. In this disaster, asphyxiating carbon dioxide was released from an active volcano underneath Lake Nyos. The gas enveloped nearby villages and caused approximately 1,500 deaths.

Public health issues associated with floods extend beyond concerns for mortality due to drowning. In Bangladesh, the flooding that followed the 1991 tropical cyclone reduced the potability of water from wells and caused widespread outbreaks of diarrheal disease. Flooding may result in increased numbers of breeding sites for mosquitoes and their associated diseases, such as malaria or dengue fever. Immediate public health actions following floods usually include the provision of potable water, food, vector control, and the restitution of vital environmental health services. However, early warning systems, improved evacuation plans, and discouragement of settling in flood-prone areas may have much greater potential to save lives than activities associated with external emergency response to flood disasters.

Earthquakes typically cause destruction of structures and traumatic injuries and deaths. The 1976 Tangshan earthquake, for example, caused more than 200,000 sudden trauma-related deaths. In contrast to floods, the morbidity and mortality of earthquakes is much more immediate. Deaths are primarily due to crush injuries and other trauma resulting from unstable, collapsing, or crumbling buildings. Earthquakes are not usually followed by long-term public health problems such as famine or epidemic diseases, although following the Northridge earthquake (1994) a wide range of external primary care services were required by the population for up to 4 weeks. Other public health issues associated with earthquakes include concerns for the health of persons in shelters, occupational health protection for rescue workers, and the provision of mental services for survivors.

Sudden onset natural disasters have been the traditional model for understanding and organizing emergency relief services for disaster-affected populations in this country. For example, external medical services may be urgently needed after earthquakes to treat injured persons and to extract survivors trapped in collapsed buildings. This led to the development of specialized emergency services in many countries such as Urban Search and Rescue teams, which are designed to extract and treat entombed victims. Disaster response at the federal level has included the development of Disaster Medical Assistance Teams (DMATs), designed to provide emergency curative medical services primarily in response to natural disasters.

While this paradigm has been valuable, effectively coping with disasters involves much more than the timely delivery of external emergency resources. Local vulnerabilities in a community such as population density, lack of disaster planning, and poverty may enhance the risk to a population to disasters. For example, the 1988 earthquake in Armenia resulted in more than 30,000 deaths, while an earthquake of similar force, the 1989 Loma Prieta earthquake in California, resulted in less than 500 deaths. The low mortality associated with the Loma Prieta earthquake was thought to be due to enforcement of local building codes, better local emergency medical services (EMS), and superior local disaster management services, and other community-based prevention and mitigation activities.

3. Conflict-Related (Complex) Emergencies

These disasters are largely a phenomenon of the post Cold War world. In the late 1970's there were approximately five conflict-related disasters per year, but by the late 1980's there were 10 to 15 per year, and today there are an average of 25 to 30 per year. The increase in conflict-related disasters closely relates to the number of armed conflicts in the world, which also have increased dramatically in recent years, and particularly in this decade. Since 1980, there have been over 150 major armed conflicts, and in 1995, there were an estimated 26 ongoing wars.

War has always been destructive, but in recent years the nature of armed conflict has become more devastating than ever before. In many conflicts today, for every death in a combatant there are 8 to 9 deaths among civilians. Toole and Waldman have described the insidious cycle of armed confrontation, famine, and population displacement. In 1980 there were approximately 5 million refugees in the world, but largely as a consequence of this cycle, today there are approximately 23 million. In addition, today there are another 25 million internally displaced persons.

Many of the public health problems of refugees and displaced persons have been well described. Crude mortality rates among refugees and displaced populations often rise dramatically above baseline levels, principally due to nutritional shortages, environmental problems, and preventable infectious diseases. Conflict-related disasters also have similar effects on those who do not flee when the infrastructure of society is destroyed or severely damaged, which causes problems in having access to food, potable water, refuse disposal, and basic medical services. International humanitarian law in many conflicts today is unknown or disregarded, and human rights abuses are common. As a result, in some disasters, violence may be a direct, and the primary cause of morbidity and mortality. For example, in the former Yugoslavia, while morbidity and mortality due to infectious diseases increased to some extent, deaths due to fighting or so-called ethnic cleansing operations were by far the principal cause of death. Areas of increasing focus in complex emergencies are mental health women's health issues, and coping with chronic medical conditions.

Coping with these disasters is one of the great public health challenges of our time. There are a multitude of technical and logistical issues involved in providing life-sustaining services to large populations. Events may not progress in a clear linear fashion; public health needs often evolve substantially. For example, priorities for refugees who have just arrived in a location - usually shelter, food, water, basic medical care - are different from what this population may need a few months after a camp has been established, such as family planning, medical care for more chronic problems, and rehabilitation. As with natural disasters, increasing attention is devoted toward prevention, early warning, and preparation activities. Because complex emergencies are the result of many years of deeply rooted social problems, effectively dealing with them requires that relief efforts be closely integrated with political, social, economic, military, cultural, and other activities.

4. Technological Disasters

Public health problems resulting from technological accidents, or the unregulated and unsafe use of industrial technologies, are increasingly recognized as an important and increasingly common type of disaster. The extensive environmental pollution in former Soviet block nations, the nuclear reactor accident at Chernobyl, and the toxic gas leak at Bhopal, India, are examples of the disastrous consequences that can ensue from these disasters. The potential for harm from improper management of industrial technologies is a major concern in developed nations where at any given moment there are a myriad of complex industries in operation and tons of hazardous materials in transit through populated areas. In developing countries, these problems are exacerbated when rapid industrialization exceeds the development of counterbalancing safety controls.

Technological disasters are usually the result of poor engineering, improper safety practices, or simple human error. However, natural disasters can be an important factor in precipitating a technological disaster. For example, the gasoline fires that killed over 500 persons in Durunka, Egypt, in 1994 were the result of flash flooding that ruptured a fuel storage tank and carried burning petroleum into the nearby town. Such synergistic disasters have been termed NA-TECHs (natural-technological). In many places in the world, chemical plants, nuclear reactors, or other potentially dangerous industry are seated in geological regions that are highly vulnerable to natural disasters.

Dealing with the consequences of a technological disaster or a NA-TECH presents many challenges. Recognizing the hazardous material involved, evacuating citizens after an accident, providing appropriate medical care for victims, and protecting emergency responders against hazardous exposures are a few of the many challenges to emergency responders. In addition, because industrial disasters may leave toxic residues in the environment that pose ongoing threats to the health of populations, the initiation of chemical exposure and disease registries to track adverse health effects of disaster victims over time may be a fundamental component of the emergency response. Clinical investigations after technical disasters may require assistance from laboratory scientists, toxicologists, and environmental epidemiologists. Public health prevention efforts include sound plant design and operation, safe disposal of waste products, thorough safety occupational programs, linkage to local emergency management operations, and proper site selection for industrial facilities.

5. Injuries from Disasters

a. Introduction

Injuries from disasters have a major adverse impact in certain areas of the world; human activities contribute to or greatly exacerbate the effects of many disasters. The impact of disasters on human populations is much more severe in countries with environmental degradation, poorly constructed buildings, adverse climatic conditions, and large poverty-stricken populations. The effects of a disaster are also much more serious in countries that lack the skilled personnel, organization, communications, transport, and other resources to manage the disaster rapidly and effectively.

b. Classification and Reporting of Injuries from Disasters

The most basic classification involves coding the type of disaster. Individual deaths or morbidity from technological disasters mat. be coded as due to a specific toxic chemical, explosion, or radiation. For natural disasters, the following categories are provided for in the ICD-10 under the heading natural forces of nature:

1. Earthquake
2. Volcanic eruption
3. Avalanche, landslide, and other earth movements
4. Cataclysmic storm, such as a cyclone, hurricane, tornado, tidal wave from storm, torrential rain, or blizzard
5. Flood, as a direct or remote effect of storm, or from resulting ice or snow
6. Other and unspecified forces of nature.

c. Injury Pattern by Type of Disaster

Injury patterns depend upon the type of disaster and the part of the world affected. Earthquakes are one of the most dramatic sources of deaths and injuries from disasters, and vulnerability may be increasing as populations become concentrated in crowded urban areas with poorly constructed multistory housing. Droughts and floods may, however, be the disasters with the greatest potential for future morbidity and mortality, mediated by starvation and drowning. The threat of deaths from droughts and floods is increasing as ecological damage mounts, in part from population pressures on fragile tropical soils. Deforestation can lead to rapid run-off of rain and consequent flooding, while poor land management can cause landslides.

Earthquakes cause many deaths and large numbers of severe in juries requiring extensive care. Multiple fractures are a common pattern of injuries after earthquakes. Earlier studies of large earthquakes found a ratio of injuries to deaths of approximately 3:1, and suggested that the number of deaths may be a useful guide to predict the number of injured persons requiring treatment. However, a more comprehensive analysis found that this ratio only applied to a limited number of earthquakes. In the recent earthquake in Armenia, an estimated 25,000 people were killed and 31,000 injured. Thus, there were almost as many dead as injured. This was attributed to inadequate construction of buildings. It could be that large buildings constructed of heavy materials with inadequate reinforcement lead to higher ratios of fatalities to injured. It has been estimated that about 75 percent of fatalities from earthquakes result from collapse of buildings. The majority of deaths occur in masonry buildings constructed from materials such as adobe, rubble stone, rammed earth, or unreinforced brick or concrete.

High winds cause few deaths and moderate numbers of severe injuries. Tidal waves and flash floods cause many deaths and few injuries, whereas other floods generally result in relatively few deaths or injuries. Certain areas, such as the Bangladesh delta, have been subject to regular massive floods after cyclones, resulting in high fatality rates. In addition to injuries, another effect of many natural disasters that has significant public health implications is the widespread disruption of reticulated systems of water and sewage supplies.

Technological disasters such as the massive release of poisonous gas from a pesticide plant at Bhopal, India, the explosion of a butane plant in Mexico, and the explosion of the nuclear reactor at Chernobyl, USSR, are becoming increasingly common. The worst of these, such as Bhopal, can cause thousands of deaths and hundreds of thousands of injuries, including permanent disabilities.

d. Examples of Mortality and Morbidity

Most of the deaths, casualties, and damage from disasters occur in the poorer countries of the world. The true burden of nonfatal injuries from disasters is often difficult to determine, in part because there is no consistent definition for an injury in most published data.

The greatest numbers of fatalities from earthquakes during this century have occurred in developing countries. The two earthquakes with the largest number of fatalities in the past half-century were the Tangshan, China, earthquake of 1976, which resulted in 242,469 fatalities, and the 1970 earthquake of Ankash, Peru, which caused 66,794 deaths. Almost half of the total number of earthquake deaths in the world have occurred in China, and about 80 percent of all deaths from earthquakes have occurred in China, Japan, Iran, Peru, Turkey, the former USSR, Chile, and Pakistan.

Floods cause more damage than any other natural disaster and account for about 40 percent of the total damage from all disasters. The Hwang Ho, or Yellow River, in China is the most flood-prone river in the world. There have been at least three major floods in the past 100 years, including one in 1969, with estimated losses in each flood ranging from several hundred thousand to 900,000 lives.

The Pan American Health Organization compiles records of all disasters in the Americas. This gives an overview of the impact of various types of disasters in the region. In the Americas from 1970-90, nearly 150,000 persons died from natural disasters, about 500,000 were injured, millions of people were affected, and economic losses of many billions of dollars were sustained. Two major sources of injuries during this period were the 1985 volcanic eruption in Colombia with 23,080 deaths and 4,420 injuries, and the 1985 Mexico City earthquake with 10,000 deaths and 30,000 injuries.

The Asian Disaster Preparedness Center (1990) has summarized information about disasters in Asia between 1964-86. During this period, the largest numbers of deaths resulted from earthquakes and cyclones/typhoons/storms. In contrast, the largest numbers of persons were affected by drought and floods. Earthquakes and floods caused the greatest economic losses. Earthquakes, floods, and wind storms often leave a majority of affected persons homeless.

Nur (1990) has compiled from multiple sources a list of the effects of recorded disasters in African countries from 1980-89. It is evident that in Africa the numbers of deaths and persons affected are much smaller for acute disasters, such as earthquakes and cyclones, than for long-term disasters, such as drought and famine.

The volcanic release of massive quantities of carbon dioxide gas asphyxiated more than 1,700 persons near Lake Nyos in the Cameroons. Another disastrous source of enormous loss of life in many African countries has been widespread civil unrest and population movements due to ethnocentricity and civil unrest.

In the explosion of the pesticide plant at Bhopal, India, methyl isocyanate gas caused over 4,000 deaths, and immediate medical attention was required by between 50,000 to 200,000 persons. While there were about 3,000 immediate deaths, 1,700 deaths were expected from late effects. In Mexico, the explosion of five million liters of butane gas resulted in 400 deaths, 1,000 people unaccounted for, and 5,000 injured. Nuclear mishaps, such as the 1986 Chernobyl explosion in the former USSR, can result in massive acute casualties, as welt as delayed effects in areas adjacent to the facility, and widespread contamination of populations in other countries.

For technological disasters that result in many permanent disabilities and delayed deaths, if the initial registration and follow-up of exposed victims are inadequate, immense suffering can result from delayed compensation. Ten years after the Bhopal disaster, only 1 percent of the 615,000 death and injury claims had been settled and only $3 million of the $470 million compensation settlement with Union Carbide had reached the victims. Delays were attributed to poor communication between the excessive numbers of doctors and the different hospitals involved with the victims, as well as failure of the government to release funds to victims. However, many victims have been denied compensation because of a tack of documentation proving their status as victims. Bhopal represents a tragic example of the importance of organizing and providing sufficient resources for a meticulous and complete registration of all exposed victims in the immediate post-disaster period and a coordinated follow-up to document and promptly compensate permanent disabilities.

For disasters such as the Bhopal chemical plant explosion, the public health impact and costs of permanent disability among the survivors can greatly exceed the impact and cost of immediate deaths. While the explosion of the Bhopal chemical plant killed about 4,000 people in 1984, estimates of the number of survivors with long-term damage ten years later ranged from 200,000 to 500,000. The total number of persons affected is even greater, since many brain-damaged parents with memory loss are unable to provide for their children.

H. PUBLIC HEALTH TOOLS FOR DISASTER RESPONSE

Depending on the magnitude of the disaster and its extent, disasters can overwhelm the health care system in the area and disrupt the operations of fire, transportation, and rescue services. In the first few hours following a disaster, the first priorities are to identify and provide medical care to the injured, locate and rescue missing persons, and identify and control physical hazards, such as ruptured gas lines. In the case of chemical or radiation incidents, decontamination is a high and urgent priority to prevent further exposure. Subsequently, the provision of basic services, including shelter, food, potable water, sanitary facilities such as latrines, and psychological intervention become an urgent priority if the disaster has disrupted services in the community. Burial of the dead, provision of warm clothing, and evacuation of the injured or vulnerable may become health priorities, depending on circumstances. The risk of infectious disease increases in the days following the disaster, as water supplies may be interrupted and sanitation becomes an increasing problem. Over the long term, rehabilitation and reconstruction become increasingly important as the community comes to terms with the devastation.

Prior to mobilizing an emergency response on behalf of a disaster stricken population, the initial step is to obtain information regarding the extent of their immediate needs and the status of their supporting public health infrastructure. This task is accomplished through an organized needs assessment. The purpose of initial assessments is to rapidly obtain objective, reliable, population-based information that describes a population's specific needs for emergency relief services. These assessments should identify the extent of the needed response and technical areas where specialized assistance is needed and should suggest other areas where more focused health surveys or surveillance should be conducted (e.g., the nutritional status of the population, status of water and sanitation).

It is often impractical to evaluate the needs of all affected persons at the disaster site due to the size of the population and resource limitations. Relief personnel must sample representative cross-sections from the affected population through a statistically valid sampling process using standardized assessment protocols. Such an activity requires knowledge of the geographic distribution and size of the population, which may be obtained through census information, aerial photos, rapid surveys, and other sources. During sudden-impact disasters such as hurricanes the initial assessments of the affected population should be completed as soon as possible, ideally within 24 to 48 hours. Slow-onset disasters such as endemic warfare and famines that persist for years may require repeated emergency health assessments.

Public health surveillance is the logical continuum of the initial epidemiological task of emergency health assessment. Surveillance systems need to be established after disasters in sentinel sites such as clinics to monitor the health of the population and gauge the effectiveness of ongoing relief programs, particularly during the implementation of emergency programs that are likely to continue beyond the immediate aftermath of the disaster. New technologies such as e-mail, computers, and epidemiological software permitted the rapid implementation of a statewide system surveillance in Iowa following the Great Flood of 1993. Among refugees, in developing countries, critical public health events for surveillance include deaths, appearance of malnourished children, and the occurrence of vaccine preventable infectious diseases. When establishing surveillance after a disaster, it is likely to be more effective to re-establish a pre-existing system than to build a new system with external resources.

Targeted investigations and surveys complement initial assessments and surveillance. For example, in some situations, the rapid assessment of the nutritional status of a population is a critical aspect of developing appropriate relief programs. Investigation of outbreaks, surveys of vaccine coverage, and surveys for the prevalence of certain diseases are other common areas of more focused investigation. As public health information is collected through assessment, surveillance, and special surveys, relief interventions should be modified accordingly. In the absence of current data to evaluate the health of the target population, relief priorities and resources may easily become skewed.

I. PUBLIC HEALTH INTERVENTIONS IN DISASTERS

1. Introduction

A well-designed and well-executed emergency plan is essential to coping wit any type of disaster. Such a plan can ensure quick and effective mobilization to respond to the immediate health-care needs of the people affected and to restore disrupted services. The plan should be clear, concise, and complete. It should also be dynamic, flexible, and subject to frequent evaluation and update. It should designate precisely who does what and when, and everyone involved should be familiar with it. Its top priority should be to provide an immediate response to the event, by locating and providing emergency medical services to the victims, controlling fires, removing downed power lines, and controlling leaks of natural gas. On a longer-range basis, the goals should be to provide health care and shelter for victims, and to restore important services such as a safe water supply and basic sanitation. Next in importance are arrangements to provide a safe food supply and to meet needs for personal hygiene.

In general, there are two types of emergency plans. One is **national** or **regional** in scope and defines the responsibilities and mobilization procedures of personnel in key public and environmental health departments and emergency preparedness agencies. Planning at this level frequently includes coordination of civil defense and military services. The other level, which is local in scope, is much more definitive and includes detailed listings of the personnel involved, their individual responsibilities during an emergency, and the range of countermeasures available for implementation. The local plan should be closely coordinated with the national or regional effort. Together the two can provide a cadre of well-trained personnel to cope with natural disasters or industrial accidents of almost any size.

In an analysis of the costs and benefits of responses to natural disasters, it was concluded that for developing countries, as for developed countries, prevention is economically and politically preferable to recovery, and can be justified on the basis of cost-effectiveness. In Bhopal, for example, the lack of basic industrial safety measures resulted in far more costly human damage.

As part of the International Decade for Natural Disaster Reduction proclaimed by the General Assembly of the United Nations in 1987 and initiated in 1990, it was recommended that special attention be given to assisting developing countries with assessment of the potential for damage from disasters, and in establishment of early warning systems and disaster-resistant structures. The objective of the Decade is to reduce, through concerted international action, the loss of life, property damage, and social and economic disruption caused by natural disasters, especially in developing countries.

Most disaster plans have four phases: the **years before the event** (the pre-event phase); the **warning or alerting period**, just before the occurrence of events that can be predicted; the **response phase**, immediately following the event; and the **recovery (rehabilitation) phase**.

Pre-event phase - The objectives during this phase are to anticipate that accidents and disasters will occur and to plan for responding to them. Specific steps should be taken to identify all available organizational resources; inventory the types and locations of available supplies and equipment, including hardware and medical supplies; identity private-sector contractors and distributors who can provide otherwise-scarce specialized personnel and equipment; review essential community and industrial facilities to identify those that may be vulnerable to a disaster; and define the responsibilities of each agency or group and establish lines of communication. In support of these activities, an emergency operations center should be designated and properly equipped.

Warning or alerting period - For certain types of disasters, particularly those caused by natural forces (hurricanes, tornadoes, floods), advance warning may be possible. If so, there will be an opportunity to alert emergency planning personnel and to have them move, where appropriate, to the emergency operations center. Timely and accurate information should be furnished to the media and the public about what to expect, including specific details on what preparations should be made.

Response phase - Usually fire, emergency medical, and police personnel are the first to arrive with help at the site of a major disaster The laypeople already present will inevitably include well-meaning volunteers. Properly managed, volunteers can be helpful; otherwise they can hinder the response. Their sheer numbers may create a logistical problem. It is important to provide security to the affected area to assure the safety of both victims arid workers. The most experienced senior person should take charge, immediately surveying the area and carefully assessing the scene, the number of victims, and their injuries. This person should relay information to the emergency operations center and make recommendations for action. Officials at the center must then determine whether the police, fire, and emergency medical personnel on-site can adequately meet the needs.

Recovery phase - During this phase substantial numbers of injured people may need follow-up care. All survivors will require food, water, shelter, clothing, and sanitation facilities. Sometimes conditions will favor rapid increases in insect and rodent populations. Floods in particular promote unsanitary conditions not only through the buildup of debris and blockage of sewer systems, but also through the creation of breeding habitats for insects, such as mosquitoes, in rain and floodwaters remaining on the soil, in empty receptacles, and elsewhere. Planners should maintain up-to-date information on the distribution of vector-borne diseases in a given area and nearby.

Earthquakes - The impacts of earthquakes on transportation systems and sources of electrical power pose significant problems in themselves, in terms of delayed rescue and medical care and food shortages. Earthquakes can also threaten human health on a massive scale by disrupting water supplies and the safe disposal of wastes. Just as it is possible to design and construct buildings that are resistant to earthquakes, it is possible to design, build, arid maintain water-supply and sewage-disposal facilities that will withstand such events.

Hurricanes - Owing to the tremendous destruction caused by several recent U.S. hurricanes, increasing attention is being given to both preventive and mitigative measures. The following **mitigative measures** can alleviate these problems.

Improved forecasting - Computer models to predict the paths and rates of movement of hurricanes have improved significantly during the past decade. Another advance has been the use of satellite-based tracking systems. However, the accuracy of the forecasts has not improved rapidly enough to offset the lengthier evacuation times now needed to accommodate the larger number of people living in the coastal areas most subject to the damaging effects of hurricanes. Additional research is needed to develop models that will provide longer-range forecasts.

Reduced evacuation time - What is needed are improved road systems, controlled residential and commercial development, better building practices, and safe in-place shelters for people who might otherwise have to leave the impacted area. Evacuation efforts are more likely to be successful if people are asked to evacuate 10 miles rather than 100.

Provision of refuge - Shelters providing a safe haven, if used properly, would minimize potential loss of life when complete evacuations are not feasible. Ironically, the location of such facilities should not be publicized in advance; otherwise people will delay evacuating, knowing that such shelters exist. Other measures that can be used to mitigate the effects of hurricanes include restricting development and redevelopment in high-risk areas; en- forcing hurricane-resistant building codes; and educating the public on successful implementation of mitigative measures, particularly steps to reduce loss of life. Technological forecasting has also proved effective in reducing the impact of other types of natural events, such as volcanic eruptions. The eruption of Mount Saint Helens in Washington State in 1980, for example, took few lives - not only because it occurred on a Sunday morning, when few loggers were in the area, and because the primary blast was toward the more sparsely populated north and northeast, but also because the National Geological Survey had forecast the approximate time and the area likely to be affected by the release.

Floods - During the summer of 1993, the once-in-a-hundred year rains that fell on the midwestern sections of the United States led to both gradual and flash flooding. Prompt response by public health and disaster-control agencies prevented the usual impact of the historic causes of death (drownings, infectious diseases, lack of accessible medical care). Nonetheless, an estimated 46 people died and an estimated $25 billion was lost because of crop and property damage. The floods carried away some entire towns and all the possessions of the inhabitants. That the loss of lives was as low is a tribute to the effective emergency response of public health and relief agencies, and the cooperative efforts of many groups, including the military services. Advanced meteorological and communication equipment permitted the National Weather Service to deliver timely information to response agencies. This allowed time for evacuation, reduced the risk of entrapment by flash floods, and enabled planners to predict where dams and levees might fail.

2. Role of Research in the Prevention of Disaster Related Injuries

The emphasis has shifted from post-disaster improvisation to pre-disaster planning and preparedness. In order to plan for prevention and even to make long-term provision for permanently disabled survivors, the relief phase needs to include an injury surveillance and research component that should be preplanned whenever possible, and be activated immediately once a disaster is known to have occurred. Careful documentation is necessary, not only to prevent future disasters, but also to ensure that, where appropriate, disaster victims are registered and promptly compensated to avoid long-term problems such as those suffered by Bhopal residents

While body counts may be available for many natural disasters, few epidemiologic studies have been conducted to determine risk factors for injury. The value of good epidemiologic information was demonstrated by a study of the 1985 cyclone in Bangladesh. On one island with no cyclone shelters, the study group lost 40 percent of its family members, while at a similar island with eight shelters, only 3 percent of the study group lost family members. Similar studies of earthquakes and tornadoes have led to useful suggestions for preventing loss of life from disasters. Disaster planning and preparedness can reduce the overall impact of disasters, but often basic planning is not done, even in countries at high risk.

The adobe construction that was such a crucial factor in the Guatemala earthquake was not traditional to the indigenous inhabitants of the affected village, but had been copied from the houses of wealthy Spanish inhabitants of Guatemala City. In a previous earthquake prior to the introduction of these houses, there had been no deaths in the village. The research documented the lethal impact of housing "development" on the inhabitants and the fact that the risk of earthquake injury had gone from minimal to maximal in the space of 40 years.

Examples of the types of epidemiologic studies needed include research to determine risk factors for death following building collapse, injury patterns in relation to building design, factors responsible for survival, the most appropriate means of rescue and emergency preparedness, and other factors that could help in planning appropriate interventions either to prevent injury in a natural disaster or to mitigate its effects. The low fatality rates in recent disasters in the United States, including hurricanes Gilbert and Hugo in 1988 and 1989 and the California earthquake in 1989, were in part the result of the application of previous research findings.

Architectural and anthropological studies should be carried out prior to disasters to determine the best type of housing to rapidly replace houses that are lost in a disaster. This will vary for different countries, regions, and ethnic groups. While architects and epidemiologists should be able to assess the resistance of structures to locally important disasters, advance surveys of inhabitants of high-risk areas by anthropologists can determine the cultural acceptability and practicability of proposed designs. This could help to avoid situations where crisis planning and political considerations lead to immense pressure for rapid construction of foreign and inappropriate house designs in the wake of a disaster.

The 1993 earthquake in India flattened more than 32,000 homes in 57 villages, damaged as many as two million more, and killed about 20,000 people, all in less than a minute. The sudden lack of housing together with offers of foreign assistance resulted in immense political pressure to construct thousands of Japanese concrete igloos and American suburban bungalows, although the designs were alien to the local culture and lifestyle. In the 1982 Yemen earthquake, foreigners built homes that were so inappropriate to local needs that they are now used as cattle sheds.

At Tonji University in Shanghai, studies of strategic systems planning for the prevention and relief of disasters have already begun. Four major research groups have been organized, including urban earthquake' engineering, wind engineering, disaster prevention in engineering structures, and urban traffic safety.

New technology will increasingly be used for disaster surveillance, both to predict the spread and extent of certain disasters and to provide advance warning to the general public. Satellite imaging has been particularly effective in mapping the effects of floods, and can be used to obtain advance warning for affected populations. Satellite communications have also facilitated the development of remarkable networks for global communication.

In both "natural" and technological disasters, many deaths result from man-made changes in the environment and habitat. For example, earthquakes themselves seldom kill; collapsing buildings do the damage. It has been reported that in an intensity IX earthquake, a person living in an adobe or weak masonry building is 20,000 times more likely to be killed than someone living in a reinforced concrete frame building that has been properly designed for a minimum seismic load of UBC2.

Such engineering problems should be amenable to intervention if technical knowledge and funds can be made available; however, the costs can be considerable. It has been estimated that an increase of investments in preventive engineering of somewhere between 10 and 1,000 times in the buildings in the worst seismic areas would cause the problem of fatalities from earthquakes to disappear. However, earthquake-safe housing in rural villages need not always be more costly than hazardous structures, since, as noted above in the Guatemala study, simple traditional houses were much safer than the newer introduced designs. Reduced insurance premiums and taxes for disaster-resistant housing have been suggested as market incentives to promote safer building construction.

Other strategies of low to moderate cost proposed for reduction of deaths from earthquakes have included the restriction of building construction on the most unsafe land, better forecasting of earthquakes to allow evacuation of buildings before collapse occurs, and effective rescue. Creative solutions are urgently needed to avoid further massive losses of life, since many of the highest-risk areas have limited resources and high population densities.

Simple multipurpose buildings that can function as cyclone shelters have been effective in preventing loss of life in the Bangladesh delta, and should be built in other flood-prone areas. Other obvious preventive strategies, such as not rebuilding in areas subject to frequent disasters such as floods, are often not observed because of land shortages and the fact that the land in flood-prone deltas is often the most fertile.

Injury prevention in disasters can be considered at a local microlevel and at a national or international macro-level.

Unfortunately, in many countries national disaster preparedness programs are established on an ad hoc basis with limited staff and funding or not at all. The larger problems of overpopulation, environmental degradation, and settlements on marginal unsafe habitats are even more challenging to deal with. Exceptional multi-sectoral, political, and international cooperation and leadership are needed. Failure to act leads not only to local impact, but also to long-term political violence that can affect neighboring countries. In some situations, a point of no return has been reached and irreversible environmental degradation of renewable resources is now an independent variable, rather than a dependent one.

3. Environmental Health Control

Populations affected by disasters often require emergency environmental health services. Potable water is often the most important immediate relief commodity necessary for ensuring the survival of disaster-affected populations. Some water is necessary for drinking and cooking, but decreased water supplies also lead to inadequate personal hygiene. As a baseline, persons should have access to at least 15 to 20 liters of potable water per day.   Heat stress and physical activity can substantially increase the human daily requirements for potable water to levels that are many times normal. Health authorities at disaster sites must plan for additional allotments of water to support clinical facilities and feeding centers, and other public health activities.

The proper management of human waste is also an important environmental health priority, particularly during disaster conditions.   The principal public health thrust of sanitation measures in emergency conditions is to reduce fecal contamination of food and water supplies.   Communicable diseases that can be transmitted through contact with human feces include typhoid fever, cholera, bacillary and amoebic dysentery, hepatitis, polio, schistosomiasis, various helminth infestations, and viral gastroenteritis. Temporary latrines can be established in a disaster site in a variety of ways, including pits and trenches, or more permanent methods.

Apart from access to water and food, shelter is often the most immediate need of disaster-stricken populations, particularly in cold weather. High mortality rates, particularly among the young and elderly, can occur when displaced populations are suddenly subjected to severe cold stress. In some situations, control of insect vectors can be an important measure to prevent or control infectious disease.   Other types of environmental measures may be necessary after disasters when, for example, in a technological disaster, industrial chemical compounds are swept into the water sources used for drinking or soil used for agriculture.

4. Communicable Disease Control

When infectious diseases occur after a disaster, they were almost invariably endemic before the disaster occurred. However, disaster conditions often serve to facilitate disease transmission and increase individual susceptibility to infection. Infectious diseases sometimes occur in a population that moves to a new location where an unfamiliar disease is endemic. For example, devastating malaria epidemics have occurred in no immune populations who were displaced to a malaria endemic area.

The principal infectious disease problems in conflict-related disasters have been measles, diarrheal diseases, acute respiratory infection, and malaria. For example, during the Somali famine (1991-1992), measles and diarrheal diseases accounted for the vast majority of the deaths among persons in temporary camps. Disease outbreaks in complex emergencies are usually the result of many factors, including breakdowns in environmental safeguards, crowding of persons in camps, lack of appropriate immunization programs, malnutrition, inadequate case-finding, and limited availability of appropriate curative medical services.

Despite the more limited potential for disease outbreaks following natural disasters, notable exceptions have occurred. For example, following Hurricane Flora in 1963 a malaria epidemic occurred within the Haitian population. During the recent Northridge earthquake of 1995, the emergence of coccidioidomycosis infections among emergency responders as a result of environmental contamination was a public health concern. Due to such threats and the propensity for epidemics to occur when the normal public health infrastructure has been damaged, following a natural disaster it may be necessary to expand surveillance for certain diseases and rapidly institute appropriate disease control efforts.

Coping with infectious diseases after disasters involves a number of fundamental public health strategies applied to disaster settings. For example, in some settings, emergency measles vaccination programs along with the administration of vitamin A are critical and highly effective measures to prevent cases of measles and to reduce morbidity and mortality caused by this infection. In regard to diarrheal diseases, for which there are not effective immunizations, a combination of basic environmental measures to provide clean water and sanitation, plus rapid case-finding and aggressive treatment (rehydration and appropriate antibiotics) can substantially reduce the consequences of diarrhea outbreaks.

5. Nutritional Rehabilitation

After some disasters, particularly conflict-related disasters, there may be substantially decreased availability of food, which can result in specific nutrient deficiencies, overall under nutrition, or outright starvation. Poor nutritional status increases susceptibility to communicable diseases such as measles and diarrhea. Indeed, the immediate cause of death in most malnourished persons is not usually starvation per se but infectious diseases.

Emergency nutritional rehabilitation efforts for a starving population may involve a number of different types of programs to distribute food. In a food crisis, decisions must be made regarding whether emergency-feeding programs should focus on widespread distribution of general food rations, targeting specific food supplements to select high-risk groups (such as pregnant or lactating women), or on preparing food for consumption on-site in feeding centers. The type of food distributed is an important concern as well. Food must be culturally acceptable and must be nutritionally balanced. Donor-provided food has resulted in iatrogenic micronutrient deficiencies in some long-term relief operations. Sound program decisions should be based on information from rapid nutritional surveys as well as analyses of economic indicators that provide more detail on the nutritional status of the population and the context of the specific food shortage.

During emergency famine relief, it is not the mere delivery of food to the disaster site that saves lives. The most rapid reduction in morbidity and mortality will occur when improvements in environmental health and communicable disease control accompany the restoration of proper nutritional resources. Because the lack of sufficient food in disasters is usually the result of many factors such as economic collapse, disruption of production, inadequate distribution, and other socioeconomic conditions, rather than a true lack of food, the long-term solution is in restoring an indigenous food economy, not in maintaining emergency feeding programs.

6. Public Health Challenges in Disaster Relief Today

Coping with Violence - Relief organizations that wish to be neutral and impartial can have tremendous difficulty operating in settings of armed confrontation. Unfortunately, the provision of humanitarian relief can easily be perceived as a partisan act, or it can be manipulated for the benefit of different warring factions. In situations of conflict, traditional medical and public health interventions may not be very effective in preventing injury and death. Indeed, some have argued that in some situations emergency relief has served to exacerbate and prolong the conflict. Development initiatives, weapons control, conflict resolution, and other such measures may be more effective ways of preventing mortality in these situations. The role of relief organizations in preventing and coping with human rights abuses, including torture and genocide, is still complex and uncertain. Also, increasingly today, the provision of emergency relief is very dangerous. Many relief workers have been killed in recent years; how to adequately protect them is a major dilemma.

Improved Emergency Public Health Response - Many problems still remain in the effective implementation of emergency relief programs. In the Kurdish refugee crisis, despite a massive international relief effort, many deaths occurred due to preventable diarrheal disease. This was in large part due to a failure to implement basic environmental health interventions and diarrhea control programs early enough in this crisis. During the 1994 Goma, Zaire, refugee emergency as many as 50,000 persons died from cholera within the temporary camp system in only a matter of weeks. The Goma (Zaire) Epidemiology Group reported after the Rwanda refugee crisis that there is an urgent need for more intensive and focused training of relief workers to develop relevant expertise in the prevention and management of diarrheal diseases, as well as other essential elements of relief programs, such as measles immunization, public health surveillance, community outreach, and nutritional rehabilitation. A review of public health assessments and surveys conducted in Somalia demonstrated a lack of consistency in methodology, which led to difficulties in interpreting and acting upon critical public health data. Few training programs in schools of public health have curricula that cover the broad range of knowledge needed to cope with the public health issues associated with disaster-affected populations.

Vulnerable Populations - Disasters do not affect all persons evenly; identifying and focusing on populations with special needs after disasters is a critical issue. For example, the unique concerns of women in disasters have become a greater focus in disaster relief in the last few years. Recent data suggests that in some disasters women have less access to medical care and other relief services. Additionally, while data is limited pregnancy, sexually transmitted diseases, sexual abuse, and human immunodeficiency virus (HIV) infection are believed to be common issues among women in some disaster-affected populations, especially refugees. Few relief programs have sufficiently addressed these issues. The special problems of children in disasters are increasingly recognized. Children are much more vulnerable to many of the adverse health effects of disasters, such as malnutrition and infectious diseases. Additionally, the plight of unaccompanied children in Rwanda illustrated a problem common to many complex emergencies today. In disaster situations there are many other Potentially vulnerable groups, such as members of a particular ethnic group, the elderly, and immigrants.

Land Mines - One of the most extensive public health catastrophes today is the extensive worldwide dissemination of land mines. It is estimated that 65 to 110 million land mines are scattered throughout more than 60 countries. Land mines persist for decades. They impede the resettlement of displaced populations and serve to remove land from cultivation. Worldwide, land mines are responsible for more than 15,000 fatalities each year. However, many land mines are designed to maim. The survivors require emergency surgical services and prolonged rehabilitation largely related to lower limb amputation. This has had devastating impact on the individuals, the economy, and the health care system. Countries affected by severe land mine problems in the wake of endemic warfare include Afghanistan, Mozambique, former Yugoslavia, Angola, and Rwanda.

Terrorism - Terrorism is regarded by many as an increasing and evolving threat. Terrorists of today have unparalleled access to highly destructive technologies. In addition to conventional explosives, nuclear devices, chemical weapons, and biological weapons are believed to have potential as terrorist weapons. The release of the nerve gas sarin in the Tokyo subway system illustrates the emerging threat from such weapons of mass destruction and the complex public health issues that arise from an intentional technological disaster. Such issues include the need for rapid characterization of the offending agent, mass decontamination, ready access to antidotes, specialized medical training, and proper protective equipment for emergency responders.

Mental Health - In addition to traditional public health concerns, disasters may present medical responders with patients who are suffering from complaints that are predominantly psychological in nature. Consequently, mental health issues may predominate the health concerns during the acute phase of disaster response. Such concerns may include the need for specialized psychological triage and treatment programs for victims. Emergency response personnel are also subject to short- and long-term effects as a result of stress imposed by the disaster, particularly among persons required to be involved in post disaster management of decedents. The psychological impact of disasters on children has only just begun to be documented but is clearly profound. The appalling use of children as soldiers in many countries of the world may have long-term mental health consequences of unprecedented proportions.

Conclusion - The public health consequences of disasters are wide ranging, and their effects on populations are long lasting. Knowledge and experience from many health disciplines is needed for effective emergency response. Such skills include epidemiology, community health and primary care, environmental science, communicable disease control, and international health. Research is needed to develop standardized and valid assessment tools, reliable surveillance programs, low-technology environmental health interventions, and more effective intervention strategies. Unfortunately, the reality today is that many relief workers in the health sector, though well-intentioned, are often recruited and deployed on short notice with little public health preparation or training. Schools of public health must continue to expand their training in the emergency skills that practitioners will need to deal with the public health needs of disaster-affected populations if we are going meet this challenge.

VII. **BIBLIOGRAPHY**

Agency for Toxic Substances and Disease Registry. (1992). Case Studies in Environmental Medicine, Lead Toxicity, Revised September 1992, US Department of Health and Human Services.

Agency for Toxic Substances Disease Registry. (1989). Toxicological profile of lead. U.S. ATSDR.

Alperstein G, Reznik R & Duggin G. (1991, September 16). Lead: Subtle forms and new modes of poisoning. The Medical Journal of Australia Vol 155.

American Academy of Pediatrics Committee on Environmental Health. (1993, July). Lead Poisoning: From Screening to Primary Prevention, Pediatrics Vol. 92.

Barss, P., Smith, G. S., Baker, S. P., & Mohan, D. (1998). Injuries from Disasters. Injury   Prevention: An International Perspective. Epidemiology, Surveillance, and Policy (pp. 233-244). New York, NY: Oxford University Press.

Bellinger, O. & Needleman H. L. (1992). Neurodevelopmental effects of low-level lead exposure in children. In: Needleman, HL, (Ed.) Human Lead Exposure. CRC Press: Boca Raton, FL.

Berry M, Garrard J, & Greene D. (1994). Reducing Lead Exposure in Australia. Common wealth Department of Human Services and Health, Canberra.

Billick, I.H., & Gray, V.E. (1978). Lead based paint poisoning research: Review and evaluation 1971-1977. Washington, DC: U.S. Department of Housing and Urban Development.

Bornschein, R.L., Succop, P., Kraft, K.M., Clark, C.S., Peace, B., & Hammond, P.B. (1987). Exterior surface dust lead, interior house dust lead and childhood lead exposure in an urban environment. In: D.D. Hemphill, (Ed). Trace Substances in Environmental Health, (pp. 322-332). Proceedings of University of Missouri's 20th Annual Conference, June 1986. University of Missouri, Columbia, MO.

Brody, D.J., Pirkie, J.L., Kramer, R.A, et al. (1994). Blood lead levels in the US population. Phase 1 of the Third National Health and Nutrition Examination Survey (NHANES III, 1988 to 1991). J Am Med Assoc ; 272:277-283.

Castellino, N., Castellino, P. & Sannolo, N. (Ed). (1995). Inorganic lead exposure. Lewis Publishers: Boca Raton, FL.

Centers for Disease Control and Prevention. (1997). Update: Blood Lead Levels-United States 1991 – 1994. Morbidity and Mortality Weekly Report, U.S. Department of Health and Human Services/Public Health Service, Feb 21; 1997, 46(7): 141-146 and erratum July 4; 1997, 46(26): 607.

Centers for Disease Control and Prevention. (1991). Preventing Lead Poisoning in Young Children: A Statement by the Centers for Disease Control. CDC, US Department of Health and Human Services, Report No. 99-2230: Atlanta: GA.

Chemwatch Database. (1996). Lead Arsenate.

Chilsom, J.J. Jr. (1986). Removal of lead paint from old housing: The need for a new approach. Am J Public Health 76:236-237.

Clark, C.S., Bornschein, R., Succop, P., Roda, S., & Peace, B. (1991). Urban Lead Exposures of Children in Cincinnati, Ohio. Journal of Chemical Speciation and Bioavailability 314:163-171.

Clark, C.S., Bornschein, R.L., Succop, P., et al. (1985). Conditions and type of housing as an indicator of potential environmental lead exposure and pediatric blood lead levels. Environ Res 38:46-53.

Clark, H.R. (1995). The cure for all diseases. Pro Motion Publishing, San Diego: California.

Davis, T.G. (1997). Environmental Safety. In M. Morgan (Ed), Environmental Health 2nd Edition (pp.199-215). Englewood, CO: Morton Publishing Company.

EPA. (1986). Air quality criteria for lead. U.S. Environmental Protection Agency, Office of Research and Development, Office of Health and Environmental Assessment, Environmental Criteria and Assessment Office. EPA 600/8-83-028F: Research Triangle Park, NC.

EPA. (1988). Code of Federal Regulations. 40 CFR 261, Appendix VIII. U.S. Environmental Protection Agency.

EPA. (1994). Method 6020: Inductively Coupled Plasma-Mass Spectrometry, revision 0 (1994), SW-846, Test Methods for Evaluating Solid Waste, Volume 1A: Laboratory Manual, Physical / Chemical Methods, United States Environmental Protection Agency, Office of Solid Waste and Emergency Response, Washington, DC.

EPA. (1983). Methods for chemical analysis of water and wastes. Methods 239.1 and 239. 2. U.S. Environmental Protection Agency, Office of Research and Development, Environmental Monitoring and Support Laboratory. EPA Report No. 600/4-79-020: Cincinnati, OH.

EPA. (1990). Neurotoxicity Review in US Environmental Protection Agency, Air Quality Criteria for Lead: Supplement to the 1986 Addendum, Office of Health and Environmental Assessment, Environmental Criteria and Assessment Office, EPA Report No. EPA/600-8-89-049F: Research Triangle Park, NC.

EPA. (1995). Report on the national survey of lead based paint in housing - base report. U.S. Environmental Protection Agency, Office of Pollution Prevention and Toxics. EPA 747-R- 95-003, 1995. http://www.hud.szov/lea/leadwnlo.html.

Fergusson, O.M., Hurwood, L. J., & Lynskey, M.T. (1997). Early dentine lead levels and educational outcomes at 18 years. In Journal of Child Psychology and Psychiatry Vol 38 No 4. pp.471-478.

Fischbein, A. (1992). Occupational and environmental lead exposure. In Environmental and Occupational Medicine, 2nd Edition. Ed W.N. Rom. Little, Brown, & Co.

Flegal, A.R., Smith, R.D. (1992, May). Lead Levels in Preindustrial Humans. New England Journal of Medicine. Vol. 326.

Gatsonis, C.A., & Needleman, H.L. (1992). Recent epidemological studies of low-level lead exposure and the IQ of children: a meta-analytic review In: Needleman HL, ed. Human Lead Exposure. CRC Press: Boca Raton, FL.

Gibson, J.L. (1904). A Plea for Painted Railings and Painted Walls of Rooms as the Source of Lead Poisoning Amongst Queensland Children. Australasian Medical Gazette 23:149-153.

Goldstein, G.W. (1992). Developmental neurobiology of lead toxicity. In: Needleman HL, ed. Human Lead Exposure. CRC Press: Boca Raton, FL.

Hayes, J. A. (2001). Swimming Pools and Spas. In L. Williams, & R. Langley (Eds.), Environmental Health Secrets (pp. 142-144). Philadelphia, PA: Hanley & Belfus, Inc.

Jacobs, D.E. (1995). Lead paint as a Major Source of Childhood Lead Poisoning: A Review of the Evidence. In: E.B. Michael, S.D. Iske, (Eds.) Lead in Paint, Soil and Dust: Health Risks, Exposure studies, Control Measures and Quality Assurance, ASTM STP 1226, American Society for Testing and Materials. Philadelphia, PA.

Langley, R. L. (2001). Natural Disasters. In L. Williams, & R. Langley (Eds.), Environmental Health Secrets (pp. 219-225). Philadelphia, PA: Hanley & Belfus, Inc.

Lanphear, B.P., Dietrich, K., Auinger P., & Cox, C. (2000). Cognitive Deficits Associated with Blood Lead Concentration < 10 µg/dL in US Children and Adolescents. Public Health Reports November / December Vol. 115, No. 6: 521-529.

Lanphear, B.P., Emond, M., Jacobs, D.E., Weitzman, M., Tanner, M, Winter, N., Yakir, B., Eberly, S.A. (1995). Side by Side Comparison of Dust collection Methods for Sampling Lead-Contaminated House Dust. Environ Res 68:114-123.

Lanphear, B.P., Matte, T.D., Rogers, J, Clickner, R.P., Dietz, B, Bornschein, R .L., Succop, S., Mahaffey, K.R, Dixon, S., Galke, W., Rabinowitz, M., Farfel, M., Rohde, C., Schwartz, J., Ashley, P., & Jacobs, D.E. (1998). The Contribution of Lead-Contaminated House Dust and Residential Soil to Children's Blood Lead Levels: A Pooled Analysis of 12 Epidemiological Studies. Environ Res 79:51-68.

Lanphear, B.P., & Roghmann, K.J. (1997). Pathways of lead exposure in urban children. Environ Res 74(1):67-73.

Last, J. M. (1998). Housing and Health. In R. Wallace (Ed), Public Health & Preventive Medicine (pp. 777-780). Stamford, CT: Appleton & Lange.

Lipton, D. (2001). Environmental Odors and Intensive Livestock Operations. In L. Williams, & R. Langley (Eds.), Environmental Health Secrets (pp. 33-37). Philadelphia, PA: Hanley & Belfus, Inc.

Luginbuhl, R. C. (2001). Migrant Housing. In L. Williams, & R. Langley (Eds.), Environmental Health Secrets (pp. 193-196). Philadelphia, PA: Hanley & Belfus, Inc.

McElvain, M.D., DeUngria, E.G., Matte, T.D., Copley, C.G., & Binder, S. (1992). Prevalence of radiographic evidence of paint chip ingestion among children with moderate to severe lead poisoning, St. Louis, MO, 1989-90. Pediatrics 89:740-742.

McMichael, A.J., Kjellstrom,T., and Smith, K.R. (2001). In M. Merson, R. Black, & A. Mills (Eds). International Public Health Diseases, Program Systems, and Policies (pp. 404-407). Gaitherburg, MD: Aspen Publishers, Inc.

Mielke, H., Burroughs, S., Wade, R., et al. (1984/1985). Urban lead in Minnesota: Soil transect results of four cities. Minnesota Academy of Science 50:19-24.

Mielke, H.W., Adams, J.L., Reagan, P.L., et al. (1989). Soil-dust lead and childhood lead exposure as a function of city size and community traffic flow: The case for lead abatement in Minnesota. Environ Chem Health (Supp) 9:253-271.

Mielke, H.W., Anderson, J.C., Berry, K.J., et al. (1983). Lead concentrations in inner-city soils as a factor in the child lead problem. Am J Public Health 73:1366-1369.

Mielke, H.W. (1992). Lead dust contaminated U.S.A. communities: Comparison of Louisiana and Minnesota. Applied Geochemistry 6:1-16.

Mielke, H.W. (1999). Lead in Inner Cities. American Scientist 87(1).

Moeller, D.W. (1997). Disaster Response. <u>Environmental Health</u> (pp.383-409). Cambridge, MA, and London, UK: Harvard University Press.

Morris, T. (2001). Recreational and Environmental Infections. In L. Williams, & R. Langley (Eds.), <u>Environmental Health Secrets</u> (pp. 179-188). Philadelphia, PA: Hanley & Belfus, Inc.

National Academy of Sciences. (1993). <u>Measuring Lead Exposure in Infants, Children, and Other Sensitive Populations,</u> Committee on Measuring Lead in Critical Populations, Board on Environmental Studies and Toxicology, Commission on Life Sciences, National Academy of Sciences, National Academy Press, Washington, DC.

National Research Council. (1993<u>). Measuring Lead Exposures in Infants, Children, and Other Sensitive Populations.</u> National Academy Press: Washington, D.C.

Needleman, H.L., and Gastonis, C.A. (1990, February). Low-Level Exposure and the IQ of Children. <u>JAMA Vol 263, No.5.</u>

Needleman, H.L. et al. (1979, March). Deficits in Psychologic and Classroom Performance of Children's with Elevated Dentine Lead Levels. <u>New England Journal of Medicine Vol. 300, No.13.</u>

Needleman, H.L., Riess, J.A., Tobin, M., Biesecker, G., & Greenhouse, J.B. (1996, February 7). Bone Lead Levels and Delinquent Behavior. <u>Vol 275 No5. JAMA. pp 363-369.</u>

Rabinowitz, M., Leviton, A., Bellinger, D. (1985). Home refinishing: Lead paint and infant blood lead levels. <u>Am. J Public Health 75: 403-404</u>.

Repko, J. (1976, February). Behavioural toxicology of inorganic Lead. In: Carnow, W, ed. <u>Health Effects of Occupational Lead and Arsenic Exposure - a symposium.</u> US Dept of Health, Education and Welfare Public Health Service Division of Surveillance Hazard Evaluation and Field Studies.

Rice, O.C. (1992). Behavioural Impairment produced by developmental lead exposure: Evidence from primate research. In: Needleman HL, ed. <u>Human Lead Exposure</u>. CRC Press: Boca Raton, FL.

Rosen, J.F. (1992, April). Effects of Low Levels of Lead Exposure. <u>Science Vol. 256.</u>

Rosen, J.F. (1992, November). Health Effects of Lead at Low Exposure Levels. <u>Am J of Diseases of Children. Vol. 146.</u>

Royce, S.E. (1993, September). <u>Lead toxicity</u>. US Dept of Health and Human Services Agency for Toxic Substances and Disease Registry.

Schwartz, J., & Otto, O. (1987, May). Blood lead, hearing thresholds and neurological development in children and youth. <u>Arch of Environmental Health, Vol 42 No 2.</u>

Schwartz, J. (1994). Low-Lead Level Exposure and Children's IQ: A Meta-Analysis and Search for a Threshold. <u>Envir. Res. 65:42-55.</u>

Schwartz, J. (1992). Low level health effects of lead: Growth, developmental and neurological disturbances. In: Needleman HL, ed. <u>Human Lead Exposure</u>. CRC Press: Boca Raton, FL.

Shannon, M.W., & Graef, J.W. (1992). Lead Intoxication in Infancy. <u>Pediatrics 89(1):87-90.</u>

Silbergeld, E. K. (1992). Neurological perspective on lead toxicity. In: Needleman HL, ed. <u>Human Lead Exposure</u>. CRC Press: Boca Raton, FL.

Smith, M.A., Grant, L.O., & Sors, A. (1989). Lead exposure and child development: an international assessment. Kleeven Academic Publishers.

Turner, J.A. (1897). Lead Poisoning Among Queensland Children. Australasian Medical Gazette 16:475-479.

U.S. Department of Housing & Urban Development. (1990). Comprehensive and Workable Plan for the Abatement of Lead Paint in Privately Owned Housing: Report to Congress, Washington, DC.

U.S. Department of Housing & Urban Development. (1997, February). Moving Toward a Lead-Safe America: A Report to the Congress of the United States, Washington, DC.

Wedeen, R.P. (1992). Lead, the kidneys and hypertension. In: Needleman HL, ed. Human Lead Exposure. CRC Press: Boca Raton, FL.

Werbach, M.F. (1997). Foundations of nutritional medicine. Third Line Press: Tarzana, CA.

World Resources Institute. (1997). CIESIN Report. WRI: Washington, DC.

Yassi, A., Kjellström, T., de Kok, T., & Guidotti, T. L. (2001). Risk Management: Managing an Environmental Health Emergency. In A. Yassi, [et al](Eds.), Basic Environmental Health (pp. 167-172). New York, NY: Oxford University Press, Inc.

Yassi, A., Kjellström, T., de Kok, T., & Guidotti, T. L. (2001). Water and Sanitation: Sanitation. In A. Yassi, [et al](Eds.), Basic Environmental Health (pp. 231-234). New York, NY: Oxford University Press, Inc.

Yassi, A., Kjellström, T., de Kok, T., & Guidotti, T. L. (2001). Transboundary and Global Health Concerns: Disasters. In A. Yassi, [et al](Eds.), Basic Environmental Health (pp. 394-397). New York, NY: Oxford University Press, Inc.

Yassi, A., Kjellström, T., de Kok, T., & Guidotti, T. L. (2001). Human Settlement and Urbanization: Housing and Health. In A. Yassi, [et al](Eds.), Basic Environmental Health (pp. 288-292). New York, NY: Oxford University Press, Inc.

CHAPTER

13

INJURY

I. INTRODUCTION

During the 20th century, deaths from infectious diseases have declined dramatically around the world, particularly in industrialized countries. The initial decline occurred due to improved sanitation and public health. More recently it has been due to antibiotics, vaccines, and an increasing emphasis on prevention. Deaths among humankind from injuries have also declined substantially although the decrease is far less than that for infectious diseases.

Public health is the profession dedicated to extending and improving physical, mental, and emotional health and well being for the population as a whole. By focusing on ways to control environmental risks, public health works to make the world a safer place in which to live. Much of public health's work is well established and well known, going back at least a century and including efforts to improve sanitation, screen the public for various contagious or preventable diseases, and immunize against diseases. But one of the most important public health efforts is more recent in origin and less well understood. This is the field of injury prevention.

Injuries – both unintentional and intentional – are a major threat to the public's health and well-being. Each year 150,000 Americans die as the result of injuries, and an estimated 70 million suffer nonfatal injuries. As one government study noted, injuries "kill more Americans aged 1-34 than all diseases combined." Injury ranks third among causes of death overall, and it constitutes the second most costly health problem in this country, after heart disease.

II. EXPOSURE TO INJURY

A. MECHANICAL HAZARDS

Mechanical hazards are those posed by the transfer of mechanical or **kinetic energy** (the energy of motion). The transfer of mechanical energy can result in immediate or gradually acquired injury in exposed individuals. The terms **injury** and **trauma** are often used interchangeably to refer to the harm that may result from mechanical hazards. The events and circumstances that result in injury have commonly been ref erred to as **accidents**. This term is no longer used by those working in injury control. In many languages it implies that injuries are random, unpredictable, chance types of events. Environmental health specialists believe that most injuries are predictable and preventable, and can be studied using epidemiological methods, just like any illness or health effect.

Socioeconomic factors are also important to consider when addressing the problem of mechanical hazards. Injury rates are linked with poverty within both developed and developing nations. Much of the world's population lacks the resources to provide optimal safety in their immediate environment, The necessity of obtaining food for the family by riding a broken-down bicycle through crowded, poorly maintained streets without a helmet is an example of this. Governments and industry are tempted to compromise safety for economic reasons, leading to tragedies such as the collapse of a public building. Many transportation accidents involving trains, ferries, and buses are the result of inadequate resources provided for the safe upkeep and regulation of roads, rails, and vehicles.

B. IMPACT OF INJURY ON THE INDIVIDUAL AND SOCIETY

Injury is a major cause of mortality throughout the world and has been described as the most under recognized major public health problem (Table 13.1). For example, injury is the single greatest killer of North Americans between the ages of 1 and 44; in Canada, injuries are responsible for 63% of all deaths between the ages of 1 and 24. A similar pattern exists in most developed countries. The importance of injury is becoming increasingly recognized in developing countries, as injury mortality is high in developing countries and generally decreases with development. The only exception is traffic accident deaths, which increase in line with the growth of motor vehicle use in a country. While traditional health problems of infectious diseases and malnutrition remain important causes of mortality in developing nations, increased urbanization and the influx of automobiles (often on roads not designed for them) has led to increased mortality from injury.

One way to describe the prematurity of death is the calculation of **potential years of life lost (PYLL)**. The age at which a death occurs is subtracted from a standard age (usually 65) and the difference is the number of premature or productive years of life that were lost because of the young death. For example, a traffic fatality at age 20 results in 45 years of PYLL, whereas a similar death at age 60 only results in 5 PYLL. While this approach is not intended to judge the value of a lost human life, this measure is used to describe the loss to the individual and to society of the potential contributions an individual may have made. Injuries account for an enormous amount of PYLL even in comparison to other leading causes of death (cardiovascular disease and cancer) that tend to occur in older age-groups. In the United States, the PYLL due to injury in 1985 was more than cancer and cardiovascular diseases combined.

C. VULNERABLE GROUPS

Children, the elderly, and disadvantaged groups have higher rates of injury than the overall population. Peak ages for fatal injuries are ages 1-4, 15-25, and over 70. Deaths in the 15-25 year range are mostly motor vehicle related. At all ages, males have higher injury death rates than females.

D. INJURY SETTINGS

Historically, injuries that occur at work and injuries that occur in other settings have been considered separately, more for practical reasons than for conceptual reasons. Work environments often present a high level of exposure to mechanical hazards both in terms of the magnitude of risk (working with dangerous machinery) and the length of exposure (40 hr a week for 30 years). Legislation has been passed in many jurisdictions to control and regulate the workplace for the protection of workers.

Table 13. 1. Ten Leading Causes of deaths by Age group – 1998 (Source: National Center for Health Statistics, 2000).

Age Groups

Rank	< 1	1-4	5-9	10-14	15-24	25-34	35-44	45-54	55-64	65+	Total
1	Congenital Anomalies 6,212	Unintentional Injuries 1,935	Unintentional Injuries 1,544	Unintentional Injuries 1,710	Unintentional Injuries 13,349	Unintentional Injuries 12,045	Unintentional Injuries 15,127	Malignant Neoplasms 45,747	Malignant Neoplasms 87,024	Heart Disease 605,673	Heart Disease 724,859
2	Short Gestation 4,101	Congenital Anomalies 564	Malignant Neoplasms 487	Malignant Neoplasms 526	Homicide 5,516	Suicide 5,365	Malignant Neoplasms 14,711	Heart Disease 35,056	Heart Disease 65,068	Malignant Neoplasms 384,186	Malignant Neoplasms 541,532
3	SIDS 2,822	Homicide 399	Congenital Anomalies 198	Suicide 317	Suicide 4,135	Homicide 4,565	Heart Disease 13,593	Unintentional Injuries 10,946	Bronchitis Emphysema Asthma 10,162	Cerebro-vascular 139,144	Cerebro-vascular 158,448
4	Maternal Complications 1,343	Malignant Neoplasms 365	Homicide 170	Homicide 290	Malignant Neoplasms 1,699	Malignant Neoplasms 4,385	Suicide 6,837	Liver Disease 5,744	Cerebro-vascular 9,653	Bronchitis Emphysema Asthma 97,896	Bronchitis Emphysema asthma 112584
5	Respiratory Distress Synd. 1,295	Heart Disease 214	Heart Disease 156	Congenital Anomalies 173	Heart Disease 1,057	Heart Disease 3,207	HIV 5,746	Cerebro-vascular 5,709	Diabetes 8,705	Pneumonia & Influenza 82,989	Unintentional Injuries 97,835
6	Placenta Cord Membranes 961	Pneumonia & Influenza 146	Pneumonia & Influenza 70	Heart Disease 170	Congenital Anomalies 450	HIV 2,912	Homicide 3,567	Suicide 5,131	Unintentional Injuries 7,340	Diabetes 48,974	Pneumonia & Influenza 91,871
7	Perinatal Infections 815	Septicemia 89	Bronchitis Emphysema Asthma 54	Bronchitis Emphysema Asthma 98	Bronchitis Emphysema Asthma 239	Cerebro-vascular 670	Liver Disease 3,370	Diabetes 4,386	Liver Disease 5,279	Unintentional Injuries 32,975	Diabetes 64,751
8	Unintentional Injuries 754	Perinatal Period 75	Benign Neoplasms 52	Pneumonia & Influenza 51	Pneumonia & Influenza 215	Diabetes 636	Cerebro-vascular 2,650	HIV 3,120	Pneumonia & Influenza 3,856	Nephritis 22,640	Suicide 30,575
9	Intrauterine Hypoxia 461	Cerebro-vascular 57	Cerebro-vascular 35	Cerebro-vascular 47	HIV 194	Liver Disease 531	Diabetes 1,885	Bronchitis Emphysema Asthma 2,828	Suicide 2,963	Alzheimer's Disease 22,416	Nephritis 26,182
10	Pneumonia & Influenza 441	Benign Neoplasms 53	HIV 29	Benign Neoplasms 32	Cerebro-vascular 178	Pneumonia & Influenza 506	Pneumonia & Influenza 1,400	Pneumonia & Influenza 2,167	Septicemia 2,093	Septicemia 19,012	Liver Disease 25,192

In some jurisdictions, compensation systems exist to cover the financial burden of injury on the worker through payment generally charged back, at least partially, to the employer where the injury occurred. The cost of workers' compensation to employers has added further incentive to explore preventive options. The emphasis on injury prevention has also contributed to the training of physicians, nurses, ergonomists, and other professionals with expertise in the prevention and treatment of work-related injuries. The work and research of these professionals have greatly advanced the understanding of injuries in the workplace.

E. OCCUPATIONAL INJURIES AND ERGONOMICS

Occupational injuries represent a serious cost to industry and to society, and they tend to affect people during their most productive years, when they have families to support. Injury at the workplace results in significant working time loss, disability, and fatalities. As mentioned earlier, the mechanism of injury does not differ from that of injuries sustained elsewhere, but the exposure may be great in some worksites. Forestry, construction, mining, and fishing are occupations with high rates of work-related trauma. Agricultural injuries are often very severe, occur in rural locations where medical care may not be easily accessible, and may affect family members, including children, who are working and living on the farm. Ironically, healthcare is another sector in which Injury rates are high. Back injuries are the most common type of work-related injury, musculoskeletal injuries account for the vast majority of time loss claims for workers' compensation. Injuries that result from **cumulative trauma**, known also as **repetitive strain injuries**, are particularly costly.

F. TRAFFIC-RELATED INJURIES

Motor vehicle-related crashes are by far the leading cause of serious injuries in most countries. Unfortunately, high rates of injuries are usually tolerated by society and accepted as an unavoidable cost of transportation. This is quite unnecessary as injuries can be prevented by improved design of roads, improved sign and regular maintenance of cars and trucks, education of drivers, and enforcement of traffic rules.

G. HOME- AND RECREATION-RELATED INJURIES

Home- and recreation-related injuries cover a broad range of settings and types of injury. Home-related injuries affect primarily children and the elderly and can be very serious. Other than work, the home is the most common place for fatal injuries. Recreation- and sports-related injuries tend to affect primarily young people. Although these injuries tend to be less serious in general, they are often troublesome, costly to treat, and may occasionally be fatal. They are also a common cause of lost time from work.

Drownings, burns, poisoning, and falls are critical causes of pediatric morbidity and mortality. Young children can drown in only a few centimeters of water in a matter of seconds and should never be left unattended near water or in the bath. Backyard pools and natural open water are hazards for young children who may wander unattended into the water. Pools should have adequate fencing and locks to protect against this hazard.

Young children may be the victims of fire as often they are not able to remove themselves from a burning building. Properly functioning smoke detectors are effective in alerting a family in time to remove children from a burning home. Innovative programs supplying smoke detectors to families of newborns at hospital discharge have been implemented in an attempt to make this countermeasure more widely adopted. Smoking is related to many deaths - either parents' cigarettes cause the fire or matches and lighters are within children's reach. Lighters are now required to be child resistant in some countries. Regulations prohibiting flammable sleepwear have also been adopted by some countries, thus decreasing burn injuries. Hot water scalding is a major cause of home burn injuries in young children and the elderly, who have more vulnerable skin and are often not able to remove themselves quickly enough from a situation of inadvertent exposure. Hot water tanks are often set at levels at which scalding can readily occur. It is thus recommended that hot water tanks be preset to prevent scalding, and families with young children be warned to be particularly vigilant in this regard. The practice of cooking over an open fire, common in many areas of developing nations but also a practice in many poorer communities of the developed world, can result in serious bums in young children.

H. PSYCHOSOCIAL HAZARD

1. Psychosocial Hazards and Stressors

Uncertainty, anxiety, and a lack of a feeling of control over one's own life situation or environment lead to what is popularly called **stress**. The word stress is sometimes used to describe a stimulus: a specific event or situation that causes a mental or physiological reaction. To keep the terminology straight, it is best to speak of **stressors** rather than stress in this meaning. **Stress** can thus be defined as a human response to stressors. This definition of stress indicates the state of pressure that a person experiences. Another definition emphasizes the fact that stress is a process, resulting from the interaction between humans and the environment. The stress process consists of two stages: the first it involves deciding whether an event (stressor) indeed poses a hazard; the second involves appraising the possibilities of dealing with the situation. As long as an individual can cope with the stressors, there is no problem. However, when coping strategies are no longer adequate, adverse stress reactions will occur.

For many people in both developed and developing countries, stress is a part of daily life, and it may lead to a variety of serious health effects, including depression, suicide, substance abuse, violence against others, psychosomatic diseases, and general malaise. Psychosocial hazards are those that create a social environment of uncertainty, anxiety, and lack of control. This may include the anxiety about mere survival from violence, as in the case of war-torn countries, or the uncertainty about future health effects of radiation exposure, for example, after the Chernobyl accident.

2. Health Effects of Stress

The modern perception of stress is that it is a negative or adverse reaction. The evolutionary perspective is different, in that stress is considered to be an important mechanism to prepare the human organism for urgent action, both physically and mentally. The physiological characteristics of the stress reaction include increases in heart rate, blood pressure, respiration, and blood transport to skeletal muscles and a simultaneous decrease in digestive activity. Increased production of stress hormones, such as epinephrine and cortisol, also play an important role in this reaction. All of these reactions prepare the individual for defensive actions - attack or flight. They thus improve the individual's chance of survival and can influence the success of a given species.

III. INJURY PREVENTION AND CONTROL

A. INTRODUCTION

1. Injury

The term injury is derived from the Latin term **in juris** meaning "**not right**." An injury is the physical damage to a person that occurs as a result of exposure to physical or chemical agents at rates greater than the body can tolerate or the absence of such essentials as heat or oxygen. An injury is generally considered to occur acutely after exposure. Injury and trauma are synonymous.

Injuries are considered separately from diseases, although they are part of the spectrum of diseases. The difference between an injury and a disease may be only one of the dose of the causal factor, the time course during which the causal factor operates, or the body's adaptation and response to the causal factor. Injuries and diseases are often caused by the same factors, although the amount or the rate of exposure may differ. Although the symptoms of an injury are usually immediately obvious as compared to the symptoms of disease, the duration of latency periods for injuries and diseases overlap.

2. Accidents

Injuries, especially unintentional injuries have often been referred to as "accidents." The term "accidents," however, inappropriately implies chance misfortune and lack of predictability, which inaccurately describe the epidemiology of injuries. The convention of describing the injury and the injury-causing event should be followed rather than using the term "accident," which is imprecise and unspecific.

The term "accident proneness", first used in 1926, is also inappropriate because hidden psychological impulses or motives have little to do with the cause of injuries. Although the term "accident" generally is not used in scientific communications, it continues to be used in some classification and surveillance.

B. INJURY CONTROL AND PUBLIC HEALTH

Injuries are a focus of public health practice because they pose a serious health threat, occur frequently, and are theoretically preventable. Thus, the reduction in the number and severity of injuries offers a cost-effective manner in which to improve the health status of populations. Injuries are a very broad group of afflictions, arising from many different activities and risk factors and can affect all organ systems of the body. Since injuries are so diverse in mechanisms occurrence, formulating an organized and structured approach to studying their incidence and prevention is helpful.

Injuries affect people of all ages and range from minor cuts and bruises to major catastrophes that take thousands of lives. Some injuries may result in prolonged pain or life-long disabilities that restrict an individual from performing personal and work-related activities Furthermore, injuries often affect more than a single individual, destroying families and devastating communities as seen in recent earthquakes, hurricanes, and plane crashes. These events can leave individuals and societies with enormous medical costs, extensive rehabilitation needs, major lifestyle adjustments, and depression-losses that cannot easily, if ever, be recouped.

However, the majority of injuries do not occur as a result of a catastrophic disaster; instead they are related to daily events. For example, the annual number of deaths from motor vehicle crashes in the United States far exceeds that from airline crashes and natural disasters combined. Injuries disproportionately affect the young, the frail, and the underserved populations. In fact, those in the youngest age groups are more in danger of sustaining injuries than they are of being affected by the more recognized threats to health such as infections, cancer, and cardiovascular disease. Hence, injuries account for the most years of premature productive life lost, number of school and workdays missed, and have become one of the largest components of the medical care dollar expenditure per capita.

The public is largely unaware of the preventable nature of many injuries. The most common reference to injurious events, "accidents," evokes a feeling of chance, misfortune, and helplessness. Hence, the word "accident" should be avoided in discussing injury control, and instead, the focus should be on exposures to hazards and resulting injuries, as well as their preventability. In recent years, great strides have been made in injury prevention. Modifications in vehicle design and changes of hazardous behaviors, such as drunk driving, have been effective in reducing traffic-related injuries. Preventive measures have been successful in reducing the incidence of drownings, poisonings, falls, and fires. Despite successes in many areas of injury prevention, new risks and increasing population size constantly challenge the public health community. Development of effective injury prevention strategies warrants an interdisciplinary approach that draws on public health, biomechanics, engineering, behavioral sciences, law enforcement, medicine, and urban planning. Hence, future work should involve collaborative efforts of professionals from these various fields.

As the scientific base of information concerning injuries, their causes and prevention expands, public health and preventive and clinical medicine practitioners are applying increasing attention and resources to the field of injury prevention and control.

The five principal areas of study in injury control are:

1. Epidemiology
2. Prevention
3. Injury biomechanics, which applies the principles of mechanics in studying the physical and functional responses of the human body to the traumatic impact of energy
4. Treatment, including emergency response

5. Rehabilitation, the process by which an injured person's functional capacities are restored or developed to the fullest extent possible, consistent with irreversible impairments and environmental limitations.

The Public Health model of injury prevention and control offers opportunities for decreasing the incidence of injuries using the following approaches:

1. Surveillance, including feedback from those conducting surveillance to those being studied and to those with a need to know
2. Interdisciplinary education and prevention programs
3. Environmental modifications
4. Regulatory action
5. The support of clinical interventions.

C. EPIDEMIOLOGIC CONSTRUCTS

An injury is a problem of medical ecology - that is, it is a problem in the relationship between one or more individuals and the surrounding environment, related to time. An epidemiologic web consisting of factors relating to the host or individual, the physical and social environments, the agent, and the vector can be delineated for injuries, as well as for infectious and chronic diseases.

1. Host

The host, or affected individual, has been the principal focus of the research related to injuries and preventive measures aimed at decreasing injury rates. An injury may result when the requirements of a task being performed exceeded an individual's performance capacity, which varies with the individual's physical, psychological, and cognitive abilities.

Ergonomics, or human factors research focuses on the interface between the host's capabilities and the environmental and task demands. A risk factor is an attribute, determinant, or exposure that is associated with an increased probability of a condition or outcome. Host factors that affect the risk of injuries differ according to the type of injury, as do some risk indicators. Characteristics such as race, are more appropriately called risk indicators, not risk factors. Risk indicators:

a. Age
b. Sex
c. Race
d. Alcohol use: the use of alcohol increases the risk of injuries
e. Drug use:

   (1) Medications such as tranquilizers and barbiturates, increase the rate of injuries when they interfere with adaptive performance.
   (2) Illegal drugs. The use of cocaine and other illegal rugs has been associated with fatal motor vehicle-related injuries. In addition, these drugs often are used in association with alcohol.

f.   Physical condition:

    (1)   Chronic medical conditions. Some chronic medical conditions, such as poor vision and uncontrolled seizure disorders, increase the risk of injuries.
    (2)   Physiologic status. Osteoporosis, which is often related to endocrine status, increases the risk of fall-related injuries.

2. Environment

Physical environment is the location at which the injury occurs. Examples of alterations made in the physical environment that can increase or reduce the risk of injuries include the following:

a.   Road design can decrease or increase the risk of injuries
b.   Homes can be built or equipped with safety features, such as smoke detectors and automatic sprinkler systems, in which case a fire is less likely to result in fire and flame-related injuries than a fire in a home without such devices
c.   Swimming pools with fences are safer than pools without feces.

Social environment consists of societal attitudes, laws, and regulations that control or tolerate the occurrence of events that can lead to injuries. Example of social environmental factors that increase the risk of injuries include:

a.   Tolerance of violent behavior
b.   Economic deprivation
c.   Racism
d.   Sexism.

3. Agents

The injury-causing agent is energy. A large amount of energy quickly transmitted may result in injury, while a small amount of energy transmitted over a long period of time may result in disease.

There are 5 types of energy that cause injuries:

a.   Kinetic or mechanical energy (the most common cause of injuries)
b.   Thermal energy
c.   Electrical energy
d.   Radiation energy
e.   Chemical energy

4. Vector

The vectors, or vehicles of injury, are the carriers of the energy. The design of the vector markedly alters the amount of energy available to cause an injury. Examples of vector factors that alter the occurrence of injuries follow: weapons, automobiles, electric wires.

D. MEASURES OF IMPACT

1. Morbidity

Incidence – In the United States, on an average day, 405 people die of injuries, 7,500 get hospitalized because of nonfatal injuries, and 162,000 people suffer injuries severe enough to restrict their usual activities and – in 92% of those cases – require that they seek medical attention. So, each year, about one-fourth of the U.S. population will fall victim to nonfatal injuries requiring some medical attention. More than two-and-one-half million people are hospitalized annually as the result of injuries, and 8% of all short-stay admissions are injury related. **Host factors** - Incidence of most nonfatal injuries decrease with age; hospitalization increases with age; incidence rate of injuries is higher in males than females.

2. Mortality

Each year 150,000 Americans die as the result of injuries. Injury ranks third among causes of death overall, and it constitutes the second most costly health problem in U.S., after heart disease. Mortality rates of unintentional injuries are higher in rural areas, and mortality rates of intentional injuries are higher in urban areas. Fatal motor vehicle injuries outnumber by 125 to 1 deaths from cystic fibrosis, a disease that is the object of considerable public concern.

   Years of life lost (YLL) is a measure of premature death; it is the difference between the age at death and the age of life expectancy. If the difference age at death and an arbitrary cutoff for productive or potential age is measured, it is called the **years of productive (or potential) life lost (YPLL)**. The constant endpoint methods generally emphasize the causes of death that have a greater impact on younger people, while the methods based on remaining life expectancy resemble the patterns of crude mortality. The impact of mortality is based on the age at death, with the YPLL varying inversely with the age at death. Injuries cause about **5.3** million YLL and are the leading cause of YPLL accounting for about 3.7 million YPLL annually in the Unite States.

3. Direct and Indirect Cost

Economic costs include medical and related expenses, wage losses, insurance administration costs, indirect work losses (e.g., long-term disability, premature death), and associated property damage. Pain and emotional sequelae of injured and their families are incalculable.

E. CLASSIFICATIONS

1. Intent:

Injuries are classified by the intent or purposefulness of occurrence:

a. Intentional Injuries

Purposely inflicted and often are associated with violence:

(1) Child abuse
(2) Domestic violence
(3) Sexual assault
(4) Aggravated assault
(5) Homicide
(6) Suicide
(7) Abuse of elderly

b. Unintentional Injuries

Injuries that are not purposely inflicted:

(1) Motor vehicle mishaps
(2) Falls
(3) Poisonings
(4) Drownings
(5) Fire and burns

c. Distinction between Intentional and Unintentional Injuries

It is often difficult to define the intent of an injury; thus, the distinction between intentional and unintentional injuries can be tenuous and artificial, as in the following examples. Although motor vehicle-related injuries are generally classified as unintentional, vehicular assault is not uncommon. Automobiles intentionally built without certain safety features (i.e., without air bags) could result in injury to the occupants during a crash, and while the crash may be unintentional, the result in injuries could be considered preventable, and, conceivably, intentional.

Intentional injury is a particularly difficult problem. War, civil unrest, homicide, suicide, and assault all reflect deeply rooted social problems. Although they are usually beyond the scope of the environmental health professional's duties, the control of intentional violence is a fundamental problem combining human rights, social development international cooperation, peacekeeping, and law enforcement. The decrease in CO levels in domestic gas has been accompanied by decreases in both unintentional poisonings and suicides due to domestic gas.

2. Place of Occurrence

There are four principal locations at which injuries occur:

a. Motor vehicles

Motor vehicles are an integral part of our lives. They transport people and goods, provide recreational opportunities, and are used by millions of Americans on their jobs. Although they thus provide mobility for much of our society, their widespread use and the speeds at which they travel create the potential (although not the necessity) for injury and death to their occupants and other road users. Most injuries from motor vehicles result when mechanical energy is conveyed to people in amounts or at rates that exceed their injury thresholds.

b. Workplace

The incidence of repetitive motion injuries, especially carpal tunnel syndrome, is increasing rapidly. Manufacturing jobs were associated with the greatest number of injuries.

c. Home

Home injuries occur in the house and the surrounding premises, including swimming pools. Causes of home injuries include fires, drownings, suffocation, falls, firearms, and poisonings.

d. Public place

About 29 million injuries occur in public places (e.g., parks, lakes, rivers, golf courses, athletic stadiums) in the United Sates annually.

3. Nature of Injury

The **International Classification of Diseases (ICD)** is the principal classification scheme that defines the nature of injuries (**N codes**):

a. The ICD code is the primary coding mechanism for diseases and conditions and the secondary coding mechanism for injuries after classification by external cause.
b. The ICD code provides information concerning necessary health care resources and services.
c. It is most useful when accompanied by the classifications by external cause and by severity of injury: (1) **abbreviated injury scale**; (2) **injury severity scale**; (3) **consumer product safety commission hazard index**; (4) **revised trauma score**; and (5) **pediatric trauma score.**

Injury classified by the nature of the injury are classified by the part of the body that was injured and the type of damage that occurred, including injuries resulting from infectious or parasitic agents.

4. External Cause of Injury

The ICD supplementary classification of external causes of injuries and poisonings (**E codes**) is the principal classification scheme that defines the external cause of injuries; classifies the injuries by apparent intent; provides information concerning etiology; is used in conjunction with the nature of injury codes. The most important external causes of injury are:

a. Injuries by motor vehicle are the leading cause of injury mortality;

b. Falls are the leading cause of injury morbidity for all age-groups and of injury mortality among people over 75 years of age;
c. Suffocation is the leading cause of injury mortality among children less than 1 year of age;
d. Firearms cause 60% of all homicides and suicides and result in about 30,000 deaths each year in the United States. Almost half of all deaths among young black males are firearms related. In Canada, firearms cause about one-third of all suicide and homicides.

F. SURVEILLANCE SYSTEMS

Surveillance systems for injuries measure the incidence of various injuries and their severity, describe the risk factors and indicators involved, and may measure the effectiveness of interventions.

1. Federal Agencies

CDC of Public Health Services, Division of Injury Epidemiology and Control was created to accomplish:

a. Providing epidemiologic assistance
b. Improving surveillance systems
c. Assisting state and local health departments to develop injury control programs
d. Supporting university-based injury prevention research center, epidemiologic research, and demonstration projects.

The Consumer Product Safety Commission was created in 1972 to protect the public from unreasonable risks of injuries associated with consumer products. The commission maintains the National Injury Information Clearinghouse as a repository for product-related injury information. The commission runs the National Electronic Injury Surveillance System, which obtains data from 91 hospitals emergency departments that were chosen as a national probability sample of all United Sates hospital emergency departments. Estimates of national product-related injury incidence are derived from the system.

2. State and Local Agencies

Departments of Health (DH): DH conduct surveillance of fatal injuries as part of their vital statistics function. An increasing number of state and local departments of health are conducting surveillance of non-fatal injuries and developing injury prevention and control programs. The Council of State and Territorial Epidemiologists recommended in 1987 that traumatic spinal cord injuries, which were legally reportable in 10 states, be designated the first injury condition reportable to all state health departments.

In support of this, the CDC currently maintains surveillance for spinal cord injuries using a uniform clinical case definition. **Transportation Departments** conduct surveillance of motor vehicle crashes and injuries. **Police Departments** conduct surveillance of violent and intentional injuries and motor vehicle crashes and injuries.

Departments of Labor conduct surveillance of occupational injuries. **Fire Departments** conduct surveillance of fire and flame-related injuries.

3. Other Organizations

The **National Safety Council**, a nongovernmental, nonprofit, public service organization chartered by an act of Congress, annually compiles data from many sources on injury morbidity, mortality, and costs and conducts injury prevention programs. It publishes a yearly update of data. **Researchers** in public health and medical schools, universities, hospitals, corporations, and unions conduct studies on injury epidemiology and prevention. **Numerous public health and clinical professional and voluntary organizations** provide support for the study and prevention of injuries, conduct injury prevention programs and campaigns, and educate professionals and the public.

G. MODELS OF PREVENTION

The practical approach to the prevention and control of injuries should involve strategies chosen on the basis of their actual effectiveness in reducing injuries, not on the relative importance or the time of occurrence of the causal or contributing factors they influence. Usually a combination of strategies and interventions are most effective. For example, the safest automobile restraint system incorporates both air bags and seat belts.

1. Passive and Active strategies

To approach any of the injury problems, it is necessary to understand a few key concepts in injury prevention. One such concept is the distinction between active and passive approaches to injury control. The distinction lies in the level of effort or action required on the part of individuals for the strategy to be effective. **Active strategies** are those requiring initiative (such as seat belt use) whereas **passive strategies** lie at the opposite end of the continuum - little or no action is required (such as automobile airbags). **Active strategies** are voluntary, require repetitive, individual action to be protective, and are generally less effective. **Passive strategies** are automatic, require no individual or repetitive action to be protective, and are generally the most effective. The consensus within the injury prevention field is that passive strategies should be employed wherever available, and when active strategies are necessary, they are most effective when mandated. The need for a flexible combination of strategies has been recognized.

2. The four Es of Intervention

The four Es of Intervention are the following:

    Engineering Interventions – These are aimed at the vectors and physical environments that promote or support the occurrence of injuries. These interventions, which are often passive, are among the most effective in decreasing the occurrence of injuries. For example, medicine containers were redesigned to be child-proof.

    Economic Interventions - These are aimed at influencing behavior based on monetary incentives and rewards or penalties. For example, many insurance companies have lower rates for residences equipped with smoke detectors and sprinkler systems.

Enforcement Interventions – These are aimed at influencing behavior by laws and regulations that may only be effective when enforced. For example, since 1978, every state has made the use of federally approved child safety seats mandatory for children who ride in automobiles. The enforcement of these laws, however, is variable.

Educational Interventions – These are aimed at influencing behavior through reasoning and knowledge. These interventions are usually the least effective, especially when used alone without other interventions. Educational interventions could be more effective if they were directed toward societal leaders and decision-makers. For example, because high school driver education programs are often accompanied by licensure at younger ages and by an increase in the proportion of young people who drive, populations with these programs have relatively more motor vehicle crashes among young people than populations that do not have such programs.

3. Haddon Models

Injury prevention measures, such as the use of protective clothing in warfare, existed long before injuries were systematically studied. In the early 1940s, one of the first epidemiologic studies recognize the importance of studying defined populations using comparison groups. Studies compared head injury incidence between helmeted and unhelmeted motorcycle riders in the military. These studies demonstrated a decrease in head injuries among those riders wearing helmets. In 1949, John Gordon noted that injuries were patterned by age, gender, and other demographic factors, as well as by time and place.

He recognized that "accidents" could be studied utilizing epidemiologic methods similar to those used in infectious or chronic disease prevention. In 1961, James Gibson defined the agent of injury as energy in its many forms. William Haddon Jr. placed this theory into a framework, which identified vehicles and vectors of injury occurrence, analogous to the models used for the study of infectious diseases. He recognized that injuries occur when energy delivered to a living host from a vehicle or vector exceeds human tolerance. He further categorized the energy-host interaction into (a) the energy delivered in excess of human tolerance, such as mechanical energy in motor vehicle crashes or in falls, and (b) interference with energy use in normal metabolic functions, such as occurs in drownings or poisonings. Using these basic ideas as a framework, Haddon created a comprehensive matrix of host-energy interactions, which is discussed later in this chapter.

Surviving the crash of his trainer aircraft, Hugh DeHaven found a connection between his abdominal injuries and the shape and riveting location of his safety belt. In 1941, DeHaven studied ways in which engineering could reduce the severity of injuries during motor vehicle crashes. His work bred new studies on human tolerance to energy forces during many types of impacts. His approach using biomechanical principles coupled with epidemiologic evaluation is now prominent in motor vehicle crash research.

Haddon Models, formulated by Dr.William Haddon, Jr., are useful for determining possible interventions and prevention measures for particular injuries. The Haddon Matrix (Table 13.2), or multifactorial approach, arranges intervention and prevention strategies by agent, vector, host, and physical and social environmental factors, according to the time at which the strategy would be effective in relation to the occurrence of the injury event.

Table 13.2. Matrix for the Analysis of Accidents. (Source: Moeller, 1997).

Phases	Factors		
	Human	**Equipment**	**Physical and socioeconomic environment**
Pre-event	1	2	3
Event	4	5	6
Post-event	7	8	9

This model emphasizes the time of action in reference to the injury event. Haddon Matrix provides examples of each factor- and phase-specific strategy concerning motor vehicle-related injuries. Because motor vehicle accidents account for almost half the deaths resulting from unintentional injuries in the US, they are provided as examples in the following discussion:

Pre-event Phase - The goal is to reduce the likelihood of a vehicular collision. Factors that should be considered include:

a. **Humans** involved: driver impairment by alcohol or other drugs; the thoroughness of testing procedures for licensure; the degree of enforcement of traffic rules and regulations, including mandatory use of seat belts; and the availability of mass transportation as an alternative to the use of private vehicles;
b. **Equipment**: the condition of headlights, tire treads, and brakes (and whether they include antilock features); the size and visibility of brake lights; the speed the vehicle can attain; and vehicular crash tests;
c. **Environment**: the presence of barriers and traffic lights to protect pedestrians; the design, placement, and maintenance of road signs for ready comprehension; and the design of bridge abutments to prevent or reduce impact damage.

Event phase - The goal is to reduce the severity of the "second collision," as when the victim hits the windshield or steering column. Factors that can reduce the extent of injuries include:

a. **Humans** involved: occupants' use of vehicles equipped with air bags, proper use of seat belts and child-resistant systems, and driver abstention from alcohol (which affects cell membrane permeability so that even in low-impact collisions people who have consumed alcohol are more likely to sustain severe or even fatal neurological damage);
b. **Equipment**: whether the vehicle is equipped with a collapsible steering column, high-penetration-resistant windshield, interior padding (for example, on the dashboard), recessed door handles and control knobs, and structural beams in doors; low bumpers with square fronts to reduce the likelihood of pelvic and leg fractures in

pedestrians who are hit; and, on trucks, a bar under the rear end to prevent cars from going beneath them;

c. **Environment**: breakaway sign posts, open space along the sides of the road, wide multiple lanes, guard rails to steer vehicles back onto the road, and road surfaces that permit rapid stopping.

Post-event Phase - The goal is to reduce the disabilities due to the injuries. Factors that can reduce or limit the effects of injuries include:

a. **Humans** involved: rapid and appropriate emergency medical care, followed by adequate rehabilitation; properly trained rescue personnel; and injury severity scores to help medical personnel evaluate multiple traumas and predict outcomes;
b. **Equipment**: fireproof gasoline tanks to prevent fires after an accident
c. **Environment**: public telephones along the roadway for summoning emergency help; helicopters for rapid transport of victims to medical-care facilities; trauma centers equipped to handle injured victims; ramps and other environmental changes to reduce the real "cost" to the victims of being disabled; and rehabilitation of the victims.

Successful reduction of injuries incorporates many approaches and knowledge from many types of professionals because of the nature and elements in the chain of events leading to injury. The role of human behavior, which includes voluntary risk-taking, the use of behavior-altering substances, and lack of knowledge regarding safe behavior, coupled with physical limitations in perception, reaction time, and attention, which vary by individual, creates a complex set of conditions for host response. Agents of energy and environments in which energy is transferred to the host change constantly with a technologically expanding world. The interaction of the agent, host, and environment provides many opportunities for intervention, but experience has shown that introducing change into one injury element without considering the other components will rarely be effective.

Prevention strategies should be founded on an understanding of the hazard, its introduction into the human environment, and exposure to the host. This understanding needs to incorporate the state of the physical, sociocultural, and political climate in which the hazard interacts with the host. Of the many successful injury control strategies, the majority "control" rather than eliminate energy transfer. "Control" acts by reducing the magnitude of the energy transfer, thereby reducing the severity of the injury incurred, For example, neither seat belts nor helmets prevent all injuries, but they are very effective in reducing the amount of injury transferred to the host and therefore in reducing injury sustained.

In 1962, William Haddon Sr. defined the strategies for injury control into 10 logically distinct categories. However, the 10 countermeasures are not always mutually exclusive; for certain injuries a number of the countermeasures may point to the same intervention. They evolved from the Haddon Matrix (See Table 13.2). They are injury prevention strategies based on the energy exchanges that result in injuries and the need to minimize injuries that have occurred.

The following is a list of the 10 countermeasures along with examples of successful injury-control strategies in use:

(1) Preventing Creation of the Agent - Preventing creation of the agent aims to stop the production of the agent before it can present a hazard. This approach is theoretically the most effective but is not often a realistic alternative. Although motor vehicles are known to be the cause of many fatalities and injuries, they are essential for modem living. Preventing the manufacture of motor vehicles would not only be difficult to implement but would have unfavorable economic consequences. However, it is feasible to control the production of dangerous vehicles with demonstrated mechanical failures or operating failures. An example of this approach is the recall of motor vehicles with significant hazards to safe operation. Other examples are the following: banning the manufacture and sale of inherently unsafe products or prohibiting inherently unsafe practices (e.g., stop producing firecrackers, three-wheeled all-terrain vehicles, or various poisons).

(2) Reducing the Amount of the Agent - Reducing the amount of the agent involves identifying a hazard and reducing its presence in the environment. One example of this intervention is seen in unintentional drug overdose among the elderly. In a study many years ago at the Maryland Poison Center, unintentional poisonings from oral medications were noted in the elderly population). The interventions involved better packaging and labeling to reduce the chances of ingesting extra doses of medicine due to forgetfulness or failure to understand the purpose and interactions of all medications. The agent (pills) was reduced by limiting the number in each prescription so that taking them all at once would not kill or disable an individual. Another approach could include comprehensive review by physicians of all medications prescribed and taken voluntarily so that potentially harmful combinations or overmedication can be avoided. Other examples would be the following: limit the muzzle velocity of guns and the amount of gunpowder in firecrackers; limit the horsepower of motor vehicle engines; and package toxic drugs in smaller, safer amounts.

(3) Preventing Release of the Agent - Preventing release of the agent deters it from entering the environment and hence reduces exposure. Childproof safety caps on medicine dispensers is an example of this approach because the potentially harmful substance cannot be obtained by a child. The introduction of the Poison Prevention Packaging Act in the late 1970s played a significant role in reducing by over 50 percent poisonings in children ages 0 to 4). This act incorporates engineering (through the design of the child-resistant container), education (through the need to identify and address the problem), and enforcement (through mandatory compliance by manufacturers).

Another example of this countermeasure involves falls. Among those 65 and older in the United States, 2.3 million are injured due to falls, leading to nearly 9,000 deaths, 370,000 hospitalizations per year, and aggregate lifetime costs of 9.8 billion dollars). Providing the elderly with canes or walkers and installing handrails and traction strips in stairways and bathtubs decreases the number of falls in this population. One community-based program to reduce falls in senior citizens reported a 60 percent reduction in falls following this type of intervention. Other examples would be the following: store firearms in locked containers and close pools and beaches when no lifeguard is on duty.

(4) Modifying the Rate or Spatial Distribution of the Agent - Modifying the rate or spatial distribution of the agent involves altering the mechanism by which energy is transferred to the host. Use of child restraints and seat belts in automobiles reduces the risk of injury of drivers and passengers when crashes occur. Laws enforcing the presence of safety equipment in automobiles and their use by occupants are in effect, helping increase the number of people who benefit from this strategy. Seat belt use reduces motor vehicle fatalities and serious injuries by 40 to 55 percent. The lap portion of the lap-shoulder belt protects against rider ejection from the motor vehicle and the shoulder harness portion reduces violent contact with the car interior.

The effectiveness of seat belts in reducing large numbers of fatalities and injuries nationwide, however, rests with compliance to mandated laws requiring their use. The National Highway Traffic Safety Administration (NHTSA) estimates that for 1990 more than 5,770 fatal injuries would have been averted by lap/shoulder belts if at least half of all car occupants wore them. NHTSA estimated in 1988 that 4,573 lives were saved and that 15,959 lives could have been saved if everyone had worn safety belts. The cost of introducing and maintaining a mandatory seat belt law is only $69 per life- year saved, which is considerably smaller than the costs of treating injured drivers.

(5) Separating the Host and Agent, in Time or Space - Separation of the host and agent prevents an injurious event by eliminating contact between the energy source and the host. Road designs that separate vulnerable road users from potential hazards are one type of prevention using this approach. Removing pedestrians and bicyclists from vehicle traffic through signal control, overhead crossings, and bicycle trails are other examples. This strategy can be, at times, inexpensive and easily implemented to protect children from toxic substances. One method of reducing poisonings from household cleaners and other toxic substances is placing toxic agents and poisonous substances in locked cabinets or out of children's reach. Other examples are the following: provide pedestrian overpasses at high volume traffic crossings and do not have play areas near unguarded bodies of water.

(6) Separating the Agent from a Susceptible Host by Interposition of a Material Barrier - Interposition of a material barrier separates the agent from a host, preventing or minimizing damage to the host. Use of air bags in motor vehicles is an example of this countermeasure. It is estimated that air bags are 18 percent effective in mitigating serious driver injuries, 18 percent effective in preventing fatalities to drivers, and 13 percent effective in reducing fatalities to right front-seat passengers. Other examples are the following: install fencing to enclose all four sides of swimming pools; insulate electrical cords; provide protective eyewear for racquet sports; build highway medians; and make use of bulletproof barriers

(7) Modifying Relevant Qualities of the Agent - Injuries may be lessened through modification of agent characteristics. Modification of the transfer of thermal energy is an example of this approach. Burns are extremely painful, often resulting in severe physical and psychological damage. The current average hospital Stay for a moderately severe burn is 17 days with a hospital cost of approximately $42,500. This does not include the costs for reconstructive surgery, physical therapy, and psychological counseling. Clothing ignition, once a pronounced source of burn injury, has been reduced through the legislatively mandated use of flame-retardant materials for children's sleepwear. However, the use of cotton fabrics in children's sleepwear is re-emerging without appropriate clothing warnings. Many burns occurring among young or elderly populations result from high-temperature tap water. These scalds are easily prevented by regulating hot water heater levels to no more than 120^0C. These anti-scald devices are readily available and can easily be installed on existing plumbing.

(8) Strengthening the Susceptible Host - Strengthening the host is also a possible means for preventing in. juries. Alcohol consumption not only increases the risk of all types of injuries, including motor vehicle crashes and falls, but also significantly alters physiological response after head injury by promoting secondary injury processes. Strengthening the susceptible host can also occur through health promotion activities. Regular exercise helps strengthen muscles and improve balance and coordination, which reduces the potential for injury. Nutrition programs that increase bone density in older persons can help prevent falls and injury from falls.

(9) Countering the Injury Already Caused by the Agent - This approach to injury prevention involves immediate intervention after energy transfer has occurred. Regional poison control centers are an effective approach in providing early care when poisonous substances have been ingested. Poison control centers provide a phone hotline with immediate advice on the appropriate action to take depending on the substance ingested. An evaluation of Massachusetts poison control centers found that 1 percent of parents who called the poison control center after ingestion of a hazardous substance by their child went to the emergency room, compared with 44 percent of those who did not call the centers. Furthermore, only 0.5 percent of those calling the center made unnecessary trips to emergency departments compared with 28 percent of those who did not call. Providing immediate resuscitation to injured individuals is essential to recovery. In a study of children with submersion injuries, those who received immediate resuscitation were five times more likely to have a good outcome than those not receiving resuscitation. Hence, cardiopulmonary resuscitation (CPR) certification should be required, especially of mothers with small children and others working with vulnerable populations.

(10) Stabilizing, Repairing, and Rehabilitating the Injured Host - Once damage has occurred, stabilization, repair, and rehabilitation help restore function and aid in ensuring quality of life. In the event that an individual needs therapy or is disabled, his or her quality of life is dependent upon access to rehabilitation, assistance by equipment such as wheelchairs and personal attendants, and structural access to buildings and transportation. Successful rehabilitation involves a comprehensive approach to health care and a focus on returning the injured individual to a life of quality and not just subsistence. The team approach to rehabilitation developed in the 1930s involves treatment of patients by rehabilitation specialists in conjunction with other medical providers including orthopedists, neurologists, and psychiatrists. Current efforts involve an even more comprehensive approach, which begins the process of rehabilitation soon after emergency care.

4. Clinical Prevention

A decade ago, the U.S. Preventive Services Task Force evaluated health promotion and disease and injury prevention activities applicable to primary care practitioners. Practitioners should be aware of the specific injury prevention counseling and screening activities and the signs and symptoms by patient age-group. Some injury prevention activities should be undertaken for all patients in the age-group while others are for patients at high risk.

IV. SELECTED TYPES OF INJURIES

A. LIGHTNING

1. Introduction

Lightning is responsible for between 50 and 300 deaths annually (depending on which study one reads). This number may be significantly underreported due to a lack of formal data collection. There are numerous reports of lightning strikes entering a building through electrical and telephone wires, and even through the plumbing.

In several different studies, the diameter of a lightning stroke has been measured at between 3 and 8 cm. Temperature in the arc channel rises to 8000°C then quickly falls to 1500-2000°C. These strikes last between 0.001 and 0.0001 second, although "hot lightning" strikes lasting between 0.5 and 1 second have been reported.

The most common form of lightning is the well-known forked electrical arc known as **streak lightning**. In addition, there is a shapeless flash between clouds called **sheet lightning. Ribbon lightning** is streak lightning that is blown horizontally by high winds and produces parallel lines on the return stroke. **Ball lightning** is the least understood of all forms of lightning. It takes the shape of a softball-sized globe and is characterized by bizarre & unexplained activity (such as entering the front door, chasing a homeowner thru the house, & exiting the back way).

2. Five Primary Mechanisms of Injury Due To Lightning

a. **Direct Hit**: Self-explanatory,
b. **Splash:** The electricity hits another object and 'splashes" onto a person standing close,
c. **Contact**: A person is holding onto something that is hit directly,
d. **Step Voltage**: The victim is in a position in which one foot is farther away than the other from the strike point. The current travels along the ground until it reaches the closer foot. Resistance is lower through the body than across the ground, therefore the current takes the path of least resistance up the closer leg and down the other one,
e. **Blunt Trauma**: The victim is thrown by severe muscle contractions caused by the current. Additionally, explosive and/or implosive forces associated with rapid healing and cooling of air may produce injuries similar to those caused by high explosives.

3. <u>Pathway of Lightning Current in the Body</u>

Initially the lightning energy is transmitted to the interior of the body (especially through openings in the skull in the case of a head strike) through the skin and along nerves, vessels, and tissue, as are other electrical impulses. Relatively quickly (measured in microseconds), the massive impulse overwhelms the conductivity of the skin so that the majority of energy "flashes over" the outside of the body along routes of water and minerals (sweat, rain, etc.). This "flashover" appreciably decreases the amount of energy absorbed by the body and allows survival in many victims. Lightning that enters openings in the skull seems to focus on the floor of the fourth ventricle of the brain. There, it paralyzes the cardiac and respiratory centers.

Immediate lightning injuries are the following:

a. Ventricular asystole,
b. Neurologic damage indicated by seizures, change in level of consciousness, amnesia, or blindness,
c. Contusion from the shock wave,
d. Chest pain, muscle aches, and
e. Rupture of the tympanic membrane.

Following are the different categories of injuries:

Minor Injuries - Dysesthesia, or feeling like having been hit on the head. May or may not remember the lightning or thunder. Symptoms can include amnesia, temporary deafness or blindness, and temporary unconsciousness at the scene. Usually have at least one tympanic membrane or eardrum rupture and few if any bums. Vital signs are stable although occasionally there is a transient mild hypotension. Recovery is usually rapid and complete.

Moderate Injuries - Level of consciousness marked by disorientation, combativeness, or coma. Paralysis, especially involving the lower extremities, is common. Arterial spasm may cause diminished or absent peripheral pulses and a mottled appearance of the skin. Temporary cardiac standstill may be present in this group, although the automaticity of the heart may cause spontaneous pulse. Respiratory arrest may continue for a period of time after the heartbeat resumes. Burns may not be prominent immediately but may develop over several hours. 'Toe tip' burns may be noted (punctuate burns of the tips of the toes). Ruptured eardrums should be anticipated. Improvement in the first few hours can be expected, but long-term or permanent residuals have been reported. These sequelae include sleep disorders, paresthesias, and posttramatic stress disorder.

Severe Injuries: Cardiac arrest (either ventricular standstill or fibrillation). Eardrum rupture with cerebrospinal fluid leakage is common. Prognosis is poor, especially if cardiopulmonary resuscitation has been delayed.

The different types of burns in lightning strike are the following:

Linear Burns - First- and second-degree burns beginning at the head and progressing to the chest, where they split and continue down both legs.

They generally follow areas of heavy sweat concentrations (may represent sweat heated into steam).

Punctuate burns - Multiple closely spaced full-thickness burns from a few millimeters to a centimeter in diameter, sometimes located at the point of strike, sometimes at distal toe tips.

Feathering or Ferning – This is pathognomonic of lightning strikes. Delicate imprints resembling fern fronds on the skin represent the tracks of electron showers over the skin.

Thermal burns - Burns from the ignition of clothing or heated metal (e.g., coins carried in a pocket).

B. ELECTRICAL INJURIES

Hands are the most commonly injured body part, because they are the "tool" with which humans work. Electricity causes muscles to spasm (usually in a flexion "grip"), thereby "freezing" hands to the contacted circuit. The current arcs across flexed joints, causing "kissing burns" at each flexion point. High-voltage electricity burns are characterized by deep muscle, nerve, and vascular damage, and both entry and exit wounds are commonly seen. Extensive amputations are not infrequent with these injuries.

C. DIVING HAZARDS

Commercial divers make their living diving and may be involved in underwater construction, harvesting seafood, or gathering specimens for scientific purposes. Recreational diving is a popular sport in which many people participate. Diving may cause certain medical conditions to arise, such as decompression illness, which may mimic neurologic symptoms caused by environmental toxic elements or degenerative nerve diseases.

Types of Diving and Clinical Issues - Diving may take place in very shallow water or at depths of 1000 feet or more in the open ocean. The breathing gas may be air, nitrogen-oxygen mixtures, or helium-oxygen mixtures. Recreational or commercial divers use air or nitrogen-oxygen mixtures at depths shallower than 220 feet of seawater (fsw). Commercial diving using helium-oxygen at depths greater than 220 (fsw) will usually have specialized medical personnel on scene or in close touch with diving operations.

Kinds Of Breathing Apparatus Used By Recreational Divers - The self-contained underwater breathing apparatus (SCUBA) is most common. Most SCUBA regulators are of an open-circuit demand-valve type whereby the diver inhales gas from a tank then exhales all gas into the water. Closed and semi-closed SCUBA regulators retain part oral of the inhaled gas after eliminating CO2 with a chemical absorbent. The SCUBA apparatus is carried on a diver's back, allowing free, untethered swimming.

Kinds Of Breathing Apparatus Used By Commercial Divers - Open-circuit, closed-circuit, and semi-closed-circuit SCUBA gear may be used, but only rarely. Most commercial divers use surface-supplied open-circuit hard helmets. The hard helmet is usually made of heavy- duty reinforced fiberglass containing a specially designed open-circuit SCUBA regulator. Breathing gas is supplied from a boat at the surface through a long umbilical hose, which may also contain communication lines and a hot water hose for heating the diver. A backpack gas cylinder is for emergency use.

Military divers follow procedures developed by the U.S. Navy and have direct access to the medical expertise of specially trained Diving Medical Officers.

Commercial divers are civilians who receive any form of compensation for diving (money, equipment, discounts on trips or equipment, etc.) and must follow Occupational Safety and Health Administration (OSHA), U.S. Coast Guard, and in some cases state regulations. Larger commercial companies generally employ diving medical experts to look after their divers, but some smaller companies with part-time commercial divers may end up relying on local medical care.

Recreational Divers and Self-Regulation - Recreational divers participate in diving as a sport and are largely self-regulated. In the United States, the American National Standards Institute (ANSI) sets the minimum criteria for recreational SCUBA certification. Agencies that actually train divers [Professional Association of Diving Instructors (PADI), SCUBA Schools International (SSI), National Association of Underwater Instructors (NAUI), Young Men's Christian Association (YMCA), National Academy of SCUBA Educators (NASE) etc.] must conform to ANSI standards for their certification to be recognized. Certification is usually necessary to buy life support gear (e.g., tanks and regulators), get advanced training, and fill tanks with breathing gas. Similar certification mechanisms are in place in other countries.

OSHA Regulations And Commercial Diving - OSHA regulations spell out personnel requirements, certain dive procedures, safety precautions, and types of medical equipment that must be available during diving operations. They also require that there be a safe practices manual governing all diving operations. Large commercial operations will develop their own safe practices manual, but the Association of Diving Contractors (ADC) Consensus Standards for Commercial Diving Operations, the U.S. Navy Diving Manual, or NOAA Diving Manual may form the basis of a safe practices manual.

Physical Standards - Divers should be in relatively good physical shape and able to exercise at a level of at least 13 mets (metabolic equivalents; 1 met = 3.5 ml oxygen 1kg/mm), have no condition that would impair equilibration of the ears and sinuses, and have no evidence of lung lesions, which may be prone to gas trapping. The Association of Diving Contractors (ADC) has recommended standards for commercial divers.

The most important **medical conditions associated with diving** are the following:

1. Barotrauma

Barotrauma is caused when a gas-filled cavity within the body cannot equalize with changing ambient pressure. The most commonly affected structure is the middle ear, followed by the sinuses, lungs, and (rarely) teeth. In water, the ambient hydrostatic pressure increases I atmosphere absolute (ata; 760 mm Hg) for each 33 (fsw) increase in depth.

2. Decompression illness (DCI)

DCI refers to disease that arise when there is a reduction in ambient pressure after spending some time at increased pressures. Divers, tunnel workers, and pilots are usually at risk. Divers and tunnel workers go from 1 ata to an increased pressure for a period of time and then return, or decompress, back to 1 ata after their risk is finished. Pilots are saturated at 1 ata but may be exposed to sudden depressurization at altitude. DCI includes decompression sickness, CAGE (Cerebral Arterial Gas Embolism), and Chokes.

3. Reactions to environmental conditions

There are environmental hazards associated with diving. Depending on the water temperature, hyperthermia or hypothermia may occur; increased depth leads to increased gas density, causing dyspnea because of increased respiratory load. High oxygen partial pressures may cause oxygen toxicity and increased nitrogen partial pressure may cause nitrogen narcosis. Frequent exposure to immersion can lead to otitis externa.

4. Marine animal injuries.

Diving injuries caused by aquatic life are uncommon with the exception of scrapes and bruises from coral. Divers in unfamiliar waters should consult locals to see if any peculiar aquatic life hazards are present.

V. INJURY AND VIOLENCE

A. INTRODUCTION

Public health's first, critical contribution to the prevention of violence came with the very recognition that violence – by virtue of the enormous toll it takes in lives, health, and quality of life – is a health problem. Public Health also addresses itself to the social norms and attitudes that accept violence and deter prevention.
　　Violence is defined most broadly as the use of physical force with the intent to inflict injury or death upon oneself or another. For **public health**, the fact that violent acts may result in physical injuries is the primary motivation for involvement. The **behavioral sciences** see violence as a form of aggressive human behavior that can harm individuals and their families and communities. **Criminal justice** sees it as a violation of the law, that is, criminal acts. These perspectives overlap.

B. CONTEXT OF VIOLENCE

1. Cultures and Attitudes

By the time a typical adolescent graduate from high school he or she would have been exposed to 18,000 television murders and 800 suicides. The relation between televised acts of violence and individual behavior may be controversial. Child-rearing practices that convey to children the acceptability of violence can result in aggressive behavior both within and outside the home.

2. Socioeconomic Status

Racial minorities – most particularly Black Americans – bear a disproportionately large burden of interpersonal violence and poverty. When socioeconomic status is taken into consideration, the disparity between Black Americans and the general population as both victim and perpetrators of violence become quite small. Poverty and interpersonal violence, including homicide, are intimately related.

3. Firearms

Firearms play a key role in homicides. Reports showed that in 1986, three fifths of all homicides were committed with firearms; three quarters of the victims were killed with handguns. A more recent CDC report puts the percentage of homicides committed with a firearm at more than 70%. This increase has been even sharper among 15 to 24 year olds, rising from 67% in 1985 to 87% in 1994.

4. Alcohol

The link between alcohol and violence has been demonstrated in study after study. One analysis of 588 homicides in Philadelphia, for example, indicated that alcohol has been used by the victim, the perpetrator, or both in nearly two-thirds of the cases.

5. Drugs

The belief that there is a close and causal relationship between many forms of drug use and criminality and violent behavior probably form the basis for many of our laws concerning drug use and drug users.

C. VIOLENCE PREVENTION AS A PUBLIC HEALTH CONCERN

Until recently, violence was not considered a traditional public health problem. That view is changing as people realize the extent which violence meets traditional criteria as a threat to public health and the contribution that a public health approach can make violence prevention.

First, the magnitude of the problem in terms of health consequences is great. For example, in 1994, suicide ranked as the ninth leading cause of death; and homicide, as the eleventh leading cause. Further, violence affects so many young people that each homicide suicide on the average results in many years of potential life lost. Homicide is the ninth leading cause of years of potential life lost and suicide is the eleventh leading cause. For younger age groups, violence takes an even greater toll. For African Americans 15 to 24 years f age, homicide is the leading cause of death. For all Americans in the 15 to 24-year age group, homicide is the second leading cause of death and suicide is the third leading cause of death. Moreover, these deaths represent only a fraction of the impact on the health and quality of life of the US population. For every death from assaultive violence, there are probably 100 times as many nonfatal injuries. Estimates also suggest that nearly 2 million women in the United States each year are assaulted by intimate partners, resulting in psychological as well as physical injury. The consequences of these assaults include fear, depression, and incapacitation, all of which greatly diminish the quality of the life of the women, their families, and their communities. In another example, firearm violence claims 18,000 lives from homicide and 17,000 from suicide each year. In nine states and the District of Columbia, firearm-related deaths outnumber fatalities caused by motor vehicle crashes. Firearms are the most common cause of injury deaths in the United States overall for young people ages 15 to 34. Injuries and disabilities related to violence impose a tremendous economic burden on the health sector, exceeding $105 billion annually. Firearm injuries are now the leading cause of death from traumatic brain injury (TBI), and to an ever-increasing degree, violence-related injuries are filling rehabilitation hospitals.

Second, no other sector takes responsibility for preventing these consequences of violence. The criminal justice sector has long acknowledged that, because most homicides occur among people who know each other and not in connection with any other felony, the police are not able to prevent most of these. Like suicide prevention, many violence-related injuries require societal interventions that can be planned and carried out by public health practitioners.

Third, the traditional tools of public health can be successfully applied to violence prevention, and public health practitioners can play an effective role in spearheading and coordinating prevention programs. The traditional tools of public health are rooted in the notion that ours is a cause-and-effect world and that we can both understand these causes and change this world by controlling those causes to bring about the desired effects. Violence prevention follows the four steps of the public health approach, the same approach that guides public health efforts in prevention of infectious diseases, chronic diseases, and environmental and occupational health problems. Because a common approach runs through efforts in each of these areas, it is not difficult for public health workers in any discipline to understand and work on a public health approach to violence prevention.

D. THE PUBLIC HEALTH APPROACH TO VIOLENCE PREVENTION

The public health approach to violence prevention is guided by three central concepts:

1. Prevention,

Although treatment for victims of violence is important, public health aims to prevent people from becoming injured in the first place and to prevent the perpetrators from ever resorting to violence. For example, it is important to have an adequate number of shelters for battered women, but if battering could be prevented in the first place, these shelters would not be needed. This focus on prevention does not in any way diminish the importance of providing care for victims or the importance of arresting and prosecuting perpetrators. Rather the approach complements the contributions of other fields such as the criminal justice system and emergency medical care.

2. Science

The four steps of the public health approach characterize this scientific method and provide a rational framework for examining the problems of violence. The four steps are:

a. **Surveillance** (what's the problem?),
b. **Risk factor identification** (what's the cause?),
c. **Intervention evaluation** (what works?), and
d. **Implementation** (how do you do it?).

3. Integrative Leadership or Teamwork

Violence prevention does not belong to any one field, domain, or discipline. It will require many disciplines and fields, and departments and agencies, all working together. It will require practitioners who implement programs into communities to work with researchers in designing and evaluating these programs.

E. EPIDEMIOLOGY OF FIREARM-RELATED DEATHS AND INJURIES

This same public health approach is useful in understanding the role that firearms play in contributing to death and injury. In 1994, firearm-related injuries were the eight leading cause of death in the United States accounting for 38,505 deaths, including suicides, 17,866 firearm homicides, 1,356 unintentionally. Compared to other causes of injury death in 1994, the number of firearm deaths are surpassed only by the number of motor-vehicle-related deaths (42,524). From 1968 to 1994, the number of motor-vehicle-related deaths steadily cycled downward, while the number of firearm-related deaths increased. If those trends continue, firearm injuries are predicted to replace motor-vehicle crashes as the leading cause of injury death in the United States by the year 2000. Overall firearm-related deaths are the leading cause of death for young people ages 15 to 34.

Males ages 15 to 24 years are at highest risk of being shot by another person when compared to other age and sex groups. Firearm death rates also vary by race, occupation, degree of urbanization, per capita income, and geographic area of residence, and internationally. Although firearm suicide rates are higher among Caucasians and American Indians/Alaskan Natives, firearm homicide rates are higher among African Americans. Homicide is the leading cause of occupational injury death among females and a majority of these involve the use of a firearm. Death rates from unintentional shootings and firearm suicide rates are higher in rural areas, but firearm homicide rates are highest in the largest cities. Firearm death rates are higher in low-income areas and in the Southeastern and Western regions of the United States. Among children less than 15 years of age, firearm death rates among U.S. children are 12 times higher than their counterparts from 25 other industrialized countries.

F. DEFINITION OF VIOLENCE AND BRIEF TYPOLOGY OF VIOLENCE

In May 1996, the 190 member nations of the World Health Assembly passed a resolution (WHO 49.25) declaring violence **"a public health priority worldwide."** This resolution directed the World Health Organization (WHO) to develop a plan of action for a science-based public health approach to violence prevention. The first step is to develop an operational definition of violence, which must recognize the many different forms that violence may take. It may take different forms within a single culture, where it may present as child abuse, youth violence, sexual assault, domestic violence, elder abuse, or child sexual abuse. And it may present in very different forms or manners in different cultures or countries.

The definition of violence will continue to evolve, but a good starting point is the definition adopted by the World Health Organization in **Violence: A Public Health Priority**, a working paper developed by the WHO Global Consultation on Violence and Health in December 1996: Violence is the intentional use of physical force or power, threatened or actual, against oneself, another person, or a group or community, that results in or has a high likelihood of resulting in injury, death, psychological harm, maldevelopment, or deprivation. The WHO working document identified three major types of violence which are the following:

Self-inflicted violence, which encompasses intentional and harmful behavior directed at oneself, with suicide being the most severe manifestation. Other forms are suicide attempts, mutilation, and behavior whose intent is self-destructive but not lethal.

Interpersonal violence, which consists of violent behavior that occurs between individuals, but is not organized or planned by social or political groups in which they participate. This type of violence can be classified by the victim-offender relationship, which distinguishes domestic violence (involving family and intimates) from violence among acquaintances and between strangers.

Organized violence is behavior that is planned to achieve, or motivated by, specific political, economic, or social objectives of an organized social or political group. This includes, for example, political violence in which efforts to violently intimidate an opposing political faction may be carefully planned and executed. War may be considered the most highly organized type of violence, and gang or mob violence is another category of organized violence.

In assessing the health impact of violence, it is useful to look at the problem globally. Although the United States has high rates of homicide and assaultive violence compared to those of other industrial countries, the problem of violence in many pans of the world greatly eclipses the dimension of violence in the United States. Estimates of the relative and absolute contribution of assaultive violence to the global health burden have recently become available through a project that provides a comprehensive assessment of mortality and disability from disease and injuries in 1990 and projected to 2020. The burden of assaultive violence is quantified by measures of two general types of health consequences:

1. Premature mortality as measured by numbers, rates, and years of life lost due to homicide, and
2. Combined burden of fatal and nonfatal health outcomes, as indicated by a new measure called disability-adjusted life years lost (DALYs).

Clearly violence is a global health problem of major and increasing proportions. The magnitude of the health consequences of this problem and its social and economic sequelae point to the need for effective prevention strategies, as well as strategies to mitigate the severity of the physical and emotional consequences of violence. In recognition of the magnitude of this problem and the power of the public health approach, the World Health Assembly passed its resolution in May 1996, declaring violence to be a public health priority worldwide.

G. ASSAULTIVE VIOLENCE

Each of the behaviors: assaultive violence, child abuse and child sexual assault, domestic violence, elder abuse, and rape and sexual assault – can result in death as well as nonfatal injury. One group of researchers has argued persuasively that "homicide represents the final common outcome of assaultive behaviors that are both very diverse in their characteristics and many times more common than homicide."

1. Definition of the Problem

In 1994, almost 25,000 people in the United States died from homicide, making this type of assaultive violence the eleventh leading cause of death and the fifth leading cause of premature mortality. In 1994, homicide ranked as the second leading cause of death among persons 15 to 24 years of age and was the leading cause of death for black males 15 to 24 years of age. The lifetime risk of death from homicides is 1 in 28 for black males compared with 1 in 164 for white males. And while homicide is the fatal outcome of assaultive behavior and the ratio of nonfatal assaults to homicide is probably far greater than 100:1. There are about 60,000 firearm-related assaults, treated in U.S. hospital emergency departments each year.

Assaultive violence includes both nonfatal and fatal interpersonal violence in which physical force by one person is used with the intent of causing harm, injury, or death to another. Homicide is death caused by injuries inflicted by one person with intent to injure or kill another by any means. Homicide can be classified as criminal or non-criminal. Non-criminal homicide includes deaths caused – by negligence and those & committed in self-defense.

2. Causes and Risk Factors

There are many types of assaultive violence, and for each type the causes are complex and diverse. It is helpful to examine various disciplinary approaches to aspects of the problem because each contributes valuable perspectives. However, these separate approaches can obscure the complex interaction of different types of factors that contribute to assaultive violence. Ultimately, what is needed are "causal" explanations that combine biological, psychological, and sociological factors in ways that explain the occurrence of assaultive violence involving different perpetrators, victims, and circumstances. And, indeed, various disciplines have begun to converge in their quest for an explanation for assaultive violence, examining the issue from a multifactorial perspective.

Biological explanations of assaultive violence have examined sex, age, and certain psychiatric illnesses as important risk factors for homicide victimization and perpetration. For example, greater numbers of males among perpetrators and victims may reflect the influence of male sex hormones on aggressive behavior, and the decreasing numbers of victims and perpetrators with increasing age may be a result of biological transformations associated with aging.

Psychological approaches to violence address factors in four general areas. **Biobehavioral factors** encompass the biological influences on a person's proclivity for violence, including aeuroanatomy and brain chemistry. **Socialization factors** address the process by which children learn "rules" for social behavior. In this context, young children are believed to be influenced by aggressive and violent behavior of others in their environment, including family members, peers, and role models. **Cognitive factors** include the ideas, beliefs, and patterns of thinking that emerge as a child develops. Research suggests that aggressive and violent people process information and think about social situations in different ways than do nonviolent individuals, for example, tending to perceive hostility in others where it does not, in fact, exist. They also may be less adept at managing nonviolent ways to resolve conflict. **Situational factors** also contribute to a propensity for violent behavior. Aversive situations such as stressful life events, violence in the family or neighborhood, presence of the means to carry out violence, such as guns- all these may have a role in stimulating violent acts. Overall, through the perspective of these four conceptual groupings, psychology contributes to our understanding of violence by underlining that human aggression is learned behavior and thus can be prevented or minimized.

Four major sociological approaches to understanding are cultural, structural, interactionist, and economic. The **cultural approach** views violent behavior as the result of learned and shared values and behavior specific to a given group that are applied in recognizable situations and transmitted across generations. Certain subgroups exhibit higher rates of assaultive violence because they are in a subculture that has violence as a norm. However, critics point to the frequency of violence in groups where violence is clearly not a norm (e.g., the middle class) and to the fact that this theory tends to "blame the victim."

The **structural approach** holds that rates of assaultive violence are largely influenced by broad-scale social forces, such as poverty or lack of opportunity. In one widely known formulation, violence and other "illegitimate" behaviors arise when persons are deprived of "legitimate" means and resources to realize culturally valued goals. This theory does not adequately explain, however, why conflicts arising from structural deprivation lead to violence in one situation and to other behaviors, passivity for instance, in other situations.

The **interactionist approach** focuses on the nature of the interaction sequence as it escalates into violent behavior. For example, one investigator describes it as a series of offender and victim "moves" as they relate to each other and to the reaction of the audience. From this, he derived a set of time-ordered stages that most of the transactions followed. Other research has shown that violence grows out of a series of provocative arguments that escalate to murder. The arguments often are threats to identity (especially sexual identity) and self-esteem. Still another team of investigators posits that people engage in violence to "control others' behavior, to achieve retribution, or to preserve self image. For example, a young person may resort to violence in retribution for a perceived wrong or to save face. This aspect of social intervention theory may help illuminate problems of violence among young minority youth who are "quick to fight over what many adults would consider to be trivial matters.

The **economic approach** is the basis for many current policies aimed at reducing homicide and assault. This theory posits that decisions to engage in criminal behavior are based on a person's perception of what outcome appears more valuable. Thus, some people commit assaults not because their motivation differs from that of other people but because their perceived benefits and costs differ. In order for the desired choices to be made, people must be aware of the benefits and costs of the alternatives available to them. This assumes that people have equal capability of making rational decisions under all conditions and circumstances, but the ability to make a rational judgment may be impaired, for example, if the person is under the influence of alcohol or drugs.

H. WOMAN BATTERING

1. Definition of the Problem

In addition to its impact on the public health of women and families, woman battering presents a challenge to public health because its parameters are not well defined, its severity is highly subjective, its causes are poorly understood, and its psychosocial consequences are often linked to physical events in very complex ways. Equally important, perhaps more than any other health problem, battering raises political concerns about which medical care and public health officials may have ambiguous feelings, including the implications of sexual inequality for health, the competing rights of husbands and spousal victims, and public intervention in private lives.

2. Definitional Issues

The terms **domestic violence, spouse abuse, partner or intimate violence, family violence,** and **woman battering** are often used interchangeably. State statutes and service providers often subsume battering under the category of domestic or family violence. It is useful to examine these terms separately. **Domestic violence, spouse abuse,** and **partner or intimate violence** refer to the use of threats or physical force in family or other intimate relationships among adults. **Family violence** is a broad term that encompasses domestic violence (the use of force among partners in marriage or other intimate relationships) and abuse of children, the elderly, or the disabled. **Abuse** is defined as the violent exploitation, mistreatment, or neglect of persons who are dependent because of their age or physical incapacity. Although state statutes define both domestic violence and abuse as criminal, state protective service agencies handle abuse of children, the frail elderly, or handicapped persons, except in the most severe cases. By contrast, in almost half the states – and the U.S. military-police are mandated to arrest offenders in cases of domestic violence. Four characteristics differentiate family violence crimes from assaults between strangers or acquaintances. In family violence:

a. Force is used in close or blood relationships.

b. Perpetrators usually have continued access to their victims and repeat their assaults, often multiple times.

c. The perpetrator controls numerous aspects of his victim's life.
d. Acts of force are rooted in norms about how certain persons (parents, males, lovers, husbands) should behave, given various occasions or provocations. For example, because of social norms that equate manliness with exclusive possession of a woman, many men may feel that they are not "macho" unless they use force to control or possess their partners.

3. Causes and Risk Factors

a. Vulnerability Factors and High-Risk Populations

Although there are statistical associations between a risk of battering and marital status, pregnancy, age, substance use, and exposure to violence in childhood, the only factors consistently linked to future risk of battering are a history of violence, fear of violence, and control.

The confusion that surrounds population-based research on battering means that all generalizations about battered women and of fenders should be approached skeptically, including demographic profiles suggesting that some groups are more susceptible than others. Furthermore, research on domestic violence fails to establish the clear temporal sequence needed to show that personality or behavioral characteristics are risk factors, rather than outcomes of spouse abuse. Therefore it is best to view associations as vulnerability factors rather than as causal or risk factors for spouse abuse. These factors may interact with the situational dynamics in domestic conflict to increase the likelihood that violence will result.

b. Demographic Factors

Research has failed to identify clear demographic patterns in domestic violence by race, social class, or age. Population surveys suggest that battering is two to three times more common among blacks than whites; however, among groups with similar income, blacks are less likely than whites to experience spousal violence. There may be significant racial differences in outcome, however. Domestic violence appears more likely to prompt a suicide attempt in black than in white women for instance. One survey also reported higher rates of abuse among poor, unemployed, or working-class groups and showed that drinking, approval of violence, and blue-collar status had a cumulative relation to violence, with the highest rates appearing when all three elements were present. But occupational class itself was not predictive. The difference between low-income and middle-income women may be smaller than for almost any other health problem, and extensive abuse has been identified in relatively affluent communities. For example, in a survey to which 786 medical students and faculty responded, 17 percent of the women and 3 percent of the men reported physical abuse or sexual abuse by a partner in their adult life. As the control facets of battering are incorporated into research, its inverse relation to social class may disappear altogether.

c. Personality and Behavioral Factors

Victims - Studies with the most reliable designs report few, if any, significant personality differences between battered and non-battered women, and no personality profile identifies certain women as "violence prone. A more controversial view suggests that battered women become trapped in abusive relationships by a "cycle of violence" (buildup of tension, explosion, and a "honeymoon" phase), which elicits a battered woman's syndrome (BWS) characterized by learned helplessness, depression, and delayed or reluctant help-seeking. Although some victims evidence both the cycle and the BWS, in the majority of cases, battered women are aggressive help-seekers (with help-seeking increasing as abuse escalates) and employing a range of strategies, including frequent separations, to minimize or end abuse.

Perpetrators - Based on offenders' self-reports on various psychological tests, researchers have identified a number of personality disorders among batterers, including borderline and schizoidal disorder, narcissistic/antisocial personality, and passive/dependent compulsive disorders. A comparative study of batterers and non-batterers established a strong correlation between abusive behavior (as measured by the CTS) and elevated scores on a measure of borderline personality organization, suggesting to some that woman battering is the result of psychopathology and casting serious doubt on the theory that all or most sexual violence against women is gender motivated. Some form of childhood exposure to violence (child abuse, severe physical punishment as a child, or witnessing parental domestic violence) occurs in the background of 60 to 70 percent of batterers in treatment, leading many policymakers to support therapeutic intervention to break the cycle of violence. In contrast to clinical samples, population data fails to support the belief that most batterers were exposed to violence as children. Meanwhile, other clinical studies show that batterers are psychologically indistinguishable from non abusive men. Increasing evidence suggests that offenders are men with diverse personalities, family histories, and behavioral profiles who typically use several strategies, as well as physical abuse, to establish control, extract obedience, and secure such tangibles as sex, money, and feelings of power.

The Role of Alcohol - Although the reported violence rates among men who use alcohol are 2 to 15 times higher than rates among abstainers, a causal role for alcohol cannot be supported. Among women, alcohol is typically the consequence, rater than the cause of victimization. Although drinking is associated with higher rates of wife abuse, alcohol is not typically an immediate antecedent, nor does cessation of alcohol use appear to affect abusive behavior. Alcohol appears to be involved in only 6 to 8 percent of the family disputes in which police are involved. Moreover, abuse is unaffected by recovery. Neither length of sobriety nor membership in Alcoholics Anonymous (AA) are linked to any reduction in male violence.

Violence in the Family of Origin - Childhood victimization increases the risk that a boy will abuse his adult partner, but neither the typical batterer nor his victim come from a violent home. Survey and case-control studies report significant correlations between 'current victimization' and a woman's abuse as a child. But two well-designed studies using multiple comparison groups and collecting data from men and women found no significant effect of childhood violence. Studies demonstrated that men from violent childhoods (5 percent of the population) are 10 times more likely to abuse their wives than are men who had nonviolent childhoods. However, a consideration of the relative size of the groups exposed and not exposed to childhood violence shows that a current batterer is seven times more likely to come from a nonviolent than a violent home. Even 80 percent of the children from families classified as most violent do not become batterers.

High-Risk Populations - Although the typical victim of battering is a young woman (under 30) with a child, battering is a problem at every point in the life cycle. It may be initiated during adolescence, escalate during pregnancy, present through problems among children, and continue into old age. Special treatment issues relate to the age, developmental stage, and lifestyle of the individuals and families involved in battering. Children, adolescents, and older women are often unrecognized as populations at high risk for battering. Additional high-risk populations about whom there is little research include disabled women, homeless women, and women with human immunodeficiency virus (HIV) infection.

Children whose mothers are battered are exposed either to arts of violence, coercion, and control or to the consequences of these acts. As a result, children may be co-victims who are also are at risk for severe injury as well as short and long-term physical, medical, and psychological problems. As co-victims, children are injured in an estimated 17 percent of all battering episodes. The estimated 8 to 80 percent of the children of batterers who witness their father's behavior may be more damaged psychologically than victims of child abuse. The estimated 3.3 million to 10 million children who are exposed to battering each year are forced to cope with high stress, including fear of injury to their mother and themselves. The medical and psychological effects of exposure flow directly from the developmental age of the child, the dynamics in particular relationships, and the nature and extent of exposure.

Adolescent girls are also at high risk for battering. Nineteen to 31.5 percent of young women are threatened or assaulted during dating relationships, with 45 percent of these incidents resulting in injury. Thirty-four percent of injuries brought to the emergency department by girls between the ages of 16 and 18 are the result of partner violence. Partner violence is also a major context for sexual assault, unwanted pregnancy, depression, attempted suicide, addiction, and a range of somatic complaints among female adolescents. Presentations frequently associated with partner abuse among adolescents include injury, teen pregnancy, malnutrition, isolation, depression, anxiety or suicidality (among males as well as females), truancy, homelessness, and the use of addictive substances. The battered adolescent may fall between the cracks, as she is too old for child protective services and too young for adult protective services, including domestic violence shelters.

Partner violence poses a major threat to the health of **older women**, accounting for 18 percent of the injuries presented to the hospital by women over 60. In addition to injury, partner violence also may account for depression and other psychiatric disorders among the elderly, as well as attempted suicide, physical disability, addiction, chronic pain syndromes, and a range of somatic complaints. In general, physical injury is a less prominent feature of battering among the elderly than is a complex psychosocial profile reinforced by chronic mental abuse, isolation, and control over social life and resources in the relationship. Common presentations of domestic violence among the elderly include recent onset of substance use, noncompliance with medical regimes, chronic anxiety, malnutrition, depressive symptoms with no supporting history, and complaints of pain with no clinical evidence of disease. This profile often subjects the older battered woman to the dual stigma associated with age discrimination and with pseudopsychiatric labels that obstruct her access to health and other services. Although most domestic violence among the elderly is long-standing, in certain cases, the onset or intensification is linked to developmental milestones such as aging, dependence on medication, retirement, loss of sexual function, or another sudden change in social, medical, or mental health status.

I. RAPE AND SEXUAL ASSAULT

1. Definition of the Problem

Part of the problem inherent in understanding rape and sexual assault is derived from its equivocal definition. From a legal perspective, rape is a criminal act. Old laws viewed rape as an act of illicit sex; more recent legislation defines rape as a type of assault. As defined by the Federal Bureau of Investigation (FBI) Uniform Crime Report (UCR), forcible rape "is the carnal knowledge of a female forcibly and against her will." Although some variations among states exist, rape is generally legally defined as forced sexual penetration of a victim by an offender who is not the victim's spouse. Some state laws attempted after the FBI's definition limit the term "rape" to incidents in which the victim is female and vaginal penetration has occurred. Many statutes have a marital exclusion rule, which states that criminal sexual conduct cannot legally occur if the offender and victim are married. This rule stems from the historical legal theory that a wife is the property of her husband.

Because the legal definition of forcible rape is so restrictive, the term "sexual assault" has been used to cover a wider range of sexual crimes, including any manual, genital, or oral contact with the victim's genitalia without consent and obtained by force, threat, or fraud. Most states define as illegal any type of sexual behavior with a child. Statutory rape may also be charged in cases where the victim cannot give consent because of mental deficiency; psychosis; or altered consciousness induced by sleep, drugs, illness, or intoxication. Reformed legislation with its increased emphasis on force, threat of force, and coercion comes closer to capturing the psychological dimension of rape.

2. Causes and Risk Factors

Broadly conceptualized, research on sexual offenders falls into two categories: studies that focus on offender characteristics and studies that view social/cultural factors as causative.

The first approach (i.e., the psychopathology model) focuses on known offenders, typically incarcerated rapists. Early research in this area resulted in a large number of descriptive studies that attempted to differentiate rapists from other non-sex-offending criminals. Attempts to identify discriminating characteristics have been largely unsuccessful to date, with the general consensus that convicted rapists represent a heterogeneous group. Research in this domain continues with the goal of developing typologies among rapists.

Studies examining social or cultural factors have generally relied on male subjects (typically, college students) who self-report engaging in sexual violence. Available research indicates that between 15 and 25 percent of male college students admit to sexual aggression.

The social/cultural model maintains that perpetrators adhere to a belief system that both allows them to engage in and justify rape. This belief system is viewed as the result of a society that legitimizes violence against women, of which sexual aggression is one form. Viewed from this perspective, sexual aggression is not the result of any diagnosable individual pathology, but rather is the result of acceptance of societal attitudes that foster male dominance and dehumanize females. The results of numerous studies have lent support to this model by showing a relationship between certain attitudes (e.g., acceptance of rape myths, sex role stereotyping) and various measures of aggression.

Current research in this area appears driven by the view that neither approach adequately explains sexual violence and that there may not be just a single etiological factor. The recent literature encompasses the gamut from bisocial theorizing, including evolutionary and neurohormonal variables, to quadripartite models, incorporating physiological, cognitive, affective, and personality variables.

J. CHILD ABUSE

1. Definition of the Problem

Definitions of child abuse have broadened significantly in the last two decades. The commonsense meaning of the term "child abuse" is a situation where a caregiver generally a parent, sets out in a systematic way to harm a child. In 1962, Professor C. Henry Kempe and his associates published an article in the **Journal of the American Medical Association** entitled "**The Battered Child Syndrome**" that drew great attention in the professional and lay media. One of the outcomes to increased public awareness was the drafting of a model child abuse reporting statute by the Children's Bureau, the lead federal agency for children. Child abuse came to be defined in the state reporting laws as injuries inflicted by caregivers, and many believed that it could be diagnosed by physicians and medical institutions. However, Kempe's perpetrator-victim model of etiology and the notion of a syndrome of physical examination findings in the child and psychopathology in the caregiver led to several problematic consequences.

2. Causes and Risk Factors

Early efforts to understand child abuse centered on psychological problems of the parents of the victims, focusing on distorted expectations of the children, frustrated dependency needs, personal isolation, and histories of having themselves been abused as children. But many other social and cultural factors have been proposed as contributing to the causes of child abuse in addition to individual deviant behavior. The psychoanalytical approach posits that unconscious parental drives and conflicts determine abusive behavior. Social learning theory suggests that abusers learn the behavior as abused children themselves. Environmental stress theory suggests that overwhelmingly stressful factors, such as poverty, unemployment, social isolation, and inadequate housing, help cause the violence or interfere with the parent's ability to care for the child. Cognitive-developmental theory suggests that immature parental understanding of the child and of the parental role are associated with abuse. By presuming social inequality, labeling theory suggests that the interests of dominant power groups are served by defining as deviant a class of socially marginal individuals (child abusers) whose problems are the concerns of helping professionals.

All these theories individually explain some part of the problem, but all have clear limitations. Professionals and researchers have begun to integrate parts of these theories into interactive, multicausal theories that investigate how aspects of an individual's personality or environment interact with his or her particular experience.

Some researchers have attempted to integrate causal factors for child abuse from multiple levels: individual, family, and society. At the individual level, one consistent finding has been the prevalence of acute or chronic illness in the abused children. However, a number of long-held "causes" of child abuse are now viewed with skepticism; these include low-birth weight of the infant, young maternal age, and inadequate mother-infant bond formation.

A number of recent studies have pointed to the association between domestic violence and child abuse. For example, one report found that marital violence is a statistically significant predictor of physical child abuse. The greater amount of violence against a spouse, the greater likelihood of physical abuse to the child by the abusive spouse.

Behavioral and social science research have not generally produced results that are applicable in clinical settings, mostly because the predominant research approach attempts to explain child abuse statistically, factor by factor, thus ignoring the complexity of individual cases. Those studies that have considered the complexity of family interactions have focused on the formation of universal rules that govern behavior, whereas the clinician is concerned with treatment appropriate to individual cases. Interaction among clinicians and researchers is needed to develop a body of knowledge concerning etiology, therapeutic interventions, and effective intervention programs.

K. CHILD SEXUAL ABUSE

1. Definition of the Problem

Child sexual abuse is sexual contact with a child that occurs as a result of force or in a relationship where there is exploitative because of an age difference or caretaking responsibility. There is almost universal agreement that sexual contact between a child and the child's father, stepfather, mother, stepmother, another older relative, teacher, or baby sitter constitutes sexual abuse, as does sexual contact by any adult or older person, whether known or unknown. Also included are rape and forced sexual contact at the hands of anyone, even a peer.

2. **Causes and Risk Factors**

Community studies are the best sources of information about the characteristics of different types of sexual abuse. These studies suggest that abuse by fathers and stepfathers, even though it dominates reports from the child welfare system, actually constitutes no more than 7 to 8 percent of all abuse cases. Abuse by other family members (most frequently uncles and older brothers) make up an additional 16 to 42 percent. Other non-relatives known to the child make up 32 to 60 percent of offenders. Abuse by strangers is substantially less common than abuse by family members or persons known to the child.

The largest category of abuse in most studies involves groping or fondling of children's bodies on top of or underneath the clothing. Only 16 to 29 percent of the abuse involves intercourse or attempted intercourse. Another 3 to 11 percent of the activities involve attempted or completed oral or anal intercourse; and 13 to 33 percent, manual touching of the genitals.

Community studies show that the frequency of child sexual abuse seems to occur when victims are between ages 9 and 12 and then declines somewhat during later adolescent years. Most studies show that a quarter of the incidents occur before the child is 8 years of age, and some clinicians insist that this percentage would be even greater if it were not for the occlusion of memories from these early years. Approximately 42 to 75 percent of experiences reported in the surveys are single events. Repeated abusive experiences occur at older ages and are associated with abuse within the family.

In addition to community surveys, compilations of cases known to professionals have been used to generate incidence estimates and describe other characteristics of child sexual abuse. For example, the Third National Incidence Study projected that 300,000 new cases of sexual abuse became known to professionals in the United States in 1993. Incidence estimates based on reported cases such as these appear to over represent (a) abuse involving fathers and step-father (b) abuse involving intercourse and other more intrusive acts, and (c) abuse perpetrated over an extended period. The ages of the victimized children also tend to be higher in these incidence studies because reported cases record the age at the time of the disclosure rather than the age at onset. Compared with the community studies, there seems to be an underreporting of the sexual abuse of boys.

Community surveys also have provided information on the socio-demographic distribution of sexual abuse. These studies consistently fail to find differences in rates among different social classes or races. However, other factors have been associated with risk of abuse:

a. Living without one of the biological parents, unavailability of the mother because of outside employment or disability or illness,
b. Reports from the child stating that the parents' marriage is unhappy or full of conflict,
c. Reports from the child of a poor relationship with the parents or of extremely punitive discipline or child abuse, and
d. Report by the child of having a stepfather

Although few studies have examined why these factors increase risk, poor supervision, emotional turmoil, neglect, and rejection may make the child vulnerable to child molesters. With little help or support from parents, children may also find it hard to stop the abuse once it begins.

L. ELDER ABUSE

1. Definition of the Problem

Wide variation exists in the way researchers have defined the term "elder abuse." The confusion surrounding exactly what constitutes elder abuse has made it difficult to interpret the results of studies on the subject. Researchers have included some or all of the following dimensions in describing maltreatment of the elderly: physical abuse, physical neglect, emotional abuse, emotional neglect, emotional deprivation, sexual exploitation and assault, verbal abuse, medical neglect, material abuse, and neglect of the elder's environment.

Despite definitional issues, researchers agree on certain points. For example, they concur that physical assault against an elder constitutes abusive behavior. Most of the research literature also includes in the terminology the following: psychological or emotional abuse; financial abuse (the misuse or theft of an elder's property or assets); and the intentional failure of a clearly designated caregiver to meet the needs of an elder (neglect). Beyond these generally accepted categories, however, there is little consensus on definitions.

Recently, attention has shifted to learning more about the older person's perception of mistreatment and the role of culture and attitudes in defining the issue. A study of how various potentially abusive situations were perceived by African American, Korean American, and Caucasian American women revealed that African American women tended to interpret abuse more broadly; and Korean American women, least broadly. The reluctance of older Korean American women to label situations as abusive or to seek help was explained within the context of Korean culture, which "emphasizes, as desirable behavior, family harmony over individual well-being, denotes some degree of human suffering as a virtue, and dictates enduring and keeping one's problem to oneself, rather than exposing the problem to others. A study of Japanese Americans also reported similar findings of valuing group above self. Thus, cultural variations confound attempts to define elder abuse.

2. Causes and Risk Factors

Characteristics of Abuse Victims - Despite their methodological limitations, studies suggest fairly consistent findings about the abused elderly who come into contact with the human service systems. Although a number of studies based on agency samples suggest that abused individuals tend to be female, several prevalence studies have found roughly equal numbers of women and men in the victimized group. This apparent discrepancy may be due to women's greater likelihood of suffering injuries and emotional distress as a result of abuse. Many studies have found victims to be somewhat vulnerable because of illness or impairment, making it difficult for them to defend themselves or escape the situation. In addition, a shared living arrangement is strongly associated with abuse: most studies have found that the majority of physical abuse victims live with the abuser. These, however, are the only findings that emerge reliably from the studies. Results relating to the frequency with which abuse occurs and the types of abuse most often found are virtually impossible to compare because of the widely varying definitions employed.

Causal Factors - Extensive research literature in the area of child and spouse abuse and on the relations between older persons and adult children can provide important insights into elder abuse, particularly in concert with the literature on domestic violence in younger populations and with the limited literature on elder abuse. Five primary risk factors have emerged from research: intra-individual dynamics (psychopathology of the abuser), intergenerational transmission of violent behavior, dependency and exchange relations between abuser and abused, external stress, and social isolation.

Intra-individual dynamics emphasizes pathological characteristics of the abuser as the primary cause of maltreatment. Some research has indicated that abusers of the elderly are more likely to be developmentally disabled mentally ill, or alcoholic.

A number of studies of child and wife abuse have provided evidence concerning **intergenerational transmission** of violent behavior; the findings indicate that people learn to be violent in the family setting. Research evidence shows that witnessing parental violence during childhood is a strong risk factor for wife abuse as an adult, and the amount of physical punishment experienced as a child is positively associated with the rate of abusive violence to one's own children. Given the strength of this connection in other forms of family violence, it is reasonable to postulate that abusers of the elderly will also be more likely to have been raised in violent homes. Studies of this issue are, unfortunately, still lacking, so this risk factor remains to be tested.

Two competing theories relate **dependency** to elder abuse. One emphasizes the role of "caregiver stress" as a risk factor for maltreatment, and the second suggests that increased dependency of the abuser on his or her victim leads to maltreatment. Based on the literature on family care-giving, some analysts have postulated that families experience "generational inversion" when the elderly person becomes dependent on the children for financial, physical, or emotional support which leads to stress on the caregiver. As economic pressures for the caregiver grow and rewards diminish, the change is perceived as unfair. If the caregivers do not have the ability to ameliorate the situation, they may become abusive. Although this theory seems plausible, there are few firm research findings to support it.

M. SUICIDE

1. Definition of the Problem

Suicide is the result of violence directed against self. In 1994 there were 31,142 deaths from suicide in the United States, making suicide the ninth leading cause of death in this country. Unlike the rates for many diseases, suicide rates are substantial among both young and old people. As a result, in 1991, suicide was the sixth leading cause of premature death, as defined by years of potential life lost before age 65. In past decades, the rate of suicide was relatively low among adolescents and young adults and increased steadily with age. However, in the last four decades, suicide rates among younger age groups have increased dramatically. In particular, the suicide rate among persons 15 to 24 years of age has more that tripled. In 1950 the suicide rate for this age group was 4.5 per 100,000, and in 1994, this rate was 13.8. Suicide has been the third leading cause of death among persons 15 to 24 years of age in recent years and the fourth leading cause of death among persons 10 to 14 years of age. Although most suicides occur among persons younger than 40, the highest rates occur among the elderly.

2. Causes and Risk Factors

Even though it is common to hear people say that a person committed suicide because he was mentally ill or because he could not cope with stressful events in his life, in reality, many factors contribute to the causal mechanism of suicide. Certain psychiatric illnesses are, of course, both extremely important and well recognized as risk factors. In particular, affective disorders have been clearly shown, in both retrospective case-control studies and prospective cohort studies, to increase markedly the risk of suicide. For example, in a population based cohort study of 3,563 males in Sweden who were observed for15 to 25 years, the suicide rate among men with an initial diagnosis of any mental illness was almost 39 times higher than the rate for men with no mental disorder. Men with an initial diagnosis of a depressive disorder had a suicide rate 80 times higher than the rate for men with no mental disorder.

Alcoholism is the second most commonly reported mental illness, after clinical depression, associated with suicide. However many studies have lacked a control group to help assess the contribution of alcohol to suicide risk. In addition, the independent effect of alcoholism on the suicide rate is rarely estimated; rather, the diagnosis of alcoholism among the case series is often reported, in addition to the prevalence of affective illness, social isolation, and other factors that might, in themselves, account for any observed increase in the risk of suicide. Because most of the studies have been carried out among special populations, such as psychiatric inpatients or hospitalized alcoholics, their findings are not necessarily applicable to alcoholics in general. Finally, little work has been done separately to assess the effects of acute exposure to alcohol (i.e., alcohol medication) and alcohol abuse on the risk of suicide. More research is needed to elucidate the mechanism(s) underlying the observed association between alcoholism and suicide.

N. WORKPLACE VIOLENCE

1. Introduction

The scope of workplace violence ranges from offensive language to homicide and includes actions that make one person uncomfortable in the workplace; threats and harassment; and bodily injury inflicted by one person on another. NIOSH defines workplace violence as "violent acts, including physical assaults and threats of assault, directed towards persons at work or on duty." These acts may include beating, obscene telephone calls, rape, suicide, attempted suicide, intimidation, shooting, stabbing, harassment, threat, following someone, or swearing or shouting at someone.

A workplace is any location, either permanent or temporary, where an employee performs any job-related duty. It may include buildings, surrounding premises, parking lots, field locations, clients' homes, and vehicles used to travel to and from work assignments.

US BLS classifies workplace homicide according to the type of circumstance, such as business disputes (including actions of a co-worker or former co-worker), customer or client disputes, disputes involving a relative of the victim (such as spouse or ex-spouse, boyfriend or ex-boyfriend), incidents involving police or security guards in the line of duty, and incidents in which death occurred during a robbery or crime.

CA Div. of OSH has defined three types of workplace violence. Type I involves assailants with no legitimate relationship to the workplace (generally in the course of a robbery or other criminal act). Type II involves customers of a service provided by an establishment or clients, patients, passengers, criminal suspects, or prisoners. Type III involves current or former employees, supervisors, managers, and other persons with employment-related involvement with an establishment, such as an employee's spouse, boyfriend, friend, relative, or a person who has a dispute with an employee.

2. Workplace Violence, Important Occupational Health Problem

Workplace violence is a major contributor to occupational injury. Homicide at work is the second leading cause of occupation-related death after motor vehicle-related deaths. According to estimates from the National Crime Victimization Survey of the U.S Department of Justice, approximately 1 million persons per year are assaulted while at work or on duty.

Workplace violence represents about 15% of all acts of violence experienced by U.S. residents aged 12 or older. Furthermore, the epidemiology of workplace violence suggests that prevention strategies may be different from strategies to prevent violent injuries in general. For example, the circumstances of occupational homicides are different from the circumstances of homicides in general. Robbery is a factor in about 75% of occupational homicides, whereas robbery is involved in only about 9% of all homicides.

Although almost one-half of all murder victims in the general population were related to or knew their assailants, most occupational homicides involve persons not known to one another. Workplace violence also disproportionately affects certain occupations. More than one-quarter of workplace homicides and more than three-quarters of all nonfatal workplace assaults occur in retail trade and service industries. Therefore, the risk of workplace violence is associated with specific factors that largely involve dealing w/the public (e.g., clients, patients, inmates, or customers).

3. Major Causes of Workplace Homicides

NIOSH reports that over the past 10-15 years homicides have surpassed machine-related deaths as the second leading cause of fatal occupational injuries. Work-related homicides are primarily an urban problem; eight of the largest U.S. metropolitan areas account for almost one half of the total number of incidents.

The average workplace homicide rate for 1980-1992 was 0.70/100,000 workers. The majority (80%) of workplace homicides occur among men, although homicides are the leading cause (42%) of occupational fatalities among women. The risk of homicide among men is more than three times the risk among women. Most homicides among men occur in retail, service, public administration, or transportation industries; most homicides among women occur in the retail and service industries.

The largest number of workplace homicides occurs in the 25-34-year-old group, but the highest rate occurs in workers aged 65 or older. Most homicide victims are Caucasian, although African-American workers have rates 2-3 times higher than Caucasian workers. Firearms account for an increasing percentage of all workplace homicides and are now involved in over three-quarters of all fatal injuries at work. The largest number of deaths occurs in grocery stores, eating and drinking places, taxicab services, and justice/public order establishments. Taxicab services also have the highest rate of work-related homicide, followed by liquor stores, detective/protective services, gas service stations, and jewelry stores. For occupational groups, the highest rates occur among taxicab drivers/chauffeurs, sheriffs/bailiffs, police and detectives, gas station/garage workers, and security guards.

U.S. BLS reports that robbery was involved in over three-quarters of all workplace homicides; a business dispute or conflict with a coworker or associate, customer or client accounts for less than one in five deaths on the job. More limited data are available about the major causes or nonfatal violent injuries. The BLS estimates that most nonfatal assaults occur in the service and retail trades. Among service employees more than 50% occur in nursing homes, social services, or hospitals. The source of injury in most cases was a patient. Most injuries involve hitting, kicking, or beating. A survey completed by a major life insurance company estimated that 2.2 million workplace assaults occurred between July 1992 and July 1993.

A household survey by the U.S. Department of justice from 1987-1992 indicated that each year about 1 million persons were assaulted at work or on duty. Workplace assaults represented 15% of all acts of violence experienced by Americans during that period. Women workers 'were more likely to be attacked by someone they knew. Government workers accounted for disproportionately more work-related violence, suggesting a great risk in dealing with the public or delivering services to clients.

Workers' compensation data have recently been used to describe the major causes of nonfatal workplace injury. Data from California indicate that the greatest risk of nonfatal workplace assaults is among police, correctional employees, bus drivers, hospital workers, and security guards. The overall rate of nonfatal occupational assaults was 72.9 per 100,000, approximately 50 times the rate of fatal occupational injury.

When police reports of workplace assault were included for eight cities, the combined annual rate of workplace assault was 184.7 per 100,000 workers, almost twice the rate found by either source individually. Almost two-thirds of all non-fatal workplace injuries are type II-involving a customer or client. MN workers' compensation claims data show that women have an assault rate twice that of men. The greatest number of assaults occurred among nursing aides, orderlies, and attendants. Social service workers had the highest rate of injury (l69 per 100,000 workers).

Most assailants were people with whom the workers were in contact as part of their jobs (e.g., patients, clients, inmates, or customers). An analysis of 600 nonfatal workplace violence claims at a large workers' compensation insurance carrier found that over one-half of cases were caused by a criminal act (e.g., type I), whereas 38.5% of cases were caused by a patient, client, customer or student (type II). The highest percentage of nonfatal workplace violence claims were filed by school and health care employees.

4. Risk Factors for Assault

National Institute of Occupational Safety and Health has identified many factors that increase the risk of workplace assault, which are the following:

a. Contact with the public
b. Exchange of money
c. Delivery of passengers, goods, or services
d. Mobile workplace, such as taxicab or police cruiser
e. Working with unstable or volatile persons in health care, social service, or criminal justice settings
f. Working alone or in small numbers
g. Working late at night or during early morning hours
h. Working high-crime areas
i. Guarding valuable property or possessions
j. Working in community-based settings

5. Reduction of Risk Factors for Workplace Violence

The risk factors for workplace violence can be reduced by attention to environmental design, administrative controls, and behavioral strategies. For example, the use of drop safes, carrying small amounts of cash, and posting of signs that limited cash is available may help to reduce assaults in retail establishments. Bullet-resistant barriers or enclosures may be used in gas stations or convenience stores, hospital emergency departments, and social service agencies.

Other issues such as visibility, lighting, access/egress, and use of security devices also should be considered. Increasing the number of staff on duty may help to reduce the risk of assault in retail establishments or may reduce frustration among patients, customers, or clients in public service settings. Employee training in hazard recognition, nonviolent response, and conflict resolution is essential.

6. Components of a Workplace Violence Prevention Program

Specific guidelines have been published by federal and state agencies for effective workplace violence prevention programs for health care and social service providers and retail stores. An effective violence prevention program should include the following components:

a. Management commitment and employee involvement
b. Workplace security analysis

c. Hazard prevention and control measures
d. Incident reporting and follow-up procedures
e. Employee and supervisor training
f. Record keeping
g. Evaluation

One of the first steps in developing a workplace violence prevention program is to establish a system for documenting violent incidents. A written policy should specify zero tolerance of violence at work and establish a threat assessment team to which all incidents should be reported.

An existing labor-management committee or a joint committee responsible for workplace violence prevention should develop written policies and procedures. The workplace security analysis includes a step-by-step inspection of all areas in and near the workplace to identify potential hazards as well as review or records documenting past incidents.

The engineering, administrative, or work practice control measures are selected based specifically on the results of the security analysis. Prevention programs should include post-trauma counseling services for employees and supervisors.

O. NEED FOR COLLABORATION

Public health offers a new approach to the prevention of violence and adds a new voice a new and a new set of tools and techniques. Need of criminal justice, health care, social work and mental health. Collaboration is critical both to break barriers and to advance prevention and control activities. Hospitals treat more violent injuries than ever are reported to the police.

The Health Care System - Hospital personnel and medical professionals play important roles in the diagnosis, reporting, and treatment of child abuse.

The Criminal Justice System - This system and its components play a variety of roles in child abuse cases, including case finding and reporting, assisting child protective agencies, investigating cases, placing children in protective custody, arresting perpetrators/prosecuting offenders.

The Social Service System - The development of child protective agencies in every state has been society's basic response to the problem of child abuse. These agencies are the only vehicles through which social workers respond to child abuse cases.

The Mental Health System - Mental health workers are more recent participants in child abuse treatment and prevention.

Even a brief look at the overlapping roles played by health professionals and representatives of the criminal justice, social service, and mental health systems in child abuse prevention and treatment highlights the need for collaboration and the tensions that inhibit it.

VI. **PUBLIC HEALTH CONSEQUENCES OF WAR AND TERRORISM**

A. **INTRODUCTION**

The most destructive human activity is warfare. The 1960s expression "war is not healthy for children and other living things" is so understated that one hesitates to attempt to define how unhealthy war is. Not only is war intentionally destructive between the sides engaged in fighting, but when modern warfare is practiced, the environment is another casualty. The first and most tragic consequence of war is the **direct casualties**, the soldiers and civilians who die or are maimed in the fighting, and their loved ones who must carry on, with all the limitations and inaccuracies in data collection of this sort, indicate that mortality rates from war rose dramatically in the twentieth century. This was largely attributable to large increases in mortality during World Wars I and II. Prior to World War II, more war-related deaths occurred due to disease than to battlefield deaths.

The need to support a war effort and the care required by those who are wounded but survive place a burden on the society supporting the fighting. Modern warfare also strikes directly at the economic and logistical ability of the society to make war, often by targeting the environment directly. It has been suggested that civilian deaths compose 90% of all deaths in twentieth-century wars.

In **War and Public Health**, the impact of war on public health is documented and suggestions of what health professionals could do to prevent war and minimize its consequences are offered. With respect to the Gulf War, for example, studies have shown that the war and trade sanctions caused a threefold increase in mortality among Iraqi children under 5 years of age. The suggestion that by using high-precision weapons with strategic targets the Allied forces were producing only limited damage to the civilian population was shown to be false, confirming that the casualties of war still extend far beyond those caused directly by warfare.

The threat of terrorist incidents involving NBC (Nuclear, Biological, or Chemical) agents is an increasingly serious concern for the world community. Table 13.3 provides the chronology of state use and biological and chemical weapons throughout history from 429 B.C. to 1998. The public health impact of terrorism is relatively small, in the sense that terrorist attacks create only a small number of casualties compared to the much greater number of deaths and cases of disability caused by more traditional hazards. Terrorism creates a climate of fear and depends on a collective state of anxiety to achieve its ends. There are signs, however, that terrorism may become more of a direct threat to health. The 1995 terrorist attack on the Tokyo subway, with the nerve gas sarin, caused over a dozen deaths and over a thousand casualties, making it one of the most devastating such incidents on record.

Terrorist weapons can include nuclear devices, radiological material, and chemical and biological agents. Figure 13.1 contrasts the likelihood of the materials being used by terrorists with their potential impact. The conventional wisdom is that a nuclear weapon will be very difficult for a terrorist group to acquire; however, radioactive material, chemical agents, and biological agents are relatively easy to obtain, and thus pose a greater threat. Both the availability and the impact of chemical and biological threat materials are high, with potential devastating consequences.

Table 13.3. Chronology of State Use and Biological and Chemical Weapons Control. (Source: CNS, 2001).

YEAR	PLACE	INCIDENT
429 B.C.	Rome	Spartans ignite pitch and sulfur to create toxic fumes in the Pelopponnesian War.
424 B.C.	Delium	Toxic fumes used in siege of Delium during the Peloponnesian War.
960-1279 A.D.	China	Arsenical smoke used in battle during China's Sung Dynasty.
1346-1347	Crimea	Mongols catapult corpses contaminated with plague over the walls into Kaffa (in Crimea), forcing besieged Genoans to flee.
1456	Belgrade	City of Belgrade defeats invading Turks by igniting rags dipped in poison to create a toxic cloud.
1710	Sweden	Russian troops allegedly use plague-infected corpses against Swedes.
1767	U.S.	During the French and Indian Wars, the British gave blankets used to wrap British smallpox victims to hostile Indian tribes.
April 24, 1863	U.S.	The US War Department issues General Order 100, proclaiming "The uses of poison in any manner, be it to poison wells, or foods, or arms, is wholly excluded from modern warfare.
July 29, 1899	The Netherlands	"Hague Convention (II) with Respect to the Laws and Customs of War on Land" is signed. The Convention declares "it is especially prohibited...To employ poison or poisoned arms".
1914	France	French begin using tear gas in grenades and Germans retaliate with tear gas in artillery shells.
April 22, 1915	France	Germans attack the French with chlorine gas at Ypres, France. This was the 1st significant use of chemical warfare in WW I.
Sept 25, 1915		First British chemical weapons attack; chlorine gas is used against Germans at the Battle of Loos.
1916-1918		German agents use anthrax and the equine disease glanders to infect livestock and feed for export to Allied forces. Incidents include the infection of Romanian sheep with anthrax and glanders for export to Russia, Argentinian mules with anthrax for export to Allied troops, and American horses fed with glanders for export to France.
Feb 26, 1918	Germany	Germans launch the first projectile attack against US troops with phosgene and chloropicrin shells. The first major use of gas against American forces.
June 1918	U.S.	First U.S. use of gas in warfare.
June 28, 1918	U.S.	The U.S. begins its formal chemical weapons program with the establishment of the Chemical Warfare Service.
1919	Britain	British use Adamsite against the Bolsheviks during the Russian Civil War.
1922-1927	Spanish Morocco	The Spanish use chemical weapons against the Rif rebels in Spanish Morocco.
June 17, 1925	Geneva	"Geneva Protocol for the Prohibition of the Use in War of Asphyxiating, Poisonous or Other Gases, and of Bacteriological Methods of Warfare" is signed – not ratified by US and not signed by Japan.
1936	Abyssinia	Italy uses mustard gas against Ethiopians during its invasion of Abyssinia.
1937	Japan	Japan begins its offensive biological weapons program. Unit 731, the BW research and development unit, is located in Harbin, Manchuria. Over the course of the program, at least 10, 000 prisoners are killed in Japanese experiments.
1939	Nomonhan	Japanese poison Soviet water supply with intestinal typhoid bacteria at former Mongolian border. 1st use of biological weapons by Japanese.
1940	China /Manchuria	The Japanese drop rice and wheat mixed with plague-carrying fleas over China and Manchuria.
1942	Maryland, U.S.	US begins its offensive biological weapons program and chooses Camp Detrick, Frederick, MD as its research and development site.
1942	Germany	Nazis begin using Zyklon B (hydrocyanic acid) in gas chambers for the mass murder concentration camp prisoners.
Dec 1943	Bari, Italy	A US ship loaded with mustard bombs is attacked in the port of Bari, Italy by Germans; 83 US troops die in poisoned waters.
April 1945	Germany	Germans manufacture and stockpile large amounts of tabun and sarin nerve gases.
May 1945	Bohemia	Only known tactical use of BW by Germany. A large reservoir in Bohemia is poisoned with sewage.
Sept 1950-Feb 1951	San Francisco,U.S.	In a test of BW dispersal methods, biological simulants are sprayed over San Francisco.

YEAR	PLACE	INCIDENT
1962-1970	Vietnam	US uses tear gas and four types of defoliant, including Agent Orange, in Vietnam.
1963-1967	Yemen	Egypt uses chemical weapons (phosgene, mustard) against Yemen.
June 1966	New York, U.S.	The U. S. conducts a test of vulnerability to covert BW attack by releasing a harmless biological stimulant into the NY subway system.
Nov 25, 1969	U.S.	President Nixon announces unilateral dismantlement of the US offensive BW program.
Feb 14, 1970	U.S.	President Nixon extends the dismantlement efforts to toxins, closing a loophole which might have allowed for their production.
April 10, 1972		"Convention on the Prohibition of the Development, Production and Stockpiling of Bacteriological and Toxin Weapons and on Their Destruction" (BWC) is opened for signature.
1975	Geneva	US ratifies Geneva Protocol (1925) and BWC.
1975-1983	Laos and Kampuchea	Alleged use of Yellow Rain (trichothecene mycotoxins) by Soviet-backed forces in Laos and Kampuchea. There is evidence to suggest use of T-2 toxin, but an alternative hypothesis suggest that the yellow spots labeled Yellow Rain were caused by swarms of defecating bees.
1978	London, U.K	In a case of Soviet state-sponsored assassination, Bulgarian exile Georgi Markov, living in London, is stabbed with an umbrella that injects him with a tiny pellet containing ricin.
1979	Afghanistan	The US government alleges Soviets use of chemical weapons in Afghanistan, including Yellow Rain.
April 2, 1979	Sverdlovsk, Soviet Union	Outbreak of pulmonary anthrax in Sverdlovsk, Soviet Union. In 1992, Russian President Boris Yeltsin acknowledges that the outbreak was caused by an accidental release of anthrax spores from a Soviet military microbiological facility.
August 1983	Iraq	Iraq begins using chemical weapons (mustard gas), in Iran-Iraq War.
1984	Iraq	First ever use of nerve agent tabun on the battlefield, by Iraq during the Iran-Iraq War.
1987-1988	Iraq	Iraq uses chemical weapons (hydrogen cyanide, mustard gas) in its Anfal Campaign against the Kurds, most notably in the Halabja Massacre of 1988.
1985-1991	Iraq	Iraq develops an offensive biological weapons capability including anthrax, botulium toxin, and aflatoxin.
Sept 3, 1992	Geneva	"Convention on the Prohibition of the Development, Production, Stockpiling and Use of Chemical Weapons and on their Destruction"(CWC)approved by UN.
April 29, 1997		Entry into force of CWC.
1998	Iraq	Iraq is suspected of maintaining an active CBW program in violation of the ceasefire agreement it signed with the UN Security Council. Baghdad refuses to allow UNSCOM inspectors to visit undeclared sites.

Table 13.3. Continued.

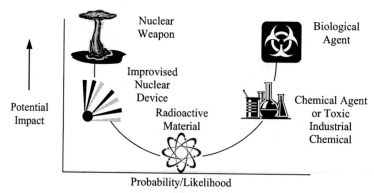

Figure 13.1. Probability of NBC Agents vs. Potential Impact (Source: CNS, 2001).

B. MODERN CONVENTIONAL WARFARE

The primary purpose of modern warfare is to defeat or debilitate the enemy's society and support systems to control a strategic resource and thereby impose or avoid political domination. This is in contrast to warfare in earlier societies, when battles tended to be fought by smaller armies with limited force and the fighting was confined to soldiers or warriors. Sometimes, such battles were really only rituals, hurting & only a small fraction of the population, and the losers were taken as hostages for ransom. Although there are many examples in history of horrific wars undertaken with crude weapons that led to great suffering, such as the Hundred Year's War in Europe, for the most part, the damage that could be done was limited.

In the eighteenth century the so-called art of war changed and by the time of Napoleon, new tactics and artillery had greatly increased the damage that one army could cause. **Scorched-earth strategies** of intentional widespread destruction were used by Russia to stop Napoleon and by General Sherman against the rebels in the American Civil War. By the time of World War I, the world had had extensive experience with a type of warfare that made all civilians targets. Such warfare did not hesitate to destroy the environment for the sake of depriving the other side of food and shelter, and it aimed at shredding the fabric of civil society to demoralize and confuse the enemy. The emphasis in modern warfare became disruption of the economy and civil society, not merely the defeat of troops and the destruction of military targets.

Displacing civilians by warfare and making them **refugees** is often part of the enemy's strategy to occupy the conquered territory (**ethnic cleansing** was the term used for this in the former Yugoslavia). Large movements of dispossessed people reflect profound human tragedy, create problems for public health and primary health care services, and add to crowding and overpopulation in the camps and communities that receive them. Children of refugees may be denied education or health services and may face growing up in an unstable, hostile, and unfamiliar society. Scavenging for food and firewood may cause local ecological damage.

As tragic as scorched-earth strategies and refugee movements are, given the opportunity, people rebuild and carry on with their lives and the land usually recovers. However, following chemical, biological, or nuclear warfare, land could be contaminated for generations to come. These acts of warfare at least have a military purpose in seeking to defeat the enemy. Armies intent on winning a war are not generally interested in their environmental impact. In addition to this largely intentional devastation, the arbitrary destruction and confusion that occurs incidental to war leads to ecological damage from air and water pollution, road building through sensitive environments, and troop movements.

C. CHEMICAL WARFARE

Chemical warfare, introduced on a large scale in World War I, involves the controlled release of toxic chemicals, usually nerve toxins or intensely irritating agents. When used in the field, these poisons are indiscriminate in their actions and may affect civilians or troops on either side, as well as wildlife and domestic animals (Figure 13.2 and Table 13.4). These chemical agents are classified as either lethal, or incapacitating and "riot control," according to their intended use. Industrial chemicals are generally respiratory agents that are exceedingly volatile and dissipate rapidly outdoors. Table 13.5 lists the four industrial chemicals (chlorine, phosgene, hydrogen cyanide and cyanogen chloride), which have been previously used as chemical warfare agents. The chemical warfare agents include blister agents and nerve agents. The first of the chemical warfare agents are classified as "blister agents" that include sulfur mustards, nitrogen mustards, arsenicals, and Nettle agents. The next three categories of agents all owe their physiological effects to a similar mode of action and are usually categorized as nerve agents which are G- agents, V- agents, and others. The nerve agents were discovered in the mid-1930s when German scientists were looking for better pesticides. A number of other organo-phosphorous compounds have been found to have potent nerve agent-like effects and could be used by terrorists. Commercial insecticides, given enough concentration and the right disseminator, could well be used as nerve agents. They are usually produced either from organo-phosphorous based compounds or from carbamates. Figure 13.3 compares the approximate lethalities of the chemical agents. They are based relative to chlorine in terms of respiration. If chlorine is used as a baseline (1.0 on the Figure 13.3), phosgene (CG) is about 6 times more toxic, hydrogen cyanide (AC) 7 times more toxic, parathion 12 times more toxic, mustard (H) 13 times more toxic and sarin (GB) 200 times more toxic.

These chemical agents can cause considerable local damage and may wipe out entire villages. As a consequence, they are often considered to be weapons of terror and civilian intimidation rather than effective military measures. The agents that have actually been used in recent years do not seem to be very persistent in the environment, perhaps because armed forces that use them know that they may have to enter and occupy the same area later. The storage of chemicals used for chemical warfare has sometimes created a hazard, particularly over many years when the containers begin to disintegrate. Although chemical weapons have been outlawed for a very long time by an international agreement known as the **Hague Declaration**, there have been many documented instances of their use and many more suspected incidents in which absolute proof has been lacking or controversial.

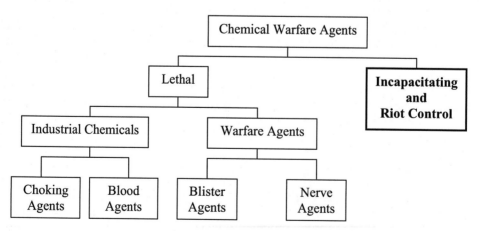

Figure 13.2. Classes of Chemical Warfare Agents (Source: CNS, 2001).

Table 13.4. Bioterrorism Hazard Classification (Source: CNS, 2001).

AGENT TYPE	SYMBOL	DOT CLASS	NFPA 704	DOT ERG	PEL*/TWA** (mg/m³)
CHEMICAL					
Nerve Agents					
Tabun	GA	6.1	421	153	.0001
Sarin	GB	6.1	411	153	.0001
Soman	GD	6.1	411	153	.00003
V Agent	VX	6.1	411	153	.00001
Blister Agents					
Mustard	H	6.1	411	153	.003
Distilled Mustard	HD	6.1	411	153	.003
Nitrogen Mustard	HN	6.1	411		.003
Lewisite	L	6.1	411	153	.003
Phosgene Oxime	CX	6.1	411	153	NS
Blood Agents					
Hydrogen Cyanide	AC	6.1	442	117	5.0
Cyanogen Chloride	CK	2.3	442	125	0.06
Choking Agents					
Chlorine	CL	2.3	300	124	1.5
Phosgene	CG	2.3	400	125	0.4
Irritant Agents					
Tear Gas	CS	6.1		159	0.8
Mace	CN	6.1		153	0.3
Pepper Spray	OC	6.1		159	NA

Airborne Exposure Limit (AEL) – The permissible time weighted average airborne exposure concentration for an 8- hour work day of a 40-hour week. AELs are expressed in either ppm or mg/m³.

* Permissible Exposure Limit (PEL) – The Time Weighted Average (TWA) concentration at which 95% of exposed healthy adults will suffer no adverse effects over an 8-hour/day shift of a 40 hour work week. PELs are expressed in either ppm or mg/m³. PELs are enforceable by law, whereas TWAs are recommended limits.

** Time Weighted Average/ Threshold Limit Value (TWA/TLV) – The Maximum airborne concentration of a material to which an average healthy person may be repeatedly exposed for 8-hours each day, 40-hours each week, without suffering adverse effects. TLV/TWA are expressed in either ppm or mg/m³.

Table 13.5. Industrial Chemicals Used as Terrorism Agents (Source: CNS, 2001).

	Choking Agents	Blood Agents
	Chlorine/Phosgene	Hydrogen Cyanide/ Cyanogen Chloride
Physical Appearance	Greenish-yellow gas/ Colorless gas	Colorless Gas
Odor	Bleach/Mown hay	Bitter Almonds
Symptoms	• Coughing • Choking • Tightness in chest	• Gasping for air • Red eyes, lips, skin
Protection	Respiratory (Skin)	Respiratory (Skin)
First Aid	Aeration	Aeration, cyanide kit

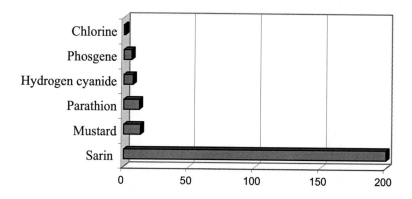

Figure 13.3. Approximate Lethalities of Chemical Agents (Source: CNS, 2001).

D. BIOLOGICAL WARFARE

Biological warfare, which is even more difficult to control, involves targeted release of pathogens such as viruses, bacteria, and toxins. In the few instances in which it has been tried, there have been limited outbreaks of disease involving local residents and wildlife. The effects of biological weapons are short term and unpredictable, but certain agents, are transmissible and could cause widespread epidemics. Because the weapons perform poorly in the battlefield and are unreliable against civilians, biological warfare has been used only rarely, although it has been often alleged. In recent years, world concern over biological weapons has focused chiefly on the testing and development of these weapons and the use of biological agents in laboratories released into the environment during studies to develop protective measures. These weapons have been outlawed by the **Geneva Protocol** since 1925. This was strengthened by a further Convention in 1972 to which 100 countries subscribe. In recent years there have been fears that terrorist groups would use biological agents.

Unlike chemical agents, most of which have an immediate effect, biological agents have a delayed effect ranging from several hours to days, and in some cases weeks. They are more toxic than chemicals by weight. Table 13.6 presents the bioterrorism agents that may or may not be transmitted to man. For example, ricin, one of the toxins is 6 to 9 times more toxic than sarin, and botulinum, another toxin, is 15,000 to 30,000 times more toxic than sarin. Anthrax and plague are two examples of disease caused by bacteria. Examples of viruses are smallpox (the mortality rate can reach 30%) and Ebola (mortality can reach 90%). Examples of toxins are botulinum (a neurotoxin) and ricin (a cytotoxin). Other biologically derived compounds, such as Q-fever, Tularemia, Staphylococcal Enterotoxin B, and Venezuelan Equine Encephalitis, have been considered candidates for weaponization or terrorist use.

E. Nuclear Warfare

The ultimate extension of ecological warfare is, of course, nuclear war, where the target is both the people and the region. The massive destructive power of nuclear weapons led to an impasse that dominated the latter half of this century: both sides held such massive military power that any attempt by either side to use nuclear weapons assured their mutual destruction. This climate of fear is thought to guarantee that neither side would use these weapons, a terrifying basis for peace but, to many, an effective one.

Since the collapse of the Soviet Union, there is little immediate prospect of total nuclear war, but the proliferation of nuclear weapons to other countries carries a grave risk that they will be used in regional conflicts. Should a nuclear exchange ever occur, the regional devastation it would bring would be inconceivable: sudden death, fire, massive destruction, and slow death by radiation sickness for those survivors at the periphery. However, this would be only pan of the impact. Release of radiation, potentially carried many miles by wind and water, disruption and contamination of food supplies, shortages of medical services and supplies, and the susceptibility to infection of malnourished and irradiated survivors would result in massive casualties well beyond the initial blast zone. It is also possible that a massive exchange would propel huge quantities of debris into the atmosphere, creating dust clouds that would block sunlight and cause a prolonged cooling of the earth's surface called **nuclear winter**.

The testing and production of nuclear weapons continue to pose a threat of accidental release and local contamination. The sites of several nuclear weapons plants are reported to be seriously contaminated and radionuclides have been detected in groundwater downstream from at least one plant in the United States, although the details are usually military secrets. Test sites in the South Pacific used by the United States after World War II have shown high levels of residual radiation and radionuclide contamination decades after the test, which is not surprising considering the long half-lives of some decay products of uranium and plutonium.

Table 13.6. Bioterrorism Agents That May or May Not be Transmissible to Man (Source: CNS, 2001).

Disease	Likely method of dissemination	Transmissible man to man	Infective dose	Incubation period	Duration of illness	Lethality	Persistance	Vaccine efficacy (aerosol exposure)
Anthrax	Spores in aerosol	No (except cutaneous)	8-10,000 spores	1-5 days	3-5 days (usually fatal)	High	Very stable spores remain visible for years in soil	2 doses of vaccine protects against 200-500 LD$_{50}$s in monkeys
Cholera	Sabotage (food & water) Aerosol	Rare	>10^6 organisms	12 hours – 6 days	≥ 1 week	Low with treatment, high without	Unstable in aerosols & fresh water, stable in salt water	No data on aerosol
Pneumatic Plague	Aerosol	High	<100 organisms	1-3 days	1-6 days (usually fatal)	High unless treated within 12-24 hours	For up to 1 year in soil; 270 days in bodies	3 doses not protective against 118 LD$_{50}$ s
Tularemia	Aerosol	No	1-50 organisms	1-10 days	≥ 2 weeks	Moderate if untreated	For months in moist soil or other media	80% protection against 1-10 LD$_{50}$S
Q Fever	Aerosol Sabotage (food supply)	Rare	10 organisms (aerosol)	14-26 days	Weeks	Very low	For months in wood and sand	94% protection against 3,500 LD$_{50}$S
Ebola	Direct contact (endemic) Aerosol (BW)	Moderate	1- 10 plague forming units for primates	4-15 days	Death between 7-16 days	High for Zaire strain, moderate with Sudan	Relatively unstable	No vaccine
Smallpox	Aerosol	High	Assumed low	10-12 days	4 weeks	High to moderate	Very stable	Vaccine protects against large doses in primates
Venezuelen Equine Encephalitic	Aerosol Infected vectors	Low	Assumed very low	1-6 days	Days to weeks	Low	Relatively unstable	TC 83 protects against 30-500 LD$_{50}$s in hamsters
Botulinum Toxin	Aerosol Sabotage (food & water)	No	0.001 µg/kg is LD$_{50}$	Variable (hours to days)	Death in 24-72 hours; lasts months if not lethal	High without respiratory support	For weeks in nonmoving water and food	3 doses efficacy of 100% against 25-250 LD$_{50}$s in primates
t-2 Mycotoxins	Aerosol Sabotage	No	Moderate	2-4 hours	Days to months	Moderate	For years at room temperature	No vaccine
Ricin	Aerosol Sabotage	No	3-5 µg/kg is LD$_{50}$	Hours to days	Hours to days	High	Stable	No vaccine

Release to the atmosphere and across long distances was a serious concern for above-ground nuclear testing and venting from below-ground testing, and low levels of radionuclides such as strontium-90 were well documented to have migrated with prevailing winds from test sites in the 1950s and 1960s, before bilateral test ban treaties were negotiated between the United States and the Soviet Union. In the current complicated world situation, there is somewhat more concern over accidental release from deteriorating stockpiles or handling accidents involving nuclear weapons.

Of the three types of threats (chemical, biological or nuclear/radiological), a nuclear weapon explosion is considered the least likely for a terrorist to be able to use. However, the potential exists for it to happen and even more potential exists for the use of radiological materials. The detonation of an improvised nuclear device (IND) would be devastating; if successfully detonated, this would cause widespread explosive damage with a large release of radioactive particles.

Historically, human anthrax in its various forms has been a disease of those with close contact to animals or animal products contaminated with **Bacillus anthracis** spores. In the mid-1800s, inhalational anthrax related to the textile industry became known as woolsorters' disease (in England) and ragpickers' disease (in Germany and Austria) because of the frequency of infection in mill workers exposed to imported animal fibers contaminated with **B. anthracis** spores. In the early 1900s, human cases of inhalational anthrax occurred in the United States in conjunction with the textile and tanning industries. In the last part of the 20th century, with improved industrial hygiene practices and restrictions on imported animal products, the number of cases fell dramatically; however, death rates remained high (>85%). In 1979, in Sverdlovsk, former Soviet Union, an apparent aerosol release of **B. anthracis** spores from a military facility resulted in the largest outbreak of inhalational anthrax in the 20th century.

Before October 2001, the last case of inhalational anthrax in the United States had occurred in 1976. Identification of inhalational anthrax in a journalist in Florida on October 4, 2001, marked the beginning of the first confirmed outbreak associated with intentional anthrax release in the United States.

From October 4 to November 2, 2001, the Centers for Disease Control and Prevention and state and local public health authorities reported 10 confirmed cases of inhalational anthrax and 12 confirmed or suspected cases of cutaneous anthrax in persons who worked in the District of Columbia, Florida, New Jersey, and New York. Epidemiologic investigation indicated that the outbreak resulted from intentional delivery of **B. anthracis** spores through mailed letters or packages.

Of the 10 inhalational cases, 7 occurred in postal employees in New Jersey and the District of Columbia who were likely exposed to letters known to be contaminated with **B. anthracis** spores. Two cases were in employees of a media company in Florida: one is believed to have received contaminated mail, the other to have sorted and distributed that mail. Case 10 was in a resident of New York, and the nature of her exposure to **B. anthracis** is currently unknown.

F. GUERRILLA WARFARE AND DELIBERATE ENVIRONMENTAL DESTRUCTION

In the twentieth century, there have been a number of regional conflicts involving **guerrilla warfare**, where one side avoids direct engagement with the enemy and instead attacks periodically and without warning, often by ambush, and seeks to escape into the surrounding countryside before an effective retaliation can be launched. Guerrilla warfare is usually undertaken by a weaker, poorly armed indigenous force against an occupying or dominant power with conventional military resources. This form of warfare rapidly escalates into environmental destruction because the dominant force finds it difficult to engage the insurrectionary force directly and so responds by destroying the villages and countryside where the insurrectionary force is concealed and supported. Indeed, destruction of the environment is often a military strategy to inflict damage on the other side in a guerrilla war. In particular, the dominant forces have sprayed tropical forests with herbicide, burned off vegetation, and employed carpet bombing of large areas, leaving craters and many unexploded bombs, and both sides have commonly planted land mines. The result has been devastated forest growth and the creation of deadly hazards that last well beyond peace or a cease-fire. In many areas of the world today, buried **land mines** are a serious hazard, particularly for people working in agriculture. It is thought that there are 100 million land mines, planted in some 64 countries. About 26,000 people, mostly civilians, are killed or injured by mines each year.

VII. <u>BIBLIOGRAPHY</u>

Baker, S.P., O'Neil, B., Ginsburg, M.J., Li, G. (1992). <u>Injury Fact Book</u>. New York, NY: Oxford University Press.

Budnick, L.D. (1992). Injuries. In B.J. Cassens (Ed.), <u>Preventive Medicine and Public Health, 2nd Edition</u> (pp.189-208). Baltimore, MD: Williams & Wilkins.

Center for Nonproliferation Studies. (2001). <u>Chemical and Biological Weapons Resource Page</u> (pp.1-7) retrieved from http: cns.miis.edu/research/cbw/pastuse.htm on December 13, 2001.

Committee on Trauma Research, Commission on Life Sciences, National Research Council and the Institute of Medicine. (1985). <u>Injury in America: A continuing public health problem</u>. Washington, DC: National Academy Press.

Compton, B., Stewart-Craig, E., and Doak, M. (2001). <u>SBCCOM Domestic Preparedness Training Program (M2-3 – M2-10)</u>. Washington, DC: U.S. Army Edgewood Research, Development and Engineering Center.

Davis, T. G. (1997). Environmental Safety. In M. Morgan (Ed), <u>Environmental Health 2nd Edition</u> (pp.199-215). Englewood, CO: Morton Publishing Company.

Fee, E. (1997). History and Development of Public Health. In F.D. Scutchfield, C.W. Keck, (Eds.), <u>Principles of Public Health Practice</u> (pp. 10-30). Albany, NY: Delmar Publishers.

Harrison, R. (1999). Workforce Violence. In R. Bowler, & J. Cone. (Eds.), <u>Occupational Medicine Secrets</u> (pp. 311-314). Philadelphia, PA: Hanley & Belfus, Inc.

Jernigan, J.A. et al. (2001). Bioterrorism-Related Inhalational Anthrax: The First 10 Cases Reported in the United States. <u>Emerging Infectious Disases,</u> (pp.933-934). Vol.7, No. 6, November –December 2001. Atlanta, GA: CDC.

MMWR. (1996).<u>Trends in rates of homicide-United States, 1985-1994</u> (pp. 460-464). Vol. 45.

Moeller, D. W. (1997). Injury Control. <u>Environmental Health Revised Edition</u> (pp.217-239). Cambridge, MA, and London, UK: Harvard University Press.

National Center for Health Statistics. (2000). <u>Chart developed by the National Center for Injury Prevention and Control, CDC.</u>

National Center for Injury Prevention and Control. (1996). <u>National Summary of Injury Mortality Data, 1987- 1994.</u> Atlanta, GA: U.S. Centers for Disease Control.

Rosenberg, M. L. & Baer, K. (1998). Injury and Violence. In R. Wallace (Ed), <u>Public Health & Preventive Medicine</u> (pp. 1207-1260). Stamford, CT: Appleton & Lange.

Rosenberg, M.L., Mercy, J.A.(1992). Assaultive Violence. In J.M. Last, R.B. Wallace (Eds.), <u>Maxcy-Rosenau-Last: Public health and Preventive Medicine. 13th Edition</u> (pp. 1035-1039). Norwalk, CT: Appleton & Lange.

Thalmann, E. D. (2001). Diving Hazards. In L. Williams, & R. Langley (Eds.), <u>Environmental Health Secrets</u> (pp. 154-167). Philadelphia, PA: Hanley & Belfus, Inc.

The National Committee for Injury Prevention and Control. (1989). Violence and Injury. <u>Injury Prevention Meeting the Challenge</u> (pp. 192-203). New York, NY: Oxford University Press, Inc.

Yassi, A., Kjellström, T., de Kok, T., & Guidotti, T. L. (2001). Nature of Environmental Health Hazards: Mechanical Hazards. In A. Yassi, [et al](Eds.), <u>Basic Environmental Health</u> (pp. 92-102). New York, NY: Oxford University Press, Inc.

Yassi, A., Kjellström, T., de Kok, T., & Guidotti, T. L. (2001). Transboundary and Global Health Concerns: Health Consequences of War. In A. Yassi, [et al](Eds.), <u>Basic Environmental Health</u> (pp. 370-375). New York, NY: Oxford University Press, Inc.

U.S. Army Edgewood Research, Development and Engineering Center. (1999). The Threat of NBC Terrorism. <u>Domestic Preparedness Defense Against Weapons of Mass Destruction</u> (M2.3-R.9). Washington, D.C.: Booz-Allen & Hamilton Inc., Science Applications International Corporation Inc., EAI Corporation, and PDI Inc.

CHAPTER

14

THE WORKPLACE

I. <u>INTRODUCTION</u>

Industrial hygiene originated with physicians identifying adverse health effects in their patients and subsequently associating these illnesses with specific occupations. Industrial hygiene has progressed from simply recognizing occupational illnesses with very little done to protect workers, to basic hygiene, to worker protection, and finally to legislation. Industrial hygiene has evolved from an abstract and undefined science to a recognized and respected profession.   Industrial hygienists are professionals with the training, education, and experience in anticipating and recognizing health standards arising from work processes and operations. Industrial hygienists evaluate work-related environmental hazards and stresses through measurement of chemical, physical, ergonomic, and biological stresses. Skilled at evaluating and measuring the magnitude of hazards, they are equally equipped to establish and implement effective hazard control methods for reducing or eliminating exposure.

Protective legislation came piecemeal and slowly (Table 14.1) in the U.S. Worker's compensation laws, passed in France, Germany, and the UK in 19th century, were one of the earliest forms of social insurance on a prepaid basis, with no direct contribution from workers. The Walsh-Healey Public Contracts Act of 1936 established safety and health standards in industries conducting work under contract to federal government. The first significant federal legislation for workers outside government projects did not come until 1969, with the Federal Coal Mine Health and Safety Act. This legislation was followed by the landmark Occupational Safety and Health Act of 1970, whose announced principle purpose was to "assure so far as possible every working man and woman in the Nation healthful working conditions and to preserve human resources." Among the provisions of this act was the establishment of the Occupational Safety and Health Administration (OSHA) and the creation of the National Institute for Occupational Safety and Health (NIOSH). Later, Congress incorporated "right-to-know" provisions in amendments to the 1976 Toxic Substances Control Act (TSCA) to require employers to furnish workers with information about the health hazards of their occupational environment. One recent law that has significantly reduced occupational exposures is the Pollution Prevention Act of 1990.   This law, which established a national policy to encourage the prevention of pollution at the source, with disposal to the environment acceptable only as a last resort, has led to the substitution of less toxic substances for those used in wide range of industrial processes. In turn, significant reductions in worker exposure have resulted.

Growth has been rapid, with at least three major phases involving the early years prior to 1930, the dramatic increase between 1935 and 1945 due to social security legislation and World War II, and the more recent phase of growth resulting from the passage of the federal OSH Act in 1970.

Over the past few years it would appear that, at least in the United States, occupational hygienists are in the midst of a fourth period of change. There are at least three major driving forces involved with this phase. The first involves the "reinvention" of much of the government, including OSHA, to focus less on a regulatory approach to problem solving and to enhance cooperation and partnerships with those considered to be stakeholders. Although OSHA remains a regulatory agency, the pace of regulation and inspection has slowed.

Table 14.1. Significant Federal Legislation Pertaining to Occupational Health and Safety. (Source: Moeller, 1997).

Year	Act	Content
1908	Federal Workers' Compensation Act	Granted limited compensation benefits to certain U.S. civil service workers for injuries sustained during employment
1936	Walsh-Healey Public Contracts Act	Established occupational health and safety standards for employees of federal contractors
1969	Federal Coal Mine Health and Safety Act	Created forerunner of Mine Safety and Health Administration; required development and enforcement of regulations for protection of mine workers
1970	Occupational Health and Safety Act	Authorized federal government to develop and set mandatory occupational safety and health standards; Established National Institute for Occupational Safety and Health to conduct research for setting standards
1976	Toxic Substances Control Act	Required data from industry on production, use, and health and environmental effects of chemicals; led to development of "tight- to-know" laws, which provide employees with information on nature of potential occupational exposures
1990	Pollution Prevention Act	Established policy to ensure that pollution is prevented or reduced at source, recycled or treated, and disposed of or released only as last resort; led to substitution of less toxic substances in wide range of industrial processes, with significant reductions in worker

The second force is the downsizing of corporate America and increased outsourcing of services, including occupational hygiene. In 1986 approximately 15% of AIHA's 6500 members identified themselves as consultants. By 1996, of the 13,000 members, 30% were listed as consultants. The other major factor affecting the profession is the shift of the American economy from a manufacturing to a service base. Although not necessarily less hazardous, service industries often have problems much different from those of a traditional manufacturing site. While service industries have many of the same chemical, physical, and biological hazards found in manufacturing, the awareness of the need for industrial hygiene services is usually low.

Recognition of the need to address occupational health problems in nontraditional workplaces is not new. Jack Bloomfield, one of the first industrial hygienists in the USPHS, noted in 1938 that "industrial hygienists have concentrated their efforts on the so-called industrial population—that group of workers engaged in the manufacture, mechanical and mining industries. Although it is probably true that the bulk of the occupational diseases occurs in these industries, nevertheless, the 10 million workers in agriculture, the 4 million persons employed in transportation and communication, and the large number of workers in domestic and personal services, all have health problems deserving attention".

To not only remain viable but also to achieve increased recognition and acceptance of their work, it is apparent that occupational hygienists must achieve two goals. First, hygienists must continue to expand the scope of their practice to include environmental health considerations, especially those arising from the workplace. The skills and knowledge involved in the recognition, evaluation, and control of air, and even water, pollution problems as well as those of hazardous wastes as they affect the health and well-being of those in the community are not dissimilar to the skills and knowledge applied to traditional industrial hygiene problems. Indeed, many of the early environmental health practitioners, especially addressing air pollution, radiologic health and hazardous waste problems, were industrial hygienists. The first air pollution disaster in the United States, the Donora, PA smog of October 1948, resulted in the death of 20 people and to some degree affected almost 6000 persons. The investigation of the incident involved a multidisciplinary team of physicians, nurses, engineers, chemists, meteorologists, housing experts, veterinarians, and dentists under the direction of a USPHS industrial hygienist - George D. Clayton. Occupational hygienists must become more effective in providing comprehensive rather than one-issue services.

Secondly, as a profession and as individuals, occupational hygienists must demonstrate that their services, in addition to preventing occupational and environmental health problems, provide a positive contribution to the individual worker, the community, and the employer.

II. PUBLIC HEALTH ROOTS

It has been postulated that the first Public Health Revolution unfolded in nineteenth century Europe as that society sought to address the adverse health effects of squalid living conditions: poor sanitation, poor housing, dangerous work environments and air pollution.

The Institute of Medicine has defined public health as "what we, as a society, do collectively to assure the conditions in which people can be healthy". Thus, when industrial hygienists implement a control measure to reduce a worker's exposure to a toxin, they are practicing the art and science of public health. Those who practice in the field of public health are well aware that throughout the history of public and especially occupational health, two major factors have shaped our solutions: the availability of scientific and technical knowledge and the content of public values and opinions. The Institute of Medicine has recognized the lack of agreement about the public health mission as reflected in the diversion in some states of traditional public health functions "such as water and air pollution control, to separate departments of environmental services, where the health effects of pollutants often receive less notice." Although industrial hygiene functions are now most often found combined with safety programs in labor rather than public health departments, the concepts of injury prevention, whether on or off the job, have strong public health underpinnings. Thus, safety and hygiene are intertwined.

The first professional journal to address industrial hygiene concerns was the Journal of the American Public Health Association. In 1914 the journal announced a new department on industrial hygiene and sanitation to put the readers "in touch with the latest information in this very recently new field of Public Health work," and a review article on industrial hygiene and sanitation was published. In the same year, the association created an industrial hygiene section, and at the annual meeting a special symposium on industrial hygiene was held. Alice Hamilton served as vice chairman of the new section and succeeded to the chairmanship in 1916.

In 1914 the USPHS established an office of industrial hygiene and sanitation, which 57 years later became NIOSH. NIOSH is part of the federal Centers for Disease Control and Prevention, which encompasses most of the public health functions of the federal government. Prior to the OSH Act of 1970, most state and local government industrial hygiene units were found in public health agencies.

Industrial hygiene graduate level academic training in the United States has since its inception been associated with schools of public health. In 1918 the Harvard Medical School established a Department of Applied Physiology, which in 1922 became the Department of Physiology and the Department of Industrial Hygiene in the School of Public Health. In the late 1930s state public health agencies used Social Security funds to train industrial hygienists in schools of public health at Harvard, the University of California, Columbia University, The Johns Hopkins University, the University of Michigan, and Yale University. Today industrial hygiene academic programs are found in at least 18 of the 27 accredited schools of public health.

There is ample evidence that the roots of industrial hygiene are in the field of public health. The public health philosophy of protection and enhancement of the health and well being of groups of people through preventive rather than curative measures applies as well to industrial hygiene.

III. **HISTORY OF THE CONTROL OF THE WORKPLACE**

A. **BACKGROUND**

1. **Introduction**

At the beginning of the twentieth century, most persons who had concerns about health matters arising in and out of industry were physicians and engineers. The physicians led the way in pointing out the conditions of health that existed in many workplaces. Several physicians in the United States made studies in the early part of the century that pointed out the appalling conditions that existed in some workplaces.

Prior to the twentieth century, physicians had made observations about the conditions of health in working persons, particularly in Europe. The physicians did an admirable job of identifying the hazardous conditions that existed in many workplaces and pointing out the effects on health caused by exposure to them. The profession that came to be known as industrial hygiene remained in this discovery mode well into the twentieth century. It was not until perhaps the 1930s or 1940s that engineers began to take an active role in finding ways to control the hazards found in industry. Hence, the industrial hygiene profession really came of age only when it began to do something about the exposures that the physicians had been discovering all along.

Interestingly, today, very few industrial hygienists come from the medical profession. Most physicians who are interested in occupational health become occupational physicians and there are relatively few of them. Similarly, relatively few industrial hygienists now come from the field of engineering. The majority of industrial hygienists come from chemistry and biology. Instead of becoming specialized as others have done in many other fields, most industrial hygienists are generalists. Once there were physicians who specialized in the recognition of diseases and engineers who specialized in the control of hazards leading to disease. Now most industrial hygienists must have a comprehensive ability to recognize, evaluate, and control occupational diseases.

In the United States and Canada the profession is known as industrial hygiene. However, in most of the remainder of the world - in particular Great Britain and such countries of the British Cornmonwealth as Australia and Kenya - it is known as occupational hygiene.

2. Occupational Health

Occupational health, a field of endeavor in which many different professional persons practice, is part of a larger field known as **environmental health**, and of an even larger field known as **public health**.

The name given to the field of occupational health is somewhat unfortunate because it causes confusion over what an industrial or occupational hygienist does. After all, industrial or occupational hygiene literally means occupational health, as hygiene and health are synonymous. In fact hygiene was used in preference to health in the common vernacular in the later nineteenth century.

There is a need to recognize the differences between occupational health (OH) and industrial or occupational hygiene. First, **OH** is only a field, a field of endeavor or an area of **practice**. Hygiene is a discipline or a profession like law or medicine. Disciplines are taught. **A discipline is an area in which one practices**. The first physicians and engineers who became interested in worker health practiced their professions in the context of occupational health. At some point, a group of engineers and physicians (with perhaps a few chemists and biologists) asked the questions, are we practicing our profession (engineering or medicine) in the field of occupational health, or have we defined a new discipline or profession? The answer was yes to the latter, and a new discipline was born, although it still struggles somewhat to be recognized as such.

Today members of many professions, including hygienists, engineers, physicians, and nurses, practice in the field of occupational health. Specialized names such as ergonomist, occupational physician, and occupational health nurse have developed. People from other professions also practice in the field of occupational health, such as chemists, toxicologists, epidemiologists, and lawyers. So long as each is called chemist, toxicologist, or the like, then each maintains an allegiance to his or her first profession. A chemist who does research on methods to detect workplace chemicals usually remains a chemist first.

However, many persons who have training (in order of frequency) in biology, chemistry, engineering, physics, and medicine have taken subsequent special training in hygiene and now consider themselves hygienists. A chemist who becomes a hygienist must look beyond the chemical aspects of occupational health and consider aspects of many other disciplines in the context that each relates to worker health. To repeat, the hygienist is a generalist.

Members of many professions practice in the context of occupational health and are part of a team, including hygienists, occupational physicians, occupational health nurses, safety professionals, ergonomists, occupational epidemiologists, occupational toxicologists, and others. Hence, the industrial hygienist is part of the occupational health team. When safety professionals and ergonomists are included in the team, it is usually termed the occupatiopal safety and health team.

The difference between occupational health and occupational safety is defined by convention. Occupational safety also is a field in which members of several professions practice. Anything that affects worker health obviously also affects worker safety, or anything that affects worker safety may eventually affect worker health. However, by convention, those agents in the workplace that tend to cause systemic illness are studied in the field of occupational health, whereas those agents or unsafe acts that may cause injury are studied in the field of occupational safety. The two important words to differentiate are injury and illness. Illness is associated with occupational health and injury with occupational safety. There is considerable overlap in these two definitions.

3. Occupational Health Prior to 1900

It is not certain who coined the phrase "industrial hygiene." However, prior to 1900 it does not appear to have been used widely. Nevertheless, there were a number of individuals, particularly physicians and engineers, who practiced their profession in the context of occupational health during this time. A few other individuals of note wrote important treatises dealing with workplace health as early as the time of Christ.

From the early 1900s back through time, very few people actually devoted their careers to working in occupational health. However, several notable individuals made observations about occupational health, most of them physicians who made observations concerning unhealthy conditions in the workplace and described the disease that they thought emanated from those unhealthy conditions. It appears that the control of those conditions, to the extent that control took place, was left to enlightened individuals, probably the early forerunners of supervisors, foremen, and engineers, who stumbled upon or in some cases systematically discovered means to make work easier or presumably more healthy.

Alice Hamilton (1881-1972) was a pioneer in industrial hygiene and industrial medicine in the United States. She stated in 1910, when she entered the field, that there was essentially no American literature to be reviewed. She spent two years reviewing German and English literature prior to beginning her studies.

The very earliest records of occupational disease would have been those of Hippocrates, who made observations about lead poisoning in the fourth century B.C. Hence, written observations concerning the unhealthiness of work have been made for at least 2,000 years. It is important to note three other points about Hippocrates work. First, his observations were concerned with lead - which down through the ages has been the most studied occupational disease hazard although we continue to find out things about its effects and continue to reduce exposure levels that are thought to be safe. Second, Hippocrates made far-reaching observations on the subject of medicine and essentially began the process of turning medicine from an art into a science. A similar process began in the early 1900s in the field of industrial hygiene. Third, in 1978, Hunter pointed out very succinctly that the medical principles and the eating, drinking, and exercise habits that Hippocrates recommended were meant for the upper class. People who worked in the "mechanical arts" were at first slaves, and once freed still were looked upon as fourth-class citizens. This social dichotomy between the haves and have-nots was and in some cases still is the biggest obstacle to improving worker health. In Hippocrates' time if a worker complained about conditions, there were many others to take his place, a situation that still exists. If management does not respect the managed as human beings with equal rights and privileges, then it will not be sincere in providing healthy working conditions, even if it complies with the "letter of the law."

Galen (l30-200), Celsus (first century), and Pliny the Elder (first century) also made references to occupational health. Galen and Celsus were physicians; but Pliny the Elder was not one. However, according to Patty in 1958, the latter wrote an encyclopedia of natural sciences in which he referred to the use of animal bladders being worn over the faces of miners to avoid the effects of mercury poisoning. It is not hard to imagine the appalling conditions that existed in many unventilated mines. Mining of metals and metallurgy were the subjects of the first thorough observations on the diseases of occupations. In 1978, Hunter pointed out that by the year 965, mines were established in regions historically associated with Germany, and mining and mining industries remained an important part of commerce for some time. This industry and its tremendously cruel effects on the health of miners, their families, and in some cases owners as well became the subject of observations on the relationship of disease and occupation.

Ellenbog in 1473 described the hazards and mechanisms for the control of mercury and lead. In 1556, almost 100 years later, **De Re Metallica** by Georgius Agricola (1494-1555) was published posthumously. It was an incredible 12-volume treatise on the mining industry that only Agricola could have written. His training was broad and included medicine. In 1526, he was appointed physician to the famous mining town of Joachirnsthal in Bohemia. **De Re Metallica** reports on every aspect of mining. Volume 6 leads with a very brief (five pages from a 600-page treatise) description of diseases and injuries of miners and methods for their prevention. What appears to be arsenical poisoning was well described. In a region of the Carpathian mountauns, it was stated that women resided "who have married seven husbands, all of whom this terrible consumption has carried to a premature death." Although Agricola recognized some of the maladies of mining, his observations were simplistic, even if advanced for his day. He blamed some cases of death on demons, regarding them to be preventable by prayer and fasting, but it is doubtful that the fasting aided the miners' already deteriorating health. Indeed, fasting causes metals to be released from body reservoirs such as bone and kidney tissue. On the other hand, Agricola showed incredible insight into the roots of poor hygiene: ". . . for we should always devote more care to maintain our health, that we may freely perform our bodily functions, than to making profits." This quote applies equally well today, if we can only determine the best way to maintain health.

Another great man of medicine plied his trade as a contemporary of Agricola. Paracelsus (1493-1541) wrote an entire treatise on diseases of mine and smelter workers. Unlike Agricola, he had no formal training, but he had experience in chemistry and metallurgy and became physician of the mining town of Villach. He is best known for abandoning the humoral theory of medicine and adopting specific remedies for diseases. Some were quite amazing, including opium, mercury, lead, and arsenic. Paracelsus said that "it is the dose only that makes the thing not a poison." He taught in German, not Latin, circulated freely among the masses, and in general did everything he could to buck the scholastic etiquette of the day. For this he was exorcised from academic medicine. He is often cited as the **father of toxicology**.

More than a century after Paracelsus, the next scientist to coalesce many years of knowledge on occupational health was Ramazzini. A physician, he went beyond Paracelsus and Agricola in his treatise of 1700, **De Morbis Artificum Diatriba** (Discourse on the Disease of Workers). Certainly other descriptions following Paracelsus' description of the diseases of scholars, seafarers, soldiers, salt workers, lawyers, and other occupations had been prepared. However, Ramazzini brought all of them together in one treatment. As a result he has been called the **father of occupational medicine**.

In 1713, Ramazzini's second edition covered 54 occupations. His descriptions of conditions, hazards, diseases, and prevention are, in some cases, amazingly accurate to this day. Hippocrates had formulated a series of questions that physicians should ask of their patients. Ramazzini added an indispensable one:

> When a doctor visits a working class home, he should be content to sit on a three legged stool, if there isn't a gilded chair, and he should take time for his examination; and to the questions recommended by Hippocrates he should add one more - What is your occupation?

From this quote, modern physicians can gain insight on more than one point. Although his book seems timeless in its ability to describe diseases and make observations about their control, it is somewhat sad to observe that after almost 300 years it is still difficult to find general physicians who will ask questions of their patients regarding their occupations. In other words, occupational medicine, and the propensity for work to cause disease and ill effects on health, still is not adequately recognized by the medical profession.

4. Industrial Revolution

Most Americans probably would be surprised to learn (or relearn) that shortly before the American Revolution for independence, the industrial revolution began in Great Britain. Historians commonly cite 1760 to 1830 as the years for that revolution in Great Britain, but in 1830 the United States was still very much an agricultural economy with little mining or manufacturing. Its cotton was milled in England. Its chemicals, what little it used, were made in Europe, as were its metal products. Not until 1860 would the United States enter the industrial revolution, a revolution that ended about 1900.

Industrialism led to several important changes in the way work was done. First, it was divided. No longer would one craftsman spend two months making a rifle. Instead, many workers would make only small parts of rifles, over and over again. Second, it was mechanized. Third, it called for mass labor - hence, children, women, and anyone else who could perform menial, repetitive, mundane tasks were acceptable and often dispensable. Hunter quoted Pierre Ramp, of this era, as saying:

We live on the sufferings of others. Everyone makes life a torment for some of his fellow men. How many people earn their living pleasantly? Many do so in unpleasant and often intolerable conditions. To love one's occupation is to be happy, but where are the occupations which one can love?

To this the current editors of **Hunter's Diseases of Occupations** have added, "Yet it might be said, in an age of unemployment, that one kind of work, however unpleasant, is better than none." Certainly, workplace conditions have changed for the better, but should work necessitate suffering in unpleasant surroundings? Are all workers entitled to safe and healthful working conditions?

The unsafe and unhealthful conditions brought on by the industrial revolution did not reach the United States until the late 1800s; and because these conditions first existed in Europe, Europeans led the way in attempts at improving them and in research. Thus physicians were employed at textile mills as early as 1789. Sir Robert Peel became the British **father of industrial legislation** when he introduced the Health and Morals of Apprentices Act of 1802 as a result of working conditions in his own textile mills. This act was followed by the 1819 and 1825 Factories Acts, which, like their predecessors, were largely child labor laws. The 1833 Factories Act added the teeth of enforcement or inspection, an important step that set up an adversarial relationship between government and industry, which has developed full strength in the United States.

Child labor laws were not enacted by most U.S. states until 1913. This meant that until then, six-year-old children in Southern mills worked 13-hour days with a 35-minute lunch break. A strong national law was not enacted until 1938.

Great Britain also produced Charles Turner Thackrah (1795-1833), who went one step further than Ramazzini. Whereas the latter realized the importance of occupation to health, Thackrah devoted his career to the prevention of diseases caused by occupation and wrote extensively on the subject, including problems of child labor, tuberculosis in tailors, lung disease in miners and metal grinders, and lead poisoning in glaze dippers. His untimely death from tuberculosis at age thirty-seven retarded the prevention movement.

By 1895 Great Britain had passed several other Factories Acts, each strengthening the former, and in that year for the first time certain occupational diseases became reportable. Every physician had to report to the government patients with diseases that he believed to be caused by lead, phosphorus, arsenic, or anthrax. Others were later added. In 1898 Thomas Legge (1863-1932) became the first medical inspector of factories, and other notable British figures soon followed, each associated with seminal research on a disease and work: Edgar Collis (silica), John Sydney Henry (coal tar pitch-skin cancer), F. R. A. Merewether (asbestos), and Ethel Browning (solvents). Interestingly, New York appointed a medical inspector in 1907, but the idea did not catch on. For whatever reason, the United States instead excelled in the area of industrial hygiene, and by the early 1900s its laws were reasonably in line with those in Europe. By 1970 it had accelerated past the rest of the world - at least in legal protection of workers' health.

There are many other contributions to the research and legislative efforts aimed at improving the conditions in the workplace. The German K. D. Lehmann did extensive studies on the toxicology of industrial gases in the late nineteenth, and the French chemist and pharmacist Jean Baptiste Alphonse Chevalier (1793-1879) made a significant contribution. No doubt there were many other contributions, such as those of F. F. Eresiman (1842-1915) of Russia.

5. <u>1910-1940</u>

Most industrial hygienists who are familiar with the work of Alice Hamilton would call her the **first hygienist**. Alice Hamilton was an American physician who vigorously promoted hygiene in industry. Early in her career, she was a physician first and industrial hygienist second. Today, most hygienists use their backgrounds (e.g., chemistry and biology) as stepping-stones toward their ultimate profession. However, the process by which industrial hygiene became a discipline and a profession took place over approximately 40 years. Its roots, at least in the United States, are in the work of Alice Hamilton and began approximately in 1910.

Prior to 1910, no federal legislation had been passed in the United States for the specific purposes of protecting workers' health. Thus, while the Reverend Charles Brigham of the Michigan State Board of Health prepared an essay entitled "The Influence of Occupations Upon Health" as early as 1875, it was not until the pioneering work of Alice Hamilton in Illinois in 1910 to 1915 and the work by Dr. Emery Hayhurst on Ohio industries in 1913 and 1914, that American society began to be awakened to the grim realities of health in the workplace.

Even though Pliny the Elder had pointed out the effects of lead mining upon health as early as the fourth century B.C., the work of Dr. Hamilton again pointed to the fact that lead was the number one cause of extremely disabling disease, or even death, in industry. In fact, the agents of disease that were studied by Dr. Hamilton continue to be agents of disease of the workplace as we enter the twenty-first century. In addition to lead, Dr. Hamilton pointed out diseases associated with mercury, carbon monoxide, phosphorus, aluminum, beryllium, cadmium, chromium, benzene, methanol, carbon disulfide, and synthetic rubber. It is interesting to point out that the diseases associated with aluminum as described by Dr. Hamilton were found in miners who were exposed to aluminum dust, not through the mining of aluminum ore (bauxite), but rather through the use of aluminum dust to cover the surface of mines for the prevention of silicosis (caused by silica). This process has now stopped, and aluminum is well controlled in other industries. This control and aluminum's lack of propensity to cause chronic disease make it the only agent studied by Dr. Hamilton that is of little hazard in today's industry.

Dr. Hamilton's studies and those of others were remarkably revealing of the extent to which disease existed in industry. Nevertheless, very little was done in terms of legislation to control exposures in the workplace. One of the most often-cited pieces of legislation for the control of a specific occupational disease is an act of 1912 that placed a heavy tax on the use of yellow phosphorus, also called **white phosphorus**. The phosphorus was used in the manufacture of matches and caused an extremely disfiguring disease of the jawbone among match workers, known as phossy-jaw. Essentially, the bone deteriorated to the point where, in some cases, workers lost their entire jawbone. However, what is interesting about this particular episode was that even though the disease itself was so disfiguring and a substitute (sulfur) was available for the manufacture of matches, the U.S. government did not choose to place an outright ban on the use of phosphorus. With the exception of food additives that cause cancer in animals (and even the relevant Delaney clause of the Food, Drug, and Cosmetic Act of 1958 is being attacked currently), this trend of restricting, as opposed to banning, substances prevails in the United States. Even highly toxic pesticides that have had effects on humans and wildlife (e.g., the chlorinated hydrocarbons) are regulated closely but are not banned from commerce.

Instead of trying to control occupational agents of disease through legislation, laws were enacted to compensate workers suffering from occupational diseases and injuries. This effort began at the federal level when limited benefits were provided in 1908 for U.S. civil service employees. In 1911, New Jersey adopted worker's compensation legislation, and in 1948 Mississippi became the last state to enact worker's compensation laws. Many of these laws were originally intended to compensate workers for injuries suffered on the job, but gradually various states began compensating workers for illnesses contracted on the job. Some states limited compensation to specific diseases such as silicosis and lead disease, whereas other states allowed compensation for any illness that could be associated with the workplace.

The worker's compensation acts had both advantages and disadvantages. This form of no-fault insurance allowed a worker to be compensated for medical benefits and time off from the job and, in some cases, given a monetary grant where disabling disease or injury occurred, but the legislation took away most other legal remedies that the worker had. Prior to workers' compensation acts, a worker could sue in court for damages due to injury or illness arising from the workplace. The employer had three defenses, which were often liberally used. The first was the **fellow servant defense**: a worker could not be compensated for an injury if another worker's (supervisor's) negligence contributed to the injury. The second defense was the **assumption of risk**. This defense was most reflective of the attitudes of society at the time. It stated that the employee assumed the risk of the hazards inherent in a job. In other words, the employee knew, or should have known, that the job was risky. Of course, at that time many workplaces were full of hazards that were largely acknowledged because they were so obvious; hence a worker would have to know about them. The third defense was that of **contributory negligence**. In this case, if the employee were negligent in any way, he or she would collect nothing, regardless of the employer's negligence.

Regardless of these three strong defenses, conditions in the workplace were apparently appalling enough that large awards began to be made to workers, and industry called for some means of controlling their compensation. Hence, while worker's compensation is a no-fault system in which industry must pay regardless of how, when, or where the accident occurs, it nevertheless gives industry a way of controlling its expenses and, in fact, predicting them.

Another phenomenon that occurred in the 1910 to 1940 period again was a function of the states rather than the federal government. During this time, many states set up industrial hygiene units within either departments of public health or departments of labor, the majority of them located in departments of public health.

By 1909 at least 21 of the states had enacted laws that attempted to regulate various working conditions. Some of the laws dealt with ventilation, whereas others pertained to dust control and general sanitation. Of course, enforcement lagged, either because there were no inspectors or industry was simply expected to comply with the laws, or because inspectors were political appointees who had no training in what they were to inspect. Consequently, as society was enlightened about hazards in the workplace and the profession of industrial hygiene gradually began to be molded, various states set up industrial hygiene units. In addition to their roles as inspectors, persons in these units also had responsibilities for conducting studies of workplace diseases and, in some cases, conducting physical examinations of workers in certain industries.

These industrial hygiene units ebbed and flowed until a point midway through the Great Depression. In 1935 the Social Security Act was passed, and one of its provisions made funds available for the expansion of public health programs, which included industrial hygiene programs. This act alone probably did more to promote industrial hygiene in the United States than any other act up until the 1970 Occupational Safety and Health Act. By today's standards the amounts of money provided were not great. For example, from 1947 to 1950, one million dollars in federal funds was allocated. Nevertheless, there were 30 states and local units established by 1939. Hence, industrial hygiene was born because of an act that allowed the states to hire personnel to investigate, prevent, and control various diseases that had long been established as some of the most debilitating human diseases.

As further testimony to the development of the industrial hygiene profession, several organizations were established in the late 1930s. In 1937, the Federal Division of Industrial Hygiene held a seminar that led to the establishment in 1939 of the American Conference of Governmental Industrial Hygienists. Until recently, members of this organization had to have government affiliation. Hence, in that same year the American Industrial Hygiene Association was established, and it was open to all persons having an interest in industrial hygiene. Thus, it is probably impossible to pick an exact point in time when engineers with an interest in hygiene in industry became industrial hygienists. This was a gradual process by which the principles for recognizing, evaluating, and controlling the agents of disease in industry gradually were developed. However, it seems likely that the establishment of the two organizations in 1939 and the impetus added to the development of the field by the Social Security Act can be cited as the beginnings of the industrial hygiene profession.

It should be noted that the British Occupational Hygiene Society was formed in 1953. One reason for the time lag may be that European countries were far more concerned with the two great wars than was the less deeply involved United States. In fact, the development of the British Industrial Health Research Board in 1918 was for the primary purpose of increasing British wartime output by finding ways to make workers most efficient through healthful conditions. Up to 1939, the Health Board published 80 reports. Nevertheless, Merewether conceded, in 1942, the American leadership in "industrial hygiene engineering."

6. 1940 to the Environmental Movement

World War II led to a tremendous expansion of industrial hygiene in the United States, in Great Britain, and probably throughout the world. One reason for this, as discovered by the British Industrial Health Research Board, was quite simply that efficiency of production was increased if workers remained healthy and did their job with the least amount of nuisance and discomfort. Some of the beginnings of the industrial hygiene movement in Great Britain can be traced to similar needs during World War I. Much of the early effort in Great Britain for improving efficiency in World War I was centered around fatigue. It was found that for women engaged in turning shell cases, their productivity could be increased by 11% by decreasing their hours of work by 12%, from 68 to 60 hours per week. Of course, fatigue is a form of discomfort and a lack of well being that is thus detrimental to health. The study of fatigue, then, in World War I led naturally to the study of other forms of detriment to health.

In the United States, the state efforts that had begun with the Social Security Act were tremendously expanded during the World War II years. The number of state and local units increased to 47 in 38 states. One million dollars was provided to the states from 1947 to 1950. During the same time, 70 federal industrial hygienists were loaned to state and local industrial hygiene agencies. As a result, all but two states (Delaware and Nevada) were engaged in industrial hygiene work, on at least a limited basis, by 1950, and the number of professional personnel in state and local agencies reached 425.

A direct result of World War II was the industrial development of the United States. Prior to World War I, the United States had no organic chemicals industry whatsoever. Because of the depression, the organic chemicals industry was slow to develop. However, after World War II, the U.S. organic chemicals industry expanded significantly. Even though industry was expanding substantially throughout the 1950s, the number of industrial hygiene professionals at state and local agencies was actually declining during the early 1950s owing to a reduction in funding under the Social Security Act. Interestingly, however, the role that industrial hygiene came to play in the fields of community air pollution and radiological health, which were receiving increased funding, caused an overall increase in the number of industrial hygiene professionals during the 1950s.

Many modern students of industrial hygiene wonder why there is at least a minor emphasis in industrial hygiene on community air pollution and radiological health when these fields are not necessarily encountered in the professional careers of industrial hygienists. The explanation for this can be traced to the 1950s when these two fields were first developing. The first Air Pollution Control Act was passed in 1952, and in addition to providing funds to the federal government for conducting research, it gave federal money to the states for setting up air pollution control programs. In general, the states used the existing industrial hygiene programs to provide these services. By the same token, with the development of the atomic and hydrogen bombs during and after World War II, increased emphasis was placed upon radiological health in the United States. Once again, it was left to state and local public health departments, and specifically their industrial hygiene functions, to study and control radiological health exposures. For example, during the 1950s the fluoroscope, a shoe-size measuring device utilizing X-rays, was banned as a result of studies done by industrial hygiene personnel.

One of the most significant developments of this period was the publication in 1948, with a second edition in 1958, of Industrial Hygiene and Toxicology by Frank A. Pany. This two-volume treatise was a milestone in the discipline of industrial hygiene. Although several other books had been published on occupational diseases and on industrial toxicology, no large works had appeared specifically on industrial hygiene since the work of Chenoweth and his colleagues in 1938. Thus Patty added the mortar to the bricks. Industrial hygiene had not only become a profession, but also a science with a set of principles and practices, which were fully described in Patty's work. J. A. Zapp, a prominent occupational physician and industrial hygienist, has stated that "science, by definition, means knowing or knowledge of the realities of nature and their interrelations". If one uses the scientific method - starting with precise observations, the collection of further observations based upon preliminary observations, the classification or organization of the facts, the stating of hypotheses based upon these relations, and testing of the hypotheses by the previously mentioned method - then one is doing science. Hygienists were doing science by the 1960s and had carved themselves a niche from the natural sciences. No longer were they engineers, chemists, and physicians; they were hygienists.

As the 1950s came to a close, the United States began an era dedicated to the establishment of laws and characterized by a social conscience regarding the adequate provision of a safe, healthful, and pleasing environment to its citizens - the environmental movement. Many laws relating to the environmental movement were passed during the 1960s, and, indeed, the overall awareness of society with respect to the status of the environment was increased many fold. The culmination of this era was the various pieces of legislation of 1970 concerning air pollution, environmental policy, and occupational safety and health.

The Occupational Safety and Health Act of 1970 was preceded by the Mine Health and Safety Act of 1969. Prior to that, the first serious effort at a national occupational safety and health code occurred in 1968, when it appeared as if the Congress would pass occupational safety and health legislation under a Democratic president and Congress. Although that legislation failed, the success of the Federal Mine Safety and Health Act, which was spurred on by a series of mining accidents claiming many lives, led to the final passage of the Occupational Safety and Health Act on the last day of 1970 under a Republican administration.

The act was largely supported by industry. Although to some this may seem odd, it has become an important lesson of American history to realize that it is much easier to answer to one boss than to many. Consequently, industry has supported legislation relative to the environment on several occasions in order to avoid regulation by the individual states, which varies from state to state. More confederate systems exist in Canada and especially in Australia, but each has far fewer than 50 states and 280 million people.

By 1968, 42 states had some form of industrial health regulation, but in many states it was quite poor. Overall there was only one state-employed health professional for every 21,000 workers. Only 14 states regulated noise, one of the most pervasive occupational health hazards. There was also a great deal of clamor from labor unions for passage of the legislation.

Passage of the Occupational Safety and Health Act has been cited as the most important event in the history of U.S. occupational health. The Health and Safety Act of Great Britain of 1974 and various acts of Australian states between 1972 and 1989 represent movements similar to the Occupational Safety and Health Act in size and scope, but much different in philosophical approach.

However, other developments that took place mainly in the 1960s had an impact on industrial hygiene that cannot be overestimated. These developments, along with the passage of the Occupational Safety and Health Act, led to the exponential growth and importance of the industrial hygiene discipline in the 1970s and 1980s.

Three of the most important developments are related to the way in which the hygienist evaluates the workplace. **By the 1960s**, approximately 40 years had passed in which the development of techniques for evaluating airborne chemical exposures had ebbed and flowed. There were **impingers, electrostatic precipitators,** and **filtration techniques** for dusts that were reasonably adequate; even so, the evolution of these techniques was relatively slow. Techniques to measure exposures to organic chemicals were particularly cumbersome and inaccurate in the 1960s and, by today's standards, seemingly archaic. The development in the **1960s** and the common usage by the **1970s** of the **charcoal tube** for collection and the gas chromatograph for evaluation of organic chemicals appear to be inevitable results of a rapidly growing organic chemical industry. Synchronously, the **development of a battery-operated portable pump** that could be worn by workers for moving air through a sampling medium (i.e., charcoal) was also a great step. Although the development of each of these three tools took place in the 1960s, each was fully developed, adequately documented in the literature, and available to hygienists by 1970. Thus, these three developments, along with the Occupational Safety and Health Act, burst open the doors for U.S. hygienists and led to exponential growth in the population of the profession. This is best shown by the growth of membership in the American Industrial Hygiene Association.

7. 1970 and Beyond

The number of hygienists in the United States, as evidenced by membership in the American Industrial Hygiene Association, has increased exponentially since 1970. Likewise, the number of educational programs throughout the country graduating industrial hygiene professionals has increased. Patty pointed out in 1958 that industrial hygiene academia had grown from the very first program in the world, developed at Harvard in 1918 (which, by the way, employed Alice Hamilton), to a list prepared by the Committee on Professional Education of the American Public Health Association in 1947 that included nine universities in North America: Columbia, Harvard, Johns Hopkins, Toronto, Yale, and state universities of California, Michigan, Minnesota, and North Carolina. The London School of Hygiene and Tropical Medicine had begun offering degrees, either at the graduate or the undergraduate level, for industrial hygienists and occupational safety and health professionals. But there could easily be over 100 institutions now offering baccalaureate, graduate, or associate degrees in some aspect of occupational safety and health. There are apparently about 30 programs that offer graduate degrees in industrial hygiene.

An important development of the 1970s, which led to high-quality education of graduate - level industrial hygienists as well as other safety and health professionals was the creation of Educational Resource Centers by the National Institute for Occupational Safety and Health. This effort has grown from the 8 resource centers originally established in 1976, to 14 current ERCs. In addition, there are 10 industrial hygiene programs that are not part of an ERC but are funded by this process. Through these federal funds, there are 22 industrial hygiene programs funded throughout the United States. These training funds are used to purchase equipment and other supplies necessary for the education of industrial hygienists, to fund teaching-faculty salaries, and to provide stipends and pay tuition and fees for industrial hygiene students. Similar funding is also available to occupational medicine, occupational nursing, safety, and ergonomics programs. In order to be classified as an Educational Resource Center, an institution or a consortium of institutions must have training established in three of the four core areas of occupational safety and health (**industrial hygiene, nursing, medicine**, and **safety**).

With the tremendous growth of the profession in the 1970s and 1980s, the passage of the Occupational Safety and Health Act in the United States, and increasingly complex technological advancements made in the evaluation and control of workplace environments have come changes in the field of industrial hygiene. The evolutionary process is not surprising; however, the changes that have occurred may not be apparent to many of the professionals in the field. Early physicians were devoted to the recognition of diseases in industry and the causes of those diseases. With time, engineers became interested in the control of agents causing those diseases. As the discipline developed, engineers and chemists became predominant in the field. Recognition of disease remained a major aspect of the profession, even though engineers and chemists often lacked adequate training in the medical and biological sciences. They usually received that "training" through experience.

However, since 1970 the practitioners in the field have gradually drifted away from an emphasis on the recognition of disease, and for a very good reason. Imagine going into a workplace in 1940 armed with meager evaluation technologies and limited knowledge of what effects the substances in that workplace might be having on the workers. In addition, written information or research in these areas was quite limited. If the hygienist determined that carbon tetrachloride was present in the workplace, he would have limited resources for determining what levels were there and what levels were safe or acceptable. If the clock is turned back to 1920, the situation becomes even more difficult. In 1920, and indeed until 1940, hygienists had very little information regarding what was an appropriate level of exposure in the workplace. Hence, hygienists had to "study" the workplace. Several workplaces with varying exposure levels to a single compound needed to be studied, and a dose-response relationship relating the workers' responses to the various exposure levels had to be developed.

A result of the establishment of the American Conference of Governmental Industrial Hygienists (**ACGIH**) in 1939 was the publication of exposure guidelines for various substances. These guidelines evolved over 30 years until they were adopted by the Occupational Safety and Health Administration (OSHA) as one of its first administrative acts in the early 1970s. The work of the American Conference of Governmental Industrial Hygienists in this area and the establishment of health standards by OSHA continued throughout the 1970s and 1980s until now there are recommended standards of presumably safe exposure levels for approximately 600 compounds or elements and their related compounds (e.g., lead and its compounds). Hence, there now are thousands of compounds for which there are airborne exposure levels established as "safe."

As a consequence, the old approaches toward research into the causes of health effects and safe exposure levels by everyday practitioners have been emphasized less. Today's practicing professionals apply the established exposure limits. Research aspects have been left largely to large research organizations such as the National Institute for Occupational Safety and Health, a few academicians, and large companies. Hence, of the more than 10,000 industrial hygienists in the United States, probably fewer than 5% are actively engaged in the activities that caused industrial hygiene to be established. Even so, this 5% (500) is equal to the total number of hygienists in 1950 in the United States.

This is perhaps the biggest change that occurred in the 1970s and 1980s - the evolution from research to application.

Evolution in this direction has been promoted by regulation. Hygienists, particulariy those in industry, more often than not find themselves constantly challenged by new regulations, for which they have the responsibility of compliance. Although this has certainly caused the numbers of professionals in the field to expand, it has also caused hygienists to take a more reactive, rather than proactive, approach to their practice.

Perhaps chief among those regulations has been the Right-to-Know or Hazard Communication standard. This standard entails the labeling of chemicals and education, requiring that all workers receive minimum training in the hazards to which they are exposed in industry; and it has been the role of the hygienist to perform these duties. Although this has been an extremely important aspect of promoting health and safety in this country, it has burdened the hygienist with a tremendous amount of paper-shuffling compliance work. In some cases, it may be the excuse needed by a hygienist to remain in the office and administer rather than go into the workplace to see exactly what is going on and determine the relationships between exposure and disease.

Another important phenomenon, which has occurred throughout the world, but is particularly important in the United States, has been the effort in the 1970s and 1980s to control asbestos. This abatement effort has required a considerable amount of industrial hygiene time, and, again, because this is purely a control effort. It has virtually nothing to do with the process of observing disease and determining its causes.

In the future, hygienists may once again turn more toward research into the prevalence and causes of occupational disease. For example, OSHA has asked for comments on a proposed standard for exposure assessment in the workplace. Currently, for the large majority of regulated and all unregulated substances, there are no OSHA requirements for evaluating worker exposures. Should OSHA require exposure assessment, not only for the compounds for which there are regulations but also for other compounds, then this could open the door to a tremendous exposure database, which would then be available for comparison to the disease states of the workers who are receiving the exposures.

However, this opportunity may not be realized for several reasons. First, it is unlikely. given its history, that OSHA will require monitoring for substances for which there are not exposure standards. Second, the monitoring that OSHA requires may be of such a simplistic nature that it does not provide an adequate statistical basis for the evaluation of exposure levels over time. Third, unless OSHA requires specific procedures for analyzing the data and somehow couples its analysis with the analysis of similarly collected medical data. The exposure data will probably go into a file cabinet and have little long-term benefit for occupational health.

Hygienists trained now and in the future must take a hard look at what role they will play and services they will provide in their professional careers. To simply learn the tools of the trade and apply those tools without questioning them or trying to improve them means that these industrial hygienists will be performing at a technician level and will be doing very little to advance their profession. The industrial hygienist of the future must continue to develop new tools and refine old ones. He or she must be adept at controlling exposures, but must be able to recognize hazards that previously were not recognized. Finally, to get management's cooperation the hygienist must be able to communicate well, orally and in writing. This latter step will be the most important one in terms of achieving our goals because good communicators, regardless of their backgrounds, are seen as peers by management. Ultimately, some are promoted to management levels outside of industrial hygiene, where their viewpoints have a wider audience and greater influence.

In 1992, Sherwood reported his thoughts on the future role of hygienists and consequent needs that educational institutions must meet. He sees a drift, by necessity, away from measurement and epidemiology of the biological and toxicological sciences toward stronger engineering backgrounds. In his words, "hygienists should provide the unique and special skills required to establish economically optimum controls systems." If our society stops making it necessary to count bodies as a prerequisite for taking action to control exposures. Then Sherwood is right, and one would hope he is right. However, these engineering-oriented hygienists still must possess a biological basis. Most likely, however, there will continue to be a need to prove cause and effect, and therefore to measure exposure and document every disease.

Since the very essence of what we are about is health, hygienists of the future must pay particular attention to the study of disease, its causes, and ways to prevent it. Professor Theodore Hatch, an eminent academician and professional of industrial hygiene, said as early as 1960, "Without attempting to become a physician or physiologist, the industrial hygienist must nevertheless acquire an independent capacity to understand and evaluate the human side of the man/environment equation in order to most wisely employ his primary skills in physical science and engineering, to recognize, evaluate, and control the work environment". In other words, simply applying the rules and using established tools can be done by anyone; however, the industrial hygienist who contributes the most to the worker and to the profession must understand the basis of health so that his or her application of industrial hygiene principles will be most effective. This not only makes mandatory the study of a biology book, but requires going to the field, observing workers and what they are doing, asking questions about their health, evaluating their exposure levels, and correlating health status with exposure levels.

Finally, this effort requires work within the occupational health team. Professor Hatch also said:

> No physical measurements of dustiness, of radiation, heat, noise, or light, of chemical fumes or vapors, no matter how precisely these are made, have direct biological meaning but are useful only in proportion to the goodness of their respective calibrations, so to speak, against appropriate biological scales of human health. Thus, standing alone on its foundation of physical science and engineering, industrial hygiene would have little meaning. Through teamwork, however, between the medical scientists and physicians on the one hand, and the physical scientists and engineers, on the other, it has developed on a base, which provides the link between environment and man. It may be noted here that progress on the medical side is equally limited without such a common base in both the physical and biological sciences. The medical diagnostic techniques, like the procedures of the industrial hygienist, when used alone, will not tell us that an observed state of ill health was necessarily caused by a particular industrial exposure. Such interpretation is permitted only when the diagnostic findings can be evaluated in relation to quantitative description of the conditions of exposure and both examined in the light of previously established correlations between similar environmental stresses and human response.

Industrial hygienists are the cement between the physical, biological, and medical sciences. We must do more than measure exposure levels and simply compare them to presumed safe exposure standards. We must go a step further and interact with the medical professionals in order to determine if effects are occurring at the levels that we have measured, no matter how safe those levels are currently presumed to be. If industrial hygienists take this latter step, then they are doing more than simply being technicians; they arc being inquisitive scientists who are doing their best to promote health. This will improve society's awareness of the important role played by industrial hygienists.

B. Essential Impetus behind the History of Occupational Health in the U.S.

Although the history of occupational health can be traced back to the ancients, in the United States the development of occupational disease was given enormous impetus by the Industrial Revolution. The advancement of occupational health and safety in the United States has typically been part of broader social reform movements, characterized by coalition politics and political compromise between labor and industry, catalyzed by tragic events, and spurred by heroic individuals. The medical profession has played an important role in disease definition and in framing the scientific debate, although ironically, and with some conscious effort, the evolution of a technically oriented discipline has resulted in the divergence of occupational health from mainstream medicine and medical care. As much as any medical and public health issue, the history of occupational health and safety provides clear evidence of Rudolph Virchow's observation that medicine is often politics writ small.

C. Social Factors that Contribute to the Recognition of Work-Related Disease

Although the sixteenth-century Italian physician, Ramazzini, is often cited as the "**father of occupational medicine**," occupational disease in the modern sense evolved in the aftermath of the Industrial Revolution of the nineteenth century. The nations' economy was rapidly transformed from dependence on small shops controlled by skilled guildsmen to a highly mechanized economy powered by an increasingly unskilled labor force with little influence over the conditions of work. Industrial growth was powered by successive waves of immigrants, urbanization, and the amassing of great fortunes in the hands of a new and influential capitalist class. This mechanization invariably generated workplace hazards that far exceeded those that were possible before wide-scale industrialization. Along with these socioeconomic developments, a new medical and public health paradigm emerged. The bacteriologic revolution led to a de-emphasis on environmental factors in health and disease in the belief that all disease could be linked to microbes. Before the spectacular successes of the bacteriologic revolution, according to medical historian Charles Rosenberg, the body was seen, metaphorically, as a system of dynamic interactions with its environment. Health or disease resulted from a cumulative interaction between constitutional endowment and environmental circumstance. Despite the ascendancy of the biomedical model, however, labor and its allies continued to view occupational disease as an indication of a flawed social welfare system, thereby setting the stage on which political debate about occupational health and safety issues has been fought throughout the twentieth century.

D. HISTORIC ROLE OF INDUSTRY IN OCCUPATIONAL HEALTH AND SAFETY

For internal reasons American industry has been involved with medicine beyond its periodic participation in larger social reform movements and coalition politics, as demonstrated by the numerous and extensive development of both medical care and occupational medicine programs in numerous corporations dating before the turn of the 20th century. The horrific injury rate in the booming railroad industry spawned a number of medical care plans and benefit associations. Similar efforts existed in many mining, manufacturing, and service companies, such as U.S. Steel, the Anaconda Mining Company, and Macy's, to name a few. The important role played by the nascent insurance industry in the control of certain high-profile occupational diseases provides a rare glimpse of the unfulfilled potential of the insurance industry in identifying and preventing occupational disease and injury. For example, in the 1920s and 1930s diligent field work by progressive actuaries working for Metropolitan Life and Prudential documented that silicosis remained prevalent despite the institution of "safe" dust levels. The epidemiologic evidence gathered by insurance company field workers helped to elucidate the complex interaction of silicosis with tuberculosis and defined a prototypical example of the multicausal etiology of chronic lung diseases among industrial workers. Throughout the 1940s and 1950s occupational medicine matured into a full-fledged scientific discipline. Corporate medical departments and residency and fellowship training programs bloomed, and ancillary disciplines such as occupational health nursing, industrial hygiene, and vocational rehabilitation continued to evolve. Momentum was increased by the remarkable growth of the military-industrial complex and the development of the nuclear industry.

E. ALICE HAMILTON

Alice Hamilton (1869-1970) was a pioneering physician who first delved into the problem of occupational disease in 1908 when the governor of Illinois asked her to investigate industrial diseases in Illinois. Hamilton was a resident of Chicago's well-known Hull House and a friend of the famous social reformer Jane Addams. Through her lifetime work of visiting industrial sites, evaluating workers, convincing management and legislators to take action, teaching and conducting research as the first woman faculty at Harvard Medical School. Hamilton played a critical role in the study and prevention of a wide range of industrial conditions, including the elimination of phosphorus in matches and the reduction of lead, mercury, benzene, trinitrotoluene, carbon dioxide, and carbon monoxide poisoning. Hamilton's profound influence on the nascent discipline of industrial hygiene (most early hygienists were, in fact, physicians and not engineers) and the importance of toxicology to occupational disease is eloquently detailed in her 1943 autobiography, "Exploring the Dangerous Trades."

F. IMPACT OF WORLD WAR II ON OCCUPATIONAL MEDICINE

The profound impact of WWII on American society and industry cannot be overstated. The wage freeze enacted by Congress, the manpower shortages caused by the war, and pro-labor legislation supported by President Franklin D. Roosevelt spurred the growth of unions, diversified the workforce, and forced industry to consider alternative means of attracting and maintaining its workforce. One consequence was the tremendous growth of employer-based health insurance, gained as part of the collective bargaining process. Although occupational health per se was not the generative force in this important development, the widespread availability of insurance - at least theoretically - has made it possible to advance the recognition and treatment of occupational diseases and injuries. Of greater importance, the severe labor shortages caused by the war forced both industry and the government to pay significantly more attention to occupational health issues than ever before. Indeed, the historical roots of current understanding of ergonomic issues can be traced directly to this period when protecting workers (be they bomber pilots or Rosie the Riveter) was at a premium.

G. IDENTIFICATION OF OCCUPATIONAL HEALTH PROBLEMS

Today well over 100 million men and women are gainfully employed in the U.S., and increasing numbers of people, particularly women, are entering the workforce. To some degree, all these workers are exposed to occupational hazards, and all risk-job related adverse health effects. Compounding these problems is the fact that more than 25 percent of Americans are employed in businesses that have fewer than 20 employees, and more than 50 percent in companies with fewer than 100 employees. These smaller companies often lack the knowledge to identify occupational health hazards and the funds to finance associated control programs; moreover, many are exempt from state and federal occupational health and safety regulations. The effects of occupational exposures range from lung diseases, cancer, hearing loss, and dermatitis to more subtle psychological effects, many of which are only now beginning to be recognized.

The National Security Council (1996) estimates that almost 500,000 cases of job-related illnesses occur per year in U.S. Large though these numbers are, the true magnitude of the health and economic impacts of occupational disease and injury remains unknown.

H. INDUSTRIAL HYGIENE AS A BRANCH OF OCCUPATIONAL HEALTH

Industrial hygiene is a branch of occupational health science devoted to preventing diseases caused by workplace exposures to chemical, physical, and biologic agents. Just as physicians diagnose and treat illnesses and injuries, industrial hygienists (IHs) recognize, evaluate, and control workplace conditions that may cause adverse health effects among workers.

As a public health endeavor, industrial hygiene attempts to solve problems before conditions cause ill health. Over the years, the focus of industrial hygiene has expanded beyond factories and mines to include service industries and offices. Thus, the terms industrial and occupational are often used interchangeably with the word hygiene.

Industrial hygiene is the science and art dedicated to the anticipation, recognition, evaluation, and control of environmental factors or stresses arising in or from the workplace. Such workplace environmental stresses may cause illness, impaired health, or significant discomfort among workers or the citizens of a community.

Physicians were the first to clearly recognize the relationship between workplace conditions and disease. During the early 20th century, Dr. Alice Hamilton was one of the first physicians in the United States to venture from the treatment room into the factories to deal with the root causes of certain diseases. She visited factories to learn firsthand about the conditions that caused the grave ailments associated with lead poisoning. She witnessed uncontrolled releases of dust into workroom air that was then inhaled by workers. Having "diagnosed" the problem, her training as a physician led her to the next step, finding a "cure". She was confident that lead poisoning could be prevented if the amount of dust released into the workroom air was reduced. She was thinking as an industrial hygienist-understanding the work process, identifying the source and magnitude of the exposure, and developing a solution to the problem.

Industrial hygiene as it was practiced in the late 20th century did not really begin until the 1930s and 1940s, when the work of pioneers such as Alice Hamilton was integrated with engineering and chemistry.

Initially, industrial hygiene was practiced in heavy industrial sectors, such as mining, metal foundries, steel, and auto manufacturing, where recognized serious health hazards existed. The field grew slowly. Between 1910 and 1940, individual states developed small industrial hygiene units in their Departments of Labor Professional associations of industrial hygiene were established in 1939. By the 1940s, a handful of universities granted degrees for industrial hygiene or related disciplines. However, until the 1970s the practice of industrial hygiene was limited and remained rooted principally in industry and only secondarily in government, including the federal Public Health Service. During the late 1960s and early 1970s, a confluence of social, political, scientific, and economic phenomena led to a great leap forward for industrial hygiene and for occupational health in general.

The 1960s were years of rapid social change. One of the unforeseen consequences of the upheavals wrought by the civil rights and anti-Vietnam war movements was a growing consciousness of environmental and occupational health issues. Organized labor, environmental, public health, and community organizations fought for federal standards to protect the environment and workers.

In 1969, Congress established the Environmental Protection Agency (EPA), and in 1970 the Williams-Stieger Occupational Safety and Health Act (OSHAct) was passed. The OSHAct guaranteed a safe and healthful workplace for all workers. With the passage of the OSHAct, the field of industrial hygiene blossomed. The federal OSHA was created to enforce health and safety standards. Field offices responsible for enforcing these standards were opened across the U.S.

The need for trained industrial hygienists to inspect workplaces and enforce regulations grew. In response to the threat of legal sanctions for violations of workplace health and safety standards, large companies began to hire industrial hygienists to ensure compliance. In addition, consulting groups flourished to meet the growing demand for workplace inspections and worker training.

The OSHAct also established the National Institute for Occupational Safety and Health (NIOSH) within the Centers for Disease Control (Department of Health and Human Services). NIOSH was assigned the task of researching the causes of occupational disease.

During the 1970s, awareness of workplace diseases and the resources to deal with them increased, and the focus of industrial hygiene expanded beyond factories and mines to service industries and the corporate world.

Industrial or occupational hygiene is now a discipline taught in many colleges and universities throughout the U. S. A bachelor degree is required, preferably in one of the basic sciences. Currently, most IHs have a Bachelor of Science (B.S.) or an engineering degree, and a Master of Industrial Health (M.I.H.) or a Master of Public Health (M.P.H.). The core curriculum for these degrees includes biostatistics, epidemiology, toxicology, principles of industrial hygiene, industrial processes, industrial ventilation, and physical hazards. In addition, IHs may acquire a Certificate of Industrial Health (C.I.H.) by the American Board of Industrial Hygiene (ABIH). To be eligible to sit for the certification examination, a candidate must have a bachelor degree with 60 credits of science and 5 years of experience as a practicing IH.

The examination takes place over two days and tests the candidate's knowledge in at least 10 areas of industrial hygiene science and practice. Since the profession of industrial hygiene is not controlled by local or federal government, (the ABIH is a private organization), nothing prevents a person from professionally designating him or herself as an "industrial hygienist," although the C.I.H. designation cannot be used legally in this context.

The majority of IHs work in private industry and for consulting firms. In private industry IHs manage health and safety programs, assess workers' exposures to hazards, recommend controls, and conduct employee training in health and safety issues. A smaller number work for insurance companies, local and federal government, trade unions, and as academics in colleges and universities.

Governmental IHs engage in a range of activities depending on the agency for which they work and their function within the agency. Their activities may range from managing health and safety programs aimed at protecting agency employees to conducting research into possible work-related disease. Of course, the largest number of IH's in government are employed by OSHA and work mainly as compliance officers.

IHs employed by trade unions conduct IH surveys for their members, develop and deliver member training, participate in contract negotiations, and represent the unions in congressional hearings and rulemaking procedures concerning relevant health and safety issues. Academic His, teach and conduct research.

To evaluate potential chemical hazards, the hygienist gathers information by reading labels and material safety data sheets (MSDSs)[Figure 14.1]. All manufacturers are required to have a MSDS on each product sold, and employers are required by OSHA to have them on file at the worksite. Although far from perfect, the MSDS provides product information, including chemical make-up, health effects, and required protective measures for handling. The information garnered from MSDSs is an important clue in hazard recognition.

When personal protective equipment must be worn in a workplace, it is important that an effective personal protective equipment program is in place so that workers are properly trained in using the equipment. Unless absolutely required by conditions, no safety and health program should be totally dependent on protective equipment.

Economic considerations also tend to delay or reduce attempts to solve occupational health problems. Another problem is that the patterns of occupational disease are constantly changing, requiring ever more refined methods to uncover the subtle injuries and disabilities resulting from low-level, on-the-job psychological stress and other nonphysical or chemical hazards.

Figure 14.1. Generic MSDS. (Source: Beck & Krieger, 1992).

Material Safety Data Sheet May be used to comply with OSHA's Hazard Communication Standard, 29 CFR 1910.1200. Standard must be consulted for specific requirements.	**U.S. Department of Labor** Occupational Safety and Health Administration (Non–Mandatory Form) Form Approved OMB No. 1218–0072
IDENTITY *(As Used on Label and List)*	*Note: Blank spaces are not permitted. If any item is not applicable, or no information is available, the space must be marked to indicate that.*

Section I

Manufacturer's Name	Emergency Telephone Number
Address *(Number, Street, City, State, and ZIP Code)*	Telephone Number for Information
	Date Prepared
	Signature of Preparer *(optional)*

Section II — Hazardous Ingredients/Identity Information

Hazardous Components (Specific Chemical Identity; Common Name(s))	OSHA PEL	ACGIH TLV	Other Limits Recommended	% *(optional)*

Section III — Physical/Chemical Characteristics

Boiling Point		Specific Gravity (H_2O = 1)	
Vapor Pressure (mm Hg.)		Melting Point	
Vapor Density (AIR = 1)		Evaporation Rate (Butyl Acetate = 1)	

Solubility in Water

Appearance and Odor

Section IV — Fire and Explosion Hazard Data

Flash Point (Method Used)	Flammable Limits	LEL	UEL

Extinguishing Media

Special Fire Fighting Procedures

Unusual Fire and Explosion Hazards

(Reproduce locally)   OSHA 174, Sept. 1985

Figure 14.1. Continued.

Section V — Reactivity Data

Stability	Unstable		Conditions to Avoid
	Stable		

Incompatibility *(Materials to Avoid)*

Hazardous Decomposition or Byproducts

Hazardous Polymerization	May Occur		Conditions to Avoid
	Will Not Occur		

Section VI — Health Hazard Data

Route(s) of Entry:	Inhalation?	Skin?	Ingestion?

Health Hazards *(Acute and Chronic)*

Carcinogenicity:	NTP?	IARC Monographs?	OSHA Regulated?

Signs and Symptoms of Exposure

Medical Conditions
Generally Aggravated by Exposure

Emergency and First Aid Procedures

Section VII — Precautions for Safe Handling and Use

Steps to Be Taken in Case Material Is Released or Spilled

Waste Disposal Method

Precautions to Be Taken in Handling and Storing

Other Precautions

Section VIII — Control Measures

Respiratory Protection *(Specify Type)*

Ventilation	Local Exhaust	Special
	Mechanical *(General)*	Other

Protective Gloves	Eye Protection

Other Protective Clothing or Equipment

Work/Hygienic Practices

Page 2 ☆ U.S.G.P.O.: 1986-491-529/45775

IV. <u>ANTICIPATION, RECOGNITION, EVALUATION, AND CONTROL (AREC)</u>

A. <u>INTRODUCTION</u>

The AIHA definition goes on to state that these areas of science are used to anticipate, recognize, evaluate, and control disease agents in the workplace. The word "anticipate" was added to the original definition. It may or may not be necessary, as it is implied in recognition; one recognizes that a hazard may exist in the future or in the present. What, then, does it mean "to recognize or anticipate a disease agent in the workplace"? In everyday life we constantly recognize agents that may cause injury and occasionally agents that may cause disease. For example, a roller skate left unattended on a floor serves as a hazard that may cause a fall. This is a mechanical agent of injury. A wary parent may recognize that playground equipment a child is using is not safe - perhaps a chain is about to break. This is recognition of a mechanical agent. We also recognize health hazards akin to those that occur in industry. For example, we may recognize that if petroleum-based paints are used in a closed room, the vapors from the paint may somehow affect our health. So, the job of recognizing health hazards in industry is easy - or is it? Would you be able to recognize that a person welding in the presence of chlorinated solvents might be exposed to a poisonous gas called phosgene? Or that a person restoring old artwork might be exposed to a gas called arsine?

There are many levels of recognition of disease agents in the workplace. In some cases, it is fairly easy to see a situation and recognize that it is unsafe. In other cases, the hygienist must use the scientific method - the consideration of multiple facts and observations leading to a hypothesis, testing the hypothesis, reformulation and retesting if necessary - in order to clearly recognize a health hazard. In other cases, the hygienist can only estimate that a hazard may exist. In many cases the hygienist will be able to spot a hazard only after sufficient experience. There are many hazards in the workplace, and most of them have not been documented.

What is evaluation? We often evaluate hazards. Stepping outside on a winter day to determine how to dress provides a qualitative evaluation of temperature. If we had a thermometer, we could go one step further and make a quantitative evaluation.

Once the hygienist has recognized that a health hazard might exist, it may be obvious that the situation is hazardous enough to warrant immediate control. The industrial hygienist immediately should do something to control the situation. However, for the most part, the leap from recognition to control (with a quick qualitative evaluation step) is not possible.

How could a hygienist, while walking through a plant, determine that worker exposures to trichloroethylene were unsafe or hazardous? With experience, there are some techniques that will allow the hygienist to make qualitative judgments about hazard. However, for the most part, the evaluation step must be quantitative. This means that the hygienist usually will need to quantitatively analyze the levels of contaminants in workplace air to determine the degree of hazard. In the case of physical agents such as noise and radiation, the types of analyses have the same principles but are based on physics rather than chemistry. In the case of biological agents, the types of analyses are based on microbiology.

The word "hazard" has been used repeatedly. 2,3,7,8-Dibenzo-dioxin is extremely toxic in mice. Strychnine and the toxin produced by the hotulinum bacterium are fatal to humans in small doses. Are they hazardous? Not necessarily. Toxicity or propensity to cause harm is certainly a component of hazard. However, there must also be a potential for exposure at a significant level. So, if a chemical is toxic and it is handled in such a way that an exposure may occur that could lead to a significant outcome, then that situation is hazardous. The word "significant," above, must be defined by the person assessing hazard. Certainly death is a significant outcome; but, in some cases, a reversible skin rash may be the outcome of concern.

What is control? We often control hazards in everyday life. The application of seatbelts to the control of injuries arising from automobile accidents is a great example of the recognition, evaluation, and control process. Undoubtedly, soon after Henry Ford, at least in the United States, drove the first automobile, someone recognized this type of transportation to be a more hazardous form of conveyance than the horse and buggy. However, it was not until accident and injury statistics from automobile accidents were analyzed that a public outcry occurred, and automobile conveyance was commonly thought of as a significant hazard. Although the automobile accident evaluation step probably took place sometime in the 1950s or earlier, it was not until the early 1960s that the control process began to take place. This scenario is not unusual, as the process of hazard evaluation is often subjective. Inherent in the hazard evaluation step is the concept of risk. No matter what we do to the process of automobile conveyance, it will probably never be risk-free. Therefore the question arises as to what is an acceptable risk. It was not until the 1960s that society put enough pressure on automobile manufacturers, through government intervention to cause seatbelts to be installed in automobiles. However, even in the presence of seatbelts, individuals still choose to take risks rather than control the hazard.

There are many techniques available to the hygienist for controlling disease agents in the workplace. An important one of these is ventilation. Essentially, the principle of ventilation is to control the disease agent at its source or its origin, and thus to remove it from the workplace. Other techniques control the hazard at the worker. These include the use of respirators or facemasks with absorbents or filters. Also included would be chemical protective clothing for controlling the exposure of skin to chemical agents. Finally. There are various types of "administrative" controls, which are ways of reducing the amount of time that the employee is exposed to a hazard, or changing the way that the employee performs a job to reduce the hazard. A very simple example of this would be rescheduling an operation that must take place outdoors, from the afternoon to the morning, in order to avoid the effects of heat stress.

B. RECOGNITION OF POTENTIAL HEALTH HAZARDS

1. Recognition

Industrial hygienists follow general principles to assist with their recognition of potential threats to workers.

Industrial hygienists must:

a. Conduct research and extensive field study to become familiar with the processes, job activities performed, and effective control measures in place, to determine hazard potential,

b. Become familiar with all work processes used in the particular workplace under scrutiny,

c. Learn what chemicals or materials are used, and what intermediate products, or byproducts are produced,

d. Physically survey the workplace under evaluation, ask questions during the survey, and collect process flow diagrams and other information on the layout of the facilities,

e. Prepare and maintain an inventory of the chemical and physical agents used in the workplace.

2. Determining if a Chemical is Toxic

Industrial hygienists research and review reference books and material safety data sheets for specific information on chemicals or products used in the workplace to determine which of these are toxic and to what degree. Information about the toxicity of chemicals can be found in the latest texts and scientific journals.

Chemical dictionaries provide the concentration at which each substance is known to be toxic, and how the chemical is formed and used. They may identify the threshold limit value (TLV) outlined by the ACGIH or the permissible exposure limit (PEL) mandated by OSHA.

3. Toxicity versus Hazard

Industrial hygienists recognize that toxicity and hazard are not synonymous. The injury produced when a chemical has reached a sufficient concentration in the body is referred to as toxicity. The hazard of a chemical is the probability that this concentration will be reached within the body.

The nature of the work process in which a potentially hazardous substance is used, its possible reaction with other materials, and the degree of effective control measures all affect the potential hazard an agent may represent. The severity of a hazard depends on many variables an industrial hygienist must consider, including how a chemical is to be used, the type of job performed, the duration of exposure, and work patterns.

4. Several Factors To Be Reviewed By Industrial Hygienist

By what route of entry will the chemical enter the body?

How much of a chemical and for how long must a chemical be in contact with cellular components of the body?

What is the likelihood that the material will be absorbed by the body and come in contact with body cells?

What is the generation rate of the airborne contaminants?

What effective control measures are in place or must be in place to minimize adverse health effects?

5. <u>Preliminary Survey</u>

Industrial hygienists conduct a preliminary survey of the work area. As a preliminary survey is conducted, many potentially hazardous work processes can be visually observed, such as:

a. Operations that generate fumes (such as welding) are easily recognized as a potential hazard and quickly indicate that further evaluation may be required,
b. Operations where chemicals are used for cleaning or degreasing work-in-process (WIP) are also easily recognized and indicate that further evaluation is necessary,
c. The presence of vapors or gases may be detected by the sense of smell,
d. Review workers' routine job requirements,
e. Visually observe how work is performed and whether all workers perform their jobs in the same manner, or if worker-to-worker variability may affect their exposures,
f. Review the types of control measures in use, and examine their effectiveness. These include local exhaust ventilation, personal protective clothing or equipment, shielding from ultraviolet radiation, etc,
g. Take notes during the preliminary survey, draw layouts of the work area, note whether housekeeping is adequate, whether workers eat or drink in the work area, if control measures are adequate but not used, etc.

6. <u>Typical Investigation Questions</u>

Typical questions that should be asked during a preliminary survey include the following:

a. What is produced?
b. What raw materials are used?
c. Are any of these raw materials regulated by OSHA or the EPA and require employee exposures to remain within permissible exposure limits (PELs)?
d. What materials are added? Are materials generated?
e. What equipment is involved?
f. What operational procedures are involved? Do these procedures minimize exposures?
g. Is there a written procedure for the safe handling and storage of materials?
h. What about dust control, cleanup after spills, and waste disposal?
i. Is there a ventilation or exhaust system in place? If so, is it adequate?
j. Does the facility layout minimize exposure?
k. Is the facility well equipped with safety appliances such as showers, masks, respirators and emergency equipment?
l. Are safe operating procedures outlined and enforced?
m. Do these include procedures for maintenance personnel and non-routine operations?
n. How many work-shifts are there? How many workers perform these job functions?
o. Do workers leave the area during their lunch break?
p. Do workers exceed 40 hours a week with extensive overtime?
q. Are all workers skilled and adequately trained?

7. Sources of Airborne Contaminants

The list of raw materials, products and byproducts used and generated, and the results of the preliminary survey, will indicate the source and type of potential airborne contaminants.

8. Forms of Airborne Contaminants

a. **Aerosol**: Suspension of liquid or solid particles in air,
b. **Dust**: Particulate material generated by a mechanical process (0.5 to 50μm),
c. **Mist**: Suspension of liquid particles in air formed by condensation from vapor or by some mechanical process (40 to 400μm). For comparison, rain=100μm,
d. **Fume**: Solid particle aerosol formed by condensation from the vapor state (0.001 to 0.2μm),
e. **Fiber**: Particle with aspect ratio (length/width) greater than 3:1 (NIOSH 5:1),
f. **Smoke**: Aerosol formed from combustion of organic material (0.01 to 0.5μm).

9. Routes of Entry

In order for a toxic agent to exert its effect, the agent must first come in contact with a worker's body. This can occur through inhalation (breathing), absorption (through direct contact with skin), or ingestion (eating or drinking).

a. Inhalation

Inhalation involves airborne contaminants that are breathed into the lungs. Airborne contaminants include gases, vapors, and particulate matter (including dusts, fumes, smokes, aerosols, and mists). Inhalation is the most rapid form of entry for a contaminant to enter the body. The airborne contaminant is inhaled, absorbed in the lungs, picked up by the bloodstream and distributed throughout the body.

b. Ingestion

Failure to follow proper hygiene practices may allow chemicals to enter the body through ingestion. Toxic compounds can then be absorbed into the blood from the gastrointestinal tract. Lead oxide is an example of a material that can cause serious physical harm if ingested.

c. Absorption

Absorption of a chemical through the skin is a much slower method of entry, but occurs very quickly if the skin is cut or damaged. Many compounds can be absorbed directly through the skin. Phenols, benzene and organic lead compounds are examples of materials that can be absorbed through the skin.

10. Sources of Occupational Exposures

Years ago, most of the people who were classified as workers were employed in manufacturing. Over the past several decades, however, this situation has changed significantly. Today only about 20 million of the workers in U.S. are employed in manufacturing; the remainder are in service industries. Both types of employment have associated occupational health problems and, as would be expected many problems are common to both. One of the most common problems in manufacturing is the presence of contaminants in the air that results from various industrial processes. Other problems include noise, vibration, and ionizing radiation. Common problems in the service industries include inadequate indoor air quality, low-back pain, and cumulative trauma disorders. In certain situations, problems not heretofore recognized are assuming importance. These include the need to protect workers from potential exposures to biological agents and to provide them with safe (nonslip) floors and stairs and comfortable, employee-friendly work–station environments.

a. Toxic Chemicals

Toxic chemicals used or generated in industry play a major role in occupationally related diseases. The two primary portals of entry for such agents are the skin and the respiratory tract.

b. Biological Agents

The presence of biological agents (bioaerosols) in the air of the workplace is increasingly recognized as a common problem. This is especially true in the health care industry, where studies have demonstrated that blood-containing, respirable aerosols are routinely produced in the operating room during surgical procedures of health care workers who are exposed to bloodborne pathogens, such as hepatitis B virus and the human immunodeficiency virus, which causes AIDS. Compounding the problem is the discovery that fungi may grow in respirators designed to protect workers from inhaling airborne contaminants. This is particularly a problem for units containing cellulose and fiberglass filters. Closely related is the presence of airborne allergenic dusts in the workplace that can cause respiratory allergies, such as asthma and allergic rhinitis. These dusts are common in the agriculture and food industries.

c. Physical Factors

Stresses can be imposed on workers by improperly designed equipment that leads to repetitive motions, forceful motions, static or awkward postures, mechanical stresses, and local vibration. Nearly 60% of the illness cases reported among workers are associated with this group of factors. The annual cost in compensation expenses for U.S. workers exceeds a half-billion dollars. Studies show that 25% of all injuries in the workplace occur in the process of lifting and moving objects. Another pervasive problem is heat stress, especially among workers who wear protective clothing. Other problems include inadequate lighting and the wide range of musculoskeletal disorders that can be caused or aggravated by improper design of equipment and work stations.

C. EVALUATION OF POTENTIAL HEALTH HAZARDS

1. Evaluation Criteria

a. Introduction

The work process must be understood in order to identify where contaminants are released. Extensive information must be obtained regarding:

(1) Types of hazardous materials used in a facility,
(2) The kind of jobs performed,
(3) How the workers are exposed,
(4) Work patterns and how they vary between employees,
(5) Levels of air contamination,
(6) Duration of exposure,
(7) Control measures used,
(8) Other necessary information.

b. Information Required

For each process, the following must be performed:
(1) Observe who performs work, how, where, how long, and how many people do it.
(2) Observe how health hazards are generated, and the control measures in use.
(3) For each contaminant, find the OSHAPEL or other recommended exposure guideline based on the toxicological effects of the material.
(4) Determine the actual level of exposure to harmful agents.
(5) Determine the number of employees exposed and length of exposure.
(6) Identify the chemicals and contaminants in the process.
(7) Determine the level of airborne contaminants using air sampling or other analytical techniques.
(8) Calculate the resulting daily average and peak exposures from the air sampling results and employee exposure times.
(9) Compare the calculated exposure with OSHA standards, the TLV listing from the ACGIH, or other toxicological recommendations.

2. Air Sampling

To effectively evaluate a potentially hazardous workplace, objective and quantitative analysis is necessary. This usually requires some form of air sampling. Air sampling instruments are categorized as follows:

(1) Direct reading.
(2) Those that remove the contaminant from a measured quantity of air.
(3) Those that collect a known volume of air for subsequent laboratory use.

a. Instrument Selection

Instrument selection depends on various factors including:

(1) Type of contaminant under evaluation,
(2) Instantaneous results or whether laboratory analysis is required,
(3) Portability (Figure 14.2)
(4) Ease of use
(5) Efficiency of the device
(6) Reliability of the equipment
(7) Type of analysis
(8) Availability of the equipment

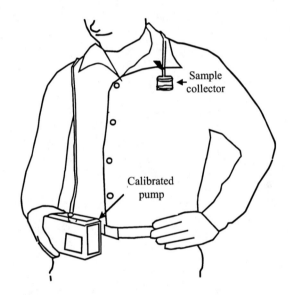

Figure 14.2.   Personal Air Sampler. (Source: Moeller, 1997).

b. Sensitivity, Accuracy, and Reproducibility

When evaluating a worker's exposure or the environment, an instrument must   be used that can provide sensitivity, accuracy, and reproducibility. Factors to consider when selecting equipment are:

(1) Whether or not the particular instrument is specific for the contaminant to   be determined,
(2) What other substances interfere with the test,
(3) The accuracy and sensitivity of the device.

c. Equipment Calibration

Calibration procedures must be used to insure that analysis of field samples accurately represents concentrations in the environment, and specifically, concentrations to which a worker is exposed. It is critical that air-sampling equipment operate at a known rate of airflow. The equipment must be calibrated against a standard airflow measuring device both before and after use in the field. The precise rate of airflow must be recorded so that when it is multiplied by the sampling time, the total volume of air sampled or collected will be known. This volume of air is used in calculating the concentration of contaminant to which the worker was exposed.

d. Standard Methods

Standard methods of analysis should always be used. The National Institute of Safety and Health (NIOSH) has developed a Manual of Analytical Methods that contains many established and recognized methods of collection and analysis. When in doubt, many industrial hygienists work very closely with the laboratory that will be performing the tests to assure that proper sample collection, storage and handling methods are utilized.

3. The Field Survey

Every effort must be made to obtain samples that represent the worker's exposure. To determine what constitutes a representative sample, an industrial hygienist must decide:

a. Where to sample
b. Whom to sample
c. How many samples to take
d. Duration of sampling
e. When to sample

a. Where to Sample

Where the purposes of sampling are to determine a worker's exposure and daily time-weighted-average, it is necessary to collect samples at or near the breathing zone. Actual exposure levels can be documented by combining the proper number of personnel samples with the results from stationary sampling points.

b. Whom To Sample

Monitoring different job tasks in a suspect area is best accomplished by personnel exposure monitoring. Properly attaching personal monitors to workers directly exposed should provide a representative sample of actual breathing zone exposure.

c. How Many Samples to Take

No set rule exists to determine the number of samples that are necessary to evaluate a worker's exposure. It is necessary to take enough samples to truly characterize the exposure for the particular job. A single sample is never enough. Samples should be taken for a number of workers over several days to reflect a typical exposure.

d. Duration of Sampling

When determining the volume of air to sample and the duration of sampling, it is necessary to consider:

(1) Sensitivity of the analytical procedure.
(2) Estimated air concentration.
(3) The TLV of the particular contaminant.
(4) The best results can be obtained (when analytical methods will permit) by allowing the worker to work a full eight-hour shift with a personal breathing zone sampler attached for the duration of that shift.
(5) Full-shift integrated personal sampling is preferable to that of short term or general area sampling if the results are to be compared to standards based on time-weighted average concentration.

e. When to Sample

Sampling strategies should be repeated every few months to determine if seasonal or production schedule variations affect exposure. It has been found that individual exposures may be different for each shift. If multiple shifts are used, sampling employees on each shift should be considered. If production schedules are non-linear, sampling at the end of the month or during peak production periods may also affect personnel exposures, therefore sampling during low and high production schedules is critical to assessing accurate exposure levels.

4. Interpretation of Results

a. Introduction

The final step in evaluating the workplace environment is the interpretation of analyses. Prior to determining that a group of workers has been exposed to an injurious hazard, the following must be established:

(1) Nature of substance or physical agent involved.
(2) Concentration of exposure.
(3) Duration of exposure.
(4) Air sampling results are expressed as time-weighted averages (TWAs) for an 8- hour day & 40-hour work week.

b. Comparing Results to Standards

Results of the environmental study must be compared with exposure limit standards before control methods can be recommended. Exposure limits are the crux of most occupational health codes, regulations, and standards. The toxicity of a substance expressed in terms of a threshold limit value (TLV) is an important component in evaluating the presence of a health hazard. Typically, if there is no exposure to a harmful agent, it is concluded that its presence does not create a health problem. Legislative exposure limits, referred to as permissible exposure limits (PELs), can be found in the Code of Federal Regulation (CFR), Title 29,

Part 1910, Occupational and Environmental Standards. Recommended exposure standards, referred to as threshold limit values, can be found in the TLVs and BEIs, Threshold Limit Values for Chemical Substances and Physical Agents, Biological Exposure Indices, published by the American Conference of Governmental Industrial Hygienists (ACGIH).

5. Occupational Exposure Standards

a. Introduction

The late 1930s brought the first organizations of occupational health professionals, and with them the first occupational health and safety standards. The American Conference of Governmental Industrial Hygienists (ACGIH) established in 1938, has played a major role in developing limits for exposures in workplace. These TLVs now exists for more than 750 chemical substances. Early on, it established "threshold limit values" by providing biological exposure indices (BEIs) for about three dozen chemicals. By establishing both TLVs and BEIs, the ACGIH offers a two-step approach to assessment of the importance of chemicals in the workplace: first monitoring of the air being breathed; second, monitoring of the chemicals themselves or their metabolites in biological specimens (such as urine, blood, and exhaled air). TLVs have been established for physical agents, including heat and cold, noise, vibration, lasers, radiofrequency/ microwave radiation, magnetic field, and ultraviolet and ionizing radiation. The TLVs are based on the best available information from the industrial experience, from experiments involving humans and other animals, and, when possible, from a combination of both.

Most industrialized countries use occupational exposure levels (PELs, also called permissible exposure levels in the United States and maximum allowable concentrations in Europe), which are either peak or average concentrations that must not be exceeded in the workplace over a particular period of time. The usual times are either 8 hr or 15 min, depending on the rapidity with which health effects can occur.

The 8-hr PELs are average concentrations over this time period. A system of averaging called the time-weighted average (TWA) simplifies calculation; an 8-hr TWA is the average of each measured concentration weighted by the length of time it lasted during the work shift. Sometimes toxic effects can occur with short exposures to high concentrations, regardless of the overall average. In such cases, 15-min short-term exposure levels (STELs) or instantaneous ceiling levels are used as absolute maximum concentrations that cannot be exceeded under any circumstances.

The most influential single body in recommending and promoting these levels has been the American Congress of Governmental Industrial Hygienists (ACGIH), which, despite its name, is international in its membership, has no relationship to Congress or the U.S. government, and includes many occupational health professionals who are not hygienists. The ACGIH, through its committees, establishes threshold limit values (TLVs), which are recommended occupational exposure levels set to protect all or most workers (excepting those with particular susceptibility). The ACGIH also establishes biological exposure indices (BEIs), which are special tests that detect a chemical or its metabolite in the blood, urine, or expired air of a worker and that can be used together with, or instead of, workplace measurements.

b. Permissible Exposure Limit (PEL)

The maximum time-weighted average exposure allowed by OSHA for an eight-hour workday during a normal 40-hour workweek is called the permissible exposure limit (PEL). This is the regulatory synonym for the TLV, which is a recommended exposure limit.

c. Threshold Limit Value-Time Weighted Average (TLV-TWA)

The Threshold Limit Value is based on a time-weighted average (TWA) concentration for a normal eight-hour workday and a 40-hour workweek, to which nearly all workers may be repeatedly exposed, day after day, without adverse effect. It is referred to as the threshold limit value, the TLV, or the TLV-TWA.

d. Threshold Limit Value-Ceiling (TLV-C)

The concentration that should not be exceeded during any period of the working exposure is called the Threshold Limit-Value-Ceiling (TLV-C). In conventional industrial hygiene practice, if instantaneous monitoring is not feasible, then sampling over a 15-minute period (except for those substances to which even short exposures may cause immediate irritation) can assess the TLV-C.

e. Threshold Limit Value-Short Term Exposure Limits (TLV-STEL)

The Threshold Limit Value-Short Term Exposure Limit (TLV-STEL) is the concentration to which workers can be exposed continuously for a short period of time without suffering from:

(1) Irritation
(2) Chronic or irreversible tissue damage
(3) Narcosis of a sufficient degree to increase the likelihood of accidental injury, impair self-rescue, or materially reduce work efficiency, provided that the daily TLV-TWA is not exceeded

The TLV-STEL is not a separate, independent exposure limit. It supplements the time-weighted average (TWA) limit where there are recognized acute effects from a substance whose toxic effects are primarily of a chronic nature. STELs are recommended only where toxic effects have been reported from high short-term exposures in either humans or animals. A TLV-STEL is defined as a 15-minute TWA exposure that should not be exceeded at any time during a workday even if the eight-hour TWA is within the TLV-TWA. Exposures above the TLV-TWA up to the STEL should not be longer than 15 minutes and should not occur more than four times per day. An averaging period other than 15 minutes may be recommended when this is warranted by observed biological effects. There should be at least 60 minutes between successive exposures in this range.

f. Understanding the Limitations of Exposure Standards

When comparing sampling results to regulatory or recommended exposure limits, the following must be considered:

(1) The dose-response relationship of the agent and the worker.
(2) Hypersusceptibility that some workers may experience despite levels within the TLV or PEL.
(3) A TLV does not definitely determine a safe versus dangerous condition.
(4) Skin absorption potential.
(5) The impact of ceiling limits.
(6) The biological effects of some agents.
(7) Time-weighted- averages for specific substances, unless designated by special categories or ceiling limits, permit limited excursions above the TLV-TWA.
(8) The additive or synergistic effects produced in the presence of multiple chemicals.

(1) TLVs and Dose Response

Threshold values are based on a dose-response relationship between the agent and the worker. The application of this knowledge to assure that workers are not exposed to concentrations above these threshold values is an important concept in the prevention of occupational diseases.

(2) Hypersusceptibility

Despite maintaining levels of exposure below a designated TLV, there is no assurance that an individual worker may not show some deleterious effects if hypersensitive to the substance. Individuals may be hypersusceptible to some   chemicals due to genetic factors, age, personal habits, medication, or previous conditions.

(3) Safe Versus Hazardous

Threshold limit values (TLVs) refer to airborne concentrations of substances and represent conditions under which it is believed that nearly all workers may be repeatedly exposed day after day without adverse effects. The TLV of a material is not a fine line between safe and dangerous concentrations. Due to individual variations in susceptibility and the many unknown factors in the working environment, some workers may not be adequately protected from adverse health effects from exposures to certain chemicals at concentrations below the TLV.

(4) Biological Effects

Biological Standards, i.e., the concentration of a specific substance in the urine or blood, represent the body's burden of that agent and may be used as a monitor of the exposure of a worker to a specific agent. Biological exposure indices can be found in the TLVs and BEIs, Threshold Limit Values for Chemical Substances and Physical Agents, Biological Exposure Indices, published by the American Conference of Governmental Industrial Hygienists (ACGIH).

(5) Additive and Synergistic Effects

When multiple chemicals, or mixtures of toxic substances are present in the absence of other information, their effects are considered additive. The combined effect of multiple chemicals or mixtures should be given primary consideration, rather than the effect of any of them individually.

6. Evaluation of the Severity of a Problem and Quantification of Exposures

Quantification is accomplished by exposure assessment. There are many ways to assess exposures, and many kinds of exposures to assess. More frequently, the IH is interested in assessing the exposure that a worker receives while he or she is performing his or her daily job during the total time spent on the job or performing a particular task. In order to measure exposure, the area surrounding the worker's mouth and nose (the "breathing zone") are assessed. Such measurements are referred to as personal monitoring or assessment.

Monitoring is accomplished with the use of several simple devices: a small, belt-mounted, microprocessor-controlled sampling pump, which continuously draws air at a precalibrated flow rate through a sampling medium attached to the pump by means of a length of tygon tubing. The sampling medium, typically an adsorbent for gases and vapors such as activated charcoal and a filter for dusts, is sent to a laboratory for analysis of the particular contaminant(s) of interest.

Over the past several decades, instrumentation for chemical analysis has improved greatly: it is possible to quantify contaminant concentration down to parts per billion. IH's also have at their disposal a broad array of instruments that both sample and analyze a volume of air for contaminants.

Direct reading instruments generally use a physical or chemical property of a contaminant to determine its concentration in air, such as its ability to conduct a current in solution, to absorb radiation of a particular wavelength, or to change color upon chemical reaction. Some direct reading instruments are used to obtain quick approximations of worker exposures during the walk-through investigation in order to determine if longer-term monitoring is necessary. Other direct reading instruments may be connected to alarms that alert workers to dangerous situations. They may be designed to test for one chemical or many. Some are so small that they can be herd in the palm of the hand, whereas others require a large cart to be moved.

Hygienists also may rake other types of samples that may reveal important potential sources of exposure by means other than inhalation. For instance, wipe samples are used to assess contamination on work surfaces or on skin. Workers may ingest contaminants if their hands come in contact with settled dust or if they eat food contaminated from contact with dusty surfaces. Additionally, settled dust may become airborne by air currents. Wipe samples of skin may help assess the presence of substances such as organic compounds (solvents) that are readily absorbed through the skin and into the systemic circulation. Occupational exposure limits refer only to airborne concentrations of substances and do not consider the potential for skin absorption. Therefore, it is important to characterize if and how much of a chemical may he deposited on the skin in order to fully assess a worker's exposure. In addition to testing the air for contaminants, exposures, or more precisely, absorbed doses, may be assessed by measuring the quantity of contaminant (one of its metabolites) in the body.

Most commonly, chemicals are measured in blood, urine, or exhaled air. For example, exposure to carbon monoxide may be measured by carbon monoxide in exhaled air or by measuring carboxyhemoglobin in a venous blood sample. Exposure to mercury may be assessed in urine, and exposure to benzene may be measured by phenol in urine. Although the measurement of biologic dose to assess exposure has its advantages, there are very few chemicals in common industrial use for which so-called biologic exposure indices have been developed. Also, it is not always practical or legally possible to obtain a biologic sample from a worker.

D. CONTROL OF POTENTIAL HAZARDS

1. Control Methods

Reducing or eliminating harmful exposure can control health hazards. Control methods for health hazards in the workplace are classified into three basic categories: engineering controls, administrative controls, and personal protective equipment (PPE).

2. Engineering Controls

Engineering controls limit hazards by implementing new design specifications or by applying methods of substitution, isolation, enclosure, ventilation, and work practices. Engineering controls are the primary and most desirable method of control, especially for environment hazards.

a. Substitution

Substitution, or replacement of a toxic material with a harmless one, such as using solvent with a lower order of toxicity or flammability, is a very common strategy for minimizing solvent exposure.

b. Changing a Process

Changing a process or how a job is performed is a very effective control method. Degreasing an aerospace part by dipping into a solvent tank is preferable to spraying the erospace part with an atomized solvent.

c. Isolation

Isolating employees from a high noise source (either by providing a sound barrier around the noise source or by providing a sound proof booth for workers to be isolated from the noise) is ideal.

d. Enclosure

Enclosure is another method of minimizing the escape of air contaminants into the workroom atmosphere.

e. Work Practices

Work Practices: Wetting an operation is an effective method for minimizing the source of dust. This can be accomplished by washing down work areas rather than sweeping or dusting off a work area.

f. Ventilation

Ventilation is one of the most beneficial methods for minimizing the release of airborne contaminants into the workplace. A local exhaust system that traps and removes the air contaminant near the generating source is more effective than general ventilation.

3. Administrative Controls

Administrative controls reduce employee exposures by alternating work schedules or by scheduling reduced work times in contaminant areas. Whenever engineering controls to reduce air contaminants are not feasible, administrative controls may be applied.

Caution must be used when applying administrative controls, as they have been criticized as a means of spreading exposure to more workers rather than resolving the exposure problem. Examples of administrative controls include arranging work schedules and the related duration of exposures so that the employees are minimally exposed to health hazards, and transferring employees who have reached their upper permissible limits to an environment where no further exposure will be experienced. Where exposure levels exceed levels the PEL for one worker in a single day, the job can instead be assigned to two, three, or as many employees as are needed to keep each one's duration of exposure within the PEL.

4. Personal Protective Equipment

When effective engineering control methods cannot render a work environment safe, personal protective equipment (PPE) may be required (Figure 14.3). PPE is specific clothing, gear, or protective devices worn by workers to protect them from a contaminated environment. PPE is the least effective method of control and does nothing to reduce or eliminate the presence of the hazard. PPE is the least desirable method of control since it relies heavily on human implementation or intervention. If the barrier fails, or if the worker refuses to use the equipment, exposure occurs.

5. Control of Specific Hazards

A complete and effective control program requires process and work place monitoring systems and education and commitment of both workers and management to appropriate occupational health practices.

Full-facepiece, dual cartridge   Half-mask, facepiece-mounted cartridge

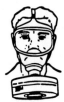

Full-facepiece,
chin-mounted canister

<u>Figure 14.3</u>. Several Types of Respirators Used to Protect Workers from Airborne Contaminants (Source: Moeller, 1997).

Ideally, protection is provided not only under normal operating conditions but also under conditions of process upset or failure, particularly in systems for controlling airborne contaminants. To assure that occupational health specialists apply the best methodologies, one must keep in mind the full range of possibilities available.

a. Toxic Chemicals

Emphasis in recent years has been on designing each element in process to eliminate generation of contaminant. If this aim proves impossible to achieve, the second defense is to prevent dispersal of the contaminant into the workplace.

In a generic sense, there are six basic approaches for controlling toxic airborne chemicals:

(1) **Elimination or substitution**: This approach involves control at the source by completely eliminating the use of a toxic substance or substituting a less toxic one.
(2) **Process or equipment modification**: Older processes that do not meet existing or proposed occupational health standards can be modified and upgraded.
(3) **Isolation or enclosure**: Operations involving highly toxic materials can be isolated from other parts of the facility by constructing a barrier between the source of the hazard and the workers who might be affected.
(4) **Local exhaust ventilation and air cleaning**: Airborne gases or particulates produced by essentially all industrial operations can be captured at the point of generation by an exhaust ventilation system. Two possible types of equipment are a glove box and a laboratory hood.
(5) **Personal protective equipment**: Controls can also be applied to individual workers, the fundamental concept being to isolate the worker rather than the source of exposure. For these and other reasons, personal protective equipment should

generally be considered a last resort, particularly when controlling the inhalation of airborne contaminants through the use of respirators.

(6) **Paper work practices and housekeeping**: Correct work practices and housekeeping are also important control strategies. The first step involves proper equipment design coupled with operating and maintenance procedures that minimize exposures and emissions. Appropriate housekeeping practices include chemical decontamination, wet sweeping, and vacuuming.

b. Biologic Agents

One of the best approaches to controlling airborne biological agents in the workplace is limiting the types of environments, namely, wet spots and pools of water, that promote the growth of organisms. Another key step is proper maintenance of the air handling system, especially the humidifier. Other approach include careful housekeeping with specific requirements for discarding contaminated needles and other sharp instruments, and proper handling of accompanying wastes.

c. Physical Factors

Control techniques for physical factors differ those for toxic chemicals or biologic agents. People who apply this technique must take into account human/machine interface and promote the use of industrial equipment design to reduce both physical stresses and accidents. One specific example is heat stress. As with various airborne contaminants, noise can be controlled at the source by damping, reducing, or enclosing the vibrating surface that produces it. Reducing or controlling stresses associated with the interface between human and machine often involves redesigning equipment to conform to ergonomic principles.

E. ENVIRONMENTAL FACTORS OR STRESSES

The diverse environmental factors that cause illness, impaired health, or significant discomfort in workers can be classified as chemical or physical.

1. Chemical Hazards

Most occupational health hazards are a result of inhalation of chemical agents in the form of gases, vapors, mists, fumes, and dusts, or by skin contact with these agents. Risks associated with exposure depend on the magnitude and duration of exposure. To effectively evaluate and measure a worker's potential exposure, the chemicals in use in any work process must be known. A working knowledge of the physical properties, nomenclature, and effects of exposure are critical to making a proper chemical hazard assessment. To learn about chemicals used in a work process, review the raw materials and the nature of the products and by-products manufactured by referring to the products' material safety data sheets (MSDSs). The severity of a chemical hazard depends on many factors, including how a chemical is to be used, the type of job performed, duration of exposure, and work patterns.

a. Inhalation Hazards of Chemicals

When reviewing workplace chemicals for possible inhalation hazards, industrial hygienists must determine whether the chemicals used are soluble or insoluble, asphyxiants, systemic toxins or poisons, irritants, corrosives, teratogens, mutagens, or carcinogens.

(1) Carcinogens

A carcinogen is a substance or chemical capable of inciting or producing cancer. Benzene is an example of a chemical carcinogen identified as a leukemogenic agent and is notorious for its effects on the blood-forming tissues of the bone marrow.

(2) Solubility

The solubility of a chemical determines where the chemical deposits become trapped in the respiratory system. The inhalation of highly soluble chemicals, such as sulfur dioxide, may irritate the upper respiratory tract. The inhalation of highly insoluble chemical hazards, such as nitrogen dioxide, may irritate the lower respiratory tract by penetrating the terminal passages of the lungs and the air sacs.

(3) Asphyxiants

Asphyxiants are classified as simple or chemical. Some chemicals, such as nitrogen gas or Halon, are considered simple asphyxiants and may dilute the atmospheric oxygen below the level required to sustain the normal blood saturation level. Gases and vapors considered chemical asphyxiants, such as hydrogen cyanide and carbon monoxide, prevent the blood from carrying oxygen to the tissues or interfere with its transfer from blood to tissue.

(4) Systemic Toxins

Systemic toxins may enter the body through the respiratory system, then enter the bloodstream and produce adverse health effects in a specific organ of the body. Lead is an example of a systemic toxin that can be inhaled and can damage the blood-forming bone marrow and the urinary, reproductive, and nervous systems.

b. Contact Hazards of Chemicals

When reviewing workplace chemicals for possible skin contact hazards, determine whether the chemicals used are irritants or corrosives, or whether they are capable of penetrating the skin by absorption. Petroleum-based solvents are examples of skin irritants. Contact may cause the skin to appear white as it defats the skin's oils, but long term damage is minimal. Corrosive chemicals may destroy the skin's surface and internal tissues. Hydrofluoric acid is a particularly dangerous corrosive when in direct contact with the skin. Some chemicals can directly penetrate the skin, be transported throughout the body, and produce a systemic reaction. Benzene and carbon tetrachloride (CCl_4) are two examples of chemicals with skin absorption potential.

c. Physical Propoerties of Chemicals

Some chemicals or products used in the workplace may, under specific circumstances, cause injury to persons or damage to property because of their reactivity, instability, spontaneous decomposition, flammability, or volatility.

(1) Explosives

Explosives: A mixture, substance, or compound that is capable of entering into a combustion reaction so rapidly and violently as to produce an explosion.

(2) Corrosives

Corrosives: Corrosives are capable of destroying living tissue and have a ruinous effect on other substances (especially on combustible materials, which can result in a fire or explosion).

(3) Flammability

Flammability: Flammable liquids are liquids with a flash point of 100°F or less.

(4) Oxidizing Agents

Oxidizing Agents: Oxidizers are chemicals that produce oxygen when they decompose. They may create a fire when in contact with a combustible substance, can react violently with water, and can react violently in a fire.

(5) Pressurized Chemicals

Pressurized Chemicals: Chemicals stored under pressure, such as compressed gases used for welding, create unique physical hazards. These compressed gases are usually stored in compressed gas cylinders. Extreme caution must be practiced to store these cylinders upright and locked in place.

2. Physical Stresses

To effectively evaluate a workplace, the physical stresses, as well as the chemical hazards, of the work environment, must be understood. Workplace problems associated with noise, temperature extremes, ionizing and non-ionizing radiation are examples of physical stresses or physical hazards

a. Noise Hazards

High noise levels in the workplace are physical stresses that may produce psychological effects by annoying, startling, or disrupting the concentration of the worker. High noise levels interfere with human speech, job performance, and safety. Physiological effects of noise include tinnitus, aural pain, and noise-induced hearing loss.

b. Thermal Stress

Temperature extremes in the workplace affect the amount of work employees can perform and the method by which they perform their work. The body can only operate effectively within a very narrow range of temperature. In high temperature environments, the body must rid itself of excessive heat as quickly as possible to maintain its normal temperature range. In extremely cold environments, the body uses other mechanisms to maintain adequate core body temperatures.

c. Ionizing Radiation

Five types of ionizing radiation-alpha, beta, x-ray, gamma, and neutron- may be found or produced in the in the workplace, subjecting workers to ionizing radiation exposure. These radioactive materials emit energy that can damage living tissue. Different types of radiation require different control methods and can cause various external and internal hazards. External hazards come from certain chemicals that can be hazardous even when located some distance away from the body. Internal hazards enter the body through inhalation, ingestion, or injection.

d. Non-Ionizing Radiation

Non-ionizing radiation is a form of electromagnetic radiation with varying effects on the body, depending on the wavelength of the radiation involved. Non-ionizing radiation includes extremely low frequencies, radio frequency, microwave, ultraviolet light, visible light, and infrared radiation. The predominant adverse health effect from non-ionizing radiation is thermal stress, or heating of the body tissues, related to the wavelength, power intensity, and exposure duration. Generally, longer wavelengths produce a greater penetration and more significant temperature rise in tissues than shorter wavelengths.

e. Ergonomics

The human body can endure significant discomfort and stress. However, when awkward conditions or motions continue for prolonged periods, they can exceed a worker's physiological limitations. Ergonomic considerations include the total physiological and psychological demands of a worker's job, rather than just productivity, health, and safety. Ergonomics includes the biomechanics, workplace design, and behavioral components of a job. Benefits include minimizing physical stress on workers by reducing repetitive motion injuries, reducing injury rates, more efficient operations, lower operating costs, reducing training times, and more effective uses of human resources.

f. Workplace Design

Workplace design considers the job and the equipment used by workers, and uses a workplace survey to identify ways to minimize human injury, increase worker efficiency, and decrease human error.

g. Biomechanics

Biomechanics deals with the structural elements of the body and the effects of the external and internal forces on various parts of the body. This includes reviewing flexion and extension positions of the hand, elbow joints, and shoulders while performing work. Flexing motions of the joints repeated rapidly over a long period of time results in inflammation of the tendon sheaths, which may cause tendonitis, trigger finger, carpal tunnel syndrome, epicondylitis, and thoracic outlet syndrome, among other illnesses.

(1) Mechanical Vibration

Mechanical Vibration: Vibration to the extremities caused by using vibrating power tools, such as jackhammers, reduces circulation in the hands and causes Raynaud's Syndrome, or "white fingers."

(2) Lifting

Lifting: When reviewing jobs that require lifting consider task variables, human variables, and environmental variables.

(3) Static Work

Jobs that require very little movement of the major muscle groups in the body can be as discomforting and fatiguing as highly repetitive jobs. For example, a cramped working posture generates excessive static muscular loading.

3. Biological Hazards

Where biological hazards are a concern, familiarity with work environments is essential. Examples include:

a. Workers in wood processing facilities exposed to endotoxins,
b. Workers exposed to allergenic fungi growing on timber,
c. Workers associated with birds exposed to Chlamydia psittaci,
d. Agricultural workers exposed to anthrax.

There are more than 200 biological agents known to produce infections and allergenic, toxic, or carcinogenic reactions in workers. These include:

a. Microorganisms such as viruses, bacteria, and fungi capable of producing infection, exposure, and allergies.
b. Allergens and toxins generated from plants that produce dermatitis, rhinitis, or asthma.
c. Protein allergens from vertebrate animals such as dander, hair, and saliva.
d. Arthropod-induced illness such as allergic reaction or inflammation caused by a bite or sting from an insect.
e. Parasite-induced illness such as schistosomiasis caused by the protozoa schistoma or roundworm infections caused by ascaris.

F. MONITORING THE WORKPLACE

Workplace monitoring can be done to assess exposures of workers under routine conditions, to alert workers to abnormal (accident) situations, or to design a control strategy. The type of monitoring programs depends to a large extent on the nature of the stress being evaluated.

1. Airborne Chemicals

If the problem is an airborne contaminant, monitoring can be restricted to collecting samples of air. The goal here is to provide data for estimating the concentrations and quantities of contaminants likely to be breathed by the exposed workers. Essentially all air samples consist of a filter or sorbent collector, an air mover or fan to pull the air and associated contaminants through the collector, and a means of controlling the rate of flow. A variety of samplers are in use. They include small, lightweight units that are battery powered and can be worn by individual workers to obtain what are called personal air samples. A second major type of air sampler is the fixed-location sampler. The objective in this case is to determine the concentrations of airborne contaminants within a given space or area. An airborne monitoring program may be supplemented by a variety of measurements of biological indicators of contaminants within bodies of the exposed workers.

2. Biological Agents

Because of the many different types of bioaerosols that must be evaluated, no single sampling method or analytical technique is optimal. Usually, culturing is required in the case of microrganisms, and microscopic examination in the case of contaminants such as pollen grains, fungal spores, and house dust mites.

3. Physical And Pyschological Factors

For certain physical factors such as heat and noise, a variety of measuring instruments is available for collecting real-time data in the workplace. Complicating the assessment of ergonomic factors is the multitude of settings in which workers are employed, the large number of interfaces between them and the equipment they use, and the increasing recognition that organizational and psychological factors - as important as physical factors may be as important as physical factors in terms of the resulting impact on health.

G. MAJOR CHEMICAL CONTAMINANTS OF CONCERN IN THE GENERAL ENVIRONMENT AND THE WORKPLACE

1. Toxic Metals

The principal toxic metals of concern in industrial pollution are lead, mercury, cadmium, and arsenic, although chromium, zinc, copper, and other metals may be of concern in some areas. It should be pointed out that human exposure to these metals is common both in the workplace and the general environment. In addition, families of workers can be exposed through dust brought home on dirty work clothes.

2. Solvents

Solvents can be categorized according to physical properties or chemical structure. Many solvents have essentially identical toxic effects on the central nervous system. They act as anesthetics and intoxicants at high concentrations (ethyl ether and chloroform were the first anesthetics used in surgery) that may cause a complete loss of consciousness if the fumes accumulate in confined spaces, but often lead to a clinical condition sometimes called **painter's syndrome** because it often affects painters. In this syndrome, the worker feels lightheaded then euphoric, loses coordination and acts intoxicated, and finally becomes sleepy or very fatigued (acute central neurotoxicity). Certain compounds exert their toxic effect on peripheral nerves, causing a loss of sensation or a burning sensation in the feet and hands. This condition is called **peripheral neuropathy** and it can also occur as a result of alcohol abuse.

3. Bulk Raw Materials

Any type of bulk materials that can induce adverse health effects after human exposure needs careful handling to prevent accidental releases of large amounts to the environment, fires, and long-term low-level emissions. Examples of bulk materials that can cause major hazards are chlorine gas, flammable liquids and gases (oil, petrol, solvents, raw materials for plastics production, such as vinyl chloride or acrylonitrile), and cyanides used in metals extraction and finishing.

4. Chemical Poisoning In The Community

Exposure in the home is perhaps the leading means by which children come into contact with toxic substances.

V. WORLDWIDE SITUATION OF OCCUPATIONAL HEALTH AND SAFETY

A. SOCIAL CONTEXT

Occupational health primarily deals with hazards of a chemical, physical, or biological nature; occupational safety primarily addresses hazards of a mechanical nature.

B. THE INTERNAL RESPONSIBILITY SYSTEM

Many government regulatory bodies for occupational health and safety have adopted the policy of internal responsibility for larger enterprises. This policy holds these companies responsible for controlling hazards and ensuring compliance with occupational exposure standards. A key feature of this system is the joint health and safety committee, a committee that consists of representatives from both management and workers who meet regularly to discuss occupational health and safety problems.

C. WORKERS' COMPENSATION

Workers' compensation is a no-fault insurance system funded by employers that compensates workers for health care and lost earnings from work-related injuries or illnesses.

D. WOMEN IN THE WORKPLACE

The role of women in the workforce is more complicated than that of men. The continued role of women in rearing children, however, places a double burden on women who are also wage earners in developing societies, and the risks of occupational injuries may jeopardize their ability to provide primary care to their children.

E. DIMENSIONS AND TYPES OF OCCUPATIONAL HEALTH PROBLEMS

The Global Estimates for Health Situation Assessments and Projections has suggested that there were 32.7 million occupational injuries and 146,000 occupational deaths in 1990. In practice, the distribution of occupational diseases in developed countries is thought to be approximated by the rule of halves, which states that the distribution of occupational diseases in a large working population in a diversified economy tends to be divided as follows, skin disorders account for roughly half of all occupational illnesses; eye disorders, roughly half of the remainder (or 1/4); lung disorders, half of that (or 1/8); and half of the residual are systemic toxicity problems.

1. Occupational Chemical Hazards

Occupational exposures to toxic metals, solvents, and bulk raw materials are much greater than exposures that occur generally in the environment.

2. Occupational Physical Hazards

Physical hazards are also very common at worksites. Noise is by far the most widespread of the occupational hazards.

3. Occupational Mechanical Hazards

Mechanical hazards may be of two general types: unsafe working conditions and ergonomic hazards.

4. Occupational Biological Hazards

Biological hazards are most obvious in health care and agriculture but may occur in many other industries.

5. Occupational Psychological Hazards

Stress at work is associated with lack of control over the working environment and with high workplace demands. Generally, it is difficult to separate out stress at work from stress in daily life.

6. Occupational Psychosocial Hazards

The Karasek model is used to document how jobs with a low degree of decision-making authority (low control) and a high degree of physical or mental demands are particularly stressful. Five categories of potential sources of work-related psychosocial stress can be distinguished: factors intrinsic to the job, the role of the worker in the organization, career development, interpersonal relationships at work, and organizational structure and climate.

F. APPROACHES TO PREVENTION

Prevention of injuries and diseases from occupational health hazards is based on two basic concepts:

1. The work environment and the production technology itself should be designed so that health risks are reduced to a minimum
2. The worker should be educated and encouraged to behave safely and use protective equipment.

G. THE OCCUPATIONAL ENVIRONMENT

1. Introduction

Industry information about the specific health hazards and preventive approaches for each industry can be found in publications of the International Labor Office (ILO) particularly the Encyclopedia of Occupational Health and Safety, as well as documents from the United Nations Environment Program (UNEP) Industry and Environment Office in Paris.

The workplace environment is generally more dangerous to health than the ambient external environment. Machinery, chemicals, dusts, ergonomic hazards, and the fact that much work is carried out with the body at its peak performance all contribute to the overall level of risk. Nevertheless, many of the same specific hazards occur in the workplace and the general environment, and hence there are many similarities in how their effects can be monitored and managed.

An important phenomenon in the workplace environment of low- and middle-income countries is the specific problems occurring at the time of rapid industrialization. Agricultural societies are transformed often without the infrastructure for environmental and workplace health protection that was built up in industrialized countries over decades of industrial development. Sometimes the new industries replace existing cottage industries, and the conditions may improve. In other cases industries with outmoded dangerous technology are moved from developed countries, creating new hazards in the receiving country. The term export of hazards has been used to describe this problem.

2. Agriculture

Agriculture is the most common occupation in rural areas of low- and middle-income countries, where most of the world's population lives. Most workers are engaged in subsistence agriculture, in which the boundaries between work and other aspects of daily life are fluid. Workplace hazards in this type of situation include the generally poor and unhealthy living environments, with unsafe drinking water, poor sanitation, and inadequate shelter.

Further, there are specific hazards, such as injury hazards from tools used in tilling the soil, vector-borne diseases related to walking in water or mud, bites from insects and animals, and falls or drownings from working on hillsides or riversides. The health risks are further increased because subsistence farm work involves the whole family, including children and the elderly. Epidemiologic evidence of these types of health risks is scanty.

3. **Mining and Extraction**

This type of industry is sometimes called **primary industry** and represents the first step in the process of creating manufactured products. It includes mining for metals and minerals, coal and oil extraction, forestry, agriculture, and fishing. Outputs of this type of industry include ore or metal concentrate, coal, oil, sand, wood, fibres (cotton, wool, hemp), grains, and fish. These primary industries can be found in all countries, but as countries develop they usually tend to represent a decreasing proportion of the overall economy.

The types of pollution and hazards related to the mining industry include dust in air and water pollution from the processes that use water to transport, wash, or concentrate the raw materials. Mines and quarries also create physical scars in the local environment and can cause major emergency pollution risks when tailings dams (accumulations of debris that trap water behind them) burst or overflow. Often processing plants for concentration or refining of metals are located together with the mine itself, and these plants can cause major sulfur dioxide or metals pollution, as has happened in a number of places. The sulfur dioxide pollution occurs because the ores of many metals contain large amounts of sulfur. Special problems accompany uranium mining as radioactive compounds can be released to the environment.

Mining is inherently dangerous to the mine workers, and most countries, including low- and middle-income countries, have recognized this by developing specific legislation and systems to protect mine workers. There are two major types of mining with somewhat different patterns of health hazards: underground mining and open-cast mining. Ergonomic hazards and physical (accident-inducing) hazards occur in both, but underground work includes the added hazards of being crushed by falling rock, poisoned by gas or dust build-up, or affected by heat or radiation. Each type of mine entails specific hazards associated with the rock from which the ore is excavated. Most types of rock contain high levels of silica, leading to high levels of silica dust in the air of a mine and the risk of silicosis in workers. Certain types of rock (particularly uranium ore) contain radioactive compounds that emanate as the gas radon, which increases the risk of lung cancer. Other types of rock contain metals that are inherently poisonous (for example, lead and cadmium), and which in certain conditions can cause dangerous exposures.

4. **Processing Industries**

Industries that process extracted raw materials into concentrated intermediate products are potentially large sources of environmental impact because of the scale and nature of their operations. The metals industries, including iron and steel production, transform metal ores to metal ingots, sheets, and pipes, and can generate considerable air, water, and land pollution. Some metals, such as lead and cadmium, are very toxic, and many incidents of poisoning in populations living around such industries have taken place. Particular problems occur in industries that recycle scrap metal products, as the content of the scrap is not always well known, and a mixture of toxic chemicals may be emitted to the air or water. Lead has been a particular problem in this regard.

5. Construction

Construction work is another dangerous occupation with potential exposures to a variety of hazards. This includes injuries from falls and falling objects, and injuries from machinery or related to excavation or underground work. As much construction work is carried out in the open, weather conditions create hazards of heat, cold, UVR, and dust storms. Construction work involves heavy lifts of materials and activities in awkward body positions leading to ergonomical hazards. Injuries, strains, and sprains are common. Many injuries are severe, leading to the high rate ratio of construction workers in the occupational mortality statistics.

Construction work also involves exposures to noise, chemicals, and biological hazards. Much of the machinery used is noisy, and this problem has increased with increasing mechanization of the industry. Demolition is a common aspect of construction work and demolition activities are inherently noisy. Noise-induced hearing loss is therefore common among construction workers. Another aspect of the noisy environment is the increased safety problems due to masking of warning calls or other alarms.

Chemical and dust exposures are related to the composition of the building materials. Asbestos, which was used as insulation and as a component of asbestos-cement pipes and sheets, has been a prime example of a hazardous material. Asbestosis (a form of pneumoconiosis), lung cancer, and mesothelioma (another cancer) have been found in many construction workers reduced in most industrialized countries and banned in some, but asbestos-cement building products are still widely used in low- and middle-income countries because these materials have attractive technical qualities and alternatives may be more costly.

Other chemical and dust exposures include cement dust among bricklayers and concrete workers. This dust causes dermatitis. Sand-blasting or rock drilling creates silica dust in the air, which can lead to silicosis in the exposed workers. Construction work often involves welding, which adds further health hazards such as inhalation of welding fumes that lead to bronchitis. Paint fumes often contain organic solvents that may cause neurologic disorders. The hazards of dusts and fumes are increased inside confined spaces, where these concentrations can reach extremely high levels.

6. Manufacturing

In this type of industry, often called **secondary industry** and common all over the world, raw materials and processed materials are used to create various consumer and industrial products. The largest plants are those that make automobiles, trains, airplanes, ships, and machinery. Occupational hazards are often the main health problems, but air and water pollution can develop in relation to processes that use toxic chemicals. There is a problem of storage and disposal of toxic wastes that are produced in manufacturing processes. In the production of paper, one of the most hazardous processes has been the chlorine-bleaching of paper to achieve a snow-white color. The presence of chlorine and organic compounds has led to the formation of toxic chemicals in effluent from the plant into water, including dioxins and furans. These chemicals have potentially serious environmental effects even though they are only produced in small quantities. They are also suspected to cause reproductive and carcinogenic effects in humans. Fortunately, new technologies in pulp and paper manufacturing do not require chlorine and thus avoid this problem. In the past, mercury has often been used as a catalyst in the production of chlorine. This mercury further contributes to water pollution.

Of the various manufacturing industries, some with particular health risks are worth highlighting. In electrical appliance manufacturing a major problem is lead-acid battery manufacture, which produces batteries for cars. Since such batteries are too heavy to transport over long distances, local production is usually established at an early stage of the "motor car society." The operation of these factories typically involves many workers who receive unacceptably high lead exposures. The usual approach is to monitor workers' blood lead levels; if the levels exceed the national standard, the worker is excused for a few weeks. Indeed, this type of risk management is enshrined in occupational health law in many countries. This approach displaces the exposure problem to the individual rather than analyzing the workplace environment as a whole.

Another manufacturing industry common in industrializing countries is metal processing and metal working. Smelting and refining of any metal provides a major potential for occupational exposures to many types of hazards, and a particular risk of exposure to toxic metal dusts, sulfur dioxide, and other fumes. As these industries are often of very large scale, even small concentrations of toxic compounds in the processes can yield substantial emissions into the workplace and the surrounding environment. The experience from lead smelters in many countries is similar: high lead exposures to workers and contamination of the local environment. Often the workers and their families live in the vicinity of the industry, and high lead exposures in children from dust emissions are found. These exposure situations have been studied in detail in the United States and Australia, and epidemiologic research there has produced some of the most valuable quantitative data on the health risks of lead in children and workers.

7. Service Occupations

An increasing proportion of overall economic activity is based on the provision of services, contrast to the production of goods. This is often referred to as **tertiary industry** and includes restaurant and hotel services, health services, personal services (such as hairdressing), entertainment, travel, tourism, public administrative services, telecommunications, and the new high-tech industries (such as software production). Generally they do not produce much environmental pollution, although all establishments at which large numbers of people are assembled create increased pressures on sanitation and waste management, e.g., tourist resorts create greater needs for sewage treatment. Hospitals and medical laboratories have particular problems with medical waste, which can contain infectious agents and radioactive materials. Another issue related to concentrations of people is disturbing noise.

A major concern in service industries is the widespread continuous work at computer keyboards or grocery store check-out counters, which in some countries has lead to "epidemics" of a number of painful hand and arm conditions called occupational overuse syndrome (OOS), cumulative trauma disorders (CTD) or repetitive strain injury (RSI).

Another occupational hazard in these types of industries is psychological stress from the demands of person-to-person contact and the economic demands for more rapid decision making and action, verbal and even physically abusive incidents are of increasing concern in the service sector, especially the health and social service sector.

Fire fighting involves exposure to carbon monoxide and toxic fumes, as well as the heat from the fire itself Injuries from falling debris, falls, or working in awkward positions are also of concern. Protection of workers depends on protective equipment, which in low- and middle- income countries may be in short supply. Law enforcement is another high-risk occupation, which involves hostile contacts with other persons who may be armed.

Garbage collection exposes workers to risks of cuts and other injuries from the garbage itself, as well as heavy lifts. A particular risk group in low- and middle-income countries is the people who scavenge on garbage dumps for recyclable materials from which to glean a meager existence.

Health care workers face other hazards, such as infections from patients, transmission of HIV or hepatitis from needle pricks, allergies to drugs given patients or to cleaning and disinfection chemicals.

8. Other Occupations

Among the other occupational exposure situations of particular importance, especially in low- and middle-income countries, are cottage industries of various types. At an early stage of industrialization, small-scale operations based on family members may be the mainstay of certain industries. This may be in the form of work contracted out from a larger enterprise, or it may arise directly in relation to the local market. The production of handicrafts, clothing, and consumer items for local households may be the starting point. However, more hazardous activities, such as recycling car batteries, may also develop initially as a cottage industry. This may entail extreme exposures to toxic chemicals, with little or no protection either for the workers or other family members. Ergonomic hazards, injuries, noise damage, and all other occupational hazards are likely to be a greater danger in these cottage industries than in more organized enterprises.

H. SURVEILLANCE, MONITORING, AND SCREENING IN OCCUPATIONAL HEALTH

1. Types and Purposes of Workplace Health Examinations

Health examinations are performed in workplaces for several distinctly different purposes. For example, the most common purpose of the preplacement medical examination, which occurs after an offer of employment has been made but before an individual is placed on specific job, is to determine if the individual has significant physical or mental impairment that would preclude the individual from performing specific essential duties related to a particular job. While this is one of the principal functions of the preplacement examination, the examination itself may be comprehensive, except in Minnesota due to a state law. One of the most common purposes of workplace health examinations and one that is most relevant to improving the health of the workforce is to identify toxic health effects at an earlier stage than they would be detected without the examination. This type of screening program is often initiated with a baseline examination and then followed with periodic follow-up examinations. The goal of this type of program is secondary prevention.

2. Ethical issues in health examinations in the workplace

One of the important differences between medical examinations in the occupational setting and those in other settings is that the relationship between the health care provider and the examinee is not, from a legal point of view, the traditional physician-patient relationship. In the traditional physician-patient relationship, the health care provider serves only the interests of the patient and the health care provider's only loyalty is to the patient. When the employer hires or contracts for the occupational health care provider, the provider may have difficulty resolving conflicts of interest between the employer and the employee-patient. This conflict is one of the most important ethical concerns of occupational health. Ethical codes have been developed by both the American College of Occupational and Environmental Medicine and the International Commission on Occupational Health. Rothstein has proposed a Bill of Rights of Examinees. ICON codes explicitly deal with many of the issues related to screening and surveillance activities, and the ACOEM has a position on medical surveillance in the workplace. All of these codes recognize the need to maintain the confidential nature of most medical screening information.

This concept is reinforced by the Americans with Disabilities Act (ADA). All medical information must be collected and sorted in separate medical files. Under ADA, management may be informed of workers' restrictions that limit theft ability to perform the job duties. In addition to ADA, other federal and state laws or regulations such as the Occupational Safety and Health Act, Department of Transportation examinations for interstate truck drivers, or state laws on human immunodeficiency virus (HIV) or drug testing deal with the issue of medical confidentiality. While the Occupational Safety and Health Administration (OSHA) mandates various preplacement and periodic medical examinations that employers must offer employees, the employees have the right to refuse to participate in these OSHA-mandated examinations unless this is part of the specific employee-employer contract.

3. Selecting the Components of Periodic Examinations

OSHA standards require periodic examinations for approximately 30 agents. Several common occupational exposures, such as asbestos, benzene, cotton dust, ethylene oxide, formaldehyde, lead, and noise, are covered by these specific OSHA standards. Generally, these examinations are required if a worker is exposed above a specific level of exposure, which is often one-half of the 8-hour permissible exposure limit (PEL). For example, OSHA requires baseline and annual audiometry testing in employees exposed to noise at an average of 85 dBA or above for a typical 40-hour work week. The National Institute of Occupational Safety and Health (NIOSH) recommends periodic testing on a larger list of agents.

Table 14.2. OSHA's Medical Surveillance Program for Lead. (Source: Fein, 1998).

Initial evaluation: Examination with attention to the teeth, gums, hematologic, gastrointestinal, renal, cardiovascular, and neurological systems; blood pressure; blood sample for blood lead; hemoglobin and hematocrit, red cell indices and peripheral smear morphology, zinc protoporphyrin (ZPP), blood urea nitrogen (BUN), serum creatinine; routine urinalysis (U/A). **Periodic evaluation:** Biological monitoring of blood lead and ZPP every 6 months or every 2 months if last blood lead at or above 40 µg/100 g of whole blood; monthly during medical removal; examinations usually for any employee with blood lead at or above 40 µg /100 g during the preceding 12 months. **Physician's written statement:** To include recommended special protective measures or limitations to be placed upon employee. **Special requirements:** Allows for multiple physician review of mechanism; provides medical removal protection.

Table 14.3. Components of a Medical Surveillance Program. (Source: Fein, 1998).

Exposure assessment and identification of most likely adverse health effects Selection of medical tests based on evaluation of test characteristics Identification of employees to be tested and testing frequency Training of testing staff Analysis arid interpretation of individual and group test results Actions based on test results Verification of test results Notification of employees and the employer while protecting confidentiality Additional tests or treatment and steps to reduce an individual's exposure Exposure evaluation and reeducation of hazardous exposures Maintenance of records Evaluation for adequate quality control and revise based on the program performance

Table 14.2 illustrates the medical surveillance features of the OSHA Lead Standard 1910.1025. The components of a medical screening program have been proposed (Table 14.3).

4. Surveillance

a. Definition

The previous discussion is focused on the role of screening and of periodic examinations in occupational health. One of the potential roles of these examinations is to supplement other occupational surveillance. Occupational surveillance is the ongoing and systematic collection, analysis, and interpretation of data related to either occupational exposures (hazard surveillance) or adverse health outcomes (injuries, disorders, or diseases). Hazard surveillance should be an important part of occupational surveillance activities. The identification of occupational exposures (hazard surveillance or exposure assessment) before work-related diseases or injuries have developed or occur should trigger further evaluation of the workplace. If high or unsafe levels of exposure are found, then these exposures can be reduced by implementation of either administrative or engineering control activities. The primary goals of surveillance are different from the goals of screening programs. The classic purpose of screening is to identify patients who have asymptomatic disease in order to initiate therapy   early in the natural course of the disease.

b. Goals

The goals of health or injury surveillance are ideally related to prevention activities. The first goal of surveillance is the identification of new or previously unrecognized problems. Identification will occur with the association of an injury or disease with a specific work process or occupation. This generally happens through two types of surveillance data: either the identification of cases without definite information about the size of the population (the cases are drawn from the sentinel health event); or from a surveillance source of cases that include some information both on the number of cases and the size of the population at risk. An example of the first type of surveillance is a recent report of cases of hypersensitivity pneumonitis with exposure to metalworking fluids. An example of the second type of surveillance is the elevated rate of workers' compensation claims for carpal tunnel syndrome in certain industries in the state of Washington. These two examples illustrate that surveillance activities often involve data such as workers' compensation claims that are collected for other purposes and may be conducted at the level of individual worksite or at a state or national level.

The second goal of surveillance is to determine the magnitude of the problem either at the national, state, or local level. This is one of the most important goals of surveillance from the perspective of prevention. Surveillance data can be used to determine where to focus prevention efforts.

At the national level, surveillance data can be used to identify which industries are at high risk. One of the few sources of national data is collected by the Bureau of Labor Statistics (BLS) in the Department of Labor, which surveys a representative sample of private sector employers with more than 11 employees each year.

The magnitude of the occupational injury or disease problem can be estimated at the national, state, or facility (local) level. Local surveillance systems we typically based on one or more of the following data sources: (a) OSHA 200 log, an important source of data for the BLS surveillance system; (b) in-plant medical records or logs; or (c) workers' compensation records. Analyses of surveillance data for the purpose of determining the magnitude of a problem sometimes also suggest a possible cause for the problem.

The third goal of surveillance systems is to track trends in the number of workers exposed to occupational hazards, or the number of workers with injuries, disorders, and diseases over time. One of the major uses of this trend data is to qualitatively evaluate the effectiveness of prevention activities. However, an important limitation of surveillance data is that changes in the rate of disorders may be due to changing levels of exposure or changes in the reporting of disorders independent of their level of occurrence.

c. Hazard Surveillance

The most effective workplace surveillance system will have a health and a hazard or exposure component. While hazard surveillance may be less common than health surveillance, it is vital. Hazard surveillance provides the opportunity to identify and intervene on hazardous exposures before an injury or disorder develops. When hazardous exposures involve only small groups (less than 25) of workers, most serious work-related health problems will be infrequent. The determination that a disease is work related will often be difficult based on health surveillance alone. In contrast with hazard surveillance data, hazards may be readily identified regardless of the number of exposed workers.

The ability of a hazard surveillance system to identify hazardous exposures is less dependent on the number of exposed workers but rather depends on the overall accuracy of methods used to identify the nature and the intensity of the exposures. As with health surveillance information, hazard surveillance information will frequently need validation with more precise data. Hazard surveillance information can be collected by worker interview, walk-through inspections, or environmental sampling. As a result of hazard surveillance and other health surveillance information, jobs can be prioritized for more sophisticated or intensive evaluation to identify hazardous exposures. The purpose of the more sophisticated evaluation is to precisely assess the nature of the exposures and to evaluate possible methods to reduce exposures. Sometimes hazardous exposures identified by the hazard surveillance activities will be so clearly hazardous and ways to reduce the level of exposure will be so obvious that the more sophisticated evaluation will be unnecessary.

d. Characteristics of Successful Health Surveillance

One of the features of an effective surveillance program is the use of a standard coding system for recording health outcomes. Standardized coding leads to more homogeneous disease categories. Surveillance systems generally have to be as cost effective as possible to be widely used. The principal advantage of using existing data sources such as workers' compensation records is low cost. Supplementing an existing surveillance system with an additional component such as symptom questionnaires should be considered when observations of the workplace suggest that there are potentially hazardous common exposures, but the existing surveillance data suggests that there are no problems.

The absence of problems will commonly occur for two reasons: the exposures are not high enough to cause any health complaints and underreporting. Underreporting of problems is likely to be more common where there are obstacles or discentives to the re-porting of a possible disorder to supervisors or health professionals. For example, if an organization gives awards to departments without lost time injuries or work-related disorders, either supervisors or coworkers may discourage reporting. In the second situation, more active collection of surveillance data is indicated when there is simply no existing health surveillance information to determine if a problem exists but substantial exposures are common. For example, in many sectors of the economy, OSHA logs are not required.

I. OCCUPATIONAL HEALTH PROBLEMS OF SPECIAL WORKING GROUPS

1. Workers with Disabilities

a. Framework for Defining Disability

The term disability is defined in various ways. In some contexts it is defined in terms of health conditions; in other contexts it is defined in terms of functional limitations; and in still other settings it is defined in terms of activity and role limitations. These varying definitions of disability have in some cases been codified into law, into standardized data collection instruments, and into the practice framework of professionals and organizations that serve people with disabilities. One consequence of the different ways in which disability is defined is that, before the characteristics and needs of people with disabilities can be discussed, the parameters of the disability definition being used must be addressed. Whatever the specific components of the definition there does appear to be some consensus that a person with a disability is someone who experiences a permanent physical or mental impairment or a chronic health or mental health condition. The health condition or impairment may be one that is visible or it may be invisible. Onset may occur at any age or it may be present at birth. Finally, the severity of disability may vary, even among people with the same condition or impairment, such that some individuals may find it difficult to participate in many life activities, while others experience the effects of disability in a single area.

Among the many definitions of disability used by professionals, government programs, service agencies, and individuals with disabilities, there are three that are most dominant. The first definition involves the extent of limitation in the Activities of Daily Living (ADL) and Instrumental Activities of Daily Living (IADL). The second definition is embodied in the International Code of Impairments, Disabilities, and Handicaps (ICIDH) of the World Health Organization. The third construct for defining disability is based upon a model developed by Sand Nagi that defines disability in terms of the interaction of environment, functional limitation, and impairment. As a result of the Disability Rights Movement of the 1970s and 1980s and the passage of the 1990 Americans with Disabilities Act, there appears to be growing consensus in the United States for the use of this third paradigm.

(1) ADL and IADL

The ADL scale measures disability in terms of limitations in the Activities of Daily Living. This scale was developed by Katz and coworkers in the 1950s and has been used extensively by researchers studying the elderly. The ADL scale asks about the need for assistance in the activities of eating, bathing, dressing, transfer, and toileting. A related measure, developed by Lawton and Brody in 1969, is the IADL scale - Instrumental Activities of Daily Living. The items in this scale ask about the need for assistance in such activities as everyday household chores, managing finances, shopping, and getting around outside one's home. More recently, these scales have been used to define levels of disability among adults in general. Both the ADL and IADL approach measuring disability by examining tasks or activities tat are limited or prevented by an impairment or healt condition. The items do not directly address work, although people with ADL and IADL limitations report low rates (approximately 25 percent) of employment.

(2) ICIDH

In 1980 the World Health Organization issued its first edition of a classification of impairments and disabilities, called the International Classification of Impairments, Disabilities, and Handicaps. The intent was to offer a framework comparable to that of the international Statistical Classification of Diseases, injuries, and Causes of Death (ICD) that would be a tool for describing the consequences of disease (as well as injury and other disorders). This disability code, referred to as the ICIDH, uses a framework consisting of four main categories: disease, impairment, disability, and handicap. Disease is not really defined in the ICIDH, but is implicitly based upon the definitions contained in the ICD. Impairment is defined as any loss or abnormality of psychological, physiological, or anatomical structure or function, and disability is any restriction or lack of ability to perform an activity in a manner or within the range considered normal for a human being. The final category, handicap, refers to a disadvantage resulting from an impairment or a disability that limits or prevents the fulfillment of a normal role.

While the ICIDH is similar to the Nagi model because it separates the medical condition from its functional and social consequences, it has not been as well accepted. Part of the reason is the lack of conceptual clarity of the different classifications and categories. An additional reason is the objection by many people with disabilities and by disability researchers in the United States to the term, handicap. The Institute of Medicine report explains this by noting that to many people handicap has a negative connotation because it implies "an absolute limitation that does not require for its actualization any interaction with external social circumstances". A revision of the ICIDH has been undertaken and is nearly complete. Representatives of the U.S. Public Health Service have played an active role in the revision process. It is likely that handicap and its related concepts will not be present in the new version. In its place will be a term that identifies the social and environmental barriers that mediate between an impairment and its disabling impact. To date, however, disability research in the United States has generally proceeded without use of the ICIDH framework, especially research focused on disability and work.

b. Civil Rights

People with disabilities are protected from discrimination in employment under Title I of the 1990 Americans with Disabilities Act (ADA) and Sections 503 and 504 of the 1973 Rehabilitation Act. While the provisions in the Rehabilitation Act were the first to a measure of protection against employment discrimination, the coverage was restricted to people employed in the public sector or by federal contractors and grantees. Much broader coverage is now available under the Americans with Disabilities Act, which applies to employers of 15 or more employees. While the definition of disability in the ADA is modeled after the Rehabilitation Act, the enforcement structure relies on the

Equal Employment Opportunity Commission (EEOC) and the methodology developed to enforce the 1994 Civil Rights Act.

c. Prevention and Wellness

With disability ranking among the nation's largest public health problems, application of the prevention model is appropriate. Primary prevention of unintentional injuries, occupationally related injuries or exposures, and other medically or health-related etiologies of disabilities are a part of the national agenda. However, primary prevention of other health issues or secondary conditions of persons with disabilities should be acknowledged. This requires use of traditional public health prevention strategies and the clinician's index of suspicion regarding possible secondary conditions. Secondary prevention is aimed at early recognition of disability or disability-producing activities, with reduction of risk factors for work disabilities and improvement in the quality of life. Disability-related legislation reflects efforts to reduce environmental and social risk factors for worker disability. Appropriate modifications of the workplace for a worker with a disability who has initiated or completed a return to work also is a secondary prevention strategy. Tertiary prevention is centered on the rehabilitation aspects of a return-to-work plan.

Despite the medical complications and implications of disabling conditions, workers with disabilities are not ill or in poor health. There has been a paradigm shift from illness and disease to health and wellness. It is important to recognize health promotion for the worker with a disability, in spite of the disabling condition.

2. Minority Workers and Communities

Environmental and occupational hazards do not affect all communities equally. Members of ethnic and racial minorities, whether as working people or as community residents, sustain disproportionate risk from chemical, physical, and biological hazards. It presents evidence for increased exposure, increased susceptibility, and increased resulting illness and injury among members / of minority groups.

The U.S. population is becoming more diverse, with minority groups accounting for a growing proportion of the overall population. According to the U.S. Census Bureau, the U.S. population is approximately 280 million, of whom 71.6 percent are white, 12.8 percent black, 0.9 percent Native American/Eskimo/Aleut, 4.4 percent Asian and Pacific Islander, and 11.3 percent Hispanic (of any race).

Members of minority groups live and work in patterns that distinguish them from the general population and from each other. Minority workers, on average, have less education, lower income levels, inferior housing, worse health status, and less access to services such as health care, compared with white workers. For example, according to 1990 Census Bureau data on the civilian labor force, the proportion of workers who had not completed high school was 14.0 percent for whites, 26.2 percent for blacks, and 44.5 percent for Hispanics. Similarly, the proportion of workers who had completed college was 23.6 percent for whites, 13.1 percent for blacks, and 9.2 percent for Hispanics. The per capita income was $15,265 among whites, $9,017 among blacks, and $8,424 among Hispanics. These and similar data signal persistent disparities in economic opportunities, residential patterns, and other important determinants of health.

a. Mechanisms of Increased Risk among Minority Workers

Members of minority groups may be at increased risk from occupational and environmental exposures through one or more of several mechanisms. First, they may be disproportionately exposed to hazards. Second, they may be more susceptible to the effects of these exposures. Third, they may receive inferior health care once injured or made ill following an exposure. In discussing these risks, the primary focus will be on blacks, since more data are available than for Hispanics, Native Americans, Asian American, and other minority groups.

(1) Increased Exposure to Occupational Hazards

There is ample evidence that members of minority groups have been, and continue to be, concentrated in jobs with lower pay, lower status, and, all too often, higher risk. This is exemplified by one of the watershed occupational health disasters in U.S. history, the construction of the Hawk's Nest Tunnel near Gauley Bridge, West Virginia in 1930-1931. This tunnel was drilled through a mountain rich in silica to transport river water to a power plant. Several hundred tunnel workers lost their lives, some from injuries, but most from acute silicosis. Although the local population was over 80 percent white, the workers hired for the most hazardous jobs - inside the tunnel - were 75 percent black. Accordingly, of over 700 deaths from 1930 to 1935 attributed to work on the tunnel construction, 76 percent occurred among black workers. As the nearby Fayette Journal noted in February 1931, "This is a great deal of comments [sic] about town regarding the unusually large number of deaths among the coloured labourers at tunnel works of the New Kanawha Power Company".

In numerous industry-specific studies, similar patterns of disproportionate exposure have continued to be documented. In the chromate industry in the 1940s, 41 percent of the black workers, as compared with 16 percent of the white workers, were assigned to the "dry end of the process, where exposures to chromate dust were highest. In the steel industry, one of the most hazardous jobs is in the coke plant, due to exposure to carcinogenic polycyclic aromatic hydrocarbons. Among coke plant workers in the 1950s, 89 percent of blacks and 32 percent of whites worked directly at the coke ovens. Among these coke oven workers, 21 percent of blacks and only 8 percent of whites were assigned to the most heavily exposed "full topside" jobs. As a result, 74 percent of full topside workers were black, and black workers were over five times more likely than white workers to be in one of the highest exposure categories. In the textile industry in the 1970s, black workers were concentrated in the dustiest areas of the plants, with a substantially higher risk of byssinosis than their white coworkers. In the rubber industry, black workers were conceatrated in the compounding and mixing job categories, where exposures to various carcinogens were highest.

Agricultural work deserves special mention because it is overwhelmingly a minority occupation. Seasonal farm workers are 71 percent Hispanic, and migrant workers are 95 percent Hispanic. Farm work is one of the most dangerous occupations; it employs less than 3 percent of the U.S. workforce, but accounts for 13 percent of workplace fatalities. It is estimated that pesticide toxicity causes 313,000 cases of illness and 1,000 deaths annually among farm workers.

Another employment-related health hazard, ironically, is the absence of employment. Black unemployment has for some time been approximately twice as high as white unemployment. In 1994, 11 percent of blacks and 5 percent of whites were unemployed. In turn, unemployment is a well-established risk factor for morbidity and mortality. The causal chain operates in both directions. While some of this association occurs because ill people are more likely to become unemployed - the inverse of the "healthy worker effect," well known to occupational epidemiologists - unemployment and its consequences play an important role in contributing to poor health.

(2) Increased Exposure to Environmental Hazards

The association of minority status with hazardous exposures extends beyond the workplace to the general environment as well. Members of minority groups live near more environmental hazards, such as polluting factories and hazardous waste sites, than do whites. A considerable body of work in recent years, much of it in the form of correlational studies, small area case studies, and ecological studies using Geographic Information Systems or similar techniques, has demonstrated this pattern. This evidence has stimulated further research, government action, and an active community-based **"environmental justice"** movement.

Minorities sustain disproportionate exposure to air pollution, independent of income and urbanization. For example, blacks and Hispanics are more likely than whites to live in air pollution non-attainment areas.

Hazardous waste exposure demonstrates a similar pattern. Early work by the United Church of Christ showed that race predicted the presence of a hazardous waste facility better than any other community variable. Communities with one hazardous waste facility averaged 24 percent minority population, and communities with two or more hazardous waste facilities averaged 38 percent minority population, compared to a 12 percent minority population in communities without such a facility. In a case study of Houston, six of eight municipal incinerators and all five municipal landfills were located in black neighborhoods. In a case study of Baton Rouge, the 10 largest white Zip codes contained five hazardous waste sites, while the 10 largest black Zip codes contained 15 hazardous waste sites. Total waste generated was estimated to be 663 times greater in the black neighborhoods than in the white neighborhoods.

Water pollution exposure also varies by race and ethnicity, although fewer data are available than for other media. Exposures to both microbial and chemical contaminants appear to be higher for minority groups. This is well documented in specific situations, such as in migrant worker camps (whose residents are primarily Hispanic), on Indian reservations, and in rural poor counties, whose residents are disproportionately black and Native American.

Lead paint poses the major environmental source of lead exposure to children, now that lead has been removed from gasoline. Black children face substantially greater exposure to lead paint than white children, through living in older, more poorly maintained housing stock. Over 50 percent of black children in poverty enter the first grade with blood lead levels above 10 µg/dL, the level at which neurotoxicity has been demonstrated.

Even dietary exposures vary by racial and ethnic background. A well-established example is fish consumption. Since compounds such as dioxins, dibenzofurans, and organometals bioconcentrate in fish, excessive fish consumption may be hazardous. In a study of Michigan anglers, the average daily fish consumption was 17.9 g among whites, 20.3 g among blacks, 19.8 g among "other minorities" (including Hispanics), and 24.3 among Native Americans. While whites tended to fish for recreation, nonwhites fished both for recreation and for food. Among Mohawk Indians in New York State, Mohawk women ate significantly more polychlorinated biphenyl (PCB)-contaminated fish than white women, although the Mohawk women successfully limited their fish consumption during pregnancy thanks to local fish advisories. This pathway is especially worrisome among indigenous and/or poor populations, for whom subsistence fishing may represent a principal source of food).

Exposures to hazards in the ambient environment may be aggravated by problems related to substandard housing, such as absence of air conditioning and appropriate ventilation, and microbiological exposures. Overall, there is a consistent trend that extends from the workplace to the general environment. Members of minority groups are disproportionately exposed to hazards through working in the most dangerous jobs and living in the least wholesome environments.

(3) Increased Susceptibility to Occupational and Environmental Hazards

Independent of increased exposure to occupational and environmental hazards, members of minority groups may be especially susceptible to the effects of hazardous exposures. This could occur through one or more of several mechanisms: increased baseline risk of certain diseases to which occupational and environmental exposures further contribute; increased probability of other exposures that may combine with workplace or environmental exposures to harm health; increased genetic susceptibility; and increased general susceptibility to disease through stress, poverty, and decreased social supports.

(a) Increased Baseline Risk of Certain Diseases

Common illnesses are multifactorial in etiology. While occupational and environmental exposures may contribute to illness, so may a range of genetic, social, environmental, and lifestyle factors. If members of minority groups carry an increased baseline risk for some of these illnesses, then workplace and environmental exposures could pose special hazards for these groups. Several examples are discussed below.

Lung cancer is a leading cause of cancer incidence and mortality for both men and women in the United States in the 1990s. Lung cancer incidence is approximately 50 percent higher in black men than in white men, although black women and white women have comparable incidence rates. Lung cancer mortality is 61 percent higher in black men than in white men, and 13 percent higher in black women than in white women. Other minority groups generally have lower lung cancer incidence and mortality than whites. The black excess is not fully explained by differences in smoking; although the prevalence of smoking is higher among black men than among white men, blacks initiate smoking at a later age and smoke fewer cigarettes compared to whites. Possible explanations include dietary differences genetic and/or metabolic differences, and differences in environmental and occupational exposures to lung carcinogens. Based on this increased risk, blacks may be especially susceptible to the effects of further exposures to lung carcinogens in the workplace or general environment.

Asthma is steadily increasing in all U.S. subpopulations, and now affects approximately 13 million Americans. Asthma prevalence and mortality are higher in blacks than in whites; the cumulative prevalence is 122 per 1,000 in blacks and 104 per 1,000 in whites, and asthma mortality is approximately three times higher in blacks than in whites. Similarly, asthma prevalence is more than three times higher among Puerto Rican children than among non-Hispanic children. Asthma prevalence and mortality are especially high, and rising, in inner cities, where minority populations are concentrated. The reasons for the increase in asthma are not fully understood; they may include changes in diagnostic practice, health care access, medication use, environmental exposures and/or immune status. Whatever the reasons, the racial disparity may imply that minority populations are especially susceptible to the effects of any of the hundreds of environmental agents known to cause or aggravate asthma. Moreover, minority workers are concentrated in several occupations, such as health aides and textile workers, with frequent exposure to asthma-causing agents and with elevated asthma mortality. Similarly, since those with asthma are especially susceptible to the effects of certain air pollutants, especially ozone and acid aerosols, 42 and since blacks are disproportionately likely to be asthmatic, excessive exposure to air pollutants may have a disproportionate impact on blacks.

Hypertension continues to cause excess morbidity and mortality among U.S. blacks. Hypertension is between 33 and 50 percent more prevalent in blacks than in whites, and severe hypertension occurs three to seven times more commonly in blacks than in whites. Hypertension has important end-organ effects, contributing to the occurrence of renal failure, congestive heart failure, myocardial infarction, and stroke, all conditions that occur at higher rates among blacks. The nature of this increased risk is complex and multifactorial. There is evidence of racial differences in salt sensitivity, neurogenic response, and other physiological factors, as well as in diet and social stressors. Again, whatever the reasons for the increased risk among blacks, they may place blacks at yet further risk when exposed to workplace and environmental factors that contribute to hypertension.

Two such factors are relevant. The first is social factors such as workplace stress and powerlessness, prominent features of the employment experience for minorities. Numerous studies demonstrate that episodes of discrimination on the job and elsewhere contribute to hypertension among blacks. Job insecurity and job loss, which are disproportionately common among blacks, also contribute to hypertension. Second, a variety of chemical and physical factors may contribute to hypertension directly, or to the end-organ damage caused by hypertension. For example, lead and noise contribute to hypertension. Chronic exposure to neurotoxins such as lead and organic solvents can cause encephalopathy, affecting many of the same functions as multi-infarct dementia. Nephrotoxins such as metals and hydrocarbons may impair kidney function, compounding the effects of hypertension. These exposures, both social and physicochemical, may therefore pose special risks for blacks.

Diabetes disproportionately affects major minority populations in the United States. The prevalence of diagnosed non-insulin-dependent diabetes mellitus (NIDDM) in adults is currently 1.4 times higher in blacks than in whites; by the age of 65 one in six blacks carries the diagnosis. The prevalence of NIDDM is two to three times higher among Mexican Americans than among non-Hispanic whites. Similar findings of increased prevalence have been published for Native American populations, while limited information is available for Asian/Pacific Islanders. Racial and ethnic differences in diabetes mainly reflect genetic and dietary factors, although one or more environmental exposures such as arsenic may play a role. As for hypertension, workplace exposures may pose a special risk for persons diagnosed with diabetes, because of a pattern of common end-organ effects. Peripheral neuropathy may be caused by metals, pesticides, and organic solvents. Kidney damage may result from exposure to metals and hydrocarbons. Retinopathy may result from carbon disulfide exposure. Therefore, worker populations with a high prevalence of diabetes, including several minority groups, may face special risk from these occupational exposures.

Infectious diseases have emerged as important occupational disease concerns and exert a disproportionate impact on minorities in varied ways. Tuberculosis increased from the 1980s through the mid1990s, when the incidence finally began to decrease. Minorities have been disproportionately afflicted. In 1992, tuberculosis incidence was elevated 4-fold among Native Americans, 5-fold among Hispanics, 8-fold among blacks, and 11-fold among Asian Americans, compared with whites; 71 percept of new cases occurred among minorities. In fact, some evidence suggests that blacks may be especially susceptible to Mycobacterium infection. Since tuberculosis is well recognized as an occupational hazard among health care workers and certain other occupations, black workers in these professions may carry an especially elevated risk of infection. Another infectious disease that bears mention is pneumococcal pneumonia. This is not usually considered an occupational disease. However, pneumonia may increase a person's susceptibility to the effects of air pollutant exposure, such as further respiratory illness and mortality following exposure to particulates. Pneumococcal pneumonia is vaccine preventable, but blacks are much less likely than whites to have been vaccinated. Therefore, blacks may again bear disproportionate risk following such exposures, in this case because of relative lack of a preventive intervention.

(b) Increased Probability of Other Exposures that may Combine with Workplace or Environmental Exposures to Harm Health

Members of minority groups may be excessively exposed to risk factors that aggravate the effects of workplace or environmental exposures. Examples include behavioral factors such as alcohol consumption and exposures in the home environment. Patterns of alcohol use vary across ethnic and racial groups, as do the health consequences of alcohol abuse. While blacks and whites have generally similar drinking patterns, a recent study using large probability samples showed that 17 percent of Hispanic men, 10 percent of black men, and 7 percent of white men were heavy drinkers. The high prevalence of alcohol abuse among Native Americans has long been recognized. Alcohol-related mortality is higher among Native Americans and Hispanics than among whites, and the recent decrease among whites has not been seen in these minority groups. Alcohol abuse may aggravate the effects of workplace and environmental hazards in two ways. First, alcohol intoxication increases the risk of injuries. Second, chronic alcohol exposure may combine with the effects of workplace toxins to cause end-organ damage such as liver dysfunction.

Housing patterns also vary across racial and ethnic groups, with members of minority groups bearing an increased risk of living in substandard housing. As noted above, such housing poses an increased risk of exposure to lead dust. Substandard housing has also been implicated in the etiology of asthma, through exposure to cockroach, dust mite, and other antigens, cooking fuels, and secondary tobacco smoke, compounded by inadequate ventilation. Again, such home exposures could aggravate the effects of workplace and environmental exposures to respiratory hazards.

(c) Increased Genetic Susceptibility

It has long been recognized that several single-gene disorders vary in frequency among different racial and ethnic groups. Among blacks, disorders that are relatively prevalent include glucose-6-phosphate dehydrogenase (G6PD) deficiency, hemoglobinopathies (HbS and HbC), and α and β-thalassemias. Moreover, differences in the ability to metabolize certain drugs, related to polymorphisms of one or more gene loci, have been associated with racial and ethnic backgrounds. One example is debrisoquin hydroxylase (also known as CYP2D6), a cytochrome P-450 enzyme that catalyzes the oxidation of more than 30 drugs. Compared to whites, blacks and Asians have fewer abnormalities of this enzyme. Mephenytoin metabolism is also controlled by an enzyme for which polymorphisms have been demonstrated, with a much higher frequency in Asians than in whites. Increasingly, with growing success at mapping the human genome, individual genes have been identified that are more common in specific racial or ethnic groups and are associated with specific diseases. Cancer risk is a special area of interest with respect to genetic polymorphisms. Some oncogenes have been reported to vary by race. For example, mutations of the CYP1A1 gene, which is involved with the metabolism of polycyclic aromatic hydrocarbons, are thought to increase the risk of lung cancer among smokers; this abnormality is more common among blacks than among whites.

(d) Increased General Susceptibility to Disease Through Stress, Poverty, and Absent Social Supports

An extensive literature documents the consistent relationship between poverty and poor health. In addition to poverty, members of minority groups are likely to encounter other forms of stress, such as discrimination, uncertainties of income, employment, and housing, and absent social supports. These experiences, of course, vary in nature and intensity among individuals and groups.

Stress has been relatively well studied in this regard. The role of stress, specifically including racial discrimination, is now well established in the etiology of hypertension among blacks. Stress is also thought to act more generally, increasing susceptibility to a number of diseases through general effects on immune and other functions. Although the medical effects of poverty and stress are not completely understood, it is reasonable to hypothesize that in the aggregate minority groups have heightened susceptibility to adverse health effects, including the effects of workplace and environmental exposures.

(e) Artifacts of Clinical Testing

Finally, minority groups may differ from whites in their clinical test norms, creating the appearance of racial differences in particular health outcomes following exposures. The best recognized example is pulmonary function testing; for a given height, age, and gender, blacks have lower lung volumes compared to whites. Another example is the white blood cell count, which is lower among blacks than among whites. Hence, a study of laboratory workers in a petrochemical plant showed no effect of exposure on the white blood cell count, but black workers had significantly lower counts than white workers. Such results may reflect disproportionate exposure or susceptibility, but they may simply reflect different laboratory norms. Therefore, clinical data must be carefully evaluated with attention to possible racial differences in test norms.

(4) Inferior Health Care for Occupational/Environmental Injuries/Illnesses

A final source of increased risk for members of minority groups is inferior medical care. Tertiary prevention consists of limiting morbidity, disability, and mortality caused by illnesses or injuries, usually through medical care and/or rehabilitation. When services available to members of minority groups are deficient, tertiary prevention cannot be optimally achieved.

The inferior health care available to minority communities is well documented. In general, members of minority groups are less likely to have health insuranc, less likely to have a regular source of medical care, less likely to have received cancer screening, and more likely to present with more advanced disease. Once under treatment, they are less likely to receive a wide range of services, including cardiovascular interventions, renal transplants, aggressive colon cancer treatment, asthma care intensive care for severe pneumonia, appropriate human immunodeficiency virus (HIV) treatment, and others. When the need arises, minority patients are less likely to gain access to long-term care. These inequities are reflected in a recurring pattern of black-white mortality differences that exceed black-white incidence differences for most major diseases. Members of minority groups receive less medical care, and die earlier and more often of their diseases, than do whites.

3. Migrant and Seasonal Farmworkers

Harsh social, economic, and political conditions combine to make migrant and seasonal farm workers - predominantly people of color - arguably the most at-risk of American workers. These same factors render the traditional analyses of occupational health status made adequate to the task of describing the impact of hazardous working conditions on the health of farm workers. Discriminatory partial or total exclusions of migrant and seasonal farm workers from labor and health and safety protections mean that their illnesses and injuries are undercounted in government databases such as workers' compensation data or Occupational Safety and Health Administration (OSHA) 2000 logs. In the case of pesticide poisoning, there is no national reporting system to document the extent of the problem or to monitor rends in response to statutory or regulatory changes.

Over the last decade, agriculture has ranked consistently among the three most hazardous U.S. industries. In 1994, agricultural workers ranked second in the rate of work-related fatalities and third in the rate of disabling injuries. Although agriculture accounts for less than 3 percent of the total workforce, it accounted for 18 percent of workplace fatalities that year. In 1994 the death rate in agriculture was 26 per 100,000 workers, 6.5 times greater than the national rate across 11 industries (4 per 100,000), and a 7 percent increase over 1993. In comparison, the worker mortality rate in mining was 27 per 100,000 workers and 15 per 100,000 in construction. The disabling injury rate a 1994 for farm workers was 41 per 1,000, behind the 48 per 1,000 for construction workers and 43 per 1,000 for transportation and public utilities workers, respectively, and almost 1.5 times the rate of 29 per 1,000 for all industries combined. In addition to safety hazards, poor sanitation, infectious agents, pesticides, and excessive heat jeopardize the health of farm workers. Economic necessity for migrant families dictates that children often must work and play in the fields alongside their parents, exposed to an array of potentially life-threatening health and safety hazards such as farm machinery and toxic chemicals.

a. Demographic Profile

The U.S. farm labor system is characterized both nationally and regionally by an oversupply of workers. Thus, migrant and seasonal farm workers face both unemployment and underemployment. Agricultural labor demand is structured into short-term work opportunities, with over half of farm jobs lasting fewer than 13 weeks (one quarter). The extensive use of temporary jobs is largely due to deliberate labor management decisions. Politically, the industry supports expanding the supply of temporary foreign guest workers, which replaces domestic workers with a compliant workforce subject to deportation at the employer's will. The chronic oversupply of farm workers has led to a pattern of replacement of one group by another. Farm workers cannot achieve and maintain improved pay and working conditions while employers and intermediaries can recruit newly arrived immigrants willing to work for less. Workers without legal work authorization (about 10 percent of the overall farm work force and nearly one-fourth of migrants) are the most vulnerable to employment abuses and the lowest wages.

By virtue of their mobility, geographic and linguistic isolation, seasonal employment, and, for a segment of the labor force, their undocumented status, migrant and seasonal farm workers defy accurate census and demographic description. Enumeration difficulties are compounded by definitional differences among government agencies, e.g., whether nonmigratory seasonal workers, undocumented foreign workers, and accompanying dependents are included in counts. Generally, seasonal farm workers are distinguished from migrants in that the former live and harvest crops in their own communities, whereas the latter travel various distances to find employment. Because many workers shift back and forth between seasonal and migrant status, depending on political, economic, weather, and other conditions, this distinction becomes artificial. The inability to count accurately the farm worker population is significant because underestimations translate into reduced funding for desperately needed health, education, legal, and other service programs targeted to these groups.

b. U.S. Agricultural Production

Increasing consolidation and mechanization, along with intensive chemical usage, have characterized U.S. agricultural production over the last 50 years. While the average fruit, vegetable, and horticultural specialty (FVH) farm is small in comparison with other farms in the United States, intensive production means that profits are more likely to be higher. Corporations control a higher percentage of the land in the FVH sector and account for most of the value of agricultural products sold. The FVH sector is the most labor-intensive, with labor accounting for over 25 percent of total farm expenses, compared to 11.5 percent for all of agriculture. Over 50 percent of hired farm-workers on farms employing more than 10 workers are located in California and Florida, two states with a predominance of high-value, labor-intensive crops. In California, there are approximately 18 farm-workers for every farmer, and over 80 percent of farm work is performed by hired labor. FVH farm workers - male and female alike - work in a variety of settings, including orchards, vineyards, vegetable farms, nurseries, greenhouses, mushroom sheds, and packinghouses. Workers perform a variety of tasks such as picking, cutting, hoeing, thinning, pruning, weeding, sorting, grading, wrapping, packing, potting and tending ornamental plants, laying and moving irrigation pipes, operating farm machinery, and mixing and applying pesticides.

c. General Health Status

Serious deficiencies in sanitation, housing, education, nutrition, and access to health care operating synergistically with hazardous occupational exposures, notably to pesticides and communicable diseases, create a bleak health status picture for the farm worker population. A study of farm worker medical encounters in migrant health centers in Texas, Indiana, and Michigan concluded that migrant farm workers have different and more complex health problems from those of the general population. Migrant farm workers suffered more frequently from infectious diseases than the general population and had more clinic visits for diabetes, medical supervision of infants and children, otitis media, pregnancy, hypertension, and contact dermatitis and eczema. Almost half (44 percent) of all farm workers who visited migrant health clinics had more than one illness. The patterns of significant comorbidity indicate the potential for substantial disability in this population.

d. Farmworker Women's Health

Farm worker women total more than one-quarter of the hired agricultural work force. In recent years, farm worker women have formally organized around issues of family, community, and personal health and are collaborating with researchers, clinicians, and advocates on a range of issues and projects, including prevention of domestic violence, acquired immunodeficiency syndrome (AIDS), and mental health problems such as depression and substance abuse; the promotion of maternal-child health; prevention of pesticide poisonings; and the development of public policy to protect farm workers.

AIDS is now growing more rapidly in rural than urban areas, and the fastest increase in new cases is among women and children of color. Human immunodeficiency virus (HIV) infection has been increasing dramatically among Hispanic and African American women in the United States, two groups to which the majority of farm worker women belong. Studies show that the rate of HIV infection between migrant and seasonal farm workers may be as much as 10 times the national rate.

e. Work-Related Health Problems

Agricultural health and safety was given a boost in 1990 when Congress granted monies to the National Institute for Occupaonal Safety and Health (NIOSH) for a national agricultural program. Part of this initiative included establishment of six NIOSH regional enters (in California, Colorado, Iowa, Wisconsin, Kentucky, and New York) for agricultural research, education, and disease and injury prevention. More recently, NIOSH centers have been added in Texas and Washington state. Information about the work of all centers is accessible through the Internet. During the first 5 years of funding, these centers predominantly focused on studying the health and safety of farm owner/operators and their families. In 1995 NIOSH convened an ad hoc advisory committee of migrant health clinicians, farm workers, researchers, and policymakers to identify priorities for farm worker surveillance and research. The group ranked ergonomic/musculoskeletal conditions, pesticides, and traumatic injuries as the three most important subjects for both surveillance and search.

(1) Pesticide-Related Illnesses

The primary route of farm worker exposure to most pesticides is through dermal absorption. Inhalation and ingestion are secondary avenues of exposure. Fieldworkers who cultivate and harvest crops are exposed to pesticide residues on foliage, on the crops themselves, odin the dusty soil and decaying organic material that collects in the fields. Aerial and ground pesticide application exposes workers rough direct spray and through drift of pesticides sprayed on adjacent fields.

Deficiencies in sanitation in the fields and in nearby labor camps exacerbate pesticide exposures. Pesticide residues contaminate irrigation water that may be used for drinking, cooking, and bathing. The increasing use of fumigation, putting pesticides in the irrigation water, underscores this problem. The lack of adequate toilet and hand washing facilities in the fields means that workers may eat and smoke with pesticide-contaminated hands, use pesticide-contaminated leaves or twigs as a substitute for toilet paper, and contaminate the genitals even after elimination because they are unable to wash their hands. Even when children do not accompany their parents to the fields, they can be exposed to pesticide residues via contact with contaminated work clothes.

(2) Effects of Inadequate Sanitation

The basic public health principle that poor sanitation increases the prevalence of disease has been well understood and universally accepted for over 100 years. Nevertheless, U.S. migrant and seasonal farm workers have lived and worked under conditions analogous to those faced by third world populations.

(3) Dermatitis

Dermatitis has increased in agriculture and may contribute significantly to workplace morbidity, although it is rarely a cause of death. Farm workers face nearly four times the risk of developing skin disease as workers in other industries. Occupational skin disease accounts for 30 percent of all occupational illnesses nationwide but approximately 70 percent of occupational illnesses in agriculture in California. Pesticides and allergenic plants and crops are the primary culprits. Their effects are exacerbated by constant exposure to the sun, sweat, chapped or abraded skin, and the lack of appropriate protective gear and adequate hand washing facilities. Patch testing generally is necessary to determine whether a rash is chemical-or plant-related. Most pesticide-related skin problems are primary irritant, or contact, dermatitis. Pesticides also can be sensitizers, causing allergic dermatitis. Some workers can be permanently disabled because they cannot tolerate exposure even to minute amounts of pesticides. Sunlight can aggravate the dermatitis, adding to the disability, even leading to convulsions and comas.

(4) Musculoskeletal Problems

Farm workers face many of the hazards traditionally associated with musculoskeletal problems, including forceful exertions such as lifting, carrying, and hoisting heavy loads overhead; fast-paced, repetitive work; and awkward positions such as stooping, bending, twisting, and leaning over. Redesign of tools or work processes, changes in crop production, regulatory actions, and worker and employer education are some methods to address these problems. For example, the short-handled hoe, el cortito, requires the worker to labor in a doubled-over position and is linked with development of back strain and other ailments. The ban on its use in California was associated with a 34 percent decrease in the rate of sprain and strain injuries among relevant California farm workers. No national ban on its use has been issued. In 1995 OSHA held a series of stakeholder meetings with employer and worker representatives before publishing a proposed ergonomic standard to cover all industries. Intense employer opposition forced OSHA to halt the rulemaking process.

(5) Injuries

Farm workers suffer a wide variety of injuries, including acute pesticide poisonings, fractures in falls from ladders, strains from heavy lifting, eye injuries from chemicals and debris ejected by machinery, cuts and lacerations from knives and machetes, and a host of crush, contusion, fracture, and amputation injuries associated with heavy equipment use. Piece work, heat stress, the effects of mild pesticide exposure, long hours, and awkward work positions contribute to the risk of injury. Farm workers are also at high risk for work-related transportation deaths and injuries because they are often transported by farm labor contractors from central locations to the fields in substandard buses, vans, or pick-up trucks. In 1990, 41 percent of Florida farm worker deaths were transportation-related. Often large distances separate the fields from the nearest health care facility and frustrate the receipt of prompt and appropriate treatment. Lack of health insurance and exclusion from coverage under the state's workers' compensation system contributed to delayed or no care for 65 percent of injured North Carolina migrant farm-workers, including those with more serious injuries. Employers covered medical expenses for only 38 percent of injured workers, and only 20 percent were compensated for lost work. Washington state workers' compensation data showed that farm work accounted for half of the total number of severe or disabling injuries among claims filed by children under 14 and those aged 14 or 15. Researchers noted that these findings indicated underreporting because only those injuries or illnesses that resulted in the filing of a claim were counted.

4. Women Workers

About 70 percent of American women are in the paid labor force. Although, overall, women's employment has a positive effect on their health and employed women live longer than unemployed women and housewives, risk factors present in some jobs may adversely affect women's health. Action to improve women's occupational health has been slowed by a notion that women's jobs are safe and that any health problems identified among women workers can be attributed unfitness for the job, hormonal factors, or unnecessary complaining. However, the rise in the number of women in the labor force has sensitized public health practitioners, workers, and scientists to the necessity to include women's concerns in their occupational health activities.

Although it is too soon to speak of convergence of research directions, certain occupational groups have excited the interest of searchers: factory workers in repetitive tasks, hospital workers, and solvent-exposed workers. Particular industries (clothing manufacturing, food-processing) have received attention because health problems have been identified and/or because they employ a large number of women (health care). Methodological questions are emerging: how to analyze data by gender; how to take into account the different age patterns of women and men; and how to identify health problems that arise in women's traditional work and for which strategies may have been developed. Related social issues arise and must also be dealt with: how to ensure that recognition of health hazards in women's work does not lead to denial of employment opportunities for women; whether men and women should be distributed in a more random way across employment categories or if each gender is more suited to a specific type of work.

Despite considerable progress in integrating women into the work force, women are still found in specific jobs where employment conditions are relatively unfavorable. This sexual division of labor affects women's health in six ways:

a. Women's jobs have specific characteristics (repetition, monotony, static effort, multiple   simultaneous responsibilities), which may lead over time to deleterious effects on physical and mental health;

b. Spaces, equipment, and schedules designed in relation to the average male body and lifestyle may cause problems for women;

c. Segregation may cause health isks for women and men by causing task fragmentation and thus inreasing repetition and monotony;

d. Sex-based job assignments may appear to protect the health of both sexes and thus distract from more effective occupational health promotion practices;

e. Discrimination against women is stressful in and of itself and may affect mental health; and

f. Part-time workers are excluded from many health promoting benefits such as adequate sick leave and maternity leave.

a. Gender Implications of Pathology-Based Approaches

Occupational health researchers trained in medicine have often limited their interest to pathologies rather than to indicators, signs, or symptoms of deterioration in physical or mental states, reasoning that the presence of pathology guarantees that the problem examined is worthy of serious consideration. However, a requirement for diagnosed pathology may be premature when studying women's occupational health. Since the aggressors present in women's traditional work have been understudied, and the effects of even well known conditions on women workers are often unknown, identification of occupational disease in women's work is embryonic. For example, women who handle money report unusual-looking and painful red streaks on their hands. A literature search revealed one article on nickel allergy among cashiers, but no other reference to skin disease among those handling money. It may be years before sufficient research enables us to decide whether to define it as an industrial disease.

b. Women's Occupational Health Problems

Women's most common health problems are musculoskeletal problems, skin problems, and hypertension. Women are also more likely than men to be hospitalized for mental disorders. Some of these differences can be attributed to specific jobs. One approach has been to examine health problems reported by women according to the sector of the economy where they work. Although the employment sector is a poor indicator of job content, this type of gross analysis does suggest a need to study women's jobs. Musculoskeletal problems emerge as a specific risk associated with sales, restaurant, and cleaning work. Psychological distress is found among those in sales, restaurant work, and teaching. Allergies and skin conditions are common in white collar work, especially teaching, and also in personal services such as hairdressing. Heart disease is found among cleaners, personal service workers, saleswomen, and managers.

(1) Musculoskeletal Disorders

The major research area in women's occupational health is probably musculoskeletal problems, the majority of cases of compensated occupational diseases. Although women live longer than men, women and men in many countries can expect to live a similar number of years in good health. Put differently, women spend about twice as long as men being disabled. One cause of disability is muscle and joint problems, more often found among women. Women are twice as likely as men to have chronic backache.

(2) Health Effects of Stress

Any discussion with women (and often men) workers tends to identify "stress" as an important occupational health problem. We can ask whether women "really" have more such problems, but it is undeniable that women consult more health practitioners and take more medication for mental problems than men. Women service workers were particularly likely to experience stress. Secretaries have also been identified by the

National Institute for Occupational Safety and Health (NIOSH) as a group particularly prone to stress).

(3) Occupational Cancers

Women have been traditionally excluded from studies on occupational cancer, either to keep samples uniform or because data on their professional exposures is lacking. Recently, women have been increasingly included in studies, and risks are becoming apparent, for example, among cleaners, hairdressers, and health care workers. Exposures to industrial chemicals such as solvents and metals are associated with breast cancer.

5. Health Hazards of Child Labor

Child labor is defined in the United States as the paid employment of children younger than 18 years of age. According to data from the U.S. department of labor, more than 4 million American children were legally employed in 1988, a substantial increase from a decade earlier. Illegal child labor is also widespread, and at least 1 million children are employed under unlawful and often exploitative conditions. Despite the common belief that the problem of illegal child labor was remedied long ago, the practice has in fact persisted in the United States and appears to be on the rise.

Child labor is also a major problem internationally. According to the International Labour Office (ILO), at least 200 million children under age 14 are employed worldwide. In some countries, children constitute 15 to 25 percent of the total workforce. Children are employed as rug weavers in the Middle East, as underground tin miners in South America, and as metal workers, fireworks makers, textile weavers, and glass blowers.

Child labor is associated in virtually all countries, industrialized and developing, with poverty, high unemployment, inadequate educational opportunities, and failure to enforce relevant laws and standards. Particularly severe abuses have been documented in so-called free enterprise zones, special industrial areas that have been established in many countries, such as along the Mexico-United States border, where relaxation has been permitted in the enforcement of labor and environmental laws.

a. Resurgence of Child Labor in the United States

A series of economic and social factors similar to those that produced the major increases in child labor at the beginning of the Industrial Revolution has produced the current resurgence of child labor:

(1) **Increased poverty**: More American children live in poverty today than 20 years ago, and the number below the poverty line increased especially rapidly during the 1980s. For the 20 percent of American children who live in poverty, financial need constitutes a compelling reason to seek employment.

(2) **Unstable world conditions**, particularly war and poverty in Central America, the Caribbean, and Southeast Asia, have led increasing numbers of immigrants, both legal and undocumented, to enter the United States. These immigrants, particularly children without parents, are highly vulnerable to exploitation in the workplace. Their vulnerability is compounded by their lack of access to health care.

(3) **Relaxation** since 1981 in enforcement of federal child labor law, including relaxation of provisions limiting maximum permissible hours of work and prohibiting use of dangerous machinery.

b. Children's Vulnerability to Toxins in the Workplace

Children are uniquely vulnerable to toxins encountered in the workplace. This heightened susceptibility stems from several sources:

(1) Children have greater exposures to toxins than do adults. Pound for pound of body weight, children drink more water, eat more food, and breathe more air. In consequence, children have substantially heavier exposures pound for pound than adults to any toxins that are present in water, food, or air.
(2) Children's metabolic pathways are immature compared with those of adults. Children are less able than adults to detoxify and excrete most toxic chemicals and thus are more vulnerable to them.
(3) Children are undergoing rapid growth and development, and their delicate developmental processes are easily disrupted. Many organ systems in young children - the nervous system in particular - undergo very rapid growth and development in childhood. If cells in the developing brain are destroyed by chemicals encountered in the workplace such as lead, mercury, pesticides, or solvents, or if vital connections between nerve cells fail to form, there is high risk that the resulting neurobehavioral dysfunction will be permanent and irreversible.
(4) Because children have more future years of life than do most adults, they have more time to develop any chronic diseases that may be triggered by early environmental exposures.

c. Risks of Child Labor

(1) Health Risk

Work is a major, but insufficiently recognized, contributor to the continuing epidemic of childhood injury in the United States. The number of American adolescents killed each year in work-related injuries (110) is comparable to the number killed in falls (103), in fires (126), on bicycles (129), by poisoning (191), and by unintentional firearms injuries (266).

(2) Toxic Hazards and Chronic Illness

Little information is available on the incidence or severity of work-related illness caused in children by toxic occupational exposures. Children are, however, known to experience a variety of toxic exposures at work. These include formaldehyde and dyes in the garment industry, solvents in paint shops, pesticides in agriculture plant nursery work and lawn care, asbestos in building demolition, and benzene in pumping unleaded gasoline. It appears likely that some still undefined fraction of adolescent asthma might be related to occupational exposures to dusts or formaldehyde, that some cases of neurotoxicity and developmental impairment may be caused by occupational exposure to solvents or pesticides, or that some cases of leukemia and lymphoma in children and adolescents may be the consequence of occupational exposure to benzene.

(3) Health Risks of Agricultural Child Labor

Agriculture is the least regulated and consequently the most dangerous sector of industry for American children. Rural children are employed extensively in agriculture, both on family farms and in commercial farming operations. The hazards to health associated with agricultural work include lacerations, amputations, and crush injuries from farm machinery; blunt trauma from large animals; motor vehicle accidents involving farm vehicles on public roads; suffocation in grain elevators and silos; and exposures to pesticides, fertilizers, and solvents. Small physical size and inexperience may superimpose additional risk for young workers.

(4) Risks to Education and Development

Interference with school performance is another serious consequence of child labor. Working children risk having too little time for their school homework and being overtired on school days. Teachers in areas where employment of children is common or industrial homework is escalating have reported declines in the academic performance of previously successful students. These children are described as falling asleep at their desks, and they are unable to learn. Even if they maintain their academic standing, working children are able to participate less than their peers in after-school activities and sports. Child labor also interferes with play, which is important for children's normal development; relaxation and freedom from fatigue are necessary for children to grow and learn.

6. Workers in the Global Economy

The increasing integration and globalization of the world economy has been widely noted and debated. In the occupational safety and health field, these global trends refocus attention on a long-recognized fact: workers in developing nations face more dangerous conditions, and enjoy fewer protections, than workers in wealthier nations.

The term "**developing countries**" is used to include the poorer nations of the world. These include most of the nations of Latin America and the Caribbean, Africa, Asia, and Oceania, often grouped under the term "**third world**" or, more recently, "**the South**." Also included are the transitional economies of the former Soviet block in central and Eastern Europe. Some countries, such as the "Asian tigers" (Singapore, South Korea, Taiwan, and Hong Kong), Mexico, and Brazil were "developing" a generation ago and have since made rapid strides toward industrialization, but many of the trends discussed here continue to apply to these countries as well. The common features are relatively low economic indicators such as gross domestic product and per capita income; relatively low per capita consumption of energy and goods, and relatively undeveloped infrastructures. Many developing countries also have limited traditions of democracy and labor rights.

Economic integration has increased rapidly in recent years, due to advances on electronic telecommunication and communication, liberalization of banking and trade laws, and changes in investment practices. This process has manifested itself in several ways that have a direct impact on occupational health: the growth of multinational companies, the development of free trade zones, and the promulgation of multilateral free trade agreements.

a. Multinational Companies

Multinational companies have increased in size, wealth, and international reach over recent decades. The 200 largest corporations now account for more than a quarter of the world's economic activity, with combined sales that exceed the combined gross domestic product of all countries except the "big nine" (the United States, Japan, Germany, France, Italy, the United Kingdom, Brazil, Canada, and China). The trend toward consolidation of economic activity is continuing; in 1982, the top 200 firms accounted for 24.2 percent of global GDP, and by 1996 this figure had increased to 28.3 percent.

b. Free Trade Agreements

Multilateral free trade agreements have developed throughout the world during the second half of the twentieth century. These agreements aim to facilitate international trade by lowering and in some cases removing trade barriers. Increasingly, free trade agreements define the rules of international commerce. To the extent that these agreements incorporate related social issues such as working conditions, they may help advance occupational safety and health. On the other hand, trade agreements that ignore labor standards may have a negative impact. Several major free trade agreements serve trade as important examples.

The General Agreement on Tariffs and Trade (GATT) arose in the years after World War II as a global attempt to regulate trade and limit trade barriers. It has evolved over the last 50 years through a series of eight renegotiation "rounds". The Uruguay Round (1986 to 1993) created a successor organization to GATT, the World Trade Organization (WTO), which broadened its scope from trade in goods to include trade in services and intellectual property as well. GATT and the WTO have been generally silent on issues of worker safety and health, restricting their domain to problems that bear directly on trade. Article XX (b) of GATT authorized nations to enact legislation that is "necessary to protect human, animal or plant life or health," but this clause was never used to support trade challenges based on worker health issues. During the Tokyo Round of negotiations, which began in 1978, Sweden proposed adding a social clause to GATT, which would have acknowledged "the freedom of association, trade union rights, [and] adequate health and safety precautions, social standards and social welfare schemes." However, objections from the United States and certain developing nations blocked the adoption of this clause.

c. Export of Hazards and the Race to the Bottom

Scholars, public health practitioners, and labor advocates have for some years recognized that increasing international trade might threaten worker health and safety. In the 1980s, considerable attention was devoted to the "export of hazard". Concern grew out of observations of double standards; 26 industries from developed nations would relocate plants in developing nations due to lower labor costs, more lax regulatory environments, and in some cases, proximity to raw materials and/or markets. In doing so they would fail to follow the same standards of workplace safety and health that were required in their countries of origin, exposing workers in developing nations to relatively greater risks. Case studies of products such as asbestos, pesticides and hazardous wastes and high-profile disasters such as the Bhopal explosion and the observations of professionals from developed nations who visited and worked with colleagues in developing nations all fed concern that workers in developing nations faced serious risks from rapid industrialization.

7. Special Problems of Occupational Health and Safety In Developing Countries

Occupational safety and health faces a range of challenges in developing countries. These can be divided into several categories: **working conditions, the social organization of work, the workforce, and human resources.**

Working conditions in developing nations may present special hazards to workers. The tropical climate that often prevails poses risks of heat exhaustion and heat stroke, especially in hot facilities such as textile plants. The workweek is often well in excess of 40 hours, so exposures to chemical and physical hazards, even if regulated to an intensity considered safe in industrialized nations, may exceed anticipated levels because of duration. Much of the production machinery used in developing nations is imported, sometimes after it is deemed obsolete for use in developed nations. As such the machinery may be old and dangerous, and modifications, replacement parts, and technical backup difficult or unavailable. Moreover, alternatives such as safer machinery may be unavailable or prohibitively expensive on local markets.

The **social organization of work** may also contribute to workplace hazards. In many developing nations, the predominant employment setting is the small firm. These firms have even less access to safe technologies than their larger counterparts and tend to he riskier. In fact, large portions of the workforce in developing countries may work in the informal sector, which consists of smaller, often family-based production units, remote from registration and other government controls and from occupational safety and health services. Moreover, many developing countries lack a significant independent labor movement and a tradition of labor rights, without which one of the major forces for occupational safety and health is absent.

Developing nations also face important occupational safety and health challenges related to the **workforce**. Low literacy rates are an obstacle to effective worker training and risk communication. Workers may be especially susceptible to the effects of workplace hazards due to relative nutritional deficiencies. In Islamic countries, workers who fast during Ramadan may be at increased risk of dehydration while working at hot jobs. Biological features of the workforce may increase susceptibility to various hazards. For example, Asian workers on average have a smaller stature than the European and North American workers for whom much industrial machinery was designed, which may lead to ergonomic risks. African workers have a high prevalence of glucose-6-phosphate dehydrogenase deficiency, which increases susceptibility to certain oxidizing chemicals, and Asian workers have a high prevalence of hepatitis B antigenemia, which may increase susceptibility to hepatotoxins. Endemic parasitic disease in some settings reduces work capacity and immunocompetence and increases susceptibility to a range of diseases. Many of these workforce features can be addressed through modification of jobs.

Finally, developing nations face severe **shortages of trained personnel** essential to occupational safety and health practice. Adequately trained industrial hygienists and safety professionals, who would be able to recognize, assess, and control hazards in the workplace, are scarce. Epidemiologists with skills in surveillance, who would be able to monitor disease and injury trends and identify problem areas, are also scarce. Finally, health care providers such as occupational physicians and nurses are scarce, preventing adequate diagnosis and treatment of work-related illnesses and injuries.

VI. <u>BIBLIOGRAPHY</u>

Beck, C., & Krieger G.R. (1992). Hazard Communications and Material Safety Data Sheets. In J.B. Sullivan, & G.R. Krieger (Ed.), <u>Hazardous Material Toxicology: Clinical Principles of Environmental Health</u> (pp. 239-253). Baltimore, MD: Williams & Wilkins.

Davis, T.G. (1997). Environmental Safety. In M. Morgan (Ed), <u>Environmental Health 2nd Edition</u> (pp.199-215). Englewood, CO: Morton Publishing Company.

Fein, L.J. (1998). Surveillance, Monitoring, and Screening in Occupational Health. In R.B. Wallace (Ed.), <u>Public Health and Preventive Medicine 14th Edition</u> (pp.669-673). Stamford, CT: Appleton & Lange.

Frumkin, H. (1998). Workers in the Global Economy. In R.B. Wallace (Ed.), <u>Public Health and Preventive Medicine 14th Edition</u> (pp.698-707). Stamford, CT: Appleton & Lange.

Frumkin, H., & Walker, E.D., (1998). Minority Workers and Communities. In R.B. Wallace (Ed.), <u>Public Health and Preventive Medicine 14th Edition</u> (pp.682-688). Stamford, CT: Appleton & Lange.

Goldberg, M., & Nagin, D. (1999). Principles of Industrial Hygiene. In R. Bowler, & J. Cone. (Eds.), <u>Occupational Medicine Secrets</u> (pp. 21-27). Philadelphia, PA: Hanley & Belfus, Inc.

Grey, M.R. (1999). A Short History of Occupational Health in the United States . In R. Bowler, & J. Cone. (Eds.), <u>Occupational Medicine Secrets</u> (pp. 29-33). Philadelphia, PA: Hanley & Belfus, Inc.

Herrick, R. & Dement, J. (1994). Industrial Hygiene. In L. Rosenstock, & M. Cullen (Eds), <u>Textbook of Clinical Occupational and Environmental Medicine</u> (pp. 169-193). Philadelphia, PA: W.B. Saunders Company.

Landrigan, P.J., Pollack, S.H., Belville, R., & Godbold, J. (1998). Health Hazards of Child Labor. In R.B. Wallace (Ed.), <u>Public Health and Preventive Medicine 14th Edition</u> (pp.697-698). Stamford, CT: Appleton & Lange.

McCunney, J.M. (1994). Industrial Hygiene. In R. McCunney (Ed.), <u>A practical Approach to Occupational and Environmental Medicine, 2nd Edition</u> (pp. 321-332). Boston, MA: Little, Brown and Company.

McMichael, A.J., Kjellstrom,T., & Smith, K.R. (2001). In M. Merson, R. Black, & A. Mills (Eds). <u>International Public Health Diseases, Program Systems, and Policies</u> (pp. 407-413). Gaitherburg, MD: Aspen Publishers, Inc.

Messing, K. (1998). Women Workers. In R.B. Wallace (Ed.), <u>Public Health and Preventive Medicine 14th Edition </u>(pp.693-696). Stamford, CT: Appleton & Lange.

Moeller,   D.W. (1997). The Workplace.   <u>Environmental Health</u> (pp. 52-76). Cambridge, MA, and London, UK: Harvard University Press.

Mudrick, N.R., Weber, R.J., & Turk, M.A. (1998). Workers with Disabilities. In R.B. Wallace (Ed.), <u>Public Health and Preventive Medicine 14th Edition </u>(pp.675-682). Stamford, CT: Appleton & Lange.

Pearson, R., & Morgan, S.L. (1997). Occupational Health. In M. Morgan (Ed), <u>Environmental Health 2nd Edition</u> (pp. 233-256). Englewood, CO: Morton Publishing Company.

Perkins J. L. (1997). Industrial Hygiene-Historical Perspective. In <u>Modern Industrial Hygiene: recognition and evaluation of chemical agents</u> (pp. 11-45). New York, NY: Van Nostrand Reinhold.

Plog, B.A. (1996). Overview of Industrial Hygiene . In B.A. Plog, J. Niland, & P.J. Quinlan (Eds.), <u>Fundamentals of Industrial Hygiene</u> (pp. 9-10). Itasca, IL: National Safety Council.

Rose, V.E. (1997). History and Philosophy of Industrial Hygiene. In S.R. Dinardi (Ed.), <u>The Occupational Environment: Its Evaluation and Control</u> (pp. 13-14). Fairfax, VA: AIHA press.

Wilk, V.A. (1998). Migrant and Seasonal Workers. In R.B. Wallace (Ed.), <u>Public Health and Preventive Medicine, 14th Edition </u>(pp.688-693). Stamford, CT: Appleton & Lange.

Yassi, A., Kjellström, T., de Kok, T., & Guidotti, T. L. (2001). Industrial Pollution and Chemical Safety: Hazards by Industry. In A. Yassi, [et al](Eds.), <u>Basic Environmental Health</u> (pp. 340-344). New York, NY: Oxford University Press, Inc.

SECTION

IV

ASSESSMENT AND MONITORING METHODOLOGIES

CHAPTER

15

RISK ASSESSMENT

I. INTRODUCTION

A. RISK CHARACTERISTICS

Risk has several defining characteristics. The two characteristics that most embody risk are uncertainty and the unknown. Risk can be defined as the likelihood of an unwanted occurrence coupled with an element of uncertainty about when the risk might occur. Many other definitions of risk exist, all varying slightly, but focused on the concepts of uncertainty and the unknown. Other risk characteristics may include dread, voluntary or involuntary, immediacy or latency, catastrophic potential, threat to future generations and unknown to the exposed. Risk often encompasses the ideas of morbidity and mortality, that is, the possibility of sickness or death. Certain risk characteristics, such as involuntary, unknown and dread, generate greater fear in people than risks that are known or voluntary. As many environmental risks have the characteristics of unknown and dread, they cause people anxiety and concern about the consequences of exposure to the risk. Risk analysis is one method to address this fear and anxiety, through developing knowledge about a risk, understanding its potential health effects and devising methods to limit and manage the risk.

B. DEVELOPMENT OF RISK ANALYSIS

Risk analysis is the process of reviewing information on a hazard to characterize that hazard's impact on human health. This process involves a review of scientific studies, an understanding of the properties of a risk, an assessment of levels of human exposure and dose, and a conclusion about the likelihood, impact and extent of a risk. By employing these methods, risk analysis allows researchers to develop conclusions on the severity and consequences of environmental risks. Risk analysis developed over the past thirty years out of a need to understand modern, technologically based risks. It began with an increased interest in the environment, from the government, scientific and public sectors. Rachel Carson's 1962 book **Silent Spring** spurred concern about environmental issues, specifically pesticide use. Environmental crises such as Love Canal, Three Mile Island, and the chemical accidents in Seveso, Italy and Bhopal, India encouraged research into the effects of these environmental risks. The purpose was to assess the potential health impact of these hazards and to develop methods to cope with these risks.

The field of risk analysis developed as a response to several changes in the modern world. First, the number of risks society faces today has increased dramatically compared to times past. For example, over 100,000 synthetic chemicals are used today in industrial and manufacturing processes and in many consumer products and household items. Little detailed risk information is available for most of these substances. Second, technology has improved our ability to measure risk. Today, exposures are measured in the parts per million, billion, and even trillion, greatly increasing our capacity to accurately quantify exposure levels. Third, the number of government agencies directly or indirectly monitoring environmental risk have increased, such as the Food and Drug Administration, the Environmental Protection Agency and state-run Departments of Environmental Protection. Even towns and cities have agencies regulating local risks to public health. Fourth, the number of laws and regulations governing the environment, and protecting the public health, have increased dramatically over the past thirty years. Some of these laws drastically changed the management of risks and dissemination of information. The Superfund Amendments and Reauthorization Act of 1986 (SARA), also known as the Emergency Planning and Community Right-to- Know Act, ensured that communities were prepared for chemical emergencies and had access to information on chemicals at sites in the area. Other examples of regulations include the Food, Drug and Cosmetic Act, the Toxic Substances Control Act, and the Clean Water Act. Fifth, an increase in public interest in environmental risks has spurred research in quantifying risks. Special interest groups and grassroots movements have involved the public in environmental issues on both local and national levels.

A detailed qualitative and quantitative description of a risk can be created by gathering the relevant study information, considering the important factors, and developing a conclusion about the risk. Risk analysis has many applications across a variety of fields. This risk description can be used in decision-making and the development of environmental and public health policy. For instance, risk analysis can be used to estimate the likelihood of developing cancer from exposure to radiation, to determine the side effects of a medicine awaiting FDA-approval, to ascertain whether a synthetic food product, such as olestra® or saccharin®, is safe for human consumption, or if transgenically altered animals and plants pose a health risk. Risk analysis allows public groups to make informed decisions and weigh the risks and benefits in their community.

In a personal sense, risk can be defined as the probability that an individual will suffer injury, disease, or death under a specific set of circumstances. In terms of environmental health, the concept of risk must be expanded to include possible effects on other animals and plants, as well as on the environment itself. Knowing that a certain risk exists is not enough, however. People want to have some idea of how probable it is that they or their environment will suffer and, if they do, what the effects will be. Determination of the answers to these questions involves the science of risk assessment.

Risk assessment ranges from evaluation of the potential effects of toxic chemical releases known to be occurring, to evaluation of the potential effects of releases due to events whose probability of occurrence is uncertain. In the latter case, the risk is a combination of the likelihood that the event will occur and the likely consequences if it does. In essence, the process of risk assessment requires addressing three basic questions: What can go wrong? How likely is it? If it does happen, what are the consequences?

Once the risk has been assessed, it can be expressed in qualitative terms (such as "high," "low," or "trivial") or in quantitative terms, ranging in value from zero (certainty that harm will not occur) to one (certainty that harm will occur). At the same time, it must be recognized that a given risk assessment provides only a snapshot in time of the estimated risk of a given toxic agent at a particular phase of our understanding of the issues and problems. To be truly instructive and constructive, risk assessment should always be conducted on an iterative basis, being updated as new knowledge and information become available.

Once a risk has been quantified, the next step is to decide whether that risk is sufficiently high to represent a public health concern and, if so, to determine the appropriate means for control. **Risk management** may involve measures to prevent the occurrence of an event as well as appropriate remedial (protective or mitigative) actions to protect the public and/or the environment in case the event does occur. Each of these steps is accompanied by a multitude of related uncertainties. In fact, as many uncertainties are involved in deciding how to use risk assessment to make regulatory decisions as in conducting the risk assessments themselves.

A potential toxicant that may be present in air, water, food, and soil has to be defined first before undertaking any risk assessment. "Toxicant" refers to any synthetic or natural chemical that can produce adverse health effects. Several federal agencies evaluate potential health effects and establish standards of exposure. Each agency uses a variation of a methodology generally referred to as risk assessment. This process includes:

1. Characterization of the types of health effects expected
2. Characterization of exposure
3. Evaluation of experimental studies (animal and/or epidemiological)
4. Characterization of the relationship between dose and response
5. Estimation of the risk (synonyms: probability, frequency) of occurrence of health effects
6. Estimation of the number of cases expected
7. Characterization of the uncertainty of the analysis
8. Recommendation of an acceptable concentration in air, food, or water

Risk assessments are necessary for informed regulatory decisions regarding the following:

1. Worker exposures
2. Industrial emissions and effluents
3. Chemical residues in foods
4. Ambient air and water contaminants
5. Cleanup of hazardous waste sites
6. Naturally occurring contaminants

It is important to encourage diversity of risk assessment methodology. This helps to ensure that all possible risk models and outcomes have been considered and minimizes the potential for error. By the late 1980s, federal agencies had created their own standardized risk assessment methodologies. The "standardization" of the risk assessment process is almost a contradiction in terms. Each scenario of exposure has unique characteristics, which makes the application of a uniform methodology problematic. In 1990, the Environmental Protection Agency (EPA) announced that only the EPA's risk assessments were to have regulatory standing regarding the management of Superfund sites. Risk assessments are used to determine appropriate cleanup techniques and acceptable levels of residual contamination. Critics labeled EPA as having become arrogant in the area of risk assessment. This type of regulatory approach leads to isolation, mistakes, and stagnation. The process of risk assessment can only benefit from the contributions of many disciplines and viewpoints.

Risk assessment and risk management are an integral part of the contemporary regulatory scene. Risk management refers to the selection and implementation of the most appropriate regulatory action based on the following:

1. Goals
2. Social and political factors
3. Available control technology
4. Costs and benefits
5. Results of risk assessment
6. Acceptable risk
7. Acceptable number of cases

The major impetus for conducting risk assessments comes from federal legislation. Major federal health and safety statutes have included a directive to control public health risks, e.g.:

1. Food, Drug, and Cosmetic Act (1938)
2. Federal Insecticide, Fungicide, and Rodenticide Act (1947)
3. Clean Air Act (1970)
4. Occupational Safety and Health Act (1970)
5. Consumer Product Safety Act (1972)
6. Clean Water Act (1972)
7. Resource Conservation and Recovery Act (1976)
8. Safe Drinking Water Act (1976)
9. Toxic Substances Control Act (1976)
10. Comprehensive Environmental Response, Compensation, and Liability Act (1980)

None of these statutes and their many amendments defined what degree of public health risk was acceptable or unacceptable. The task of determining acceptable risk was essentially left up to the federal regulatory agencies. In the following discussion of acceptable risk, it is useful to note a type of reference risk: the U.S. lifetime risk at birth of dying of some type of cancer is 23/100. Lifetime risk refers to a risk that could manifest any time during the lifetime (as opposed to a risk at a certain age). Lifetime risk can be due to lifetime or less than lifetime exposure.

The Food and Drug Administration (FDA) was the first government agency to use risk assessment to make regulatory decisions. In 1973, it proposed a method for the regulation of carcinogenic drugs used in food-producing animals. A log-normal tolerance distribution risk assessment method was proposed along with an acceptable lifetime risk of 10^{-8}. Later, a linear interpolation type of risk assessment method was adopted and the acceptable lifetime risk was increased to 10^{-6}.

The EPA has been inconsistent in its definition of acceptable lifetime risk. In decisions regarding the regulation of carcinogenic air pollutants, the EPA has calculated the magnitude of individual risk and the number of excess cases generated per year in the exposed population. Risks in the range of 10^{-5} to 0.001 have been considered acceptable. These risks were associated with annual excess cases ranging from 0.006 to 0.08. In decisions regarding carcinogenic active ingredients in pesticides, risks ranging from 10^{-7}

to 0.02 were considered acceptable. Regarding enforcement of the Safe Drinking Act, the EPA goal for carcinogens is zero exposure. This goal implies that only zero risk is acceptable. Zero risk is very difficult to achieve. Regarding hazardous waste sites, EPA generally requires cleanup levels for carcinogens which are commensurate with a risk of $<10^{-6}$.

In setting permissible exposure limits (PELs) for carcinogens, the Occupational Safety and Health Administration (OSHA) is guided by a 1980 Supreme Court definition of significant risk. The Court found a risk of 1/1000 to be significant. Neither the Supreme Court nor OSHA have stated what they consider to be an insignificant (acceptable) occupational risk. In order to place a worker lifetime mortality risk of 1/1000 in perspective, it is necessary to review work-related death rates (mostly due to accidents) for various occupations. The average lifetime risk of a work-related death in the private sector is 2.9/1000. Assuming 45 years of employment in a particular industrial sector, lifetime mortality risks are presented in Table 15.1:

Table 15.1. Lifetime Mortality Risks among Different Occupations

TYPE OF OCCUPATION	RISK
Mining	19/1000
Construction	10/1000
Transportation and Public Utilities	8/1000
Agriculture	7/1000
Average (private sector)	2.9/1000
Manufacturing	2/1000
Services	2/1000
Wholesale and retail trade	1/1000
Finance, insurance, and real estate	1/1000

Since 1980, OSHA has revised several PELs. It appears that OSHA is exceeding the Supreme Court guideline for the definition of significant risk. The estimated lifetime cancer risks associated with these PELs are found in Table 15.2.:

Table 15.2. Estimated Lifetime Cancer Risks Associated with Selected Chemicals

CHEMICAL	RISK
Inorganic arsenic	8/1000
Ethylene oxide	1-2/1000
Ethylene dibromide	0.2-6/1000
Benzene	5-16/1000
Acrylonitrile	39/1000
Asbestos	6.7/1000

The International Commission on Radiological Protection (ICRP) recommends limits for radiation dose limits for workers and the general population. These limits are usually adopted by most nations, including the U.S. Nuclear Regulatory Commission. Assuming 45 years of employment in the nuclear industry, the ICRP recommended worker annual dose limit translates into a lifetime cancer mortality risk of 4/100. The general population annual dose limit translates into a lifetime cancer mortality risk of 4/1000 (assuming 70 years of exposure to the limit). In setting acceptable exposure standards, regulatory agencies (e.g., FDA, EPA, and OSHA) usually do not take into account additive or interactive effects from exposure to multiple toxicants. For example, if a worker is exposed to 10 carcinogens and each exposure conveys a risk of 10^{-3}, the additive risk is 10^{-2}. In contrast to the EPA, FDA, and OSHA, the ICRP dose limits do take into account the additive effect of exposure to all radionuclides.

Many individuals and groups need a usable treatment of the basic methodologies required to assess the human health risks caused by exposure to toxicants. This need is shared by industrial hygienists; environmental, occupational and public health professionals; toxicologists; epidemiologists; labor leaders; attorneys; regulatory officials; and manufacturers and users of chemicals. Most interested parties do not have the expertise to evaluate risks due to exposures to toxicants. Furthermore, many of the published treatments of risk assessment are confusing due to incomprehensible mathematics. This leaves interested participants suspicious of each other and with no recourse except to let the "experts" arrive at some acceptable level of exposure for the general population and/or workers. There is no justification for basing public policy decisions on obscure methodology.

A basic knowledge of biology and algebra is needed in order to utilize the methodology presented. In addition, a basic knowledge of toxicology, epidemiology, and statistics is desirable for a full understanding of some aspects of risk assessment. Sophisticated computer programs are not required. All the computations can be carried out with a pocket calculator capable of executing simple statistical analyses.

Risk assessment is a relatively new and rapidly developing science. Indeed, most federal agencies for which risk assessment is an important tool for decision-making or a subject of research were established only within the last quarter of the 20th century. Among those are the Environmental Protection Agency (EPA), Occupational Safety and Health Administration (OSHA), National Institute of Environmental Health Sciences (NIEHS), Consumer Product Safety Commission (CPSC), National Institute for Occupational Safety and Health (NIOSH), Food and Drug Administration (FDA), and Agency for Toxic Substances and Disease Registry (ATSDR). Mantel and Bryan published in 1961 the first paper on estimation of low-dose risk based on data obtained from tests in which animals were exposed at high doses; formal procedures for performing animal bioassays, which are critically important for gathering information for risk assessment, had been standardized only in the 1960s and 1970s; and formal risk assessment began to be conducted regularly in the late 1970s. It was not until 1983, when the National Research Council (NRC) committee that prepared **Risk Assessment in the Federal Government: Managing the Process** defined the steps in risk assessment, that a generally accepted nomenclature for risk assessment was established.

Expert practitioners of risk analysis have a wide spectrum of activities to analyze. Risk is associated with any object, such as the risk that a boiler will explode or that an earthquake will occur. The content may change between applications, but the techniques and ideas are surprisingly similar. In this chapter, the emphasis is on practical outcomes, or "risks in the real world," mostly from health and safety examples. Much regulatory attention focuses on health and safety particularly human health risks.

Predicting an event that commonly occurs, like a cold, that you expect soon, but that usually leads to small losses, intuitively differs from forecasting a rare event, far off in the future, that might lead to a huge loss, such as a meteor striking the earth and eliminating most biological species. The differences become more understandable, when you break the comparison into smaller pieces: the probability, the outcome, and the amount of time until the outcome of each event.

II. STRUCTURE OF RISK ANALYSIS

There is no uniform terminology in the field of risk analysis. Engineers use the term **risk assessment** very differently from scientists. Many confuse the practice of safety assessment with risk assessment. Suppose that you have a specific problem involving risk. You might want to obtain an in-depth understanding of the risk, figure out some ways to control it, and learn how to explain what you know to others. The overall process of risk analysis is divided into three components: **risk assessment, risk management, and risk communication.**

A. RISK ASSESSMENT

To us, **risk assessment** is the process of characterizing a risk. It involves estimating the probability, usually a mathematical process, and specifying the conditions that accompany the outcome. It usually incorporates descriptive data and scientific theories. So, it resembles policy analysis. Some risk assessors even think that it is a branch of policy analysis. Others describe risk assessment as science-based inference or fact-based opinion. It is put into the same category as forecasting earthquakes or bankruptcies. Risk assessors ask what can go wrong, how likely is the bad outcome, how long will it take before it occurs, and what might be the importance of the loss, if it does. Risk assessment provides us with useful information about risks. Risk management involves merging the results of risk analysis with social factors, such as socioeconomic conditions, political pressure, and economic concerns (Figure 15.1).

B. RISK MANAGEMENT

In contrast to the process of risk assessment, **risk management** is the process of deciding what to do about risk. A risk manager looks at the available options to control the probability of loss, the time until the loss, and the magnitude of the loss. The risk manager always has options of doing nothing, involving stakeholders, publicizing the risks, or obtaining more information. Risk managers usually attempt to make decisions that will reduce risks.

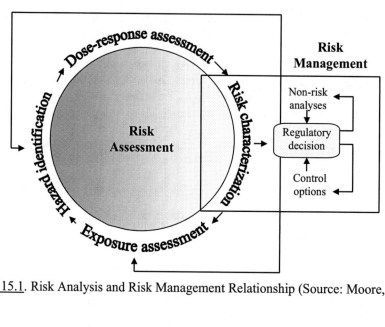

Figure 15.1. Risk Analysis and Risk Management Relationship (Source: Moore, 1999).

Risk assessment provides us with useful information about risks. Risk management involves merging the results of risk analysis with social factors, such as socioeconomic conditions, political pressures, and economic concerns. Three avenues of risk management are **educational, economic,** and **regulatory.** These are not mutually exclusive, but can be used together to manage a risk. **Educational risk management** can include use of the media to inform the public about risk, or may be the strategic placement of warnings to provide people with risk information. The risk information may be on environmental hazards, drugs and other chemical products. **Economic risk management** is accomplished through pollution taxes and permits that emphasize risk reduction through monetary incentives or disincentives. **Regulatory risk management,** also called command-and-control, is evident in the numerous laws governing potential environmental and health hazards in the United States. The Clean Water Act, the Safe Drinking Water Act, and the Toxic Substances Control Act are examples of regulatory risk management, where laws restrict and limit pollution, chemical exposures, and releases.

A risk manager will ask what we can do about a risk, and what tradeoffs do the different control options involve? The process usually begins by determining the options and estimating the risks under each option, but the risk manager must evaluate a wider array of information, including economic costs, technical feasibility, social acceptance, legal conformance, political perceptions, regulatory objectives, and enforceability. Balancing these different concerns, especially when the information is uncertain or incomplete, is a difficult task. Some analysts describe risk management as science-based decision-making under conditions of uncertainty.

Usually, the risk manager has an array of tools to support this difficult task. One of the tools is **decision analysis,** a mature branch of operations research, and risk analysts can apply this highly structured, coherent approach. Given opportunity and information, a risk manager can balance the risk of one option against the risk of another. Still another tool the risk manager may use is an analysis of the economic costs and benefits of each option, giving preference to the option with the lowest cost-benefit ratio. In addition, the risk manager may select the option with the lowest ratio of risk to benefits, by directly comparing risks with economic data. Theoretically, a risk manager could use any or all of **risk-risk, cost-benefit,** and **risk-benefit** approaches to explore the best way to manage a risk.   Practically, many constraints may prevent full exploration, including the unimportance of the decision, lack of time, legal restrictions, and sparseness of data and funds to support the process.

C. RISK COMMUNICATION

Risk communication is the process of explaining risk. To exchange information, the risk communicator has to begin by understanding the nature, assessment, and management of a risk, but other understanding is needed. The risk communicator also has to decide whom to engage in the process, how to engage them, and at what point in the process to engage them, as well as what information to exchange and how to exchange it. Most risk communicators aim for open, two-way interactions that will enable people outside the risk analysis process to understand risk assessments and accept risk management decisions.

These definitions of the components of risk analysis are commonly, but not universally, used. For example, most risk analysts in the private sector, the states, and the federal civilian agencies accept these definitions. However, the U.S. Department of Defense reverses the meanings of risk analysis and risk assessment.

When scientists estimate the chances of getting lung cancer from radon gas in homes, they are engaged in risk assessment. When transportation experts estimate the annual chances of death from driving automobiles at different speeds, they are engaged in risk assessment. When the Environmental Protection Agency (EPA) requires a certificate of radon levels for every home sold, EPA is engaged in risk management. When Congress sets a maximum speed limit of 55 miles per hour on federal highways, Congress is engaged in risk management. If a realtors' association issues a press release explaining EPA's requirement for radon certificates, it is engaged in risk communication. When a Department of Transportation official appears on television to explain why Congress has reduced the speed limit, the official is engaged in risk communication.

Risk analysis encompasses much more than a description of a risk and an accompanying risk assessment but the process begins with them. For example, good risk management requires an understanding of how the public views a risk, which may differ dramatically from the way that risk assessors evaluate it. **Risk perception** is a separate area of research, and understanding it is crucial for good risk communication. Perceiving a highly probable, but slight, loss expected in the near future is inherently different from thinking about a huge, but rare, loss that will only occur in the distant future and that may never occur Our efforts to avoid a huge potential loss will color our intuitive feelings about a very low-probability event.

Procedurally, decision analysis separates probabilities from outcomes, and for this reason, many think it improves risk management. An understanding of how society will perceive a risk, and accept risk management decisions, is important. Good risk management requires a diversity of information about costs, feasibility, enforcement, legal authority, and so forth.

D. RISK POLICY

Some add **risk policy**, a kind of meta-topic, as a fourth component of risk analysis. They have in mind issues such as guidelines for risk assessment (often different guidelines for different kinds of risks, such as guidelines for carcinogen risk assessment or guidelines for neurotoxicity risk assessment).

The structure of risk analysis is helpful, just in sizing up the nature of regulatory tasks. Suppose that you become responsible for complete risk analyses of two different subjects: common colds and large meteorites striking the earth. How would you approach assessment, management, and communication of each of these risks?

In the past several decades, formal risk analysis has played an increasingly influential role in public policy, from the community to the international level. Although its outputs and uses are often (even usually) contentious, it has become a dominant tool for energy, environmental, health, and safety decisions, both public and private. While critiques abound, few scholars and practitioners would dispute the notion that an understanding of some essential tools of the trade is invaluable.

Risk analysis in one form or another has been used for centuries (Figure 15.2). In the early 1970s, as risk analysis evolved into a major policy decision tool, Alvin Weinberg proposed that it falls into a special category of "transscience . . . questions which can be asked of science, yet which cannot be answered by science." Individuals and society need to make decisions on issues for which there are no certain outcomes, only probabilities, often highly uncertain.

Due to the "trans-scientific" nature of risk analysis, there will always be disputes about methods, end points, and models. Individual and societal values may not be separable from the quantitative analysis, determining what we choose to analyze. Tension over the use of quantitative analysis will be amplified by distributions of gains and losses, as well as prior commitments. Key goals of the risk analyst include extracting the good data from the bad, deciding which model best fits both the data and the underlying process, as well as understanding the limitations of available methods.

In some ways, risk analysis is a mature field, and a number of methods and techniques have become institutionalized. Yet in many profound ways, risk analysis remains immature. To some, the subject amounts to many fascinating case studies in search of a paradigm! The risks of contracting human immunodeficiency virus, of acquiring cancer from pesticides, of nuclear accidents, or of space shuttle disasters are regarded as important but idiosyncratic cases. To the extent that generalized lessons are not learned, science, technology, and environmental policy research has yet to find a common language of expression and analysis.

Despite a number of attempts to rationalize the use of risk analysis in the policy process, its role continues to be controversial. A 1983 National Research Council (NRC) project, **Risk Assessment in the Federal Government: Managing the Process**, generally referred to as the "Red Book," sought to establish a risk assessment paradigm in the environmental context. It envisioned a sequence of Hazard Identification, followed by parallel Exposure and Dose-Response Evaluations, which are then combined to generate a Risk Characterization. Under this paradigm, once the hazard has been characterized, it can be used to inform risk management.

About 3200 B.C.: The Asipu, a group of priests in the Tigris-Euphrates Valley established a methodology:

1) Hazard identification
2) Generation of alternatives
3) Data collection* and analysis
4) Report creation

*Note that "data" included signs from the gods!

Arnobius, 4th century A.D., came up with decision analysis and first used the *dominance principle*, whereby a single option may be clearly superior to all others considered. Arnobius concluded that believing in God is a better choice than not believing, whether or not God actually exists. Note that Arnobius did not consider the possibility that a different God exists.

	State of nature	
	God exists	No God
Believe	Good outcome (heaven)	Neutral outcome
Alternative		
Don't believe	Bad outcome (hell)	Neutral outcome

King Edward II had to deal with the problem of smoke in London:

1285: Established a commission to study the problem.
1298: Commission called for voluntary reductions in use of soft coal.
1307: Royal proclamation banned soft coal, followed by a second commission to study why the proclamation was not being followed.

Figure 15.2. Some Historical Highlights on Risk Analysis (Source: Kammen and Hassenzahl, 1999).

III. <u>ASSESSING HUMAN RISK</u>

A farmer stands in his field, staring in horrified awe at the stream of black waste flowing onto his land from an adjacent river. This scene occurred on April 29, 1998, when a waste reservoir in Southern Spain burst, releasing toxic sludge into waterways and onto surrounding farmland. The reservoir served as a holding area for zinc, lead, iron, and cadmium wastes from a nearby Canadian-owned zinc mine. The dangerous waste posed both an immediate and long-term threat to the health and livelihoods of locals and to the environment. Crops were mined and land contaminated by the toxic mess. Locals complained of burning eyes and throats. Ten tons of dead fish and shellfish were carried away from the acidic waters. With shock and dismay, people wondered at the odds of this unexpected event. A shift in the Earth apparently sent the reservoir wall tumbling, releasing millions of cubic feet of metal waste into the surrounding region. This event typifies the multitude of environmental risks facing the world today. These types of risks are uncertain and unexpected, and the consequences can be severe, even deadly.

Risk is an integral part of life, permeating every aspect, from eating, breathing, sleeping, and socializing, to working and playing. Risk can be of a financial, personal, social, health, or environmental nature. Some industries, such as insurance, gambling, and finance, are based on risk.

The word "risk" describes a range of activities, situations, and concepts, from drinking a glass of red wine daily to skydiving and extreme skiing, to chemical exposure. Risk can imply chance, consequence, danger, and opportunity. In everyday language, risk is commonly used to describe types of people or situations. For example, the term "risky business" implies shady dealings, a "risk-taker" suggests a brave, confident, perhaps foolhardy individual. "Risk-averse" describes someone who shies away from risk. "Risk-free" describes an activity that contains no uncertainty or negative consequences. A comparison of some of life's risks are shown in (Figure 15.3).

Many of the risks in our lives are voluntary, such as our diet, sunbathing, and smoking. People accept certain risks because they enjoy the benefit they receive from the behavior or activity. People risk money in the stock market in the hopes of making a profit; people live in earthquake and hurricane prone areas in exchange for the lovely climate often found in those regions. We accept many risks in our lives, because they seem both mundane and remote. We cross streets, take pharmaceuticals, drive in cars and fly in airplanes, under the assumption that these activities are safe. However, even these everyday activities carry some level of risk. But because these activities are familiar and routine, they do not appear threatening.

However, not everyone is content with life's daily dose of risk. Some people seek out extraordinarily high levels of risk, engaging in skydiving, bungee jumping, rock and ice climbing and other extreme sports (Figure 15.4). People choose these activities because they enjoy the element of danger from the risk, and the adrenaline rush. They have defined their own "acceptable" level of risk, which might be too high for most people who reach their risk threshold more easily.

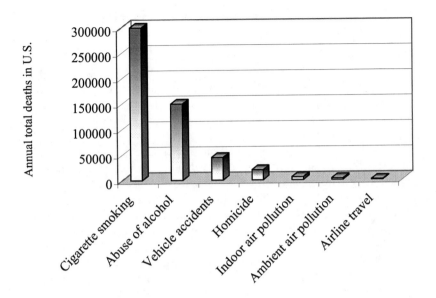

Figure 15.3. A Comparison of Some Common Risks. (Source: Moore, 1999).

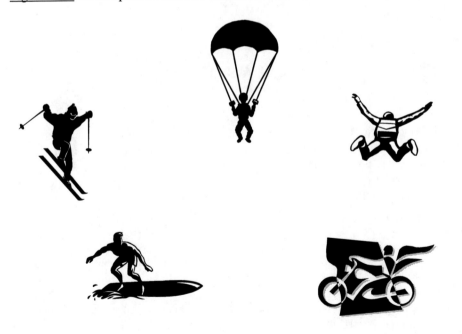

Figure 15.4. Extreme Sports are Popular because of the Excitement Associated with High Risk.

IV. <u>ENVIRONMENTAL RISK</u>

Some risks are well understood, such as driving and smoking. The vast quantity of information and statistics on automobile accidents allow us to draw conclusions about the risk of dying in a car crash. Similarly, voluminous data on smoking and disease demonstrates that smoking poses a health risk. However, some risks remain shrouded in uncertainty. Many environmental risks fall into this category. Environmental risk is a reality of today's world.

The seemingly endless supply of synthetic chemicals, consumer goods, energy, and waste creates new risks through chemical contamination, pollution and environmental degradation. Environmental disasters such as chemical spills or explosions threaten millions of people living in the vicinity of manufacturing or storage facilities. The uncertain risks of global warming and ozone depletion loom ahead. A central factor of environmental risk is that it is usually involuntary. People do not choose to ingest chemical pollutants such as pesticides or industrial solvents in their food and water, to undergo workplace exposures to dangerous chemicals, to breathe polluted air, or to experience radiation exposure from nuclear fallout or faulty nuclear power plants. These environmental risks pose a unique problem to regulators charged with protecting the public's health. Limited information may be available on the health effects of these risks. Consequently, in an effort to protect the public's health, various government agencies study these potential hazards to determine the levels of risk they pose. The effort to understand these risks, and to quantify their impact on human health, is the field of risk analysis.

V. <u>TOOLS OF RISK ANALYSIS</u>

Risk analysis employs several scientific disciplines in its goal to characterize a risk (Figure 15.5). Significant amounts of information, both quantitative and qualitative, are needed to develop an adequate picture of a risk. Toxicology, epidemiology, clinical trials and cellular studies provide some of the information for a risk analysis. The types of information reviewed include characteristics of the chemical, type and length of exposure, dose, animal response, and human response.

A. Toxicology

Toxicologists study chemicals to determine their physiological and health impacts on humans. Risk analysis relies heavily on toxicological studies and findings. A particular branch of toxicology, regulatory toxicology, aims at guarding the public from dangerous chemical exposures. For example, the health effects of nicotine, saccharin, and benzene have been explored and defined through toxicology studies. Toxicological studies usually involve controlled laboratory animal studies. The animals are evaluated for their responses to different doses of a substance. These controlled research conditions are crucial for procuring accurate information.

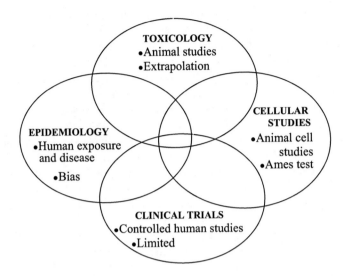

Figure 15.5. Tools of Risk Analysis. (Source: Moore, 1999).

Prior to a toxicology study, little may be known about a chemical, such as what amount causes minimal adverse health effects or death. In a study, scientists follow a series of steps to learn about a substance's activity in a living organism. A study can delineate both the lower and upper limits of a chemical's potency, that is, the amount that causes no effect in any animal and the amount at which all animals die. After these limits are established, scientists can work within this range to discover additional information about a chemical's health effects. As a chemical may have a myriad of health effects, the researchers will focus their interests on certain health responses. These specific physiological changes are called endpoints. Some common endpoints frequently studied include the effective dose of a chemical, named the No Observable Effect Level (NOEL), the No Observable Adverse Effect Level (NOAEL), the Lowest Observable Adverse Effect Level (LOAEL) and death. All of these endpoints provide valuable information on the doses and effects of a chemical. This information can be incorporated into a risk assessment.

B. DOSE

When studying a chemical agent, toxicologists use different doses to elicit different animal responses. They ascertain the threshold dose, the dose at which no effects are seen in the study animals. As the administered dose increases above the threshold amount, animals wilt begin to show adverse effects and some animals will die (Figure 15.6). The dose at which fifty percent of all the test animals die is called the lethal dose or the LD_{50}. Similarly, the ED_{50}, or effective dose, is the dose at which fifty percent of the animals demonstrate a response to the chemical. A very toxic chemical will have a low LD_{50}, signifying a low dose sufficient to kill 50% of the test animals. A less toxic chemical will have a higher LD_{50}. The Maximum Tolerated Dose (MTD) is a common level of chemical exposure in animal studies. At this dose, researchers expect to see only up to a 10% loss in weight and no death, clinical toxicity or pathologic lesions in the animal population. Some critics of the MTD believe it is too high a dose, because chemicals that cause cancer at the MTD in test animals may not cause cancer at lower doses.

Animal studies occur under controlled conditions. This control refers to exact doses, and specific lengths and times of exposure. By controlling the amount, the timing, and the duration of exposure, scientists can obtain increased quantity and quality of information on a chemical's health effects. For example, altering the amount, timing or duration of a dose in a study can alter the chemical's opportunity to inflict damage. Large doses may cause one type of response, small doses, another. Timing of a dose may also be critical. For example, if exposure is timed to occur during a "window of vulnerability" in a fetus, minuscule amounts of an agent may cause severe damage. Outside this "window", this amount would be harmless to the fetus. Clearly, control of the dose provides tremendous influence over the types of health effects seen. In addition, this control allows for variability in study design. Toxicology studies can occur over short, medium, or long periods of time. Short term, or acute exposure studies, occur over two weeks and generally involve high doses of the chemical substance. Medium length or subchronic studies involve lower chemical doses over a longer time period, from 5-90 days. Long term or chronic studies can last two years and use much smaller doses of chemicals. This variability improves understanding of a chemical's activity under different conditions. For comparison purposes, animal studies establish a control group not exposed to the agent under consideration. This group provides the researchers a level of certainty that the physiological responses seen after exposure are in fact due to exposure and not to some unrelated, uncontrolled variable.

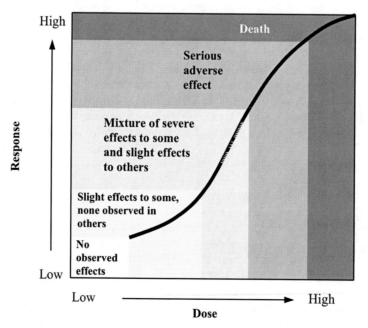

Figure 15.6. Dose Response Curve (Source: Moore, 1999).

C. EXTRAPOLATION

Extrapolation can be defined as using known information to infer something about the unknown. In risk analysis, the term extrapolation refers to the use of animal data to predict human response to chemical exposure. Extrapolation is widely used in toxicology, to deduce the risks humans face. The use of extrapolation is a vital tool of toxicology since human exposure studies are not widely accepted. Different types of animals can be used during laboratory studies, depending on the agent under consideration. While dogs and monkeys have been used for animal studies, the most common laboratory animal is the rat. During laboratory studies, animals generally receive high doses of the chemical of interest for a measured span of time, often their lifetimes. Laboratory animals have shorter life spans than humans, allowing studies to document a full lifetime of exposure, from infancy to maturity to death. The results from these high-dose, short duration studies are used to extrapolate human response to the longer term, lower-level exposures we generally receive. The difference in dose level and duration of exposure generates some doubt about the validity of extrapolation. Furthermore, biological and metabolic differences between the test animal and humans may undermine the validity of extrapolations. For instance, the test animal may have one method for detoxifying a substance, whereas a human may use a different metabolic pathway. Alternatively, a test animal may lack an adequate detoxification pathway, whereas humans may be very effective at detoxifying a substance. Because of these differences, a substance that causes cancer in one animal may not cause cancer in another animal, or vice versa. This fact limits the accuracy in extrapolating from animal data to human response. Despite these drawbacks, extrapolation is a crucial method in studying potential human outcomes based on the results of animal studies.

D. ACCEPTABLE DAILY INTAKES

The purpose of toxicology studies is often to establish an acceptable level of exposure or dose of a substance that is considered "safe." This level, which poses little risk, is termed the acceptable daily intake (ADI). In extrapolation from animals to human studies, scientists incorporate safety factors when determining acceptable exposure (dose) levels. The No Observable Effect Level (NOEL) established by the threshold dose in test animals is translated into the acceptable daily intake or the reference dose for humans. These levels include safety factors from ten to ten thousand, depending on the protected group. The safety factor is added by dividing the threshold dose by some factor of ten, thereby reducing the acceptable level of exposure and risk from exposure and increasing safety. Again, which factor of ten is used depends on the level of protection sought, the uncertainty inherent in the study data and who is being protected. Lower safety factors are used when high quality human data is available. Higher safety factors, up to ten thousand, are used as the uncertainty level goes up and the quality of the data diminishes. Although the ADI's are based on scientific studies and include a margin of safety, these numbers are not foolproof. As more data becomes available about a substance, the ADI's may change, either lower or higher. For example, as we have gained knowledge about the dangers of exposure to lead, the minimum level of exposure considered harmful to human health has decreased, as adverse health effects are seen at extremely low concentrations of lead.

E. EPIDEMIOLOGY

Epidemiology is "the study of the distribution and determinants of disease frequency in the human population." In an attempt to determine causality between an exposure and a disease, epidemiology study human response to various environmental agents, such as tobacco smoke, pharmaceuticals, exercise, and even hair dye. These are not controlled laboratory studies, but in the outside world, subject to fluctuating conditions.

VI. QUALITATIVE RISK ASSESSMENT

Although most regulatory agencies attempt to develop "quantitative" risk assessments, the number of facilities having the potential for release of toxic chemicals makes universal quantitative assessment impossible. For this reason the common approach is to apply as an initial step some type of "qualitative" or "semiquantitative" risk assessment.

Possibilities include the following:

1. Qualitative characterization where health risks are identified but not quantified (for example, hazard evaluations and carcinogen classification schemes).
2. Qualitative risk estimations where chemicals are ranked, or classified by broad categories of risk (for example, chemical potency classification schemes)
3. Semi-quantitative approaches where effect levels (for example, "no observable effect") are used in combination with uncertainty factors to establish "safe" exposure levels.

Each of these approaches can and has been used to assess risks and, in a broad sense, constitutes a form of risk assessment.

One example of the qualitative approach is the procedure developed by the EPA for assigning each toxic agent to 1 of 5 categories, depending on its potential for causing cancer in humans:

Group A: Carcinogenic to humans;
Group B: Probably carcinogenic to humans;
Group C: Possibly carcinogenic to humans;
Group D: Not classifiable as to human carcinogenicity;
Group E: Evidence of noncarcinogenicity for humans.

Simply knowing which of these categories applies to a given toxic agent can be very useful in assessing risks.

Perhaps the best example of a qualitative approach to risk assessment is the "Public Health Assessment" (PHA) methodology that has been developed by the Agency for Toxic Substances and Disease Registry (ATSDR), primarily for evaluation of the potential health hazards of toxic waste (Superfund) sites. Public health assessments are also used to identify conditions of exposure to hazardous substances that, when reduced in severity, will prevent morbidity and mortality. Although public health assessments are basically quantitative in nature, ATSDR officials responsible for conducting them use a large amount of data. On the basis of their experience, ATSDR officials have identified 10 key substances that are specifically considered in the evaluation of any hazardous waste site. These are the following:

1. Lead,
2. Arsenic,
3. Mercury,
4. Vinyl Chloride,
5. Benzene,
6. Cadmium,
7. PCBs,
8. Chloroform,
9. Benzo(b)fluoranthene, and
10. Trichloroethylent (TCE).

For each of these, and a host of other substances, ATSDR has developed a toxicologic profile that describes what is known about the related toxicity and human health effects. In a similar manner, ATSDR has identified several priority health conditions that receive specific attention in the evaluation of a waste site. The following are the 7 priority health conditions:

1. Birth defects and reproductive disorders,
2. Cancers,
3. Immune dysfunction disorders,
4. Kidney dysfunction,
5. Liver dysfunction,
6. Lung and respiratory diseases,
7. Neurotoxic disorders.

Based on the public health assessment, each site is placed in one of five categories in terms of its overall significance to public health and as a guide for follow-up action:

1. Urgent public health hazard,
2. Public health hazard,
3. Indeterminate public health hazard,
4. No apparent public health hazard,
5. No public health hazard.

VII. <u>QUANTITATIVE RISK ASSESSMENT</u>

The ultimate goal of studying the relationship between environmental hazards and health is to take some action to reduce or eliminate those hazards or to reduce the harm that may result from their effects. This is called **risk management**. But before anything can be done, the risks themselves must be identified and thoroughly characterized. This process of analyzing the possible effects on people of exposure to substances and other potential hazards, such as radiation, is known as a form of **risk assessment**. Because of different laws and approaches to regulation in different countries and different institutions, the terminology used in various reports on risk assessment varies, even in the same countries. The one used here is commonly found in WHO, ILO, and UNEP documents.

The first step in risk assessment is to identify hazards based on results from the relevant toxicological and epidemiological studies. This hazard identification step may also involve describing how a substance behaves in the body, including its interactions at the organ, cellular, and molecular levels. Such studies may also identify toxic effects that are likely to occur under experimental conditions. **Hazard identification** may be considered a qualitative description of potential health effects.

In the next step of risk assessment, research data have to be used to describe and quantify the relationship between exposure or absorbed dose and its related health risk. This second step is known as a **dose-response assessment**. It is vital that the methods used to extrapolate data (e.g., from high to low exposure levels, from animal studies to humans, or from short-term to chronic exposure) are appropriate. The dose-response assessment should describe and justify the methods of extrapolation used. It should also describe the statistical and biological uncertainties of these methods.

The third step, called **exposure assessment**, is to measure the exposure itself, identifying the sources of exposure, estimating intake into the body by the various routes, and obtaining demographic information to define the exposed population. Field measurement data provided by monitoring and surveillance systems are obtained, when possible, to assess the environmental quality. If no measurement data are available, emissions may be calculated or estimated at the source and exposure levels may be estimated on the basis of mathematical models showing how these emissions are carried by air, water, or in the ground. Integration of these data provides an estimation of the most likely exposure levels for individuals who may come into contact with the contaminants.

Risk characterization is the integration of the first three steps in the risk assessment process. Ideally, it should produce a quantitative estimate of the risk in the exposed population, or estimates of the potential risk under different plausible exposure scenarios. Typically, a range of estimates is developed, using different assumptions and statistical methods that determine how sensitive the estimates are to basic assumptions in the model. If different health effects are likely to occur, the risk of each should be characterized. Other exposures or factors contributing to the health effects should also be characterized.

The literature on environmental health risk assessment can be confusing, as the same terms are used to refer to both generic risk assessments (often regulatory agency-based) and specific field risk assessments. Generic risk assessments characterize a hazard in general scientific terms on the basis of anticipated exposures and hypothetical population characteristics. However, when there is suspicion of a risk in a specific situation, it must be ascertained if people really are sufficiently exposed for health effects to occur.

Risk assessment has its limitations. In practice, crucial data are frequently lacking, and reasonable assumptions are made to arrive at a quantitative risk estimation. Most risk assessments contain one or more of the many sources of uncertainties that may accompany a risk assessment, and it is essential to evaluate their impact on the assessment. This process, usually referred to as **sensitivity analysis**, may be quite complex.

In many situations, only a qualitative risk assessment may be appropriate. In this approach, reasoned judgment is used, taking into account what information is known. When there is little likelihood that an exposure could be harmful, a qualitative risk assessment may be all that is necessary. If it is possible that a serious adverse effect may occur and that people may be affected, a quantitative risk assessment is usually preferred.

Sources of Uncertainty In A Risk Assessment are the following:

1. Use of an experimental study involving an inappropriate route of exposure,
2. Differences in bio-kinetics and/or mechanism of toxicity between species,
3. Poor specification of exposure in experimental study, i.e., concentration, duration, route, chemical species,
4. Extrapolation of high-dose to low-dose situations,
5. Difference in age at first exposure or lifestyle factors between experimental data and a risk group,
6. Exposure to multiple hazards in epidemiology studies,
7. Potential confounding factors,
8. Misclassification of the health outcome of concern.

When the health risk of a specific environmental hazard or situation has been characterized, decisions must be made regarding which of the various control actions should be taken. Regulatory agencies may develop regulatory options, evaluate the public health, economic, social, and political consequences of the proposed options, and/or they may implement agency decisions. These actions and decisions form the core of the **risk management** process.

A. HAZARD IDENTIFICATION IN THE FIELD

From toxicological and epidemiological data, potential health effects of hazardous substances can be estimated. Recognizing hazards in a specific industrial pollution situation, however, requires a different approach. This is commonly done by conducting **health hazard evaluations** and **hazard audits**, both of which involve walking through the plant (or community facility) and investigating all operations. The difference between the two is that in a health hazard evaluation the walk-through is intended to identify the cause of a particular problem but in a hazard audit all potential hazards are systematically examined.

1. Occupational Environment

In the workplace it can be relatively easy to make an inventory of all potential hazards. This is made easier by an accurate registration or tracking system of all chemicals that are frequently used or stored, which unfortunately is not always available. To make an inventory of chemical hazards, product identity is, of course, crucial. From knowledge of which product is used, one may then learn what is in it and what constituents are hazardous. Identifying the chemicals in a product may be difficult if the manufacturer is not required by law to list ingredients or if the material is not labeled properly, or if the composition of the product is protected as a trade secret.

2. General Environment

When a point source of pollution is suspected, such as a specific industrial plant, the hazards may be established on the basis of the type of materials used and the industrial processes involved. The identity of chemical hazards is usually difficult to determine in uncontrolled environments, such as illegal dumping sites or abandoned industrial locations. For example, the chemical hazards at a suspected soil contamination may be from almost anything. One approach is to check whether there is information within the community regarding former industrial or other activities at the suspected location. Depending on the results of such an inquiry, further research can be streamlined in a specific direction. However, if no records exist or no industrial activities can be described by former workers, the situation becomes far more difficult. In such a situation, chemical analysis of samples will have to be conducted to determine the nature of the contamination. Since it is too costly to screen for all possible contaminants, chemical analysis has to be concentrated on specific marker components. For instance, analysis of benzopyrene may be used as a marker for contamination with polycyclic aromatic hydrocarbons, dieldrin for pesticides, and toluene for volatile organic compounds. All such screening methods have their limitations.

B. RELATIONSHIP BETWEEN DOSE AND HEALTH OUTCOME

1. Dose-Effect and Dose-Response Relationships

The terms dose-response and dose-effect are occasionally used interchangeably. Strictly speaking, however, a **dose-response** relationship is one between the dose and the proportion of individuals in an exposed group that demonstrate a defined effect. A **dose-effect** relationship describes that between the dose and the severity of a health effect in an individual (or a typical person in the population). A hierarchy of effects on health can be identified for most hazards, ranging from acute illness and death to chronic and lingering illnesses, from minor and temporary ailments to temporary behavioral or physiological changes. Dose-response relationships are considerably different for non-carcinogens (thought to have a threshold) and carcinogens (thought to be non-threshold).

2. Calculating Risks for Threshold Effects

Many environmental hazards have a specific effect on individuals only when the dose reaches a certain level, i.e., a **threshold** for that effect. Figure 15.7 illustrates the dose-response relationship for various health effects of lead concentrations in blood in children. Sometimes the number of years of exposure has to be used as an indicator of dose, when duration and levels of exposure are not known. When concentration and dose are known, a dose index can be calculated. This was done for workers in a Swedish battery factory.

Dose-response relationships can also be obtained for physical hazards (relationship between sound levels at work and the percentage of those with impaired hearing according to the age of the workforce).

Dose-response relationships also apply to injuries. Speed is used as an indicator of dose. With an increase in speed there is an increased risk of nonfatal injury in car drivers in a collision.

The concept of the dose-response relationship extends to psychological distress as well. The greater the noise level, the greater the percentage of people annoyed by it. At a given noise level, a higher level of annoyance was found in a U.S. Environmental Protection Agency (EPA) study, than that found by another investigator.

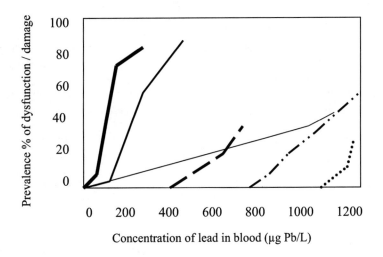

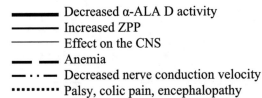

Decreased α-ALA D activity
Increased ZPP
Effect on the CNS
Anemia
Decreased nerve conduction velocity
Palsy, colic pain, encephalopathy

Figure 15.7. Dose-Response Curve for Various Health Effects of Lead in Children (Source: Yassi, 2001).

3. Thresholds and Other Important Benchmarks

A **no observed adverse effect level** (NOAEL) is the point on a dose-effect curve at which a threshold is reached. Before this level, there are either no symptoms or our technology is not sufficient to detect a problem (depending on the situation). These levels are often determined in animal studies. Similarly, a **lowest observed adverse effect level** (LOAEL), is the lowest level at which some symptoms are found (Figure 15.8). **A no observed effect level** (NOEL) is the level at which no effect, either good or bad, is detected.

Because all individuals are constantly exposed to certain levels of environmental chemicals, the question to address is what levels of exposure to these chemicals are likely to affect human health. This analysis is usually done by official agencies (e.g., the Environmental Protection Agency in the United States), by applying animal and epidemiological studies. From these studies, an **acceptable daily intake** (ADI), or **tolerable daily intake** (TDI) (depending on the jurisdiction), is calculated. These values indicate the maximal daily intake of a chemical that is not expected to result in adverse health effects after a lifelong exposure. The ADI is usually the NOAEL (or LOAEL) divided by uncertainty factors (UF).

$$ADI = \frac{NOAEL \ (or \ LOAEL)}{UF}$$

The ADIs can then be used as reference values in establishing guidelines to protect individuals. Note that time and dosimetry factors (such as body weight, surface area, and absorption rate) must be specified for an ADI. For example, an ADI is often prepared for a person of 70 kg who is exposed to a chemical for 3 hr/day. The ADIs and TDIs are often revised over time, as new information is discovered through further studies.

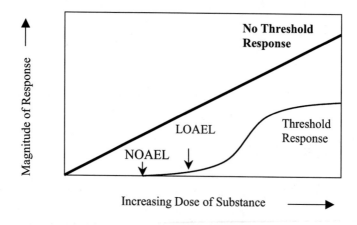

Figure 15.8. No Observed Adverse Effect Level (NOAEL) and Lowest Observed Adverse Effect Level (LOAEL) (Source: Yassi, 2001).

4. Uncertainty Factors in Establishing Thresholds

Generally it is not possible to specify an exact threshold for any substance, for a variety of reasons: the vulnerability of individuals varies; there is considerable physiological diversity in human populations; measuring techniques have their limitations; study methods are often limited; at very low exposures, the effects may not be easily detectable; and data relating to the upper end of the curve may also be difficult to obtain because massive exposures are relatively rare. Nonetheless, the principal use of dose-response curves is to predict the consequences of very high and very low exposures.

The extrapolation of animal data to humans has a number of fundamental problems. First, the effect on the animal studied may simply not apply to humans because of physiological differences between the species. Second, projections from a higher-dose response range to a lower-dose range involve various assumptions that may not prove to be accurate. Third, animal studies are often conducted using routes of administration that do not correspond to the routes of human exposure.

The **safety (or uncertainty) factor** (UF) reflects the degree of uncertainty that must be incorporated into the extrapolation from experimental data to the human population. When the quality and quantity of dose-response data are high, the safety factor is low. When the data are inadequate or equivocal, the safety factor must be higher. (Safety factors are not relevant to carcinogens.) The National Academy of Sciences (NAS) Safe Drinking Water committee and the EPA in the United States have developed the safety factor guidelines shown in Table 15.3. Risks at the lower levels of exposure may be estimated by extrapolating from middle-range observations.

Table 15.3. Safety or Uncertainty Factors (Source: Yassi, 2001).

Factor	Comments
10x factor	Applied to data from valid experimental studies on prolonged human intake. This protects the sensitive members of the population.
100x factor	Applied when experimental results from studies of human intake are not available, or are inadequate but there are valid results from low-dose intake studies on one or more species of this accounts for species-to-species extrapolation.
1000x factor	Applied when there arc no low-dose or acute human data and only scanty results on experimental animals. This is applied to account for species to species extrapolation, from high dose to low dose, and from short-term to long-term effects, as well as protecting sensitive members of the population.

Once the threshold dose for a toxic substance has been determined for the normal and healthy population, consideration must be given to high-risk groups such as infants, young children, elderly people, pregnant women and their fetuses, the nutritionally deprived, the ill, individuals with genetic disorders, and those exposed to other environmental health hazards. There are many examples of the susceptibility of these high-risk groups. The increased susceptibility of fetuses and infants has been well documented. For example, several Japanese children born to mothers exposed to methylmercury in fish in Minamata suffered congenital malformations even though the mothers showed few or no symptoms of mercury poisoning at all. The fact that nutritional deficiencies increase susceptibility is also well documented. Dietary deficiencies of calcium and iron significantly intensify the toxicity of lead. Individuals who suffer from kidney disease, for example, will experience greater effects from exposure to toxic metabolites that require excretion trough the kidneys, and impaired liver function affects the metabolic conversion, particularly detoxification of certain pollutants or their excretion in bile. Individuals suffering from cardiovascular or respiratory disease are at greater risk from the effects of carbon monoxide or sulfur dioxide. It may therefore be necessary to apply an additional safety factor to the dose that is toxic to the general population, in an effort to protect susceptible groups.

5. <u>Calculating Risks for Non-Threshold Effects</u>

Individuals either get cancer or they do not, and the probability is of an all-or- nothing event. A higher exposure does not result in a worse cancer but in an increase in the likelihood of getting it. Likewise, a lower level of exposure does not mean that the magnitude of the effect is less, so the dose-effect curve is considered irrelevant to assessments involving carcinogens. The dose-response curve, however, is very relevant, and it is generally agreed that the dose-response curve which does not assume a threshold is thus the preferred tool for analyzing risk associated with exposure to carcinogens. The argument against a threshold is that a single point mutation of the DNA can lead to an uncontrolled growth of a somatic cell that eventually produces cancer. It can be argued that different individuals have different thresholds because of differences in DNA repair genes and immune defenses, but these are not easily testable hypotheses.

In the multistage model of carcinogenesis, a cell line must pass through several stages before a tumor is irreversibly initiated. The rate at which cell lines pass through these stages is a function of the dose rate. In the multihit model, dose relates to the number of hits to the sensitive tissue required to initiate a cancer. The most important difference between the multistage and the multihit models is that in the multihit models, all hits must result from the dose, whereas in the multistage model, passage through some of the stages can occur spontaneously. The multihit models predict a lower risk at lower doses than that predicted by the multistage model. Aside from the one-hit, the multi- hit, and the multistage models, there are other models that explain dose-response relationships between carcinogens and cancer. The different models are each associated with different dose-response curves.

Just as one can produce an ADI for threshold agents such as mercury, one can produce a **risk-specific dose** for non-threshold agents, such as radon. In the case of a threshold agent, the NOAEL can aid the agency responsible for setting the ADI. In the case of a non-threshold agent, at any concentration of the agent cancer will be caused in some individuals in the population. Thus it is usually desirable to reduce the agent to the lowest possible level, realizing that it is impossible to eradicate it entirely. In setting a guideline value, an **acceptable level of risk** (ALR) must be determined. This is essentially a judgment call, which may or may not be made with the input of the people who are concerned in the community. In some countries, one fatality in a million people at risk is considered to be an acceptable level of risk for many situations, but there may be circumstances in which a greater risk, for example, 1 in 100,000, may be considered tolerable if the risk is balanced by a very considerable benefit. It should be noted that an increase in mortality in the general population at such a small rate would be virtually impossible to detect with current epidemiological techniques. One in 10,000 would be more customary for occupational exposures.

C. HUMAN EXPOSURE ASSESSMENT

1. Human exposure

Human exposure is defined as the opportunity for absorption into the body or action on the body as a result of coming into contact with a chemical, biological, or physical agent. The various routes of exposure are presented in Figure 15.9. The units of exposure to a chemical are usually the concentration multiplied by time (e.g., mg/ml/hr). The term **total exposure** implies that an attempt is being made to take into account all exposures to the contaminant regardless of media or route of exposure. Exposures from air, water, food, and soil form the link between hazards and effects. The critical parameter with respect to health effects is actually the dose, since it directly identifies the amount of the contaminant that has the potential to attack the target organ. **Internal dose** refers to the amount of the contaminant absorbed in body tissues upon inhalation, ingestion, or absorption. The **biologically effective dose** is the amount of the absorbed or deposited contaminants that contributes to the dose at the target site where the adverse effect occurs. **Total dose** is the term used to indicate the sum of all doses received by a person of a contaminant over a given time interval from interaction with all media.

Because the dose is difficult to measure, the parameter usually considered is the exposure. Therefore, regulators usually establish rules and regulations that are directly linked to reducing exposure, as opposed to dose. Estimates can then be made of the dose, based on the exposure, various assumptions, and animal models. While such estimates often have large uncertainties, it is a more practical parameter than dose. In any case, it has to be clear that measuring exposure, not just environmental concentration, is the critical parameter since it is more directly related to health effects. To put it simply, if someone is not inhaling, ingesting, or absorbing the pollutant, there is no exposure and hence no adverse health effect is possible. In all such investigations the total exposure from all sources must be assessed and not just the concentration in the medium or circumstance of concern. Exposure is usually measured for just one medium at a time. Risk assessment that is intended to optimize mitigation strategies must establish the relative risks associated with absorption from all media and routes of entry in order to gain a clear picture of which is more important.

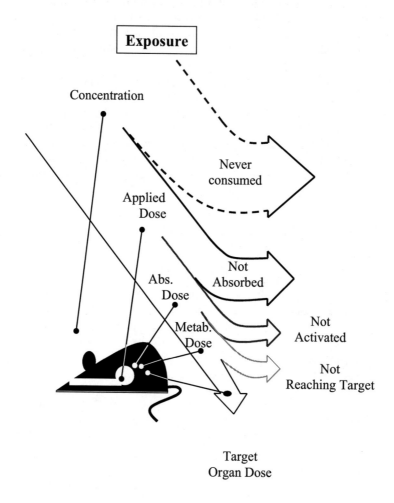

Figure 15. 9. Different Defining Levels of Exposure. (Source: Rhomberg, 1994).

2. Principles of Population Sampling

In the selection of a population sample for human exposure assessment, a **sampling frame** should be established, which should include (a) all the people in the target population, or (b) areas and the approximate number of people linked to each area. If the people in the target population are mobile, they may have to be linked to the areas where they eat or sleep.

Developed countries usually have a central statistical bureau that maintains registries or conducts a population census, which may form an ideal frame for sampling from the general population. As these listings are rarely complete, sampling frames often need to be conducted in stages with these data constituting a sampling frame for the initial stages of a multistage sample. In developing countries, where census data are generally not available, special efforts may be needed to estimate the population linked to the areas to construct a sampling frame.

If the target population consists only of people with specific characteristics, lists of these people may be available. For example, if the target population consists of lactating mothers, clinics in the area may be able to provide lists of mothers who have recently delivered babies. If available information does not provide complete enough coverage of the target population, samples from the lists must be supplemented with samples from other, possibly less efficient, frames that provide more complete coverage of the target population.

In **multistage sampling** researchers begin by sampling relatively large units and work their way down to increasingly smaller units. Using estimates of the number of people residing in each area, a sample of the geographic areas is selected. At the next stage, either the sample can be listed or smaller geographic areas can be listed within each area selected at the first stage of sampling. At the final stage of sampling, a list of the people residing in each sample area is prepared, and a sample of the people is selected from the lists. For example, to select a sample of adults living in a large city, researchers might (1) randomly select ten neighborhoods; (2) within each neighborhood, randomly select two urban blocks; (3) within each block, select ten households; (4) within each of the households, select one adult for the study. In **stratified random sampling**, an effective technique used to ensure that subgroups are adequately represented, the subpopulation of special interest (e.g., people between certain ages) is sampled at a higher rate than the remainder of the population to obtain sufficiently precise results for that group. The total estimated dose is calculated by simply adding these EDIs together. Note that the equations are very similar, except that the rate of contact varies depending on the type of exposure.

3. Errors and Quality Assurance

The potential for errors in environmental exposure assessment is large. Errors may occur with respect to the representativeness of sampling sites, the method of sample collection, the analytic procedure, and data handling.

The **representative error** refers to whether the sample collected represents the average concentration in the media under study. For example, an outdoor monitor on the roof of a multistoried building may not yield the concentration data needed to estimate average community air exposure. Even if sampling is conducted at a reasonable site, there is always a question as to how representative it is of exposure to residents at different times or when the wind blows from different directions. Portable sampling done in various directions and at variable distances from a fixed site can often provide more accurate data.

Sample collection errors (e.g., for water, soil, or food samples) can usually be minimized by simply using containers that are free of the contaminant of interest. Air samples are more difficult to properly collect and there is considerably more controversy over which instrument to use in various situations. Industrial hygienists therefore obtain considerable training in techniques of proper sample collection, and only people trained in these techniques should conduct air sampling.

Analytical errors may arise from the use of improper calibration procedures, variations in temperatures or line voltage in the laboratory, operator mistakes, as well as the intrinsic imprecision and inaccuracy of the analytical method chosen.

Finally, errors in data preparation may occur at a number of stages and often relate to the number of individuals involved in obtaining an environmental measurement. These specialists include the field person who collects the sample, the laboratory technician who does the analysis, the computer programmer who enters the data, and the epidemiologist who, often with the help of the statistician, interprets the data.

Quality assurance programs have therefore been developed and much international guidance has been provided on this subject. Effective procedures include the use of standard reference materials when calibrating instruments, monitoring of the line voltage and temperature to keep them constant, and duplicate analyses of some of the collected samples. A number of methods have been employed for quality assurance, such as interlaboratory comparisons, in which different analytical methods are used to analyze the same sample, and various statistical procedures to highlight bad data or extreme values.

4. Ensuring Adequate Sample Size

Determining an appropriate sample size requires balancing precision and cost, when the cost of a study is high, it may not be possible to obtain a very large sample size. Guidelines for calculating necessary sample sizes for accurate estimates are available in many textbooks and WHO publications, including that by UNEP/WHO. Even if the final sample sizes are determined primarily by cost constraints, rather than for desired precision, it is essential to calculate the precision that is expected for important parameter estimates and the power expected for important hypothesis tests. Studies that do not meet minimum standards for reliability of inferences are not useful - they cannot be interpreted. In general, a sample size of 50 persons is the minimum acceptable for human exposure-monitoring studies, with a range of 250 or more people considered desirable. The problems regarding inferences to the target population must be discussed in the reports of all studies but this is particularly important for studies with small sample sizes. Such problems include (1) unreliable point estimates, (2) unreliable estimates of precision, and (3) lack of normality for interval estimates and hypothesis tests.

D. HEALTH RISK CHARACTERIZATION

1. General Approach

Risk characterization (or **risk estimation** as it is also known) brings together the first three components of the risk assessment process: hazard identification, dose-response assessment, and exposure assessment. The incidence and severity of potential adverse effects are estimated as well. The major assumptions, scientific judgments, and uncertainties are described in detail to fully understand the validity of the estimated risk. Risk characterization may be subdivided into four different steps.

The **first equation** of total exposure combines the concentration of pollutants (by direct measurement through sampling and analysis, modeling, analysis of biological markers, and questionnaires) with the duration of exposure, expressed according to the health effects of concern. For carcinogenic effects, the total time (hours or days) of exposure during a person's lifetime is the principal concern (exposure every day over a lifetime would be 25,550 days, assuming a 70-year lifetime). For noncarcinogenic effects, short-term exposures at elevated concentrations are targeted, therefore a duration of hours or even minutes may be important. For chronic exposure, an average daily pollutant concentration is usually used with the assumption that it is relatively constant over a lifetime. For children, exposure periods are generally divided into age categories, e.g., 0-6 months, 6 months to 5 years, and 5 years to 12 years, because of their differing body weights.

The **second equation** combines the exposure information with dosimetry factors in a simple model to estimate the average dose per day over a lifetime. These factors include absorbed rate, average body weight, average lifetime, and others, as relevant. Dose is usually expressed as pollutant mass per kilogram of body weight per day. It should also include exposures from all media (air, water, soil, direct skin contact, etc.), such that the total dose is the sum of all of the individual doses.

The **third equation** integrates this exposure assessment with the dose-response relationship. The dose-response relationship incorporates uncertainty factors (and any other modifying factors that reflect professional judgment regarding scientific uncertainties of the entire database) with the NOAEL. This creates a benchmark against which to evaluate the significance of the dose with respect to its implication for health. The U.S. EPA has estimated potency factors that can be applied for many carcinogens. The reference dose, or **recommended maximum concentration** in some jurisdictions, is the NOAEL divided by the uncertainty factors multiplied by any modifying factors of concern. The lifetime individual risk is therefore the product of the dose multiplied by these response factors. For cancer, this is expressed as the lifetime excess risk of cancer for an individual exposed at the given lifetime exposure. For noncarcinogenic agents, it is usually assumed that there is a threshold below which there is no effect. The ratio of the exposure level to the estimated threshold dose gives some indication of the likelihood that adverse health effects will result from exposure to the toxic substance.

To generalize these average exposures and risks to the individual to an entire exposed population (consisting of many individuals, who may be very different from one another), one multiplies the estimate of average or worst lifetime individual risk by the number of individuals in the population (or each subpopulation) exposed. This final figure is the excess risk for a given effect that an exposure produces for an entire population.

2. Specific Health Risk Assessments in Field Situations

When risk assessment framework is applied to a new field situation, new or unexpected problems and pitfalls inevitably occur. In some cases it is obvious what risk factors are involved. In others the potential hazards is extremely difficult to recognize. In still other situations the ingested dose may be easily calculated from food contamination levels and average consumption data. In others the situation is very complicated because many different exposure routes are involved and dosimetry factors are not available. In such cases, the use of biomarkers may be the only effective way to come to an acceptably accurate estimate of the total dose.

VIII. <u>ACCIDENT SITUATIONS</u>

The first part dealt with the assessment of risks associated with routine releases from a facility or source. Assessments of this type require the following steps beyond those traditionally undertaken in the assessment of routine releases:

Accident scenario development and screening - The objective here is to postulate physically possible sequences of events and processes that could lead to a major disruption in a facility and the release and transport of toxic materials into the neighboring environment.

Consequence assessment - After the scenarios have been selected, a sequence of models is used to estimate the consequences of each.

Uncertainty and sensitivity analysis - Because experimental data are often not available to confirm estimates of accidental releases, the acceptability of a facility must be based largely on its predicted behavior, as derived through the input of expert judgements and the utilization of computer models.

Regulatory-compliance assessment - Because accident experience is fortunately very limited, and associated risk assessments are generally performed prior to facility construction and operation, the goal of many risk assessments is to demonstrate whether the proposed facility will comply with the applicable regulations.

In case of nuclear power plants, the Nuclear Regulatory Commission has established safety goals that serve as a gauge of the adequacy of the protective measures. In the case of low level radioactive waste disposal, the USNRC has established regulations that account for the potential long-term migration of radioactive material through the environment as well as accidental human intrusion into the waste site after loss of institutional control.

IX. <u>BIBLIOGRAPHY</u>

Aldrich, T., Drane, W. & Griffith, J. (1993). Risk Assessment. In Aldrich, T., Griffith, J. & Cooke, C., (Eds). <u>Environmental Epidemiology and Risk Assessment</u> (pp. 212-239). New York, NY: Van Nostrand Reinhold.

Byrd, D. & Cothern, C. R. (2000). <u>Introduction to Risk Analysis: A Systematic Approach to Science-Based Decision Making</u> (pp. 1-39). Rockville, Maryland: Government Institutes.

Chase, K.H. & Whysner, J. (1994). Risk Assessment. In McCunney, R.J. <u>A Practical Approach to Occupational and Environmental Medicine, 2nd Edition</u> (p. 376-382). Boston, Massachusetts: Little, Brown and Company.

Hallenbeck, W.H. (1993). Quantitative Risk Assessment For Environmental And Occupational Health (pp. 1-5). Boca Raton, FL: Lewis Publishers.

Kammen, D.M, & Hassenzahl, D.M. (1999). Introduction. In D.M. Kammen, & D.M. Hassenzahl (Eds.) Should We Risk It?: Exploring Environmental, Health, and Technological Problem Solving (pp. 3-30). Princeton, New Jersey: Princeton University Press.

Moeller, D.W. (1997). Environmental Health, Revised Edition (pp. 342-362). Cambridge, Massachusetts: Harvard University Press.

Moore, G.S. (1999). Living with the Earth: Concepts in Environmental Health Science (pp. 12.1 – 12.21). Boca Raton, Florida: Lewis Publishers.

Rhomberg. (1994).

Yassi, A., Kjellstrom, T., de Kok T. & Guidotti, T.L. (2001). Basic Environmental Health (pp. 104-142). New York, NY: Oxford University Press.

Yassi, A., Kjellstrom, T., de Kok T. & Guidotti, T.L. (2001). Basic Environmental Health (pp. 143-179). New York, NY: Oxford University Press.

CHAPTER

16

MONITORING

I. CONCEPTS AND DEFINITIONS

A. INTRODUCTION

Human populations are increasingly exposed to large numbers of chemicals that pose potential health risks. In order to understand and prevent the hazards of exposure to a chemical, precise information is required concerning its concentration in the environment and its concentration within the body in relation to its adverse health effects. It is widely acknowledged that assessment of the health risks of pollutant exposure is greatly impeded by imprecise exposure data.

Chemical exposure can be assessed in two ways: **environmental (ambient)** and **biological monitoring**. Environmental monitoring assesses exposure to a chemical agent by measuring its concentration in the environment (i.e., air, food, water). Biological monitoring assesses internal exposure to a chemical agent by measuring the chemical, its metabolites, and/or a non-adverse biological response in body tissues, fluids, expired air, and/or excreta. Biological monitoring offers a more accurate measure of individual exposure than does environmental monitoring. Each method, however, has its advantages and disadvantages. Since biological monitoring is in many ways complementary to environmental monitoring, more meaningful information is gained when both methods are used together.

Monitoring levels of pollutants in air, water, and food and identifying their emission sources is and continues to be the most important means of evaluating, reducing, preventing, and regulating such exposure.

Environmental monitoring has certain advantages. It often can be quickly applied to potentially hazardous conditions. If hazardous conditions are found, preventive measures can be instituted before severe toxicity occurs. In addition, a single environmental monitoring operation may protect many individuals. The analytic methodology needed for environmental monitoring is often less complex than that needed for biological monitoring. Because the chemicals to be tested are present in such simple media as air and water, little preparation of the sample is needed prior to analysis. Measuring chlorinated hydrocarbons in the air using infrared spectroscopy, for example, requires no isolation of the analyte, whereas extraction, trapping, and chromatographic separation are required to measure chlorinated hydrocarbons or their metabolites in the blood or urine. Because environmental monitoring has a long history, a body of information on the relationship between environmental exposure and adverse health effects is available for many chemicals. With the development of new analytic devices for measuring personal exposure to pollutants, environmental monitoring is becoming increasingly sophisticated.

The major disadvantage of measuring the ambient concentration of a chemical is that such measurements may not closely reflect the amount that is actually absorbed. Apart from differences in absorption among individuals, their varied exposure patterns, use of protective devices, activities, and life style make it impossible for environmental monitoring techniques to provide exact information on internal exposure.

Monitoring may be **direct** and **indirect**. Personal environmental monitoring and biological monitoring are considered direct approaches; environmental area monitoring as well as questionnaires, diaries, and mathematical models are considered indirect.

Environmental monitoring measures concentrations of contaminants to which individuals may be exposed. **Biological monitoring** usually measures dose, or more specifically, body burden at a point in time. Each of these can be further subdivided into **area sampling,** which measures concentrations without taking into account the extent of actual exposure, and **personal sampling,** which measures more directly the concentrations to which an individual is exposed throughout a period of time. Similarly, biological monitoring can also be further subdivided to reflect the extent to which the **biological marker** being sampled is a measure of dose, a marker of effect, or a marker of susceptibility.

B. PERSONAL EXPOSURE MONITORING

Personal air-monitoring devices provide direct measurements of concentrations of air contaminants in the breathing zone of an individual. Generally, samplers worn by subjects record time-integrated concentrations, reading concentrations directly, or they collect time-integrated samples that require lab analysis. Samplers may either be active, requiring a pump to move air, or passive, requiring no pump and collecting the airborne contaminant by diffusion.

For waterborne contaminants, a direct measurement entails sampling from the water source, such as a drinking tap, or from the water actually drunk. To measure food contaminants, duplicate meals are analyzed. In this method, an individual must collect a second portion of everything consumed. This duplicate meal is then homogenized and analyzed for the compounds of interest.

Direct measurements of skin exposure in an occupational environment have been carried out, by attaching patches on the skin. After a working day, the patches are removed, extracted, and analyzed. The effectiveness of using gloves to protect skin exposure can be established in a comparable way. Cotton gloves worn underneath latex gloves can be analyzed for specific chemical agents absorbed during handling. The results should indicate whether and to what extent the compound of interest can penetrate the gloves. These results can indicate how frequently gloves should be changed to prevent exposure.

C. BIOLOGICAL MONITORING OF EXPOSURE OR EFFECT

In biological monitoring, the contaminant of interest, its metabolite, or the product of interaction between it and some target molecule or cell is measured in the relevant body tissue. If lead is the contaminant of interest, for example, area sampling can be conducted to determine the operations associated with the greatest lead concentration; personal air monitoring for lead exposure may be conducted, blood lead levels may be drawn from exposed workers to measure dose, or a marker of effect such as free erythrocyte protoporphyrin (**FEP**) may be evaluated.

A **marker of effect** must be a measurable, biochemical, physiological, or other alteration within an organism that, depending on magnitude, is recognized as relating to the potential to cause health impairment or disease. Some markers of effect signal pre-clinical or pre-symptomatic stages in disease development, whereas others signal adaptive changes that are not themselves pathological. This often presents a difficult clinical situation - for example, with respect to workers' compensation. Workers may be told that they have an elevated leveled FEP, but they have no clear symptoms of lead poisoning. In most jurisdictions, this case would not be considered compensatable by a workers' compensation board. Also, these markers may be complicated by various interpretations and confounders. For example, FEP levels may be proportionally elevated because of iron deficiency. Or, although the presence of carboxyhemoglobin (COHb) in blood signals that carbon monoxide exposure is occurring, the source could be the inhalation of carbon monoxide or the metabolism of methylene chloride. It may also be due to hemolytic anemia with increased breakdown of hemoglobin.

Biological monitoring for susceptibility markers is a highly controversial area. Markers of susceptibility may relate to induced variations in absorption, metabolism, and response to environmental agents. For example, measurement of airway reactivity to inhaled bronchoconstrictors can be used as a marker of susceptibility to asthma.

Recently, the application of markers in a rapidly developing field sometimes called **molecular epidemiology** has attracted much interest. There has been particular enthusiasm for the study of DNA and protein adducts. However, chemical methods to detect and quantify adducts often rely on costly methods that require highly sophisticated and expensive instrumentation (such as gas chromatography and mass spectrometry) operated by highly skilled technologists. Furthermore, most of these methods still have to be validated and cannot be considered routine measurements.

D. INDIRECT APPROACHES TO ESTIMATION OF EXPOSURE

The indirect approach to estimating an individual's or a population's exposure to a pollutant combines concentration measurements in the environment with information on human activities obtained through the use of questionnaires or diaries. Exposure assessment surveys, whether they be questionnaires, telephone interviews, or measurements, usually attempt to obtain information in four areas: **demographic profile**, **health status, environmental factors**, and **time-activity**. There are three general approaches for obtaining time-activity information. One is called the **estimation approach**, in which an estimate is made of the amount of time spent by study participants in various activities during the time period of interest. The second approach uses **time activity diaries**, in which participants are asked to describe all of the activities in which they were engaged during the study period. The third approach is the **observational approach**, in which participants are monitored by outside observers. While this adds a degree of completeness and accuracy to the data, many people may refuse to participate in a study in which their activities are being monitored. Using data on concentrations in various environments and human activity data as input variables, **calculation models** can predict exposures at an individual or population level. To estimate exposures via different exposure routes, standard values for the amount of inhaled air and ingestion of drinking water and soil can be used. The standard value for total soil adhered can be used as a proxy measure for potential dermal exposure.

E. ESTIMATING INHALATION EXPOSURE

Outdoor measurements have been an integral part of environmental monitoring in many countries for several decades. Indoor air was largely ignored however, until the 1970s and 1980s. Thus, while many air pollutants are at higher concentrations indoors than outside, indoor air quality monitoring procedures are less well developed. To estimate an inhalation dose, an estimate of the amount of air a person breathes in a day is required. A person's gender, age, and amount of physical activity are major factors affecting the volume of air breathed. Other factors influencing the volume of air breathed include temperature, altitude body weight, smoking habits, history of heart disease, and possibly background air pollution. The absorbed dose is dependent on the deposition of the chemical in the respiratory tract and the absorption of the deposited chemical into the bloodstream.

F. ESTIMATING INGESTION EXPOSURE

Water - To estimate the exposure to contaminants from drinking water, the amount of water people drink and otherwise consume (for example, by bathing) must be determined. Ingestion of water includes plain water, water in coffee, tea, or other drinks made with tap water, and water in cooked food. If precise values for a community are not available, standard values can be used. To calculate the water ingestion dose, it is usually assumed that 100% of the contaminated water is absorbed after ingestion.

Soil - Soil can be eaten unintentionally when soil sticks to hands or to food. Soil can also be ingested when other objects are put in the mouth or swallowed. All children do this to some extent. The frequency that children swallow and put objects in their mouths varies. Children between the ages of 1 and 3 years, and children with iron deficiency or certain mental disorders develop a habit of swallowing objects more often than other children (known as **pica**). To calculate the soil ingestion dose, it is assumed that 100% of the contaminant ingested with soil is absorbed. The equation, however, should convert the concentration of the contaminant in the soil (C) from µg/kg of soil to µg/kg of soil, so that the units for soil concentration are the same as those for soil ingestion.

Food - To determine the amount of a contaminant eaten with food, a knowledge of eating habits of the group or population being studied is required, along with the concentration of the contaminant in different kinds of food. Eating habits - the amount of each different kind of food eaten - in a community may differ from the national average or environmental estimates. To measure the amount of contaminant absorbed into the body with food (estimated dose), a separate calculation is carried out for each kind of food or food group eaten. Although this equation looks more complicated, the extra steps are just a repetition of the basic equation used in calculating all other estimated doses (ED).

G. ESTIMATING SKIN EXPOSURE AND DOSES

The absorption of contaminants through the skin depends on a number of factors, including the following:

1. The total surface area of the exposed skin
2. The part of the body in contact with the contaminant
3. The duration of contact
4. The concentration of the chemical on the skin
5. The ability of the specific contaminant to move through the skin into the body (this is called the **chemical-specific permeability***)*
6. The type of substance through which the contaminant comes into contact with the skin (for example, whether the contaminant was dissolved in water or in soil when it came into contact with the person)
7. Whether the skin is damaged in any way before coming into contact with the contaminant.

The area of the skin that is exposed will be influenced by the activity being performed and the season of the year. To estimate the absorption of a contaminant in water through the skin, a permeability constant (P) should be used. However, such constants have been established for only a few chemicals. Even for chemicals that have been tested, the value of the constant can depend to a very large degree on the design of the experiment used to test the chemical.

H. COMPONENTS TO ADDRESSING ENVIRONMENTAL HEALTH CONCERNS

1. **Pollution Control** - To prevent the release of pollution into the environment in the first place, and the economic and regulatory structures that support vigilance in pollution control.
2. **Remediation** - To clean up polluted areas and to restore them to the extent feasible to their natural or at least an acceptable state.
3. **Resource Conservation** - Including recycling and reuse, to reduce the amount of raw materials needed by industry and increase the efficiency of use of these resources.
4. **Ecosystem Conservation** - To ensure that habitats for the world's species will be preserved in full productivity and that appropriate human uses can be sustained.
5. **Commitment to End Extreme Poverty** - With support of national efforts to achieve a sustainable economy, to provide for most of the world's peoples at least a comparable level of economic security and personal wealth to that in the developed world today.
6. **Technology Transfer** - To allow the developing world to industrialize with the advantage of the more efficient, less hazardous, and less polluting technologies.
7. **Sustainable Economic Systems -** That base their economic productivity on what can be extracted from the environment without permanent damage over the long term.
8. **Control of Population Growth** - With a concomitant commitment to improved quality of family life and individual security.
9. **Acceptance of Some Degree of Risk -** As part of daily life, along with a commitment by society to moderate the effects of risk on its citizens through education, regulation, and economic incentives so that the hazards of life are not constant preoccupations.

10. **Prevention of Conventional and Nuclear War** - To the fullest extent that human institutions can manage, and the redirection of funds spent for armaments for peaceful purposes, including environmental reconstruction.

II. ENVIRONMENTAL MONITORING

A. TYPES AND PURPOSES OF ENVIRONMENTAL MONITORING PROGRAMS.

Environmental monitoring programs were initially conducted on a local basis and had two basic objectives:

1. To estimate exposures of people resulting from certain physical stresses (such as noise and radiation) and from toxic materials that are being, or have been, released and are subsequently being ingested or inhaled, and
2. To determine whether the resulting exposures complied with the limits prescribed by regulations.

Such programs were either "source" related or "person" related. **Source-related** monitoring programs were designed to determine the exposure or dose rates to a specific population group resulting from a defined source or practice. **Person-related** monitoring programs were designed to determine the total exposure from all sources to a specific population group. The latter was particularly useful in instances where several sources were causing the exposures.

Although such programs continue to be important it is increasingly recognized that assessing risks solely to human health or focusing on problems only on a local scale is inadequate. The purposes and goals of environmental monitoring programs today have expanded far beyond these earlier objectives. Significantly, it is now accepted that certain of these programs should have an **environment-related** component, and that conditions should be examined on a regional, local, and global basis. That is, they should be designed to assess the impact of various contaminants on selected segments of the environment including ecosystems, and to evaluate factors that may have wide-scale, long-range effects. The types and purposes of current environmental monitoring programs are summarized in Table 16.1.

As a general rule, local environmental monitoring programs for industrial facilities are handled by plant personnel or environmental service contractors, whereas regional programs are handled by state and local environmental health and regulatory authorities, and the planning and coordination of national programs are handled by federal agencies. Close coordination between the facility operator and the local agencies is necessary if all objectives of the monitoring program are to be met. A well-planned program will usually involve some overlap in the activities of the several monitoring groups, including exchanges of samples and crosschecking of data.

Table 16.1. Types and Purposes of Environmental Monitoring Programs (Source: Moeller, 1997).

TYPE OF PROGRAM	PURPOSE
Based on nature of the stress	
Physical stress	To assess the impact of environmental stresses such as noise and external radiation, where the evaluation is based primarily on exposure measurements made in the field, not on samples collected and returned to the laboratory for analysis
Chemical stress	To assess exposures resulting from the ingestion and inhalation of chemical and radioactive contaminants
Based on geographic (spatial) coverage	
Local	To evaluate the impact of a single facility on the neighboring area
Regional	To evaluate the combined impact of emissions from several facilities on a large area
Global	To determine worldwide impacts and trends, such as acidic deposition, depletion of the ozone layer, and potential for global warming
Based on temporal considerations	
Preoperational	To determine potential contamination levels in the environment prior to operation of a new industrial facility; to train staff; to confirm operation of laboratory and field equipment
Operational	To provide data on releases; to confirm adequacy of pollution controls
Postoperational	To assure proper site cleanup and restoration
Based on monitoring objectives	
Source related	To determine population exposures from a single source
Person related	To determine total exposure to people from all sources
Environment related	To determine impacts of several sources on features of the environment such as plants, trees, buildings, statues, soil, water, and ecosystems
Research related	To determine transfer of specific pollutants from one environmental medium to another and to assess their chemical and biological transformation as they move within the environment; to determine ecological indicators of pollution; to confirm that the critical population group has been correctly identified and that models being applied are accurate representations of the environment being monitored
Based on administrative and legal requirements	
Compliance related	To determine compliance with applicable regulations
Public information	To provide data and information for purposes of public relations

B. MONITORING PHYSICAL STRESSES AND TOXIC MATERIALS

Because of differences in the nature of the exposures, the monitoring of physical stresses and toxic materials requires significantly different approaches. Monitoring physical stresses may simply involve identifying the sources and measuring the magnitude of the stresses. Data on the distribution of the energies of the physical stresses can be utilized to estimate the accompanying dose as a function of tissue depth and specific body organ. Monitoring toxic materials involves much more. For airborne or water-borne releases, the first step is commonly to measure discharges at the points of release. Additional steps include assessing the movement or transport of specific contaminants within given environmental media (air, water, soil), their transfer from one medium to another, and their chemical and biological transformation as they move within the environment. Data on the physical and chemical nature of toxic substances can be used to estimate their deposition and uptake by various body organs. These data, in turn, can be used to estimate the accompanying doses to people.

Because contaminants can cause exposures of people by so many avenues, most environmental monitoring specialists try to identify and trace the movement and behavior of key contaminants through several environmental pathways. They may supplement these measurements by analyzing the concentrations of selected contaminants in various ecological indicators, such as muds and biota from streams. Information on contaminants in such materials is useful in the conduct of environmental monitoring programs and in the evaluation of the resulting data.

Measurements to determine exposures from physical stresses, such as noise and ionizing and nonionizing radiation, must often be made on a real-time basis. Generally, instruments are placed near the people being exposed or in concentric rings at various distances from the source.

It is important to recognize that the mere presence of people and monitoring equipment may alter the environment in such a way as to make accurate measurements (say, of electric or magnetic fields) difficult. In addition, the position and location of the people being exposed (for example, whether they are standing on the ground or near a free, or sitting inside an automobile) can alter the resulting exposures.

During sampling to collect data on the health effects of airborne contaminants, the presence of both particles and gases is noteworthy, for they behave differently. For example, the size of airborne particles will significantly affect whether and where they will be deposited in the respiratory tract, and their chemical composition will determine their movement within the body and their potential effects on health. It is also vital to know what other chemicals are associated with a given contaminant, since certain combinations are synergistic. Sulfur dioxide, a ubiquitous acidic gas that is highly soluble and is ordinarily taken up entirely in the throat and upper airways (where its effects on health are minimal), acutely impairs the functioning of the lungs when carried to the alveoli as an acid condensed on the surface of small particles (less than 5 micrometers in diameter).

C. Measuring Waterborne and Airborne Exposures

One of the first steps in assessing potential exposures is to measure the concentrations of individual contaminants in samples of typical releases from the polluting facility. In most cases, air and water serve as the principal pathways for direct exposures (through inhalation and the consumption of drinking water) and as a vehicle for the transport of contaminants from the point of release to other environmental media (such as milk and food). Measurement of the airborne and waterborne contaminants leaving a plant can also provide advance information on impending problems in other environmental media. Since critical contaminants can be missed if only the obvious and easily measured effluents are monitored, or if monitoring ceases during key periods such as shutdowns for repairs and maintenance, sample collection and analysis should be conducted during all phases of plant operations.

1. Assessing Waterborne Releases

A range of samples can be collected to assess the impact of waterborne releases. These include the following:

Grab Samples - Collected on a one-time basis. They represent at best a snapshot in time of the characteristics of the waste. Unless the waste is uniform in composition, they will not provide useful information on the nature and characteristics of the waste.

Composite Samples – A blending of a series of smaller samples. Composites are frequently prepared by combining a series of discrete samples, each collected in individual sample bottles and each representing, as do grab samples, a snapshot of the characteristics of the waste at the time of collection.

Timed-cycle Samples - Collected in equal volumes at regular intervals. Direct averaging of data on such samples is representative of the characteristics of the waste only if its flow rate is constant.

Flow-proportional Samples - Collected in relation to the volume of flow during the sampling period. To make up a composite that is representative of the waste, such samples can be proportioned manually, when flow records are available, or the sampling rate can be set on the basis of real-time measurements of the waste flow rate.

Indicator Samples - Contaminants biologically concentrated within various living organisms and plants, most especially in the aquatic environment. Data on contaminants biologically concentrated in biota can provide information on contaminants whose concentrations in the stream itself are below the limits of analytic sensitivity; data on contaminants as a function of depth in muds can provide information on the history of the release of contaminants into a stream.

One of the primary advantages of a composite sample is that it minimizes the expense of analyzing liquid-waste streams having a relatively uniform composition. For waste streams with a wide range of characteristics, often times the collection and analysis of discrete samples is required to determine the temporal nature and concentration of various contaminants in the waste. As a general rule, the representativeness of the analytical data improves with sample-collection frequency. With highly variable conditions, samples should be collected as frequently as every five minutes to every hour.

The prime consideration is the variability of the composition of the waste at the point of sampling.

If, after collection, the sample is placed in a bottle for transport to the laboratory for analysis, care must be taken to assure that ionic species or small particles suspended in the waste do not attach themselves to the walls of the bottle. This potential problem can be avoided by an appropriate choice of bottle or by adjusting the pH or adding stabilizing chemicals to the sample prior to placing it in the container. Similar steps, including refrigeration, will assure that the sample is properly protected against deterioration due to either chemical or biological processes. Such preservation is particularly important when there is a lag between collection and analysis.

The quantity of sample collected depends on the number and nature of the parameters being tested. The quantity should be sufficient to permit all desired analyses, allowing for possible errors, spillage, and sample splitting for purposes of quality control.

2. Assessing Airborne Releases

Assessment of the impact of airborne releases will require the collection of samples from a variety of sites. As with liquid wastes, an initial step will be to sample the various release points at the polluting facility. In terms of evaluating the impact on the environment, samplers should be located in places where airborne concentrations and ground deposition of contaminants are estimated to be most likely to lead to human exposures. The selection of sites should be based on the best available meteorological information, coupled with data on local land use. Sites selected for monitoring the impact on various ecosystems will require a similar approach, the exposed entity in this case being environment, not people.

A frequently used sampling system employs a filter or electrostatic precipitator to collect airborne particles and an appropriate set of **adsorbers** to collect gaseous and volatile contaminants. Cascade **impactors** or other mechanical separation devices can be utilized to assess the size distribution of airborne particles. The choice of sampler depends on the desired sample volume, sampling rate, power requirements, servicing, and calibration. The minimum amount of air to be sampled is dictated by the sensitivity of the analytical procedure; the amount is often a balance between sensitivity and economy of time. As in any monitoring program, care must be taken to assure that the samples are representative.

As in the case of assessing occupational exposures, environmental monitoring specialists are becoming increasingly aware that it is difficult to relate the concentrations of airborne contaminants in the ambient environment to exposures to the public. Few people, for example, spend significant amounts of times at specific locations outdoors. For this reason, increasing efforts have been devoted to the development of methods to evaluate the concentrations of contaminants in the air actually being breathed by people. One of the more significant advances has been the development of personal samplers that can be worn by individual members of the public and are designed to evaluate the quantity of various contaminants being inhaled. Such samplers arc similar, in terms of the data they provide, to the personal monitoring devices available for assessing doses from external radiation sources. Personal samplers have been developed to collect airborne gases and particulates, or combinations of the two. For gaseous contaminants, the associated health effects generally are directly related to the quantity inhaled. Assessment of the potential health effects of airborne particles requires information not only on the total quantity inhaled, but also on their size distribution, chemical composition, and solubility. Personal samplers have been developed to take all of these factors into consideration.

Important characteristics of personal samplers are that they have minimal power requirements and be relatively quiet and lightweight. Although operation and maintenance costs are relatively high, they are considered worthwhile because of the amount and direct applicability of the information they provide. Table 16.2 summarizes the advantages and disadvantages of various sampling methods for the principal types of environmental contaminants and receptor media.

D. Designing a Monitoring Program

One of the first steps in designing an environmental monitoring program is to define its objective (what samples are to be collected and where and when) and how the data are to be analyzed. Not only must the program be planned so that the right questions are asked at the right time, but also so that only the data necessary to answer these questions are collected. Other attributes of a successful environmental monitoring program are that:

1. It is sufficiently inexpensive to survive unexpected reductions in supporting funds;
2. It is simple and verifiable so that it is not significantly affected by changes in; and
3. It includes measurements that are highly sensitive to changes in the environment.

Most environmental monitoring programs have at least four stages: **gathering background data**, **collecting** and **analyzing samples**, **establishing temporal relationships**, and **measuring** the **validity of the results**. Although the design depends largely on the purposes of the program, the following brief discussion (based primarily on assessment of exposures from nuclear facilities) applies in a general sense to the design of monitoring programs for pollution from all types of industrial facilities.

Although a nuclear facility can be a source of direct external exposure to nearby population groups, inhalation and ingestion of radioactive materials released into the environment are generally more important because they represent a greater contribution to dose, much the same as do toxic materials released by other types of industrial facilities. A key feature of environmental monitoring programs for such facilities is therefore identification of the potentially critical contaminants that might be released, their pathways through the environment and the avenues and mechanisms through which they may cause population exposures.

1. Background Data

Before monitoring begins, background information is needed on other facilities in the area, the distribution and activities of the potentially exposed population, patterns of local land and water use, and the local meteorology and hydrology. These data permit identification of potentially vulnerable groups, important contaminants, and likely environmental pathways whose media can be sampled.

Table 16.2. Advantages and Disadvantages of Various Environmental Sampling (Source: NRC, 1997).

TYPE OF SAMPLE	ADVANTAGES	DISADVANTAGES
Atmospheric environment		
Direct measurement Real-time field measurements of physical stresses such as noise and radiation	Monitors can be put in place to assess time-integrated exposures	Monitor often disturbs field being monitored equipment (e.g., for assessing electric and magnetic fields) expensive and complex
Airborne particulates Respirable fraction via air sampling	Direct-dose vector; provides data on potential effects on lungs	Omits larger particles that may be significant when deposited in nose, mouth, and throat
Total particulates via air sampling	Provides data for assessing doses to lungs as well as possible effects on skin and intake through ingestion	Not all measured contaminants respirable
Collection of settled particulates	Represents an integrated sample over known time and geographical area	Weathering may alter results; only large particles collected by sedimentation
Gases		
Integrated (concentrated) sample	Concentration of samples permits detection of lower concentrations in air	Samples must usually be analyzed in laboratory; chemical reactions may change nature of collected compounds
Direct measurement	Provides data on real-time basis	Lower limit of detection may not be adequate
Terrestrial environment		
Milk	Direct-dose vector, especially for children; data easily interpreted	Milk samples not always available
Foodstuff	Direct-dose vector; data easily interpreted	Samples not always available from areas of interest; weathering and process may affect samples
Wildlife	Direct-dose vector	High mobility; not always available; data difficult to interpret
Vegetation	Samples readily available; multiple modes for accumulating contaminants (by direct deposition and leaf and root uptake)	Data difficult to interpret; weathering can cause loss of contaminants; not available in all seasons
Soil sampling	Good integrator of deposition over time	High analytical cost; data difficult to interpret in terms of population exposure and doses
Aquatic environment		
Surface water (non-drinking)	Readily available; indicates contamination by aquatic plants and animals	Not directly dose related; difficult to interpret data
Groundwater (non-drinking)	Indicator of unsatisfactory waste-management practices	Not always available; data difficult to interpret because of possibility of multiple remote sources
Drinking water	Direct-dose vector; consumed by all population groups	Contaminant concentrations frequently very low
Aquatic plants	Sensitivity	Data difficult to interpret; not available in all seasons
Sediment	Sensitivity; good integrator of past contamination	Data difficult to interpret because of possibility of multiple remote sources
Fish and shellfish	Direct-dose vector; sensitive indicator of contamination	Frequently unavailable; high mobility; data difficult to interpret
Waterfowl	Direct-dose vector	Frequently unavailable; high mobility; data difficult to interpret

People responsible for the background analysis must take into account the type of installation, the nature and quantities of toxic materials being used, their potential for release, the likely physical and chemical forms of the releases, other sources of the same contaminants in the area, and the nature of the receiving environment. This last item includes natural features (climate, topography, geology hydrology), artificial features (reservoirs, harbors, dams, lakes), land use (residential, industrial, recreational, dairying, farming of leaf or root crops) and sources of local water supplies (surface or groundwater). Results from a monitoring program conducted before a facility begins operation can be used to confirm these analyses and establish baseline information for subsequent interpretation.

Contaminants released from an industrial facility may end up in many sections of the environment, and their quantity and composition will vary with time and facility operation. As a result the released materials can often reach the public by many pathways. For example, a secondary lead smelter has the potential to release elemental lead and associated compounds into the atmosphere, whereupon they may become an inhalation hazard. The same facility can also release these contaminants to the soil, either directly or through the air, whereupon they may contaminate groundwater and subsequently be taken up by fish and agricultural products.

2. Quality Assurance Requirements

To be effective, an environmental monitoring program must be supported by a sound quality assurance program. Such a program must include the following:

a. Acceptance testing or qualification of laboratory and field sampling and analytic devices;
b. Routine calibration of all associated instrumentation, including flow measurements on field sampling equipment;
c. Laboratory cross-check program;
d. Replicate sampling on a systematic basis;
e. Procedural audits; and
f. Pocumentation of laboratory and field procedures and quality assurance records.

Sampling validity and sample preservation also need to be addressed as part of the quality assurance program. Useful tools for maintaining analytic validity include duplicate sample analyses and control charts. As a general rule, 10-15 percent of the samples processed in a laboratory should be resubmitted for analysis as blind duplicates. Standard solutions (large bulk samples that have been analyzed so frequently that their chemical content is well established) should routinely be used to check the accuracy of new data.

Through services provided by the Environmental Protection Agency, the National Institute for Occupational Safety and Health, and the National Institute for Standards and Technology, laboratories conducting environmental radionuclide analyses can obtain standard and cross-check samples, as well as guidance in establishing and operating a quality assurance program. The USNRC requires all laboratories performing analyses of environmental samples from commercial nuclear power plants to participate in the EPA program or its equivalent. Whenever discrepancies are noted, follow-up action is required to determine and eliminate the causes.

E. COMPUTER AND SCREENING MODELS

Computers offer an enormous capacity for collecting, storing, and organizing information that can assist in understanding the global environment and the effects of human activities. Computer monitoring systems are being used, for example, to study and maintain records on industrial and natural processes, including documentation of trends in carbon dioxide releases and increases in atmospheric temperatures. One form of industrial monitoring in the United States that has made rapid progress is pollution tracking, that is, collection of data on the identity and quantities of toxic substances being released and their sources. The Toxic Release Inventory, for example, includes annual data on chemicals released to land, air, and water, from about 24,000 industrial facilities in this country. Public release of these data has proved to be a powerful stimulus for the application of control measures, particularly when grassroots organizations become aware of local problems.

Another major application of computers is in the development and use of models for evaluating the transport of environmental contaminants. The EPA has published guidelines for estimating doses from acutely toxic chemicals and carcinogens, and the Nuclear Regulatory Commission has published similar guidance for estimating doses to exposed individuals from radiation and radioactive materials. Using this and related environmental transport information, programmers have developed models for estimating the doses to population groups from a variety of environmental contaminants. The initial phases of this effort aimed at development of models for estimating exposures due to inhalation of airborne releases. As regulatory requirements have become more stringent and regulatory agencies have recognized the need to assess exposures through other avenues, these models have been expanded to incorporate terrestrial and aquatic food-chain pathways. The choice of model is normally based on the computer available, the type and complexity of the releases, the environmental pathways associated with the specific site or facility, and the living habits of the people being exposed.

Unfortunately, the ready availability of computers has led to models that are increasingly sophisticated and not readily applicable, particularly for operations involving small quantities of contaminants, as is the case in the release of certain radioactive materials. Recognizing the need for simpler models to assess compliance, the National Council on Radiation Protection and Measurements has developed a series of screening techniques that can be used by the operators of any facility releasing radionuclides into the environment. Although the techniques incorporate all important transfer mechanisms, exposure pathways, and dosimetry parameters, they involve only a few calculations and require a minimum of site-specific data and decisions on the part of the user. Because of their general applicability, many of these models are being modified for assessment of non-radioactive environmental pollutants.

F. COMPREHENSIVE EXPOSURE ASSESSMENT

Even if the monitoring procedures outlined above are followed, voids occur in the data- and large uncertainties in the accompanying exposure estimates - particularly in instances where it is desired to assess the total exposure of specific population groups from all possible sources. To meet these needs, environmental monitoring specialists have in recent years expanded and supplemented their procedures. One example is the **National Human Exposure Assessment Survey (NHEXAS)** currently being developed under the auspices of the EPA. It is a multiple-component program that includes:

1. The distribution of questionnaires to provide baseline information on the lifestyles, activities, and socio-demographics of population groups;
2. The collection of soil, house dust, indoor air, tap water, and diet samples.
3. The analysis of these samples for some 30 compounds, including airborne particulates in specific size ranges; and
4. The collection of samples of blood, urine, and hair, as biological indicators of human uptake of individual contaminants.

Armed with the resulting information, it should be possible to conduct detailed assessments of the exposures of the monitored groups to each and every environmental contaminant and/or physical stress in their daily lives. Although such programs are more expensive to conduct than those directed at evaluations on a local basis, they are considered essential when it is important and/or necessary to make longer-range and fuller-scale assessments of the impact of environmental pollutants.

Further enhancing the capabilities of these more comprehensive monitoring programs are data being generated through ground-based remote-sensing and fast-response instruments. It is now possible to make real-time measurements of chemical species and atmospheric conditions in both the stratosphere and the troposphere. Extension of similar capabilities to other components of the environment is enabling scientists to develop programs for evaluation of the impacts of a wide range of contaminants on the capacity of the environment to sustain ecosystems. An example is the Environmental Monitoring and Assessment Program (EMAP) being developed by the EPA. It is designed to determine the extent (numbers, miles, acres) and geographic distribution of each ecosystem class of interest; to assess the proportions of each ecosystem class that is currently in good or acceptable condition; to evaluate what proportions are degrading or improving, in what regions, and at what rate; and to appraise the likely causes of harm and methods for seeking improvement.

One of the basic premises of EMAP is that assessments of changes in the nation's ecosystems will require data collected over long periods of time (decades, at a minimum) and covering large geographical areas. Critical to the success of this program will be the selection, development and use of ecological indicators that are relevant, robust, and reliable. There must be a clear tie between the indicator, the effect it is designed to measure, and the accompanying cause-and-effect connection, particularly as it relates to possible effects on human health. If the indicators are properly selected, the resulting data will provide a broader understanding of ecosystems, help scientists anticipate emerging environmental problems before they reach crisis proportions, and assist legislators and environmentalists in addressing national and international monitoring and regulatory needs.

In essence, the data produced by EMAP will represent what might be called America's ecological report card. Some monitoring specialists have described EMAP's goal as determination of the health of an ecosystem, in much the same way as a doctor determines the health of a patient. Proponents believe that such a system, properly applied, would provide information on the point at which ecosystems begin to break down. Although analogies can readily be identified for making such a comparison, some individuals oppose the analogy because ecosystems, unlike organisms, are not consistently structured, do not behave in a predictable manner, and do not have mechanisms such as the neural and hormonal systems of organisms to maintain homeostasis.

Another weakness of such an analogy is that it contributes little to identification of the available choices for control or to the decision making process. In spite of these difficulties, essentially everyone agrees that the program will prove to be an extremely valuable tool for understanding and anticipating future problems.

As currently planned, EMAP will serve a wide spectrum of users: decision makers who require information to set environmental policy, program managers who must assign priorities to research and monitoring projects, and scientists who desire a broader understanding of ecosystems. It is hoped that the program will promote the development of more cost-effective regulatory and remedial actions.

III. BIOLOGICAL MONITORING

The aim of biological monitoring is to provide a biological marker of exposure. This may be the identification of an exogenous substance within the body, an interactive product between a xenobiotic agent and endogenous components, or other events in the body that are related to exposure. Biological monitoring provides a better measure of internal dose than does ambient monitoring. Its major advantage lies in the fact that the measurement of internal exposure is more likely to be directly related to adverse health effects than is the measurement of external exposure. In addition, the data obtained through biological monitoring are independent of such factors as the route of absorption, biovariability in absorption, variation in exposure patterns, and life styles.

Biological monitoring is used to assure that current or past exposures do not represent unacceptable health risks and/or to detect potentially excessive exposure before adverse health effects become apparent. Biological monitoring may also provide some guidance in the use and effectiveness of therapy for exposure to toxic chemicals (e.g., chelation therapy for heavy metal exposure and pharmacological therapy for organophosphate exposure). It can also be used to document exposure; such documentation may be necessary for legal and/or regulatory purposes.

The major limitations of biological monitoring of chemical exposure are the following:

1. Limited availability of valid and practical methods,
2. Insufficient knowledge of the disposition and time course (**toxicokinetics**) and the quantitative relationships among external exposure, internal exposure, and adverse effects (**toxicodynamics**),
3. Greater difficulty in obtaining biological samples and possible increased risk to the individual when invasive techniques are used (i.e., adipose tissue biopsy), and
4. High costs, particularly when individual test results may not be applicable to others experiencing similar exposure.

Biological monitoring should be distinguished from diagnostic testing and health surveillance. Diagnostic testing is used to confirm the presence of adverse health effects that are clinically apparent. Health surveillance entails the periodic medical-physiological examination of exposed individuals, primarily workers, with the purpose of protecting health and preventing disease. It should be appreciated, however, that there is a continuum between markers of exposure and markers of health status. Biological markers that define cellular, biochemical, or molecular events that are measurable in human tissues are tools that are increasingly being used to clarify the relationship between exposure to foreign compounds and adverse health effects.

We are in the era of molecular research. Between 1970 and 1990, the number of medical journals with the word **"molecular"** in the title grew from 31 to 90, signaling that the understanding of biologic phenomena has proceeded to the molecular level. This evolution resulted from advances in molecular biology, genetics, analytical chemistry, and other basic sciences. It is now possible to detect smaller amounts of analytes and contaminants and smaller biological changes, as well as to identify mechanisms at the cellular and molecular levels. Progress in the molecular approach to biology and medicine has stimulated and excited both the public and researchers, who now believe these advances can be applied to the study, prevention, and control of health risks faced by human populations. The term **"molecular epidemiology"** may be used to describe such an approach: the incorporation of molecular, cellular, and other biologic measurements into epidemiologic research.

The use of molecular markers represents a quantum leap in the evolution of epidemiologic ideas. Epidemiology has evolved through development and inclusion of many advances such as the systematic collection and analysis of viral statistics; delineation of the triad of agent, host, and vector (applied in infectious and chronic diseases); refined exposure assessments such as dietary questionnaires and job exposure matrices; clearly delineated study designs (longitudinal and case-control); and heightened computational and statistical capabilities (maximum likelihood estimators, logistic and Poisson regression). To this list now must be added technologically powerful measures of biologic variables, that is, biologic markers indicating events at the physiologic, cellular, subcellular, and molecular levels. Molecular epidemiology is the use of these biologic markers in epidemiologic research. Although use of biologic markers is not new to epidemiology, the current generation of markers enhances past approaches. The use of validated biologic markers can contribute the following opportunities and capabilities to epidemiologic research:

1. Delineation of a continuum of events between an exposure and a resultant disease;

2. Identification of exposures to smaller amounts of xenobiotics and enhanced dose reconstruction;
3. Identification of events earlier in the natural history of clinical diseases and on a smaller scale;
4. Reduction of misclassification of dependent and independent variables;
5. Indication of mechanisms by which an exposure and a disease are related;
6. Better accounting for variability and effect modification; and
7. Enhanced individual and group risk assessments.

Collectively, these capabilities provide additional tools for the epidemiologist studying questions on the etiology, prevention, and control of disease (Figure 16.1).

Molecular epidemiology is a natural confluence of powerful developments in basic biomedical sciences and the field-tested methods of epidemiology. Although "molecular epidemiology" can be viewed as an evolutionary step in epidemiology, a supplemental set of tools, or even a separate discipline, it generally does not represent a shift in the basic paradigm of epidemiology. This new approach allows for more accurate comparisons among groups, further clarification of mechanisms, and more specialized assessment of individual risk functions, all of which have been established in historical epidemiology. Molecular epidemiology does not have all of the characteristics of a distinct discipline or even of a branch of epidemiology. Rather, it is better seen as a diverse range of approaches and techniques that can supplement the field of epidemiology and boost the field to a new level of opportunity and capability.

IV. <u>DATA SYSTEMS</u>

A. <u>INTRODUCTION</u>

The interest of the American public in environmental pollution seems to be driven primarily by concerns about health. People ask, "Have we been exposed?" "Have we been affected?" "Will we be affected later?" They might well ask, also, "Do our management programs have any effect on the health of the public?" Table 16.3 outlines some epidemiologic research strategies that address these concerns. It shows that many types of epidemiologic studies and data can be used to determine the relation between the environment and human health. Although experimental studies of animals and laboratory studies of humans do provide some answers to these questions, epidemiologic research is essential to their resolution. Often, however, epidemiologic studies are neither available nor possible, and policy must be based on toxicologic evidence and animal studies.

Considerations of cost, urgency, and limited special expertise often require that officials rely on analyses of existing data that were gathered for other purposes. Epidemiologic studies of the classical kind involve the measurement of both the health status and the environmental exposure (or internal dose) of the persons being studied. However, such measurements cannot always be obtained. For instance, if historical exposures were not measured, the investigator may have to estimate them from other, less reliable, information.

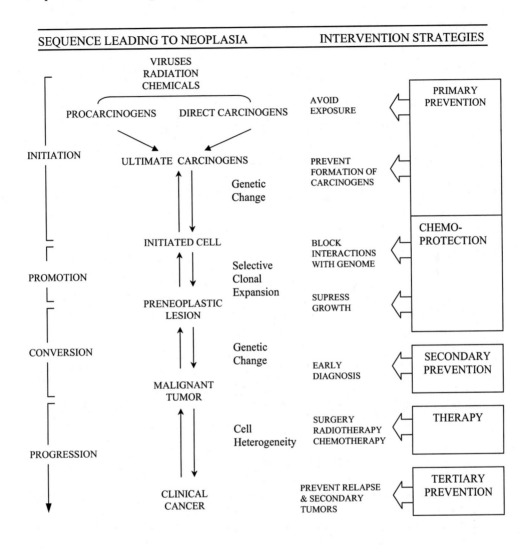

Figure 16.1. Intervention Strategies that Can Utilize Molecular Epidemiology Methods: The Example of Cancer (Source: Schulte, 1993).

On the other hand, the exposure might be so extensive that no suitable control population remains. Individualized measures of exposure and health can also be infeasible or too expensive when a health effect occurs so infrequently that adequate study would require that a large number of exposed persons be evaluated in detail; such problems require other epidemiologic methods or the use of secondary data.

Table 16.3. Issues of Major Concern to the Public and Methodologic Responses (Source: National Research Council, 1997).

	METHODOLOGIC RESPONSES						
	Exposure Assessment	Applied (Response) Epidemiologic[a]	Epidemiology Study[b]	Registries and Surveillance	Reference Surveys for Exposure	Reference Surveys for Health Effect	Risk Assessment
Are we exposed?	X				X		
Are we affected now?		X		X		X	
Did exposure cause a health effect?	X	X	X	X	X	X	X
Will we be affected later?	X		X	X	X		X
Did we improve health with a program initiative?			X		X		

[a] Applied, or response, epidemiology refers to studies designed as a quick response to concerns expressed by a group of individuals regarding the potential for exposure or health effects. These are the basis of much of the "gray" literature and many of the studies performed by public health agencies.
[b] Epidemiologic studies include classical case-control and cohort studies of targeted populations, in contrast with studies of the general population.

During development and implementation of public-health policy, analyses of secondary data are important at several stages. Intense study of selected small groups of people can provide useful information about risk that identifies a need for public policy. To determine the extent of potential exposure, the size and characteristics of the population exposed, or the background frequency of the health effect of interest, secondary data analyses are useful. Information from existing data systems is useful in program planning and development when data are needed to validate findings of earlier targeted research studies.

During implementation, data from existing systems can provide additional insights for public health policy. Existing data systems tend to reflect the programmatic and regulatory structure of government programs, so the identification of useful systems (or of their absence) might help to define the most appropriate needs for assessment and availability of the public-health response. This in turn allows for midcourse changes to reduce costs, improve response, or otherwise improve on-going programs.

Data systems are a primary mechanism for evaluating the impact of a public-health policy. For instance, a public-health program might target ozone because of its effects on several pulmonary health end points. However, the success of the program might be evaluated solely from the ambient concentrations of ozone in a polluted area. To evaluate the impact on public health, it is important to know the relation between the observed ambient concentrations of ozone and the frequency of various pulmonary health end points. Modification of public-health policies depends on knowledge of such relations, identified largely through analyses of secondary data.

B. DATA-COLLECTION SYSTEMS

Evaluation of the relationship between an environmental pollutant and human health requires data to characterize exposures to the pollutant including concentrations in the environment, the probability and characteristics of human exposure, and the distributions of internal doses, as well as trends or differences in the health status of exposed people. Determination of risk-management alternatives requires, in addition, information on the sources and distribution of the pollutant. Data Systems may address each of these needs. However, they have not necessarily been established with the goal of integration with other classes of data, and most data-collection systems collect only one kind of data or data on one aspect of the general problem.

1. Source of Pollutant

The development of systems to collect information about discharges of pollutants (apart from occupational exposures) is a primary objective of the Environmental Protection Agency (EPA) (Table 16.4). Its role as the principal environmental-risk management agency in the federal government requires data on the relative contributions of sources and on control options.

The primary objective of EPA's data systems is to provide information pertinent to regulation, so they are designed to be comprehensive with regard to polluters and pollutants that have been identified as toxic. Many pollution-related data systems have emphasized the characterization of pollutant sources, rather than the distribution and fate of pollutants in the environment or the potential exposures of humans. Representative data (as opposed to comprehensive data) have little utility in assessing compliance with regulation of individual pollution sources, though such data can be useful in assessing needs for and monitoring the success of management programs.

Other data collection systems characterize the amounts of a pollutant at its source. These include production volumes and emission inventories. These systems, too, are not directly concerned with the fate of pollutants in the environment. Data systems that contain location- and time-specific information can be used in analytic models to estimate the transport and fate of pollutants in the environment. However, few data systems contain both time-integrated information (for instance, yearly, periodic, or daily data on emissions) and geographic information (for instance, production volume at a worksite).

2. Pollutant Concentrations In The Environment

The locations covered by most pollutant-concentration data systems are chosen to be characteristic rather than representative (Table 16.5).

Table 16.4. Data-Collection Systems: Source of Pollutant (Source: NRC, 1997).

Data-System Name	Description	Primary Objective	Coverage/Sample + Design	Linking Data
Production Volume Inventories				
Synthetic organic chemicals	Annual data on production and sales of synthetic organic chemicals produced in the United Sates	Monitoring	National totals: comprehensive	None
Site Inventories				
National pollutant-discharge elimination system	Permits for worksites that specify effluent concentration limits, monitoring, and reporting requirements	Regulatory	National: comprehensive	Detailed geographic codes, pollutant limits
National Priorities List	List of the toxic-waste sites determined to be of immediate concern for remediation	Regulatory	National: based on reports from regions, comprehensive	Detailed geographic codes, environmental concentrations
Emission Inventories				
Toxic chemical release inventory	Annual estimates of releases from manufacturing facilities of minimal size and volume of chemicals per year	Informational	National: comprehensive for defined worksites	Detailed geographic codes
Integrated database	Information on spent fuel and radioactive-waste inventories for nuclear reactors, storage facilities, and mine tailings, among others	Informational	National: comprehensive for defined sites	Facility name
Sales Volumes				
Agricultural chemical use	Database of information on sales for agricultural purposes of fertilizers and pesticides, among others	Monitoring	National: characteristic farm sample	None

Table 16.5. Data-Collection Systems: Environmental Concentrations (Source: NRC, 1997).

Data-System Name	Description	Primary Objective	Coverage/Sample + Design	Linking Data
Monitoring Systems				
Aerometric Information Retrieval Systems	Ambient concentrations, emissions, and compliance data for airborne criteria pollutants	Monitoring	National: air-monitoring stations in urban areas	Detailed geographic codes/point-source identifiers
Microbiology and residue computer information system	Contaminant data from samples of meat and poultry at slaughtering establishments and from import shipments	Monitoring	National: Random sampling of meat products	No information on distribution of food
Regulatory Systems				
Permit-compliance system	Information for tracking the permit, compliance, and enforcement of permittees under the Clean Water Act	Regulatory, monitoring	National: comprehensive coverage of permittees	Detailed geographic codes, linked to Reach Pollutant Assessment System
Response Epidemiologic Studies				
Health assessments (ATSDR)	ATSDR assessments to identify potential health concerns among populations living near National Priority Lists sites	Regulatory	National: all National Priority List sites	Detailed geographic codes, linked to environmental concentration data
Microenvironment Settings				
Indoor air study	A pilot project to assess contamination in indoor air	Research	Selected sites: not sampled to be representative	None

Thus, most of the National Air Monitoring Stations or water-system quality sites of the National Stream Quality Accounting Network are in densely populated areas. These data systems contain detailed information on the location of the monitoring site, and samples are collected frequently enough to represent short periods. However, site selection is not based on detailed information about the population, the area, or the distribution of exposures among individuals, and the positioning of a station does not necessarily reflect the most likely route of human exposure. For instance, some air-monitoring stations are on the tops of buildings, and water-quality assessments are performed at the outflow pipes of water-treatment facilities, not at residential taps. Those locations might yield informative data on relative exposures, but may not represent either the distribution of concentrations in the environment or the actual exposures of people.

Pollutant-concentration data systems are probably underused for ecologic studies. These systems contain detailed geographic data, and, although few pollutants may be assessed, the analytic methods tend to be relatively stable over time, and exposure is generally measured at or integrated over short intervals.

Although most data on pollutant concentration are from monitoring systems, data from "response epidemiologic studies" are increasing. Response (or applied) epidemiologic studies are designed to respond quickly to expressed concerns regarding the potential for exposure or adverse health effects. Examples of response epidemiologic programs are the health-assessment studies of the Agency for Toxic Substances and Disease Registry (ATSDR) and the health-hazard evaluations of the National Institute for Occupational Safety and Health (NIOSH). In these studies, environmental concentrations of various pollutants are regularly assessed. However, study sites are often selected because the potential exposure is considered high or because of complaints about symptoms, so sites are not characteristic of ordinary population exposures. These studies do, however, attempt to characterize explicitly the scope or potential for human exposure in these presumably extreme settings, and they may contribute information on the relation between the environmental distribution of pollutants and human exposure or internal dose.

3. Human Exposure

Data on human exposure (Table 16.6) are the least developed of the classes considered here, and generalizations to larger groups of people or particularizations to specific exposure situations are often difficult and uncertain. Much detail is required to make this class of data useful, but few detailed data systems have been developed. Detailed information on human exposures generally requires the use of personal monitors or structured activity questionnaires, but these tools are expensive and time-consuming. Thus, most systems contain information on small populations chosen to be characteristic, but not necessarily representative, of the target population. However, systems that exist generally have substantial extent and detail over periods as long as several years.

More data of this class could be gathered by brief structured activity questionnaires in large surveys. Brief questionnaires might provide less-detailed information on human exposure patterns than personal monitors, but for a fixed total budget they can yield data on greater numbers of people. A combination of brief questionnaires for large numbers of people with validation and characterization of a subset using personal monitors might even be more useful.

4. Internal Dose

Like information on human exposure, information on internal dose is rarely collected systematically (Table 16.7). Occasional studies of biologic markers of specific agents in small, defined populations are plentiful, but broad and systematic collections of data on biologic markers in the general population are few, and surveys have yielded little information with which to characterize the subjects' exposures. Direct measures of internal dose are not usually included in health-assessment studies (conducted by ATSDR) or health-hazard evaluations (conducted by NIOSH), but these sources could be modified to include internal-dose assessments.

ATSDR conducts public-health assessments to determine where, and for whom, public-health actions should be undertaken. Each assessment characterizes the nature and extent of hazards and identifies communities where public-health actions are needed. However, the assessment is largely or entirely a compilation and analysis of existing data, which rarely include internal doses of toxicants in the population of concern. The health-assessment format does not require the collection of new data, for at least 2 reasons. First, the objective of the ATSDR health-assessment study is to determine whether there is a potential for human health effects, not to determine the extent or magnitude of actual exposure. Second, many internal-dose assessments are invasive; this decreases participation rates and increases opportunities for bias. However, when a health assessment indicates a potentially significant risk to human health, ATSDR is obliged under the 1986 Superfund Amendments and Reauthorization Act (SARA) to consider a registry as a follow-up, and registrants maybe invited to participate in biologic testing for markers of exposure or effect. There is also a need for studies that characterize a population with a well-defined sampling scheme. The National Health and Nutrition Examination Survey (NHANES), conducted by the National Center for Health Statistics, studies about 30,000 persons in the US population, chosen by random sampling (clustered, stratified, with deliberate over-sampling of some subgroups).

Table 16.6. Data-Collection Systems: Human Exposure (Source: NRC, 1997).

Data-System Name	Description	Primary Objective	Coverage/Sample + Design	Linking Data
Time-Activity Patterns and Personal Monitoring				
Total-exposure-assessment methodology	Goals to develop methods to measure individual total exposure to toxic and carcinogenic chemicals	Research	Selected sites: characteristic of urban populations	None
Surveys				
National Occupational Exposure Survey	Information on the probability of exposure to various chemicals based on job title	Research	National: characteristic of selected industries	Job-title codes
Registries				
National Exposure Registry	Identification of individuals with verified exposure to selected chemical, with followup studies to be performed on individuals in registry	Research	National: selection based on reports, not probability sampling	Job titles, personal, histories, residential geographic codes

Table 16.7. Data-Collection Systems: Internal Dose (Source: NRC, 1997).

Data-System Name	Description	Primary Objective	Coverage/Sample + Design	Linking Data
National Health and Nutrition Examination Survey	An examination survey of a probability sample of the US population, with some toxic-chemical concentrations measured in blood samples	Monitoring	National: representative of civilian, non-institutionalized	Residential geographic codes, personal histories, current job
National Human Adipose Tissue Survey	Concentrations of various toxic chemicals in adipose-tissue samples collected from autopsied cadavers and surgical patients	Monitoring	National: Characteristic of urban populations	Geographic codes

For study of general contaminants, such as lead or petrochemical oxidants, NHANES has been used as a data source. Given the follow-up capabilities of NHANES, detailed exposure data could be collected in subgroups of the entire sample that are identified as having received internal doses of particular interest. However, when the probability of exposure is small, the actual number of participants who could be studied to characterize the specific exposure would be small, possibly zero, and NHANES might not be sensitive enough. Specially designed surveys could be considered to characterize specific population exposures.

5. Health Status

Most health-status information systems are not developed for the primary purpose of studying environmental health (Table 16.8). Vital records are collected for legal reasons, hospital-discharge and cost information [e.g., Medicare provider analysis and review (MEDPAR)] is collected for economic or administrative reasons, and the National Health Interview Survey (NHIS) and NHANES are conducted for general US population health-monitoring reasons. Several other registries and surveillance systems are maintained to identify important risk factors, including environmental exposures, but in a general reporting system the amount of information that can be collected for each exposure of interest is limited. The information in such programs as the Surveillance, Epidemiology, and End Results (SEER) program of the National Cancer Institute, which collects cancer incidence and survival data from approximately 10% of the US population, and the Birth Defects Monitoring Program (BDMP) of the National Center for Environmental Health is gathered by abstractors trained in coding and abstracting from hospital records. The National Exposure Registry being developed by ATSDR will be an exception to the absence of environmentally focused health-status data systems.

The range and quality of exposure data from surveys could sometimes be expanded by data obtained as an addition to routine follow-up but at additional cost. NHANES, NHIS, SEER, and the US national vital-statistics system all have follow-up capabilities.

Table 16.8. Data-Collection Systems: Health Status. (Source: National Research Council, 1997).

Data-System Name	Description	Primary Objective	Coverage/Sample + Design	Linking Data
Vital Records				
National Vital Statistics Program	Data from birth, death, and marriage records	Monitoring	National: comprehensive	Residential geographic codes, job title
National Surveys				
National Health and Nutrition Examination Survey	Survey of a probability sample of the US population that includes interview, examination, and physiologic testing	Monitoring	National: represents noninstitutionalized population	Residential geographic codes, personal history, job title
National Health Interview Survey	Interview survey of a probability sample of the US population that includes rotating special topics, including knowledge of risk factors, such as radon, and occupational chemical exposures	Monitoring	National: represents noninstitutionalized population	Residential geographic codes, job title
Surveillance Systems				
Birth Defects Monitoring Program	Information sent by participating hospitals on birth defects diagnosed and recorded in the newborn period	Monitoring	National: covers only participating hospitals	None
Surveillance, Epidemiologic, and End Results Program	Demographic and diagnostic information on patients identified as having some form of cancer	Monitoring	Participating geographic areas	Broad geographic codes; fine detail available in special studies
Response Epidemiologic Studies				
Epidemiologic investigations	Centers for Disease Control and ATSDR; these studies in response to public concerns of potential exposures and health effects often include observational data on health status	Health-hazard detection	National: compendium, based on reports	None

Some kinds of information collected in a follow-up survey could be only qualitative, such as whether a person was exposed or not, and others will be subject to problems of poor memory and recall bias. Because of the mobile nature of the US population, collection of blood samples or examination data in a follow-up survey would require a mobile unit that would be used to assess only a few people in each location or would require transporting subjects to a central location. Tissue samples would be even more difficult to collect. These problems are magnified as the population size, geographic range, and length of follow-up period increase. Collecting good information is expensive

Comprehensive collections of data on vital events, especially birth and death, are highly accurate and nearly complete because of legal requirements to document these events. Collecting data to adequate quality standards is harder for health characteristics that change from year to year or even from day to day (such as diseases, symptoms, and use of health services) or that are thought not severe enough to warrant professional care (such as symptoms or non-life-threatening diseases). For these, accurate and comprehensive surveillance of the US population is impossible. Many of the large federal surveys collect data on representative, rather than characteristic, samples of the US population, so even large geographic areas, such as states, may not provide reliable estimates of health status.

Some systems, such as the Behavioral Risk Factor Surveillance System (of the National Center for Chronic Disease Prevention and Health Promotion), could be used to collect exposure and health-status information at the state level, but are limited to information that could be reliably solicited by the telephone interview method used.

Untapped resources that could provide systematic information on the health status of populations include routine medical examinations and school test - performance scores. However, when these data resources are not collected under common standards - as, for instance, a routine medical examination might be - the consistency of data may be poor.

C. BRIDGING ENVIRONMENT AND HEALTH

Few data systems include information on both exposure and health. Even in those with both - such as NHANES, BDMP, or SEER - the focus is generally on health, and information on exposures is minimal. Health - status data systems may have self-reported information on only a few items related to possible exposures, such as occupation. Of the 3 surveys mentioned here, only NHANES has information on biologic markers based on blood or urine samples.

1. Unidimensional Studies

Maps of cancer mortality have been used to infer environmental or occupational exposures and to identify populations at high risk for specific exposures. Clusters or trends of diseases have been used to identify populations that might have had unknown toxic exposures and that could then be studied more intensively. Conversely, emissions data from the Toxic Release Inventory, data on ambient concentrations of various pollutants, and lists of toxic-waste sites have been used to identify populations of concern for high exposures. In those descriptive studies, information or population exposure is usually inferential and based on proximity to a source of pollution.

Because chance alone will create clusters, the observation of a cluster - even one that is quite striking - often does not signal an increased probability of illness because of some risk factor. Rather, the cluster is a rare, but predictable, event in a population that is not experiencing a change in the probability of an illness. The 1-in-1,000 event will occur, by definition, one time in 1,000, and if many thousands of clusters could be defined (by time interval, geographic location, specific health end point, etc.), then the observation of even multiple clusters may have little general meaning. Because of the great number of ways a population and an outcome can be subdivided, one is nearly certain to find that some disease is more common in some segment than in others, with a low p - value.

2. Linking Data Systems

Linking several data systems can improve information on both exposure and health.

a. Studies with Information on Environmental Concentrations, Health Status, and Non-environmental Risk Factors

An environmental exposure is rarely the only potentially important determinant of risk, so a useful study must almost always include data on various other risk factors, such as certain behaviors, as well as the exposure and health status of the subjects. Such studies would involve linking data that could be used to calculate potential exposure to an environmental factor with subject-specific information on health status and behavioral risk factors. The following studies illustrate methods that could be used more widely.

In 1989, Schwartz used health data from NHANES II and air-pollution measurements from the Storage and Retrieval of Aerometric Data (SAROAD) system, now referred to as the Aerometric Information Retrieval System, to evaluate the relation between lung function and chronic air pollution. Data on individual subjects were paired with air-pollution measurements based on the census tracts of the subjects' residences and on the locations of monitoring stations within 10 miles. Lung function varies with sex, age, and body size, estimated in this case by height and body-mass index. Smoking and respiratory conditions also have major effects on lung function. Information on all these risk factors was used in a multivariate analysis.

In 1989, Ostro and Rothschild linked self-reported information on acute respiratory infections assessed in the NHIS to 2-week average air-pollution data based on metropolitan statistical areas from SAROAD. Information on other variables such as age, sex, race, smoking status, and chronic conditions was incorporated.

While outdoor monitoring provides only imprecise measures of personal exposure to air pollution, important relations may be identified if data from the monitoring stations are sufficiently correlated with exposure of the subjects. Relations might then be studied in greater detail in special studies. Broad correlations also provide indications of the impact of changes in the environment, as measured at monitoring stations, on changes in health status.

b. Studies with Information on Environmental Concentrations and Health Status, but Not Other Risk Factors

Many studies that have examined correlations between measurements and health assessments have failed to adjust for other risk factors, environmental or otherwise, often because relevant data do not exist.

Linkage with mortality data is common and generally straightforward because of the virtually complete ascertainment of deaths and the use of highly developed, standardized coding systems. Air-pollution data have been linked to mortality data on a local basis in numerous cross-sectional studies. Time-series analyses may require control for other variables, such as seasonality and autocorrelation. These approaches are ecologic; that is, a measure of the distribution of pollutant concentrations in an area is correlated with a measure of the distribution of health status in the area such as death rates.

An alternative is to study health measures in cohorts of known exposure status, such as mortality in occupational cohorts. The subjects can be persons at risk of exposure to toxic materials because they live near toxic-waste sites or for other reasons, e.g., inclusion in the National Exposure Registry of ATSDR.

Other assessments of the health of a population are based on hospital admissions, emergency-room visits, and calls for ambulances. In 1991, Pope used regression methods to study the association between hospital admissions for respiratory conditions and measurements of PM_{10} in local areas, including control for temperatures based on month of admission. Although characteristics of individual subjects were not available, Pope noted strong associations between indicators of respiratory health, particulate pollution, and the operation of a nearby steel mill.

c. Studies with Information on Health Status and Nonconcentration Measures of Environmental Status

The studies discussed above used ambient-concentration data from monitoring stations mainly as a surrogate for the probability that personal exposures were sufficient to affect health, but models can use other sources of environmental data. For instance, in 1986 Frank and his colleagues used the NHIS to evaluate the relation between chronic cardiovascular illness and exposure to carbon monoxide in the workplace. Information on occupational exposure from the National Occupational Hazards Survey was used to estimate the probability that people in specified jobs were exposed to carbon monoxide. Thus, the exposure data did not include direct measures. Information for individual subjects was linked to exposure probabilities on the basis of current occupation and humidity, based on county of residence. Additional risk factors evaluated in multivariate analyses included age, obesity, sex, demographic variables, and smoking status. Because information on health status is predicated on a subject's reporting that a medical professional had diagnosed a condition, Frank et al. incorporated economic variables-such as availability of health care and ability to afford health care-into the analyses.

The dichotomous classification of persons as potentially exposed or not is occasionally informative, as in the case of occupational exposures. However, without information on the extent of exposure, any health effects are likely to be underestimated. For instance, in 1989, Lynch and his colleagues demonstrated that misclassification of chlorination exposure could obscure a possible relation between exposure and risk of urinary-bladder cancer.

Other ambient measures of environmental status can also be informative. During NHANES II, in 1982, Mahaffey and his colleagues determined blood lead concentrations. Further analyses indicated that average exposure levels changed during the course of the study. Additional analyses quantified the relation between various sources of lead and changes in blood lead concentrations, especially in children. Exposures to leaded paint, dietary lead, and leaded gasoline were considered, and only the change in total lead used in gasoline production was correlated with the change in blood lead. The correlation was particularly strong among the youngest children.

D. MONITORING OF ENVIRONMENTAL HEALTH EFFECTS

Monitoring is the continuing and systematic collection, analysis, and interpretation of data. If monitoring is linked to specific programs designed to prevent or control health outcomes, the activity is better termed surveillance.

Many of the causes of chronic diseases are unknown, though it is clear that multiple factors affect many specific health end points, including workplace, diet, place of residence, recreational activities, and ancestry. Sorting out the relative importance of causes of disease in humans remains daunting, given the multitude of exposures and uncontrollable factors that can affect health. It is suspected that some non-communicable diseases (e.g., some cancers and diabetes) are increasing in frequency because of unknown factors in the environment. It is desirable, therefore, to monitor the occurrence of such diseases to provide a kind of early-warning system that would enable causes to be identified more readily than in the past.

Such monitoring systems must be designed in light of the problems of determining the contribution of environmental factors when some, but not all, causes are known. The problems include the following:

1. Difficulties in exposure identification and estimation;
2. Follow-up and latency (time from exposure to the appearance of disease);
3. Long-term nature of chronic diseases and the repeated use of health-care resources, such as laboratories and hospitals;
4. Size of the affected population;
5. Variable and imprecise symptomatology of some conditions.

To address those problems, monitoring systems have to be:

1. Large, i.e., cover a substantial population;
2. Of long duration;
3. Capable of producing information that can be combined with similar data systems, so as to increase sample sizes; this requires the collection of data in a standardized fashion;
4. Capable of being linked to other data sources, e.g., exposure data, which would require personal identifiers and provisions for confidentiality.

A set of sentinel health events or health-status indicators needs to be identified for use in exposure, internal-dose, and health-status data systems. Lists for this purpose have usually focused on disease or syndrome end points. For each health end point to be monitored, it is necessary to establish precise case definitions and gather baseline information on incidence and prevalence. The problems of definition and baseline determination are more complex if symptoms, rather than diagnosable disease, are considered.

Some monitoring systems for special purposes must be set up de novo, as has been the case for many cancer registries, but others can rely at least in part on existing data systems. Options include:

1. Special surveys (not designed for long-term monitoring, although surveys can be repeated periodically);
2. Disease-reporting systems focused on incidence (as exist for several infectious diseases);
3. Capture-mark-recapture systems;
4. Projects that link existing disease and exposure registries;
5. Special surveillance mechanisms based on health-maintenance organizations or health-insurance systems, such as Medicare;
6. Special record-linkage systems, such as that pioneered in Oxford, England, or under development in Manitoba, Canada. The Manitoba record-Linkage system will evaluate the extent to which census data can be linked to the provincial health-insurance scheme to provide health information. This system, built on pioneering work by Roos and his colleagues in 1979, required a special agreement between Statistics Canada and the province of Manitoba. Strict conditions of confidentiality will be observed, and no individually identifiable information will be released.

Several research methods that have been or could be used in special environmental-epidemiology studies could be extended to monitoring systems.

1. Followup (Cohort) Studies

A common example of a follow-up study is the study of health effects among individuals living near a specific toxic-waste dump. Such studies are difficult and results are often uncertain because the numbers of persons involved are seldom large enough to provide statistically powerful results. A hazardous-waste site may contain many different toxic chemicals, and it may be difficult to link a specific chemical to a specific disease. Further, of the large numbers of different chemicals, few have been characterized with respect to their ability to induce a specific disease, so such studies would have to be largely planned as **"fishing expeditions"** with extensive requirements for data collection and individual surveillance and with multiple end points. The multiple comparisons are then likely to produce some statistically significant associations by chance alone, so interpretation would be difficult.

Epidemiologic research is often expensive and time-consuming, especially where longitudinal studies of large populations are involved, so there is reason to consider "piggy-backing" needed research on other kinds of studies. For example, prospective cohort studies that are not directly related to the environment could possibly be inexpensively modified to collect additional data relevant to many of the objectives of environmental epidemiology. If this were to be done in a coordinated way for several such cohorts, a combined analysis might be informative.

2. Repeat Cross-Sectional Surveys

Cross-sectional surveys to determine disease prevalence (or cumulated incidence) could be repeated (e.g., every 5 years) in populations known to have been exposed to environmental contaminants. Although less valuable in some ways than long-term follow-up of defined cohorts, because those who move away from the area (possibly because of known exposure or illness) would not be followed, they offer an alternative when resources for a large cohort study are not available.

3. Death-Certificate Diagnoses Linked To Geographic Information

Death certificates have been used to determine whether variations in an acute, fatal disease within and between geographic areas are consistent with exposures to an environmental agent. Death certificates are especially useful for diseases with a short course, a single cause, and a high case-fatality rate, such as infectious hepatitis. They are less useful for the identification of environmental causes of chronic and multi-factorial disease.

4. Case-Control Studies

A difficulty with case-control studies is that the assessment of exposure involves extrapolation to the past. Replication of the findings in other settings is usually needed to provide the evidence required to infer causality.

5. Active Surveillance Of Emergency Rooms And Hospital Admissions

Changes in the frequency of emergency visits or hospital admissions for specific conditions can provide information about acute environmental insults. On a long-term basis, hospital admission rates measure the prevalence of serious disease in the community, though a major disadvantage is the inability of nearly all existing systems to distinguish between first and repeat admissions for the same condition. This is a strong argument for retaining personal identifiers in the basic data.

6. Outbreak Investigations

After an apparent cluster of cases is identified, investigators may go into the community to identify potential reasons for the cluster. Such investigations are often necessary to allay public anxiety, but typically they have little scientific value. It has been difficult to find direct links of environmental agents to the risk of disease, as many clusters are a result of chance, rather than an identifiable environmental agent.

Poison centers have identified acute episodes of environmental contamination. This is one type of outbreak investigation, with problems, though with the advantage that the symptoms can sometimes be related to exposure to a specific substance.

7. Health Care Financing Administration Data

Data are collected on nearly all chargeable episodes of disease in the US population aged 65 years and over by the Health Care Financing Administration. This resource is largely unexplored as a tool for disease monitoring purposes (as it is exploited in Canada, where the provincial systems cover all ages). A disadvantage in the United States is the restriction to the elderly and the fact that the elderly, especially those of higher socioeconomic status, often move away from the area where they spent most of their lives. The full impact of environmental factors on many chronic diseases may not be expressed until older ages. If diseases occurring in older members of the population can be linked to identified episodes of past pollution, they could provide information needed to prevent future disease in those who are now young, but such links are hard to discern in a mobile population.

For many chronic diseases, the time of first diagnosis may not be important. Rather, a measure of cumulative incidence (approximated by prevalence in nonfatal conditions) could be just as informative, thus increasing the usefulness of data that may mark the presence of chronic disease but not the date of diagnosis.

8. ATSDR Exposure Registries

The Agency for Toxic Substances and Disease Registry was created by Congress by the Comprehensive Environmental Response, Compensation, and Liability Act of 1980 (CERCLA) to address possible public-health effects of environmental exposures to hazardous substances from waste sites and chemical spills. CERCLA requires ATSDR, in cooperation with the states, to establish national registries of persons who have been exposed to hazardous substances and later develop serious disease or illness. While disease registries have not yet been established, the National Exposure Registry is further developed.

The stated purpose of ATSDR's Exposure Registry is "to aid in assessing long-term health consequences of exposure to Superfund-related hazardous substances". To facilitate epidemiologic research, ATSDR intends to design and create its data systems for both hypothesis generation (identifying possible adverse health outcomes) and hypothesis testing (of suspected adverse health outcomes). Other goals are to facilitate state and federal health-surveillance programs and to provide information that can be used to assess the effects of an exposure on a population.

ATSDR's data system will contain subregistries created in 4 phases:

First, it narrows down potential sites for inclusion to a workable number using criteria similar to those presented in table 16.9.

Second, site files are requested from EPA, the US Geological Survey, and agency personnel associated with a remediation project. At this time, additional secondary criteria are evaluated, including assessment of participation, existing biomonitoring data, number of secondary or potential confounding contaminants, and reported health problems.

During the **third** phase, site visits are conducted with local and state departments of health and environment and other interested officials. Affected neighborhoods are inspected, and special characteristics, including susceptible or transient populations, are evaluated.

Finally, on the basis of the above, a document presenting the rationale for selecting the site is prepared. The document is reviewed by ATSDR and, according to the resources available, the site is either approved or disapproved for establishment of an exposure registry. Final sites selected may also be based on the size of the population needed for the subregistry. An individual is said to be exposed when 3 conditions are met:

1. **Contaminated Source:** Valid information indicates the presence of the contaminant(s) of interest in air, drinking water, soil, food chain, or surface water.
2. **Route of Transmission:** Evidence for that individual of one or more routes of entry (ingestion, inhalation, topical, or other parenteral routes) exists.
3. **Indicated Transmission:** The contaminant traveled from the source via an appropriate route of entry to the body.

Table 16.9. ATSDR Criteria for Setting Priorities for Sites (Source: NRC, 1997).

Factor	Level	
	Less Concern	**Most Concern**
Level of primary contamination	Below or close to standard (if known)[a]	Exceeds standard[a]
Toxicity of primary and secondary contaminant	Not a recognized human carcinogen, teratogen, neurotoxin, immunotoxin, etc., at levels present	Recognized as a human carcinogen, teratogen, neurotoxin, immunotoxin, etc., at levels present
Size of potentially exposed population	Small (<10 persons)	Large (>100 persons)
Current potential exposure	No	Yes
Past potential exposure (length)	Short term (<1 year)	Long term (>10 years)
Other considerations: particularly susceptible population and biomonitoring data indicating body burden		

[a] The standard is the level specified for that pathway.

V. BIBLIOGRAPHY

Frank, R.G., Kamlet, M.S, & Klepper, S. (1986). The impact of occupational exposure to toxic material on prevalence of chronic illness. Pp. 59-63 in Proceedings of the 1985 Public Health Conference on Records and Statistics. DHHS Pub. (PHS) 86-1214. Hyattsville, MD: US Government Printing Office.

Lynch, C.F., Woolson, R.D., O'Gorman, T., & Cantor, K.P. (1989). Chlorinated drinking water and bladder cancer: effect of misclassification on risk estimates. Arch. Environ. Health 44:252-259.

Mahaffey, K.R., Annest, J.L., Roberts, J., & Murphy., R.S. (1982). National estimates of blood lead levels: United States, 1976-1980: association with selected demographic and socioeconomic factors. New England Journal of Medicine 307:573-579.

Metcalf, S.W. (2001). Environmental Biomarkers and Biomonitoring. In L. Williams, & R. Langley (Eds.), Environmental Health Secrets (pp. 127-129). Philadelphia, PA: Hanley & Belfus, Inc.

Moeller, D.W. (1997). Monitoring. Environmental Health (pp. 319-341). Cambridge, MA, and London, UK: Harvard University Press.

National Research Council. (1997). Data Systems and Opportunities for Advances. In Environmental Epidemiology: Use of the Gray Literature and Other Data in Environmental Epidemiology Volume 2 (pp. 94-129). Washington, D.C: National Academy Press.

Ostro, B.D., & Rothschild, S. (1989). Air pollution and acute respiratory morbidity: an observational study of multiple pollutants. Environ. Res. 50:238-247.

Pope, C.A. (1991). Respiratory hospital admissions associated with PM_{10} pollution in Utah, Salt Lake, and Cache Valleys. Arch. Environ. Health 46:90-97.

Roos, L.L., Nicol, J.B., Johnson, C.F., & Roos N.P. (1979). Using administrative data banks for research and evaluation: a case study. Eval. Quart. 3:236-255.

Schulte P.A. (1993). A Conceptual and Historical Framework for Molecular Epidemiology. In P.A. Schulte & F.P. Perera (Eds.), Molecular Epidemiology: principles and practices (pp. 3-44). San Diego, CA: Academy Press, Inc.

Schulte P.A. (1993). Design Considerations in Molecular Epidemiology. In P.A. Schulte & F.P. Perera (Eds.), Molecular Epidemiology: principles and practices (pp. 159-198). San Diego, CA: Academy Press, Inc.

Schwartz, J. (1989). Lung function and chronic exposure to air pollution: a cross-sectional analysis of NHANES II. 1989. Environ. Res. 50:309-321.

Yassi, A., Kjellström, T., de Kok, T., & Guidotti, T.L. (2001). Risk Management. In A. Yassi, [et al](Eds.), Basic Environmental Health (pp. 166- Second Paragraph). New York, NY: Oxford University Press, Inc.

Yassi, A., Kjellström, T., de Kok, T., & Guidotti, T. L. (2001). Managing an Environmental Health Emergency. In A. Yassi, [et al](Eds.), Basic Environmental Health (pp. 167-172). New York, NY: Oxford University Press, Inc.

Yassi, A., Kjellström, T., de Kok, T., & Guidotti, T. L. (2001). Action to Protect Health and the Environment. In A. Yassi, [et al](Eds.), Basic Environmental Health (pp. 399-409). New York, NY: Oxford University Press, Inc.

INDEX

A

B

F

S

T

U

V

W

Y

ABOUT THE BOOK

The book brings together the experience of more than 15 years of teaching the course entitled "**Principles of Environmental and Occupational Health Sciences**" all the way from Africa (at the Rwandan Medical School), to Chicago (at the University of Illinois), and to North Miami (at Florida International University Department of Public Health). The book is actually the result of working with the many graduate students who took that course that the author was able to compile a textbook that emphasizes the public health aspects of environmental and occupational health sciences.

ABOUT THE AUTHOR

Janvier Gasana holds an MD degree from the National University of Rwanda Medical School in 1984. He also holds an MPH degree and a PhD degree in Public Health, which he received in 1990 and in 1994 respectively from the University of Illinois at Chicago with a major in environmental health and a minor in environmental epidemiology. He has over 15 years of experience in teaching, community-based participatory research, service, and consultation in the area of environmental and occupational health sciences, epidemiology, medicine and environmental justice. He has been an educator for most of his career, including 4 years on the faculty of the Rwandan Medical School and 6 years on the faculty of the Department of Public Health of Florida International University, in Miami, Florida. He has developed and taught courses on public health and environmental management, occupational health and safety, fundamentals of industrial hygiene, environmental and occupational toxicology, environmental and occupational health monitoring, legal and regulatory aspects of environmental and occupational health, environmental and occupational epidemiology, environmental and occupational health risk assessment, epidemiology of injury control and violence prevention, epidemiologic methods, principles of maternal and child health. He also developed a *graduate certificate program in environmental health* with six courses, namely public health and environmental management, occupational health and safety, environmental and occupational toxicology, environmental and occupational health monitoring, environmental and occupational epidemiology, and epidemiology of injury control and violence prevention in the Department of Public Health of Florida International University. He has been a consulting occupational health specialist for 5 years with John Crane International Systems, in Chicago area (Morton Grove). He has been a consulting environmental health risk assessor with USEPA–Region V (Chicago). A native of Rwanda, Africa, he has been a human rights activist determined to promote and protect every human's right to a decent quality of life and health. His research addresses *environmental justice issues* such as childhood lead poisoning and environmental triggers of childhood asthma. As a result of his study findings, he formed a grass roots non-profit organization known as the Florida Children's Environmental Health Alliance (FCEHA). FCEHA is formed by concerned parents, leaders in research, education, public health, environmental protection, affordable housing and civil rights to protect Florida children from environmental hazards. The main focus of FCEHA is to identify, validate, and develop solutions to address the adverse health effects to children occurring as a consequence of exposure to environmental hazards in Florida.